Conditions of learning and instruction in nursing

MODULARIZED

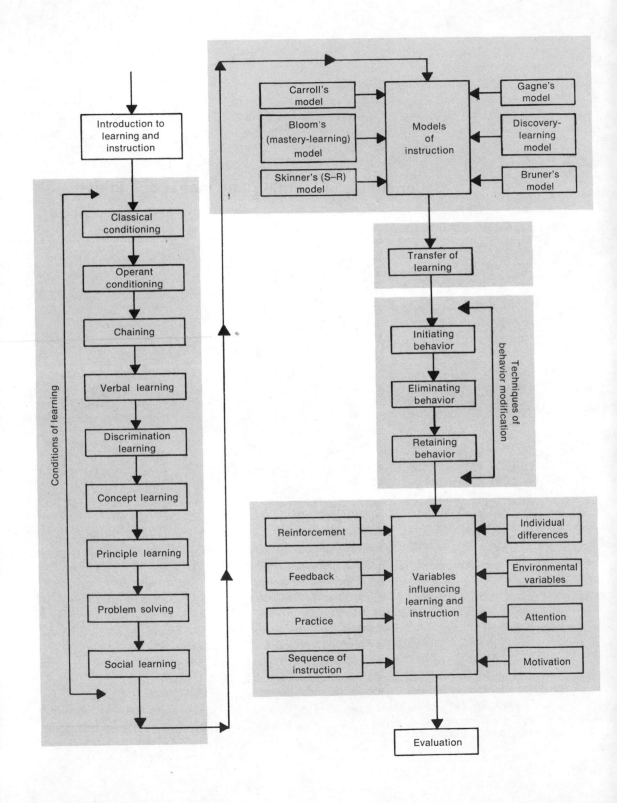

Conditions of learning and instruction in nursing

MODULARIZED

LOUCINE M. DADERIAN HUCKABAY, R.N., Ph.D., F.A.A.N.

Assistant Professor, University of California, Los Angeles, School of Nursing,
Center for the Health Sciences,
Los Angeles, California

Illustrated

The C. V. Mosby Company

ST. LOUIS • TORONTO • LONDON   1980

The C. V. Mosby Company
11830 Westline Industrial Drive, St. Louis, Missouri 63141

Library of Congress Cataloging in Publication Data

Huckabay, Loucine M   Daderian, 1939-
    Conditions of learning and instruction in nursing.

    Bibliography: p.
    Includes index.
    1. Nursing—Study and teaching. 2. Learning.
3. Teaching. I. Title. [DNLM: 1. Education,
Nursing. 2. Learning. 3. Teaching. 4. Models,
Theoretical. WY18.3 H882c]
RT71.H74   610.73′07   79-17015
ISBN 0-8016-2304-9

C/VH/VH 9 8 7 6 5 4 3 2 1   01/A/083

Preface

This book is based on the premise that theories of learning and instruction provide the nurse-teacher with a cognitive map to improve learning and to facilitate instruction.

There are four basic assumptions of this book. The first is that teaching skills are acquired behaviors; that is, they can be learned. The second is that in order to teach effectively, efficiently, and economically, one must first understand how people learn; then one can go about planning appropriate teaching strategies to produce that learning. Implicit in this statement is the proposition that knowledge of theories of learning is prerequisite to acquisition of knowledge of theories and models of instruction. Third, learning is defined in this book as a permanent change in behavior as a result of reinforced practice and experience. Instruction is defined as the manipulation of the external conditions of learning situations to facilitate learning and external conditions of learning. The last assumption is that knowledge of the subject matter is necessary but not sufficient for effective teaching.

We are now living in a time of revolution in educational process and technology. We are dealing with a new breed of students, who are more aware, are better informed, are eager to take part in their own learning at their own pace, want individualized instruction, and demand relevance in education.

These characteristics of contemporary students present a challenge to the teachers of nursing, who, for the most part, in the past have sought and rewarded conforming types of behaviors and students. In order to meet the needs of these students and the demands of the ever-changing educational technology and process, the teacher of nursing needs to be better prepared educationally in the principles of learning and instruction in order to create an environment that maximizes the potential of both the learner and the instructor.

The material in this book is of prime importance to those of us nurse-educators who want to meet the challenges and who believe that today's education ought to be concerned with tomorrow's unknowns.

The book is intended for nursing students, teachers of nursing, nurse-educators, inservice education instructors, practicing nurses, and all those who have responsibility for patient or student teaching.

The main purpose of this book is to enable the reader to achieve the following objectives:

1. To demonstrate understanding of the nature and types of human learning
2. To implement a teaching strategy utilizing an appropriate model of instruction to produce learning and transfer of learning

3. To implement behavior-modification techniques in initiating and retaining desirable behaviors in clients and to eliminate undesirable behaviors
4. To take into consideration the variables that influence learning and instruction
5. To instill in the learner intrinsic motivation for lifelong learning
6. To pace one's own learning and to take responsibility for it
7. To individualize instruction
8. To initiate research in nursing education and patient teaching, thus adding to the body of knowledge to improve practice

In order to facilitate the achievement of these purposes and objectives, the book is in a modularized format. Each topic in the book is a complete module furnished with the following ingredients to facilitate independent learning:

1. Module description with flow chart
2. Instructions to the learner that supplement those at the beginning of book
3. Objectives of each module that are to be accomplished by the learner
4. Pretest to measure the extent of knowledge the learner has prior to instruction
5. The text—the content matter about the subject under study, covering six areas:
   a. Theoretical framework
   b. Relevant research studies
   c. Issues
   d. Application to nursing education and practice
   e. Researchable questions
   f. References
6. Additional learning experiences in the form of a recommended reading list
7. Posttest to measure the extent to which the objectives of the module have been accomplished
8. Answer key to provide answers to the pretest and posttest so that the learner

can correct the tests and obtain immediate feedback about performance

The pretests and posttests have been tested for validity and reliability. Content validity of the tests was obtained by reference to appropriate literature. Reliability was obtained by two methods. The objective test items were checked by means of test-retest method. The Spearman Rho correlation between test and retest was 0.9642, p. < 0.001. The interscorer reliability test for the essay questions was done by means of item-by-item comparison. The interscorer agreement for Modules 1 to 10 was 87%, and for Modules 11 to 29 was 92%.

The book contains 29 modules. It covers four major areas. The introductory module presents an overall view of the book with the nature of learning and instruction. Part one consists of nine other modules, dealing with the types and the nature of human learning. The modules are sequenced in order of complexity with respect to the type of learning. Readers must understand how people learn before they can initiate a systematic approach to instruction.

Part two presents the different theories and models of instruction. Six specific models of instruction are presented. On completion of this section readers will be able to select a specific model of instruction and implement a teaching strategy. The readers also will be able to take an eclectic approach and utilize the strengths of each model of instruction and come up with their own models and then implement them.

Transfer of learning and behavior modification are presented in Part three. The content presented thus far will enable the learner to utilize all the principles of learning and instruction to produce transfer of learning in clients. Transfer of learning is one of the ultimate aims of education. Having understood how people learn and how to plan instruction to produce learning and transfer of learning, the learner is then introduced to the concepts of behavior modification. This section deals with initiating, eliminating, and retaining behaviors.

Part four deals with variables that influence learning and instruction. There are, of course, innumerable factors that affect learning and instruction. I have selected eight variables that are crucial for a teacher to take into consideration to facilitate learning and transfer of learning. The last module presents principles and issues in evaluation of learning and instruction.

Occasionally in this book it has been necessary to use the masculine pronoun in refer-ring to learner, nurse, teacher, or patient. This has been done for space-saving reasons alone, with no offense to any of my female colleagues in nursing or allied fields.

I would like to acknowledge the helpful suggestions of many of my graduate nursing students who utilized these modules to test the contribution of the modules to their own learning. I would also like to thank Dr. Robert Gagne, Dr. John DeCecco, and Dr. William Crawford for acting as major resource persons through their books and writings.

Loucine M. Daderian Huckabay

Instructions to the learner

The purpose of this book is to enable you, the learner, to learn the principles of learning and instruction as they apply to patient and/or student teaching-learning situations.

The content of this book is placed within the framework of modularized instruction to enable you to have control over your own learning situations by helping you learn the content with minimal or no assistance from an instructor.

A module is a self-contained unit of instruction about a topic or subject matter or a task to be learned by a student. It contains the following essential components in sequential order to facilitate learning:

1. The *description* of the module, including the nature of the module and the topic it covers
2. *Instructions to the learner* regarding the teaching strategy employed
3. The *flow chart*, depicting in a visual form where in the sequence that specific module belongs, what the prerequisites are, and its relationship to other modules
4. *Module objectives* to inform the learner about the specific tasks and the goals to be accomplished on completion of that module
5. The *pretest*—a set of test items that are composed of both objective and essay questions—to determine to what extent the learner already knows the content covered in that module, that is, to measure the entering behavior of the learner

6. The *text* of the module, presenting in detail the subject matter (content) covered in that specific module and covering five important areas:
   a. The theoretical framework of the subject matter discussed
   b. Relevant research studies in that area
   c. Issues in that specific field
   d. Implications to nursing education and practice
   e. The raising of researchable questions
7. *Additional learning experiences* in the form of a recommended reading list or other activities
8. The *posttest*, which is the same as the pretest, to enable the learner to determine the extent to which the objectives of that module have been achieved
9. The *answer key* to the pretest and posttest to enable the learner to check the answers with the correct ones in scoring the test

As you begin to study each of the modules of this book, first read the module description. It will give you an idea about what the module is all about.

Next, look at the flow chart and determine where in the sequence that specific module belongs. The modules of this book are placed in sequential order. Some are prerequisites to others; for example, the modules that deal with the conditions of learning proceed in sequential order so that the classical conditioning module is prerequisite to operant conditioning, operant conditioning, in turn, is prerequisite to chaining, and so on. The modules that belong to models of instruction are placed in cluster form. They do not proceed in sequential order. For example, you may study any of these six modules in any order. Next in line is the module on transfer of learning. The behavior modification modules, which follow the transfer of learning module, proceed in sequential order with initiating behavior to be studied first, eliminating behavior next, and retaining behavior third. The eight modules belonging to variables influencing learning and instruction are placed in cluster form. You may study any of these modules in any order that you like. Since these modules are related to both learning and models of instruction, you may read and study some of them concurrently as you are studying the conditions of learning or models of instruction. For example, after you read the module on operant conditioning you may find it helpful to read the module on reinforcement. The final module is on evaluation. It is the last module the learner should study.

After you locate the module that you are about to study on the flow chart, carefully read the module objectives. Next, take the pretest. You may want to use a separate sheet of paper for writing your answers. The purpose of the pretest is to determine your level of entering behavior—that is, to what extent you already know the subject matter covered

in that specific module. Use the answer key that is found at the end of that specific module to correct your answers. If you score 95% correct on that test, you need not study that specific module. Proceed to study the next module in line. However, if your score is less than 95% correct, study the text of the module very carefully.

Upon completion of your study of the text of the module take the posttest. Return to the pretest of that module and take it over again as the posttest. Correct your answers using the same answer key. You need to score 95% correct in order to achieve mastery at that level. The 95% mastery level is based on Bloom's theory of mastery learning in which he proposes that, given enough time and appropriate methods of instruction, 95% of a population should achieve at the "A" level, which is equal to 95% level of mastery.

If you score less than the 95% level, correct your errors and study the content of the module again. You may also want to study some of the references in the recommended reading list. Take the posttest again and score your answers. You need to study each of the modules in this fashion until you achieve the 95% mastery level or better before proceeding to the next module in line.

It is the purpose of this book that the teaching strategy of modularized instruction that is employed will facilitate your learning and initiate in you the desire and interest in further learning.

Contents

PART ONE

Conditions of human learning

Introduction to learning and instruction

DESCRIPTION OF THE MODULE

This is a self-contained unit of instruction on introduction to learning and instruction. This is the first in a series of thirty instructional modules on learning and instruction. The content of this module is presented in sequential order. The main text of the module covers five major areas as it relates to basic principles of learning and instruction: theoretical framework, research studies, issues, application to nursing education and practice, and raising of researchable questions. These five areas are presented in an integrated form. In addition to the main text, the module contains behavioral objectives for the students to accomplish at the completion of the module and a pretest and posttest to determine the extent to which they have achieved the objectives. Answers to the pretest and posttest are also provided so students can obtain immediate feedback about their degree of achievement.

MODULE OBJECTIVES

At the completion of this unit of instruction, and having studied the recommended reading list, the student will be able to accomplish the following set of objectives at the 90% to 95% level of mastery. The student will be able to:

1. Define learning
2. Define instruction
3. Define learning event and identify its elements

4. Describe the sequence of events in learning and remembering
5. Describe and give examples about the eight types of learning
6. Describe the five basic conditions of learning
7. Draw a diagram of Glaser's basic teaching model and describe each of its components
8. Write a statement of an instructional objective that contains the five criteria
9. Define entering behavior
10. Describe the theoretical framework of the role of entering behavior in learning and instruction
11. Describe the variables that influence the determination of entering behavior
12. Define:
    a. Readiness for learning
    b. Learning styles
    c. Developmental readiness
13. Apply the principles of learning and instruction as presented in this module to patient or student learning situations
14. Cite research studies to support the theoretical framework
15. Identify at least one issue
16. Raise one researchable question

PRETEST AND POSTTEST

Circle the correct answers. Each question is worth 1 point except the last question, which is worth 5 points. For this test 95% level of mastery equals 34 points. On completion of the test, correct your answers using the answer key found at the end of this module (pp. 25-26).

Multiple choice

1. Learning is defined as:
   a. change in behavior
   b. changes in behavior that are ascribable to the process of growth
   c. relatively permanent changes in behavioral tendencies that have come about as a result of reinforced practice
   d. a behavior that is retained
2. Examples of learned behaviors are:
   a. reflexes
   b. height and weight
   c. reduced responsiveness as a result of habituation
   d. temper tantrums, acquiring new vocabulary
3. Miss Smith, a nurse, watched Mr. Jones, an adult CVA (stroke) patient, develop increased skill in movement of the hand. Mr. Jones was unable to move the fingers of his right hand 3 months ago. Now he has been buttoning his pajama buttons and holding pencils in his hand. Throughout the 3 months the nurse and the physiotherapist constantly praised him for the willingness he showed to exercise correctly. Which of the following best explains Mr. Jones' change in behavior?
   a. maturation
   b. native response tendencies
   c. learning
   d. habituation
4. The elements within a learning event are:
   a. stimulus, variable, and response
   b. stimulus and response
   c. stimulus, learner, and response
   d. behavior, discriminated stimulus, and variable
5. Terminal behaviors are:
   a. same as entering behaviors
   b. observable performances that the learner is expected to achieve at the end of the instruction
   c. general goals of achievement
   d. observable behaviors that the student must possess prior to instruction

6. The sequence of events (or phases) in learning and remembering are:
   a. orienting reflex, attention, learning, and retrieval
   b. apprehending, acquisition, storage, and retrieval
   c. attention, learning, short-term storage, and long-term storage
   d. attention, stimulus, response, learner, and retrieval
7. According to Gagne (1970), there are eight conditions of learning that are hierarchically arranged. Which of the following hierarchies is correctly arranged?
   a. classical conditioning, chaining, discrimination learning, operant conditioning, verbal associations, concept learning, principle learning, and problem solving
   b. signal learning, operant conditioning, chaining, social learning, discrimination learning, verbal associations concept learning, and problem solving
   c. respondent learning, operant conditioning, chaining, verbal association, concept learning, discrimination learning, principle learning, and problem solving
   d. type-1 learning, type-2 learning, chaining, verbal associations, discrimination learning, concept learning, principle learning, and problem solving
8. When a student nurse compares and contrasts the signs and symptoms of diabetes mellitus and diabetes incipitus, what type of learning is involved?
   a. operant conditioning
   b. verbal associations
   c. multiple discrimination
   d. concept learning
9. Learning just the correct steps of nasogastric feeding (gavage) procedure demands what type of learning?
   a. operant conditioning
   b. verbal associations
   c. chaining
   d. discrimination learning
10. Behaviors that are mostly acquired by means of observation are learned by what type of learning condition?

a. signal learning
b. chaining
c. social learning
d. principle learning
11. The basic external conditions of learning are:
   a. motivation, reinforcement, practice, and contiguity
   b. contiguity, practice, reinforcement, generalization, and discrimination
   c. attention, motivation, practice, and reinforcement
   d. stimulus situation, attention, practice, and reinforcement
12. The simultaneous occurrence of the stimuli and the responses is referred to as:
   a. reinforcement
   b. contiguity
   c. conditioning
   d. practice
13. The repetition of a response in the presence of the stimulus is called:
   a. learning
   b. practice
   c. conditioning
   d. contiguity
14. In learning a specific nursing procedure (motor performances such as catheterization), which of the following plays an important role?
   a. conditioning
   b. practice
   c. concept learning
   d. generalization
15. Practice is most important in what type of learning?
   a. concept learning
   b. operant conditioning
   c. principle learning
   d. problem solving
16. A stimulus, when it is made contingent on desired behavior and when it increases the occurrence of that behavior, is referred to as:
   a. discriminated stimulus
   b. learning event
   c. reinforcement
   d. classical conditioning
17. An individual who is confronted with a new stimulus situation makes a response previously learned to another stimulus. This is referred to as making a:
   a. discrimination
   b. generalization
   c. overgeneralization
   d. contiguity
18. A nurse who observes two Italian patients on the same clinical floor overtly expressing their discomfort and "exaggerating" their pain and then, while giving a report to the next shift, states that "as usual, all Italian patient are fussy and overexpressive" is exhibiting what type of behavior?
   a. reporting objective observation
   b. verbal association
   c. overgeneralization
   d. discrimination
19. An individual who makes different responses to two or more stimuli is said to be using:
   a. generalization
   b. discrimination
   c. divergent thinking
   d. overdiscrimination
20. Entering behavior refers to:
   a. the behavior the student acquires after new learning is acquired
   b. the level of knowledge the student possesses prior to instruction, the motivational state, intellectual ability and development, and certain social and cultural determinants of learning
   c. future states of the student's knowledge
   d. the terminal behavior the student must accomplish after instruction is completed
21. The first step of a teaching process is:
   a. to determine the entering behavior of the student
   b. to assess the entering behavior necessary to accomplish the task
   c. to set up the instructional (learner) objectives
   d. to plan the instructional procedure
22. In a statement of instructional objectives, which of the following criteria should be included? Choose the correct combination.
   1—specification of entering behavior
   2—the learner, to whom the objective is directed

3—the content

4—the behavior expected after learning the content

5—the general goals of education

6—the conditions under which the behavior is expected to occur

7—the criteria of acceptable performance

a. 1, 2, 3, 5, 6, and 7

b. 1, 3, 4, and 7

c. 2, 3, 4, 6, and 7

d. all of the above

23. The differences between entering behavior and terminal performances are:

1—the list of entering behavior is longer and more comprehensive than terminal performances

2—entering behavior specifies the criteria of acceptable performance while terminal performance does not

3—entering behavior specifies where instruction should begin, while terminal performance specifies where instruction should end

4—entering behavior does not specify either the conditions under which behavior should occur nor the criteria of acceptable performance, while the terminal performance does

a. all of the above

b. 1, 2, and 4

c. 1 and 3

d. 1, 3, and 4

24. In assessing the entering behavior of the student, the teacher can use:

a. a pretest

b. a test that measures prerequisite knowledge

c. a test that measures present learning

d. a test that measures the student's level of intelligence

25. An instructor prepared a test of entering behavior on the topic of "loss of body image in patients with a leg amputation." The test specifically included three or four items to measure each terminal performance in a list of instructional objectives. The test was administered to a freshmen class of nursing students, and all obtained scores of zero. Which of the following decisions should the instructor make?

a. to prepare a new test of entering behavior

b. to adopt a new list of instructional objectives

c. to move ahead with instructional plans because it has now been ascertained that none of the students has knowledge about loss of body image in patients with leg amputations

26. There are certain preconditions of learning called "readiness for learning" that precede a learning event. They determine whether learning can occur or not. Which of the following is not a major factor in comprising learning readiness?

a. entering behavior

b. attentional set

c. motivation

d. developmental readiness

27. According to Gagne (1970), developmental readiness for learning refers to:

a. maturation of the learner

b. the stage-bound (age-bound) development of the learner, when the stages of neuro-physiological growth impose certain limitations on the kind and degree of cognitive development

c. the cumulative effects of learning and learning transfer and differences in developmental readiness that are primarily attributable to differences in the number and kind of previously learned intellectual skills

d. learning abilities

28. When given a problem situation, a learner who gives a fast answer, makes quick decisions, does not necessarily weigh the different alternative answers, and takes risks is said to:

a. have a unique learning style

b. have a fast conceptual tempo, be impulsive

c. be bright

d. be less than average in I.Q.

29. A learner who solves a problem by weighing the consequences of each alternative solution, has a slow conceptual tempo, delays answering, and does not take risks is said to be:

a. a very slow learner

b. a reflective learner

c. average or less than average in I.Q.
d. very bright

30. In conservative focusing (for solution strategy):
    a. there are some risks involved
    b. there is no risk involved
    c. opportunity for obtaining information is limited
    d. there is the strain of having to remember several bits of information simultaneously

31. Impulsive students tend to use:
    a. conservative focusing
    b. focus gambling
    c. successive scanning
    d. simultaneous scanning

Discussion question

32. Make a list of entering behaviors necessary before a hemiplegic patient is able to move from the bed to a wheelchair.

TEXT
Theoretical framework
Learning
NATURE OF LEARNING

Learning is defined as a relatively permanent change in behavioral tendency that has come about as a result of reinforced practice. The behavior learned in such a situation can be retained—it is not simply ascribable to the process of growth. DeCecco and Crawford (1974) differentiate learning from performance: learning is an inferred state of the individual; performance is an observed state.

There are some behaviors that are not considered to be examples of learning; for example, *reflexes*, such as knee jerking, eye blinking, breathing, and nausea, are natural response tendencies. Another area of behavior that is not ascribable to learning is *maturation*—growth tendencies that are relatively independent of specific learning conditions—for example, height and weight changes are not learned behaviors. A third area of behavior that is not ascribable to

learning includes those behaviors that result from *habituation,* or the influence of a drug. For example, the fatigue induced by repetition of a response disinclines its immediate repetition. Habituation changes our behavior in the direction of reduced responsiveness. Behavior changes produced or inhibited by drugs usually are temporary (DeCecco and Crawford, 1974).

There are many other factors that influence behavior, either by stimulating, controlling, or directing that behavior. For instance: (1) motivation provides vim and vigor to behaviors; (2) innate structures, such as genes, influence the direction and level of development, (3) capabilities, such as intelligence, influence a whole range of behaviors, (4) people manipulate and adapt to the external environment, and (5) learned habits control individuals to some degree (DeCecco and Crawford, 1974).

A *learning event* is perceived by Gagne (1970, p. 5) as the learning that occurs when the *stimulus situation* affects the learner in such a way that performance changes from a time *before* being in that situation to a time *after* being in it. It is this change in performance that is referred to as learning.

A learning event consists of three elements: the learner; the learning situation, or stimuli; and the response. The *learner* is the human being, for our purposes. The most important parts of the learner are the sense organs, the central nervous system, and the muscles. Events in the environment affect the learner's sense organs and send sensory impulses to the central nervous system specifically, to the brain. Gagne (1970) pointed out that "this nervous activity occurs in certain sequences and patterns that alter the nature of the organizing process itself, and this effect is exhibited as learning. Finally, the nervous activity is translated into action that may be observed as the movement of muscles in executing responses of various sorts" (p. 5). A learner's previous learning is referred to as the entering behavior, or the internal conditions of learning.

The stimuli, or the events in the environment that stimulate the learner's sense organs, are called the *stimulus situation*. When a single event stimulates the learner's sense organ, it is referred to as a *stimulus*.

A *response* is the behavior or the action that is exhibited by the learner. It results from stimulation and subsequent nervous activity. For example, the sight of a man lying unconscious on the ground is a stimulus that leads the individual (the learner) to run toward the unconscious person and provide assistance. If a nurse, the learner would turn the man onto his back or side, ensure an open airway, check the pulse (which may be another stimulus), and begin cardiopulmonary resusitation (CPR)—this entails a whole series of responses.

DeCecco and Crawford (1974) pointed out that one of the easiest ways to depict learning is as follows: when a stimulus is presented to the learner, there may be no response at first, but when it is presented the next time, there is a response. From this change in performance, one infers that learning has taken place. As in the above example, if the nurse did not know the first-aid treatment for an unconscious patient, the nurse would probably either run away from the patient because of fear or run toward the patient and, seeing the condition, yell for help. These are also responses, but they may not be as effective as the response of giving first-aid treatment. After learning the proper method of treating the unconscious patient, the nurse would respond to a second presentation of an unconscious patient by administering the appropriate first-aid treatment. If one can observe this change in behavior from a time *before* being in that situation to a time *after* being in it, one can infer that learning has occurred.

By taking the learning event into consideration, instruction can be planned. A teaching plan should foresee which stimuli will result in the students making which responses. The stimuli include all the teaching materials and media; such as films, textbooks, lectures, television, and role playing. The responses are the new performances the teacher expects the students to acquire. These performances are often referred to as *terminal behaviors*. Prior to instruction, the teacher must make it very clear which type of terminal behaviors the students are expected to demonstrate Then the teacher can write the terminal course or lesson objectives for the students to accomplish.

SEQUENCE OF EVENTS IN LEARNING AND REMEMBERING

Learning is an event or an occurrence that takes place over a period of time. Its components can be analyzed and described in terms of this time sequence. Irrespective of the type of learning, they all have this common time sequence. The total process of learning and remembering takes place in four phases: the apprehending phase, the acquisition phase, the storage phase, and the retrieval phase. In Fig. 1-1 the sequence of these phases is diagrammatically illustrated.

Following the presentation of the stimulus situation, there is a period of time, an interval, during which this stimulation is *apprehended* by the learner. This first phase is characterized by *attending, perceiving,* and *coding* of the stimulus. The learner must "register" the stimulation in order to respond to it. Most scholars agree that the initial event must be that of attending to the stimulus. However, they are not certain whether attending is a process itself containing one, two, or three stages. This topic is still being debated actively. For our purposes, attending can be viewed as a state that can be detected by observing what the learner is looking at or listening to (Gagne, 1970).

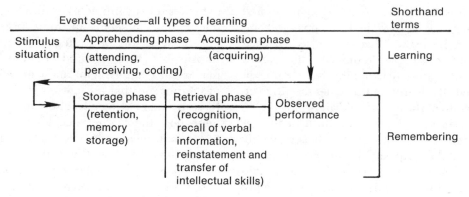

Fig. 1-1. The sequence of events in learning. (After Gagne, 1970, p. 71).

Once a learner attends to a stimulus, it leads to the *perceiving* of the stimulus. For example, one may attend to a painting on the wall and perceive it as such, or one may attend in such a way that one can perceive all the trees and birds and the number of hunters in the picture. A nurse, for instance, may look at and attend to a patient in bed and perceive the patient as a person lying in bed, or may perceive the patient's color, pupil dilation, tremors and twitching of the face, and so on. How one attends, and, therefore, what is perceived, depend on a temporary mental set of the individual, which the individual may decide or may be stimulated to adopt by means of verbal instruction. Gagne (1970) pointed out that the act of perceiving implies that the learner differentiates one stimulus from another or its parts from other parts. The learner's ability to differentiate depends on the discrimination learning that has occurred previously; that is, it depends on the level of entering behavior with regard to discrimination learning. The prior learning that determines what can be perceived is called perceptual learning (Gibson, 1968; Gagne, 1970).

The third ingredient of the apprehending phase is *coding*. There are many scholars who state that a stimulus must not only be attended and perceived but also coded. What is meant by coding is that learners apprehend any given stimulus in their own idiosyncratic ways, enabling them to use the stimulus easily. Gagne (1970) gives the example of the printed word LUX. On perceiving this word, one may code it as a detergent, another may code it as "light," another may think of it as "top of the line" (as in "deluxe"), and still another may code it as an inscription. Each person in the situation is perceiving the word equally well, but the way they are *coding* is different.

To summarize, the apprehending phase of learning is concerned with the events that "register" the stimulus situation for the learner. It includes attending, perceiving, and coding.

The *acquisition phase* follows the apprehending phase. Once the stimuli relevant to learning have been apprehended, the process can proceed. The events that take place during acquisition are the changes that occur in the central nervous system that underlie the new capability. Before the events in the acquisition phase take place, an individual cannot do some particular task; however, after the events in the acquisition phase have taken place, the learner can execute the task. This is an indication that a new capability has been *acquired.* Gagne pointed out that it is very difficult to separate completely the events that take place in each phase. For example, in order for the learner to demonstrate that a new task has been learned, the learner must remember it, even if asked to perform it immediately.

The *storage* phase is the third in the sequence of events in learning. It is generally believed that acquisition is followed by some internal activity that "stores," or "puts into memory store," the newly learned capability so that it can be retained over a period of time, ranging anywhere from a few minutes to a lifetime. Some recent evidence suggests that there may be two different kinds of storage. The first is *short-term memory,* which has a limited capacity and allows information to be retained for up to 30 seconds. The second is *long-term memory,* in which retention may persist indefinitely (Gagne, 1970, p. 74). There are also some investigators who contend that the evidence available to support the differences between the two types of memory are insufficient and unconvincing. In any case, Gagne pointed out that long-term memory is of greatest relevance to instruction in educational settings.

The fourth major phase is *retrieval.* Here, the capabilities that have been learned and stored are in some form recovered and demonstrated as performances to an external observer. Retrieval is concerned with recognition, recall of verbal information, and reinstatement and transfer of intellectual skills. According to Gagne (1970), retrieval takes place in a disorganized way. For example, an individual in a new situation may be "reminded" of a variety of related events that were originally learned in different contexts. Deliberate retrieval also takes place when an individual needs the learned items in solving a current problem or when asked a very direct question, such as "What do you remember about diabetes?" In such situations

(whether solving problems or recalling verbal information), it seems apparent that certain organizing factors or strategies are at work. As Ausubel (1968) pointed out, the learner may recall a variety of instances or categories of information that are meaningfully related to each other. Strategies also exist to determine how the learner decides what to retrieve first, what order the learner retrieves information, and how the learner "searches" for items that are related to the present purpose. Such strategies have not been systematically studied, even though their existence is accepted without doubt (Gagne, 1970, p. 76).

Gagne (1970) also stressed the fact that distinctions must be made between the recall of verbal information and the reinstatement of intellectual skills. The latter is more demanding cognitively. In order to reinstate intellectual skills, the learner must utilize the strategies that were mentioned in the previous paragraph that pertain to "how to recall" verbal information. What is observed in the retrieval of a reinstatement of intellectual skill is performance in a new situation. The elements of the stimulus situation are altered, so the learner is required to perform in a novel context. Reinstatement in this form is where the learner is asked to apply what has been learned previously to a new situation. This is a manifestation of the phenomenon of *transfer of learning.* For example, when a student nurse has learned the different techniques of sterilization in a hospital setting, one may give the nurse the new task of sterilizing syringes in the patient's home, an environment that may be entirely new. Such transfer of learned and retained capabilities are of primary importance in the design and practice of instruction in school systems.

Gagne (1970, p. 77) further pointed out that learned capabilities that can be transferred must be stored, but they are not "recalled" in the same sense that verbal information is recalled. Instead, they are applied to new situations. Therefore, one may suppose that the learner needs strategies for learning transfer and reinstatement of intellectual skills that are different from those used in verbal recall.

TYPES OF LEARNING

Gagne identified eight types of learning, ranging from the simplest form—signal learning—to the most complex type—problem solving. In this section each type of learning is described briefly. In the modules to follow, each type of learning is presented separately and in greater depth. These types of learning are also called the conditions of learning.

The first type of learning is called *signal learning*, or *classical conditioning*. The individual learns to make a general, diffuse response to a signal. An example of classically conditioned response is Pavlov's dog, who was conditioned to salivate with the ringing of a bell. Biases are learned by means of classical conditioning.

Type-2 learning is *stimulus-response (S–R) learning*, also known as operant conditioning, or instrumental learning. The learner acquires a precise response to a discriminated stimulus. What is learned, according to Thorndike (1898), is a connection, or, according to Skinner (1938), a discriminated operant, sometimes known as an instrumental response (Kimble, 1961). An example of operant conditioning is the use of token-economy systems as rewards in shaping schizophrenic patients' behaviors.

Type-3 learning is called *chaining*. What is learned is a chain of two or more stimulus-response connections. An example of chaining is skill learning, or any other motor performance, as in donning a pair of sterile gloves.

Type-4 learning is *verbal association*. It is the learning of chains that are verbal. Basi-

cally, the conditions are similar to those of chaining, but the presence of language in human beings makes this a special type of learning because the internal links may be selected from the individual's previously learned repertoire of language (Underwood, 1964). An example of verbal association may be the learning of medical terminology and abbreviations.

Type-5 learning is *multiple discrimination*. The individual learns to make different identifying responses to as many different stimuli, which may resemble each other in physical appearance to a greater or lesser degree. Although the learning of each stimulus-response connection is a simple type-2 occurrence, the connections tend to interfere with each other's retention (Postman, 1961). An example of multiple discrimination is when a nurse is able to differentiate or discriminate between a +2 and a +3 in testing a diabetic patient's urine for sugar. Another example of multiple discrimination is when a nurse is able to discriminate and differentiate between the signs and symptoms of diabetic coma and insulin coma.

Type-6 learning is *concept learning*. In concept learning, the learner acquires the capability to make a common response to a class of stimuli that may differ from each other widely in physical appearance. The learner is capable of making a response that identifies an entire class of objects or events (Kendler, 1964). An example of concept learning is when a nurse observes the following situation: a syringe being boiled, autoclaved, or disinfected; and the nurse makes the common response of "sterilization method" to this class of stimuli. The nurse is said to have acquired the idea of a "concept."

Type-7 learning is *principle learning*. The learner acquires an inferred capability to relate two or more concepts to each other. Principle learning functions to control behavior in the manner suggested by a verbalized rule of the form "if A, then B," where A and B are concepts. For example, "microbes cause infection" is a principle; when put into an "if-then" framework, one could say, "If there is an infection, then there must be microbes." However, it must be carefully distinguished from the more verbal sequence (or rote statement) of "if A, then B," which of course may also be learned as type 4.

Type-8 learning is *problem solving.* This is the most difficult and the most complex type of learning. It requires the internal events of thinking. Problem solving is the kind of learning where two or more previously acquired principles are related or combined to produce a new capability that can be shown to depend on a "higher-order" principle. For example, with the problem "infection and what to do about it," the nurse who can recall two or more relevant principles and relate them to each other and apply them to this problem is said to have acquired the skills of problem solving. For instance, if the nurse can remember the principles "infections are caused by microbes" and "antibiotics usually kill microbes" and can relate these principles to each other, then the nurse can solve the problem.

Social learning is another type of learning that Gagne (1970) does not classify separately. However, this author believes that since social learning is based mostly on the combination of the first five types of learning, as well as some of the others, it is unique. In social learning, the individual acquires behaviors and behavioral tendencies through any combination of the other eight types of learning. Examples of behaviors that are learned by means of social learning are aggressive behaviors, dependency, and affiliation. The functions of observation and modeling have tremendous effects on social learning. Most personality characteristics are developed and shaped by means of social learning.

BASIC CONDITIONS OF LEARNING

The five basic conditions of learning are: contiguity, practice, reinforcement, generalization, and discrimination. These are also often referred to as external conditions of learning. Not all of these conditions are equally important in each type of learning. In this section each of these conditions is briefly described and is related to the learning type for which it is important.

Contiguity. Contiguity refers to the almost simultaneous occurrence of the stimuli and the responses. For example, when an autistic child is taught to associate the word "milk" with the object (a carton of milk), the stimulus object (the carton of milk) must be presented at the same time the child says "milk." As nurse-teachers, we are interested in having learners (patients or students) build up associations between particular stimuli and responses. One of the important and necessary conditions for learning and developing such associations is contiguity.

Contiguity is important in most types of learning. For instance, in classical conditioning, contiguity is involved in pairing the conditioned and the unconditioned stimuli. Operant conditioning involves contiguity of the response and the reinforcing stimulus. In chaining, contiguity is involved in the occurrence of the various links in the motor chain. Concept learning involves contiguity in the presentation of examples and "nonexamples." In principle learning contiguity is involved in the recall of the component concepts. Finally, in problem solving contiguity is involved in the recall of the component principles (DeCecco and Crawford, 1974, p. 183).

Practice. Practice is the repetition of a response in the presence of the stimulus. Practice is necessary to retain stimulus-response (S–R) associations for a long period of time. In general, one learns very little from just the first response made to a specific stimulus.

Practice strengthens the bond between a stimulus and a response. Practice becomes less necessary when the student possesses a particular entering behavior that is related to the instructional objectives required.

Practice is of diminishing importance as one moves from the simpler forms of learning to more complex learning. In classical conditioning, operant conditioning, chaining, verbal learning, and multiple-discrimination learning, practice is crucial. In concept learning, principle learning, and problem solving, it is of minor importance, if the other learning conditions are properly provided (DeCecco and Crawford, 1974, p. 184).

Reinforcement. Reinforcement is one of the most important conditions of learning. One can vary the reinforcement procedure to provide different effects. The effects are the learning types the students need to acquire. In reinforcement procedure, the learner is presented with a specific stimulus, called the reinforcer, before or after a response is made. In a given situation, the learner will tend to repeat responses (R) that have been reinforced and to discontinue responses that have not been reinforced. A reinforcer is distinguished from other stimuli because it has this particular effect on behavior.

There are two main types of reinforcement: positive and negative. Each type has two components. Positive reinforcement is either the presentation of a rewarding stimulus (S) or the termination of an aversive stimulus. Examples of rewarding stimuli are gold stars, cheers, praise, and candy. Negative reinforcement is either the presentation of an aversive stimulus or the termination of a rewarding stimulus. Examples of aversive stimuli are noise, pain, and ugly sights. Skinner (1953) used a somewhat abbreviated definition; he termed a rewarding stimulus as a positive reinforcer and an aversive stimulus as a negative reinforcer. Punishment is either the removal of a rewarding stimulus, the presentation of an aversive stimulus, or both.

Extinction of a particular behavior occurs when a positive reinforcer is withheld, which subsequently weakens the response, or when two responses are made incompatible with each other.

Because of the breadth of the concept of reinforcement, a separate module has been developed that deals with this topic in detail. Briefly, the conditions of reinforcement that effect the strength of the response or the adequacy of the performance are immediacy, frequency, and amount and number.

Immediacy of the reinforcer. Experimental studies show that the reinforcer must immediately follow the response if the organism or the learner is to associate the response with the stimulus. The delay should not be longer than 1 or 2 seconds. Learning efficiency increases when students receive feedback about their performance. Knowledge of results in the form of feedback is a reinforcer.

Frequency of reinforcement. Frequency refers to the schedule of reinforcement. A learner can be reinforced for varying amounts of work, after varying amounts of time, or for fixed amounts of work or time. Responses learned using the variable schedules of reinforcement are more resistant to extinction than responses learned using the fixed schedules. Also, responses learned using a partial schedule of reinforcement are more resistant to extinction than those learned using a continuous pattern.

Amount and number of reinforcers. Response strength increases as the number of reinforcements for that response increases. However, when a limit is reached, each successive reinforcement adds smaller and smaller amounts of response strength. The amount of the reinforcer also affects behavior. The study of Wolfe and Kaplan (1941) showed that chickens ran faster to get four quarter grains of corn than to get one whole grain. This suggests that the additional activity involved in consuming the four quarter grains contributes something to the reward value (DeCecco and Crawford, 1974, p. 192).

Generalization. An individual who is confronted with a new stimulus situation and makes a response previously learned in conjunction with another stimulus is said to have made a *generalization*. Generalization gradients (curves) show that the tendency to generalize increases with the similarity of the new stimuli to the training stimulus. If we could not generalize, we would have to learn discrete responses for each discrete stimulus, and our behavior would appear to be something less than human.

Generalization is an important part of human behavior, whether it is appropriate or inappropriate. Even fear responses generalize. For instance, when an individual goes to the dentist's office and is given a small injection to anesthetize the part that is to be drilled, some pain is felt for a few minutes; but there is a tendency to generalize the fear response to other things, such as the waiting room, the smell of the office, and the white gowns. These are examples of *overgeneralization* (DeCecco and Crawford, 1974, pp. 195-196).

Discrimination. In discrimination behavior, the individual makes different responses to two or more stimuli. DeCecco and Crawford (1974, p. 197) use the designations S^D and S^Δ to indicate the different types of discrimination stimuli. "An S^D is a discriminative stimulus; the occasion on which the response is reinforced. It is the go signal, like the green traffic light. In the S^Δ situation, the response is not reinforced. It is the stop signal." Behaviors can be perceived as being under the alternate control of S^D and S^Δ.

• • •

These conditions of learning—generalization and discrimination—are important in most types of learning.

Instruction
NATURE OF INSTRUCTION

Instruction, or teaching, is the process of producing learning in the learner. In other words, it is the process of producing permanent changes in the behavioral tendency of the learner as a result of intentionally planned learning experiences.

The realm of instruction deals with: (1) the behavior of teachers, (2) the reason why teachers behave the way they do, and (3) the consequences or the effects of their behavior on the students. Since learning takes place under many circumstances (both in and out of school), instruction should also encompass the teaching of any subject, by any teacher, to any group of learners, under all situations, both in and out of school.

Gagne pointed out that as of yet, there isn't a theory of teaching that explains, predicts, and controls the ways in which the behavior of the teacher affects the learning of the students. Gagne also predicts that there probably will never be a single theory of teaching because teaching encompasses "far too many kinds of process, of behavior, of activity, to be the proper subject of a single theory" (Gagne, 1964, p. 274).

A BASIC TEACHING MODEL

Models of instruction seem to have provided a good substitute for a theory of teaching. Models demonstrate how the various conditions of learning and instruction are interrelated. Glaser's (1962) model of instruction is a basic teaching model that divides the process of teaching into four components: instructional objectives; entering behavior; instructional procedures; and performance assessment, or evaluation. In Fig. 1-2 is the diagram of Glaser's basic teaching model. The connecting arrows indicate the major sequence of events in the instructional process. Lines that connect components that are later in the sequence with earlier ones are called *feedback loops*.

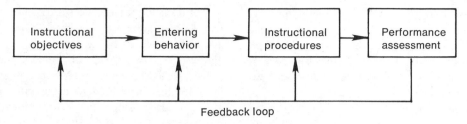

Fig. 1-2. A basic teaching model with feedback loops. (After Glaser, 1962, p. 6; DeCecco and Crawford, 1974, p. 9.)

In this next section each of the components of the model is briefly described; then the first two components of the model; namely, the instructional objective and the entering behavior, are described in more detail. Instructional procedures vary with the instructional objectives and the type of learning. Later modules describe procedures for each condition of learning. For instance, the modules on the eight conditions of learning, the different models of instruction, behavior modification techniques, and the variables within the instructional procedures are upcoming. The final module is concerned with evaluation of both learning and instruction.

The first component of Glaser's (1962) teaching model is *instructional objectives* (box A). Instructional objectives are observable or measurable behaviors or performances that the learner should attain on completion of instruction. They are the criteria that are set up prior to instruction taking place. Setting of instructional objectives is the first step in any teaching situation. *Entering behavior* (box B) refers to the level of knowledge the student possesses prior to instruction. It includes not only what the student has previously learned, but also the student's motivational state, intellectual ability and development, and certain social and cultural determinants of learning ability. *Instructional procedures* (box C) describe the teaching process; most decisions a teacher makes are on these procedures. The proper manage-

ment of these instructional procedures produces learning and achievement behaviors in students. Instructional procedures vary with instructional objectives. *Performance assessment* or evaluation (box D) is concerned with determining to what extent instructional objectives have been achieved. These are done by means of tests or observation. If evaluation shows that certain objectives have not been accomplished according to set criteria, then one or all of the preceding components of the basic teaching model may require adjustment. The feedback loops carry and feed the pertinent information provided by the performance evaluation back to each teaching component.

Setting of instructional objectives. The first step in deciding the conditions for learning is to define the objectives. Objectives are statements that specify the nature of change in behavior that is sought in the learner. Objectives make it possible to infer what kind of learning situation needs to be established to bring about this change. Objectives need to be stated in observable or measurable human performances. A number of writers (Tyler, 1949; Mager, 1962; Gagne, 1964; Arndt and Huckabay, 1975) have pointed out that utilization of such words as to know, to appreciate, or to understand in a statement of objectives is inadequate because they do not communicate reliably to any individual the set of circumstances that identify a class of human performances. A statement of objectives should include the following five criteria:

1. The observable or measurable *behavior* expected of the student; for example, to draw, identify, recognize, demonstrate, state, or describe

2. The *content* area within which the behavior is to be exhibited; for example, define the concept of discrimination, of cyanosis; demonstrate the procedure of catheterization (The content areas in these examples are discrimination, cyanosis, and catheterization.)

3. Identification of the *learner* or the *subject;* that is, who the person is for whom the objective is written (It can be any learner—a student, a child, a patient, a group of parents, or others.)

4. The *conditions under which the behavior is to be exhibited* by the learner—in other words, what are the "givens"—for example, given a diagram of the heart, the nursing student will identify the anatomical structure of the heart

5. The *criteria of acceptable performance*, which is also a very important part of the objective; for example, given a diagram of the heart, the student will identify a minimum of eight out of ten anatomical structures of the heart (The criteria of acceptable performance is eight out of ten [8:10] anatomical structures.)

When statements of objectives are as specific as possible and include these five criteria, they serve several functions: (1) inform learners exactly what is expected, (2) enable learners to determine to what extent they have accomplished the objectives, (3) provide feedback to learners from their performances that will have reinforcing, motivational, and directional value, and (4) make evaluation easier for both the learner and the teacher. Thus, having determined the learner or instructional objective, the second step is to determine the entering behavior of the learner. This is the topic of discussion for the rest of the chapter.

Entering behavior. Entering behavior refers to the behavior the student must have acquired before being able to learn and achieve a new terminal performance. In other words, it refers to the present level of knowledge, prior to instruction, intellectual ability and development, motivational level, and certain social and cultural determinants of learning ability. The level of entering behavior is the point where instruction begins. The terminal behavior is the target point where instruction concludes. Teaching, then, is the act of bringing the student from the level of entering behavior to the level of terminal behavior. DeCecco and Crawford (1974) point out that the descriptions of entering and terminal behaviors, together, define the limits of the teacher's responsibilities and expectations for each act of teaching.

Entering behavior has two characteristics: (1) statements of entering behaviors are more explicit and refer to more specific observable performances than statements of terminal objectives; (2) the list of entering behaviors as a whole is generally more comprehensive than those of terminal performances.

To illustrate the difference between the terminal behavior or performance and the entering behavior is the following example:

Terminal behavior: At the completion of instruction, given a complete hypothermia unit, the student will be able to set up and operate a unit at the 95% level of accuracy.

Entering behavior:

a. The student can state the purpose of the hypothermia unit

b. The student can state the uses of the hypothermia unit

c. The student can identify all the controls on the unit

d. The student can read and follow the written directions on how to operate the hypothermia unit

In the example provided, the statements of entering behavior do not describe the conditions under which the performance must occur, and they do not specify the criteria of acceptable performance, which is required in the statement and performance of a terminal behavior. Note also that the list of entering behaviors is more comprehensive as compared to the terminal objective or behavior.

Role of entering behavior in instruction. In this section, a brief description is given on how to use the concept of entering behavior in planning instruction. There are three important factors that have to be taken into consideration: (1) determining what entering behavior is necessary to accomplish a terminal objective, (2) assessing the entering behavior of the student, and (3) making decisions based on the results of assessment.

Determination of what entering behavior is necessary to accomplish a terminal objective. Once instructional objectives have been explicitly stated, determination of entering behaviors necessary to accomplish the terminal objective can be made. DeCecco and Crawford (1975) point out that instruction for the new objectives should begin with the recall of previously learned responses appropriate to the learning of the new material. Different entering behavior is required for different learning. Gagne's (1970) hierarchy of the conditions of learning provides a framework to follow. For example, if the learner is to problem solve, then the entering behaviors necessary to solve the specific problems are principle, concepts, verbal associations, discrimination learning, chaining, and the operant and respondent types of learning that are appropriate and relevant to the problem. Furthermore, Gagne's key question of "What should the learner need to know in order for him to be able to solve the problem given only instruction?" provides a guideline to determine the necessary entering behaviors as well. Answers to this question are the entering behaviors. By asking this question over and over again about each new entering behavior, one can come up with a hierarchy of

entering behaviors or what Gagne calls "subordinate tasks" that the learner must know in order to perform the "superordinate task" that is directly above it. An example is that the instructional objective for a diabetic patient is as follows: at the completion of instruction, the diabetic patient will be able to calculate a 1,200-calorie diet for a day (three meals) with two exchanges of protein, one exchange of carbohydrate, one fruit, and one vegetable. Gagne's strategy is utilized in determining the entering behavior necessary to solve this problem, by asking his key question, "What should the diabetic patient need to know in order to solve this problem given only instruction?" The patient needs to know the principles relevant to this problem. For instance, there are the principles of (a) the number of calories in 1 g of protein, carbohydrate, and so on; (b) the number of grams of each item that is the equivalent of one exchange; and (c) the mathematical operations of division, multiplication, addition, and subtraction.

Next, in order to know and be able to utilize these principles, what else does the patient need to know? Answers to this question may be that the patient needs to know such concepts as exchanges, protein, carbohydrate, calories, identification of food items that belong to each food category, and others.

At this stage, the instructor may want to test the patient to assess level of knowledge (entering behavior). If the patient does not have this knowledge, then it may be necessary to go through the same process, only going further down the learning hierarchy to the level of verbal association and discrimination learning where the patient is able to identify and lable the correct food item and then discriminate it from other food items. Instruction begins at the learner's present level.

Assessing the entering behavior of the learner. Once the necessary entering behavior for an instructional objective has been identified, the next step is to assess the entering behavior of the learner. DeCecco and Crawford (1974) suggest that this can be done either through an interview with the learner or a test of entering behavior. If a test is to be constructive, three or four test items have to be written for each prerequisite behavior. A pretest should be distinguished from a test of entering behavior. A pretest measures the terminal performance before instruction begins. It is often the same as, or an alternate form of, the posttest. A test of entering behavior measures previous learning rather than present learning.

In the example mentioned before, the entering behavior of the diabetic patient can be assessed either by asking the patient to explain verbally what an exchange is, how many grams of carbohydrate is equal to one exchange, and so on. One could also test entering behavior by developing a short multiple-choice type test that taps the principles that are needed to solve the problem and some of the necessary concepts, such as calorie, carbohydrate, exchange, and protein.

Assessment of entering behavior determines where the instruction must begin. Lembo (1972) cited certain advantages of starting where the learner is: (1) there is acquisition of necessary skills—a student cannot learn a complex skill if prerequisites or component parts have not been mastered; (2) enhancement of motivation—a student will persist and succeed on achieving specific goals only when the goals reflect current capabilities and concerns. Motivation to learn is inherent in the learning program, and "success breeds success."

Failure, alienation, and psychological damage occur when students do not begin at their individual levels, when they progress at a rate or in a manner not their own, or when they pursue goals and engage in activities established by others.

According to Lembo (1972, p. 37), the ultimate purpose of meeting students where they are is to "help them acquire the skills to set their own goals, to plan their own learning activities, to rely on their own resourcefulness to be successful, and to evaluate for themselves the effectiveness and relevance of their efforts and behavior."

Making decisions based on the results of assessments. If the assessment of the entering behavior of the learner reveals that there is more than enough entering behavior, the teacher may decide either to carry out the instructional plan or to begin instruction at a more advanced point and add more depth, breadth, or applications of material than originally planned. For instance, if our diabetic patient possessed all the necessary entering behaviors, the teacher could then introduce different variations of the 1,200-calorie diet with different amount of exchanges.

However, if the learner lacks the necessary entering behaviors, several alternative measures are available. First, the teacher can conduct review sessions, which will enable the learners to recall material previously learned but now forgotten, thus enabling the learners to increase their entering behavior. For instance, for the diabetic patient, the nurse-teacher could conduct review sessions on types of foods, exchanges, calorie calculations, and other topics, thus helping the patient recall forgotten material that is necessary to solve the problem. Second, the teacher can begin at an earlier point, thus increasing the amount of instruction provided than originally planned. For instance, the nurse-teacher can start at the level of discrimination learning rather than principle learning as originally planned and can ask the patient to discriminate between the food items by grouping them according to carbohydrates, proteins, fruits, and vegetables. Once the patient is able to do this, then the patient can be asked to weigh them into proper exchanges and finally to calculate their caloric value.

The third alternative that is available when learners do not have the necessary entering behavior is for the teacher either to choose a different terminal performance or lower the standard. For example, if the diabetic patient lacked much of the entering behavior, the teacher would drop this objective, instead maybe developing a simpler terminal performance. This could be that at the completion of instruction the diabetic patient will be able to weigh 120 g of protein, 50 g of carbohydrate, and one fruit, and will eat this three times daily. The other option is to lower the standard on the original terminal objective. For instance, instead of asking the patient to calculate 1,200 calories in a diet with two exchanges of protein, one exchange of carbohydrate, one fruit, and one vegetable, the teacher could give a chart that has all the items of the food labelled, with exchanges and grams per exchange specified, and then ask the patient to solve the original problem.

Therefore, it is important to keep in mind that the results of the determination and the assessment of entering behavior must become an integral part of the instructional plan and procedure.

Variables influencing the determination of entering behaviors

Readiness for learning. Learning takes place within a set of events called instruction. There are certain preconditions of learning that precede the learning event, and they determine the probability of learning taking place or not. These preconditions are collectively referred to as *readiness for learning.* The three major factors that comprise learning readiness are (1) attentional sets, (2) motivation, and (3) developmental readiness. Each of these factors refers to an internal state of the learner. These states can be established and to some degree can be manipu-

lated by management of the external environment of the individual. Gagne (1970) considered these three states to be the most important factors that can be influenced by an instructor for learning to occur.

ATTENTIONAL SET. Attentional set is an internal state of the learner. Gagne points out that it is assumed and maintained temporarily, and it enables the learner to select and apprehend the stimuli that are appropriate to the learning that is being undertaken. There are of course external methods by which to attract the learner's attention to the correct stimulus. Since every act of learning requires an apprehending phase, which is dependent on attention, the teacher can arrange for the stimulus situation to contain elements of novelty, change, variation in intensity of stimulation, and the like. To provide continuously for such external "attention getters" is a tedious job. Gagne states that there must be a means whereby attending is internally controlled, enabling the learner to select and apprehend stimuli at appropriate times. It is this internal state that is called the attentional set. There are several types of such sets available; for example, a set for attending to the source of the stimulus, another set for making appropriate responses, and still other sets for carrying out a sequence by following verbal directions and for exploring the environment. Gagne further states that these prelearning capabilities are a form of cognitive strategies that govern the learner's information-seeking behavior.

MOTIVATION. Motivation is a very large and complex topic. Module 28 covers all the aspects of motivation. In this section, motivation is treated as an internal state and a prerequisite component of learning readiness. Two motives are of particular importance here: social mastery and task mastery, or achievement. Social motives include needs for affiliation, social approval, self-esteem, and others related to these areas. These motives determine the level of the student's interaction with peers and with the teacher. Task mastery, or achievement, is perceived by many investigators to be of most importance in learning intellectual skills. The motivation of task mastery is enhanced by experiences of success in achieving the objectives of a specific learning task. Other theorists view the task-mastery motivation as a "need for achievement," "competence," or "effectance." All the theorists agree that the learner can obtain reward and satisfaction from achievement and that success in achievement perpetuates further achievement and facilitates subsequent learning. This, therefore, becomes a most dependable source of continuing motivation. Gagne further points out that such a motivation must be a strong aspect of the development of a "continuing self-learner," and this development is often stated to be the most important goal of education (Gagne, 1970, pp. 289-298).

DEVELOPMENTAL READINESS. Development is the product of inheritance and environment. The biologically determined ways of interacting with the environment are inherited (DeCecco and Crawford, 1974). Ausubel (1959) viewed readiness as the adequacy of the learner's existing capability in relation to an instructional objective. When readiness refers to a specific performance, it is viewed as the same as entering behavior. Readiness does not refer to how the learner acquired existing capacity, but it refers to the adequacy of that capacity. Readiness is often confused with maturation. Maturation refers to biological growth, which occurs under the influence of heredity. Readiness, on the other hand, is the product of both learning and maturation. Studies have demonstrated that training is a waste of time if the learner has not reached the prerequisite level of maturation. For example, the classical study on toilet training of two sets of identical male

twins (McGraw, 1940) showed that when one member of each pair of twins was given toilet training starting from the second month of life, and the other twin from each pair began toilet training at 14 and 24 months respectively, the four infants exhibited the same degree of excretory control at the end of 28 months. The conclusions that were derived from this study were that: (1) maturation of certain muscles must precede effective toilet training, and (2) training must be introduced sometime since maturation alone will not provide the necessary control. The issue at hand is not whether training should be introduced, but *when* training should be introduced. DeCecco and Crawford (1974) pointed out that what is true for physical development and training appears also to hold true for cognitive development and school learning.

With regard to cognitive development, the attainment of a state of intellectual development constitutes the third factor in learning readiness. The issue of maturation versus learning is an active one, too. One school of thought believes cognitive development is stage-bound, and that the stages of neurophysiological growth impose certain limitations on the kind and degree of cognitive development possible. Proponents of this view are Piaget (1952), Gesell (1928), Flavell (1963), Hymes (1958), and many others. For example, Piaget proposed the stages of cognitive development called sensorimotor, preoperational, concrete operational, and formal operational. These stages represent periods of development of the operations of logical thought. For instance, at a particular age, a child may be able to think logically when dealing with a concrete event because this developmental stage has been attained. However, the child may not be able to think logically when faced with a problem that involves symbolic representations of events, because the developmental stage of formal operations has not been attained.

The alternative view, which is not inconsistent with the existing evidence, is the one proposed by Gagne (1970, p. 289). He stated "Differences in developmental readiness are primarily attributable to differences in the number and kind of previously learned intellectual skills." Therefore, developmental readiness for learning is determined by the cumulative effects of learning and learning transfer. According to this view, when children learn to deal intellectually with a specific concrete problem, the resulting intellectual skills have the property of transferring to other problems that have certain commonalities. As these skills accumulate, they have the potentiality of generating other skills of increasing degrees of abstractness and generality through the process of transfer of learning. Therefore, readiness for new learning may be viewed as depending on the repertoire of intellectual skills the individual possesses that have been learned previously and that are relevant to the learning of the new task.

Bruner (1960, p. 12) also believes that the "The foundations of any subject may be taught to anybody at any age in some form." For him, readiness is practically an unnecessary concept; children are always ready.

Learning styles. Learning styles are individual or personal ways in which people process information in learning concepts and principles. Kagan (1965) has identified two types of learning styles: (1) conceptual tempos and (2) selection strategies. These are discussed here as aspects of entering behavior.

CONCEPTUAL TEMPOS. Conceptual tempos are basic dispositions of the individual either to think and reflect on the solution to the problem or to make fast, impulsive, and unconsidered responses. Kagan and his associates (1964, 1965, 1966) have conducted several classical experiments and have identified two types of conceptual tempos in children: impulsive and reflective. The child who has the impulsive or the fast tempo solves the problem quickly with little or no delay. The reflective child possesses a slow tempo and considers alternative solutions to the problem, thus delaying answering. In his experiments, Kagan used a Matching Familiar Figures test (MFF) and a Haptic Visual Matching test (HVM). In the MFF, the researcher provided the child with a drawing at the top of a page and six similar ones with slight variations at the bottom of the page. The child was asked to select from the bottom pictures the one that was identical to the top picture. The researcher then recorded the amount of time the child took to reach a decision. In the HVM the child tactilely explored a wooden figure while blindfolded. Then the researcher removed the blindfold and gave the child five other wooden figures. The task for the child was to find out which of these five wooden figures was similar to the one manipulated while blindfolded. Again, the researcher recorded the amount of time the child took to reach a decision. Results of this study (Kagan, 1965) showed that: (1) reflection and accuracy increase with age; (2) the tendency to display fast or slow decision times was more or less stable over a period of 20 months; (3) the tendency toward reflection or impulsivity shows in performance of other tasks; and (4) the disposition seems to be linked to other aspects of the child's personality.

In another study, Kagan, Pearson and Welsh (1966) showed that impulsive children can be trained to be more reflective under two specially designed tutorial conditions: (1) a normal nurturant teacher, where the tutor merely comments positively on the child's choices on two tests, and (2) an adult identification situation, where the teacher persuades the child that by taking more time and becoming more reflective, the child will be more like the teacher. The training session was for 1 hour. Results showed that all children delayed their answers for 10 to 15 seconds and answered when the teacher told them to answer. Kagan pointed out several educational implications of this study: (1) the teacher's tempo should be adjusted to that of the child, and the reflective child should not be perceived as less bright than the impulsive child; (2) the teacher should not penalize with sarcasm the impulsive child for incorrect answers, especially when correct answers given quickly are rewarded; the teacher who behaves this way handicaps the impulsive child who only has average ability (DeCecco and Crawford, 1974).

SELECTION STRATEGIES. Selection strategies comprise the second type of learning style. Bruner and his associates (1956) identify various ways in which individuals learn concepts. These methods, called *selection strategies*, control the order in which appropriate and inappropriate examples of concepts appear. Selection strategies serve three purposes: (1) to maximize the opportunity to obtain useful information about the concept that is to be learned, (2) to reduce the strain of assimilating and keeping track of the information, and (3) to regulate the amount of risk the learner takes in reaching a solution (DeCecco and Crawford, 1974).

Bruner has identified four selection strategies:

1. *Conservative focusing* is a strategy in which the learner uses an example of a concept and changes only one attribute at a time to find those attributes that are essential; for example, if the nursing student was given the task of finding a hypodermic needle, or defining a hypodermic needle. This concept has such attributes as size (length and gauge), shape (short 3/4 inch), color (steel color), and so on. The student who is said to utilize the conservative focusing selection strategy will process this information one attribute at a time until identifying the needle with all the correct attributes. This strategy guarantees success. It maximizes the opportunity to obtain useful information; it reduces the strain of remembering and holding all the information in mind at once because the student handles and processes one attribute at a time.

2. *Focus gambling* is the selection strategy in which the learner uses a focus example and changes more than one attribute at a time. Such a strategy enables the individual to acquire the concept with the use of fewer examples than those required for conservative focusing. However, if the individual uses a wrong example, the possible gain in time is lost. Kagan (1965) pointed out that impulsive children use focus gambling techniques, while reflective children use conservative focusing.

3. *Simultaneous scanning* is the selective strategy in which the student formulates several hypotheses of what the concept may be and then looks for examples. For each example encountered, the student decides which hypothesis to keep and which to eliminate. In this strategy the student has to deal with several independent hypotheses and keep them all in mind. Such a strategy involves higher risk and appeals to more impulsive types of individuals with fast tempo.

4. *Successive scanning* is the selection strategy in which the student tests only a single hypothesis at a time. For example, the student forms a hypothesis of the characteristic of a concept and tests the hypothesis against each example encountered. This is similar to conservative focusing but different in the sense that instead of testing one attribute of a concept at a time, the person tests a single hypothesis about the concept—one hypothesis at a time. Successive scanning reduces the amount of information the individual has to keep in mind and reduces the amount of relevant information each encounter may provide. Such a strategy appeals to reflective children because it carries less risk.

Travers (1963) suggested that the teacher should adjust the selection strategy to the ability of the learner. A simultaneous-scanning strategy requires more ability than a conservative-focusing or successive-scanning strategy (DeCecco and Crawford, 1974).

On the other hand, another investigator (Rosenberg, 1968) has identified four types of learning styles. An important criterion he considers for determining the learning style of an individual is the degree to which the student is aware of and open to information needed to solve a problem. The four types follow:

1. *Rigid-inhibited style* in which learners are apt to become confused and easily upset when routines are altered and manifest signs of nervousness like tic and crying; need constant supervision

2. *Undisciplined style* in which learners refuse to do what is asked and do not finish their work, have temper tantrums, and exhibit wildly destructive behavior; helped by extending their attention span (rearranging the environment to minimize competing stimuli)

3. *Acceptance-anxious style* in which learners are more concerned about outside evaluation, what others think of them, and less about the work itself; jealous of others who receive higher grades and continually looking for approval from the teacher; benefit most from the elimination of grades

4. *Creative style* in which learners are self confident, able to evaluate their own performances with objectivity, learn from their mistakes, and perform well on a wide variety of tasks.

Learning abilities. Learning abilities are the different processes by which individuals acquire knowledge. Jensen (1960) hypothesized that individuals differ in learning abilities in several ways. Some students learn better when they pace their own learning, while other learn better when the teaching machine sets the pace. Jensen (1965) also found that individuals differ in their susceptibility to factors affecting forgetting, such as retroactive and proactive inhibition and response competition. Jensen also proposed that a student's performance on any given task is the product or a function of the level of learning ability and the extent to which the new learning task involves these abilities. Research is needed to identify what the basic learning abilities are.

Jensen's study (1963) provides support for the proposition that there are several learning abilities instead of a single one and that sometimes these abilities bear little relationship to I.Q. He pointed out that I.Q. tests, which are a form of achievement test, tell us more about what the individual has learned outside the test situation than about ability to learn in a new situation. He tested this concept with mentally retarded, average, and gifted children. The task that they had to learn was to press the correct button to give a green light. Results showed that the gifted children performed better than the average children, who in turn performed better than the mentally retarded children. However, four of the retarded children were *fast learners*, and they scored above average on all tests. Even though these mentally retarded children were below average in scholastic achievement and had I.Q. scores of 65, they were *fast learners* when it came to learning this type of task. Jensen also identified another learning ability, which he called *labeling behavior*. He suggested that mentally retarded children may perform poorly in school because they lack this verbal-learning ability.

In other studies, Fleishman (1965, 1967) examined the interaction between instructional conditions and learner characteristics. He compared the contribution of the various abilities tested at the beginning of learning psychomotor skills to performance scores on successive learning trials during practice. He showed that, as practice continues, particular combinations of abilities contribute to performance change and that these different abilities, which exist prior to entering a learning situation, influence learning at different stages. The implication is that individuals with different patterns of abilities require different learning experiences at different stages.

Jensen conceives of learning abilities as being related to entering behavior because they are prerequisite capabilities for achieving instructional objectives. He also views learning abilities as occupying an intermediate position between overspecified and overgeneralized descriptions of entering behavior and believes that their identification will prove useful in designing instruction (DeCecco and Crawford, 1974).

Personality of the learner. DeCecco and Crawford (1974) pointed out that entering behavior is the product of the many personality structures. Since entering behavior refers to present performance that reflects previous learning, and this previous learning is both influenced by and influences personality structures and processes, DeCecco and Crawford also concluded that there must be a relationship between personality of the learner, entering behavior, and learning.

Spence (1956) studied the concept of anxiety and its relation to learning. He found that the level of anxiety (as measured by a personality test) characteristic of a person has a bearing on learning. It seems that people of high anxiety do well on simple tasks, but poorly on more complex problems.

Application to nursing education and practice

Within the preceeding sections of this module, a detailed application of the specific basic principles of learning and instruction was made to patient- or student-teaching situations. The following list draws attention to the highlights. Patient teaching is one of the identified functions of the nurse in areas like prevention of disease and promotion of health.

Prior to initiating any teaching to a patient, the nurse must have the following plan in mind and should implement it:

1. Identification of the instructional (learner) objective, that is, statement of the terminal behavior expected of the patient at the completion of instruction, stated in observable or measurable terms

2. Identification of the type of entering behavior necessary to achieve the objective

3. Assessment of the patient's entering behavior, taking into consideration the following variables:

   a. Readiness factors, such as the patient's level of attention, motivation, and developmental level in terms of age and level of intellectual skills relevant to the learning of the task

   b. Learning style—whether the patient is a person who has a fast or slow tempo, or is impulsive or reflective—which could be assessed by the speed and method used to answer some of the questions

   c. Learning abilities—the patient's verbal ability and level of knowledge—which can be inferred by finding out the patient's educational level, occupation, general level of knowledge, and so on

   d. Personality of the patient—such as level of anxiety, amount of inhibition, and degree of acceptance of suggestions—which is harder to assess than the others

Having done this assessment, the nurse can implement the instructional procedure. The instructional procedure depends on the type of learning that is being undertaken, whether it is a single motor skill or a higher order teaching of concepts, principles, or problem-solving situations.

Evaluation to determine the extent to which terminal objectives have been accomplished should also be done. Feedback from these evaluations should be channeled to the appropriate source if objectives have not been accomplished at the criterion level.

What is presented here is a schematic view of instruction. The same principles can be applied to any patient- or student-teaching situation.

Researchable questions

As mentioned previously, identification of the different learning abilities and accommodation of individual differences in cognitive style (conceptual tempos and selection strategies) in developing instructional procedures need further investigating. Studies are also needed to determine the methods by which attention span and level of motivation can be increased. Valid and reliable tools are needed in assessing patients' levels of knowledge in specific areas, such as diet information, knowledge about their disease conditions, and so on.

Evaluation of the entering behaviors of nurses with R.N. credentials who return to school to obtain their baccalaureate degrees needs investigation.

1. Measure the affective and cognitive consequences of an educational program that takes into consideration the entering behavior of R.N. students in a B.S. program versus programs that do not take into consideration their entering behavior.
   a. Independent variables: consideration versus no consideration of the entering behavior of students
   b. Dependent variables: cognitive and affective behaviors of R.N. students

ADDITIONAL LEARNING EXPERIENCES—RECOMMENDED READING LIST

DeCecco, J., and Crawford, W. *The psychology of learning and instruction: educational psychology.* (2nd Ed.) Englewood Cliffs, N.J.: Prentice-Hall, Inc., 1974, pp. 1-10, 47-69, 177-201.

Gagne, R. *The conditions of learning.* (2nd Ed.) New York: Holt, Rinehart, and Winston, Inc., 1970, pp. 1-31, 277-301, 325-344.

INSTRUCTIONS TO THE LEARNER REGARDING POSTTEST

You are now ready to take the posttest to determine the level of achievement of the module objectives. Return to the pretest of this module and take the same test over again as the posttest. Use the answer key on pp. 25-26 to correct your answers. You need to achieve 34 correct points (95%). If you score less than 34 correct points, correct your errors, study the content of this module again, and read some of the articles in the recommended reading list or in the references. Take the posttest again. You need to study until you achieve the 95% level of mastery or better before proceeding to the next module.

ANSWER KEY TO PRETEST AND POSTTEST

1. c (DeCecco and Crawford, 1974, p. 178)
2. d (DeCecco and Crawford, 1974, p. 179)
3. c (DeCecco and Crawford, 1974, p. 181)
4. c (Gagne, 1970, p. 5)
5. b (Gagne, 1970, pp. 325-328)
6. b (Gagne, 1970, p. 71)
7. d (Gagne, 1970, p. 35)
8. c (Gagne, 1970, pp. 47-51)
9. c (Gagne, 1970, pp. 42-45)
10. c (Bandura and Walters, 1967, pp. 47-108)
11. b (DeCecco and Crawford, 1974, p. 182)
12. b (DeCecco and Crawford, 1974, pp. 182-183)
13. b (DeCecco and Crawford, 1974, p. 183)
14. b (DeCecco and Crawford, 1974, pp. 183-184)
15. b (DeCecco and Crawford, 1974, p. 184)
16. c (DeCecco and Crawford, 1974, p. 185)
17. b (DeCecco and Crawford, 1974, pp. 195-196)
18. c (DeCecco and Crawford, 1974, pp. 195-196)
19. b (DeCecco and Crawford, 1974, p. 197)
20. b (DeCecco and Crawford, 1974, pp. 9-10)
21. c (DeCecco and Crawford, 1974, pp. 8-10)
22. c (DeCecco and Crawford, 1974, pp. 8-10; Gagne, 1970, pp. 48-49)
23. d (DeCecco and Crawford, 1974, pp. 48-49)
24. b (DeCecco and Crawford, 1974, pp. 67-68)
25. a (DeCecco and Crawford, 1974, pp. 559-560)
26. a (Gagne, 1970, pp. 298-301)
27. c (Gagne, 1970, p. 289)
28. b (DeCecco and Crawford, 1974, pp. 63-65)

29. b (DeCecco and Crawford, 1974, pp. 63-65)
30. b (DeCecco and Crawford, 1974, p. 65)
31. b, d (DeCecco and Crawford, 1974, pp. 65-66)
32. a. Ability to balance self in sitting position
    b. Ability to turn over and push up in bed
    c. Ability to follow simple directions about movement of the unaffected side
    d. Ability to bear body weight on the arms
    e. Ability to pay attention and follow directions to a series of actions and commands for the span of a few minutes

REFERENCES

Arndt, C., and Huckabay, L. M. D. *Nursing administration: theory for practice with a systems approach.* St. Louis: The C. V. Mosby Co., 1975.

Ausubel, D. P. Viewpoints from related disciplines: human growth and development. *Teachers College Record*, 1959, **60**:245-254.

Ausubel, D. P. *Educational psychology: a cognitive view.* New York: Holt, Rinehart and Winston, Inc., 1968.

Bandura, A., and Walters, R. *Social learning and personality development.* New York: Holt, Rinehart and Winston, Inc., 1967.

Bruner, J. S. *The process of education.* Cambridge, Mass.: Harvard University Press, 1960.

Bruner, J. S., Goodnow, J. J., and Austin, G. A. *A study of thinking.* New York: John Wiley & Sons, Inc., 1956.

DeCecco, J., and Crawford, W. *The psychology of learning and instruction: educational psychology.* (2nd Ed.) Englewood Cliffs, N. J.: Prentice-Hall, Inc., 1974.

Flavell, J. H. *The developmental psychology of Jean Piaget.* Princeton, N.J.: Van Nostrand Reinhold Co., 1963.

Fleishman, E. The description and prediction of perceptual motor skill learning. In R. Glaser (Ed.) *Training research and education.* New York: John Wiley & Sons, Inc., 1965, pp. 137-176.

Fleishman, E. Individual differences in motor learning. In R. Gagne (Ed.), *Learning and individual differences.* Columbus, Ohio: Charles E. Merrill Publishing Co., 1967, pp. 165-191.

Gage, N. L. The theories of teaching. In N. Gage (Ed.), *Handbook of research on teaching.* Skokie, Ill.: Rand McNally & Co., 1964, pp. 268-285.

Gagne, R. Problem solving. In A. Melton (Ed.), *Categories of human learning.* New York: Academic Press, Inc., 1964.

Gagne, R. The implications of instructional objectives for learning. In C. Lindvall, (Ed.), *Defining educational objectives.* Pittsburgh: University of Pittsburgh Press, 1964.

Gagne, R. *The conditions of learning.* (2nd Ed.) New York: Holt, Rinehart and Winston, Inc., 1970.

Gesell, A. *Infancy and human growth.* New York: The Macmillan Co., 1928.

Gibson, E. Perceptual learning. In R. Gagne and W. Gephart (Eds.), *Learning research and school subjects.* Itasca, Ill.: F. E. Peacock Publishers, Inc., 1968.

Glaser, R., Psychology and instuctional technology. In R. Glaser (Ed.), *Training Research and Education.* Pittsburgh: University of Pittsburgh Press, 1962, pp. 1-30.

Hymes, J. *Before the child reads.* Evanston, Ill.: Row Peterson and Co., 1958.

Jensen, A. Programmed instruction and individual differences. *Automated Teaching Bulletin*, 1960, **1**:12-17.

Jensen, A. Learning ability in retarded, average, and gifted children. *Merrill-Palmer Quarterly*, 1963, **9**:124-140.

Jensen, A. Individual differences in learning: interference factors. *U.S. Office of Education, Cooperative Research Project No. 1867*, Berkeley, Calif.: University of California, 1965.

Kagan, J. Impulsive and reflective children: significance of conceptual tempo. In J. Krumboltz (Ed.), *Learning and the educational process.* Skokie, Ill. Rand McNally & Co., 1965, pp. 133-161.

Kagan, J., Pearson, J., and Welsh, L. Modifiability of an impulsive tempo. *Journal of Educational Psychology*, 1966, **57**:359-365.

Kagan, J., Rosman, B., Day, D., Albert, J., and Phillips, W. Information processing in the child: significance of analytic and reflective attitudes. *Psychological Monographs*, 1964, **78**(1).

Kendler, H. The concept of the concept. In A. Melton (Ed.), Categories of human learning. New York: Academic Press, Inc., 1964., pp. 211-236.

Kimble, G. *Hilgard and Marquis' conditioning and learning.* New York: Appleton-Century-Crofts, 1961.

Lembo, J. *When learning happens,* New York: Schacher Books, 1972.

Mager, R. *Preparing objectives for programmed instruction.* Belmont, Calif.: Fearon Publishers, Inc. 1962.

McGraw, M. Neural maturation as exemplified in achievement of bladder control. *Journal of Pediatrics*, 1940, **16**:580-590.

Piaget, J. *The origin of intelligence in children.* New York: International University Press, 1952.

Postman, L. The present status of interference theory. In C. Cofer (Ed.), *Verbal learning and verbal behavior.* New York: McGraw-Hill Book Co., 1961.

Rosenberg, M. *Diagnostic teaching.* Seattle: Special Child Publications Book Co., 1968.

Skinner, B. *Behavior of organisms.* New York: Appleton-Century-Crofts, 1938.

Skinner, B. *Science and human behavior.* New York: The Macmillan Co., 1953.

Spence, K. *Behavior theory and conditioning.* New Haven, Conn.: Yale University Press, 1956.

Thorndike, E. Animal intelligence: an experimental study of the associative processes in animals. *Psychological Review Monographs Supplement,* 1898, **2**(4):(whole no. 8).

Travers, R. *Essentials of learning.* New York: The Macmillan Co., 1963.

Tyler, R. W. Achievement testing and curriculum construction. In E. G. Williamson (Ed.) *Trends in student personnel work.* Minneapolis: University of Minnesota Press, 1949, pp. 391-407.

Underwood, B. J. Laboratory studies of verbal learning. In E. R. Hilgard (Ed.), *Theories of learning and instruction.* 63rd Yearbook of NSSE, Part I. Chicago: University of Chicago Press, 1963, pp. 133-152.

Wolfe, J. B., and Kaplon, M. D. Effect of amount of reward and consummative activity on learning in chickens. *Journal of Comparative Psychology,* 1941, **31**:353-361.

Classical conditioning

DESCRIPTION OF THE MODULE

This module presents a systematic study of the theory, principles, and issues of classical conditioning and its application to nursing education and nursing practice. It is the second in a series on the conditions of learning and should be the program mastered *second* in the series. Classical conditioning is the simplest form of learning, and it is *prerequisite* to all the other conditions of learning and instruction.

This module (as all the rest of the modules) emphasizes or focuses five major areas: theoretical framework of classical conditioning, specific relevant research studies in this area, application of the theory into nursing education and practice, issues, and identification of researchable questions.

The format of the module is based on the concept of mastery, that is, each learner should accomplish the objectives of the module at the 95% level or better.

MODULE OBJECTIVES

At the completion of the independent learning module on classical conditioning, having studied the enclosed text and performed the suggested adjunctive learning experiences and formative and summative evaluations, the student will be able to (1) apply the theories and principles of classical conditioning to actual patient-teaching or student-learning situations and (2) identify a problem in nursing education or practice relative to the theory of classical conditioning and develop a proposal of study to investigate that specific problem. The student also will be able to:

1. Discuss learning theory in relation to concepts of classical conditioning
2. Give an oral or written definition of classical conditioning
3. Compare and contrast the principles and theory of conditioned reflex and unconditioned reflex
4. Identify the unconditioned stimulus, unconditioned response, conditioned stimulus, and conditioned response in a signal-learning situation
5. Identify and discuss the conditions of learning under which classical conditioning occurs
6. Identify and discuss the conditions under which extinction of classical conditioning occurs
7. Define and discuss giving one example, the phenomenon of stimulus generalization
8. Define and discuss, giving one example, the phenomenon of discrimination as it applies to classical conditioning
9. Define and discuss, giving one example, the phenomenon of forgetting
10. Identify and discuss two areas of research relevant to classical conditioning
11. Identify and discuss two applications of

classical conditioning theory to nursing education or practice
12. Discuss two issues that relate to the principles, theory, or practice of classical conditioning
13. Raise two researchable questions relative to the principles, theory, or practice of classical conditioning; identify the independent and dependent variables

PRETEST AND POSTTEST

Circle the correct answers. Each question is worth 1 point. The 95% level of achievement for this test is 26 points. On completion of this test correct your answers utilizing the answer key that is found at the end of this chapter.

True or false

1. Signal learning is categorized as a diffuse, emotional type of learning. True or False
2. It stands to reason that since classical conditioning is so susceptible to extinguishing techniques, it also has little resistance to forgetting. True or False
3. The external conditions necessary for classical conditioning to occur are contiguity and practice. True or False
4. In classical conditioning the entering behavior is a learned one. True or False
5. The unconditioned stimulus must precede the conditioned stimulus by 0 to 1.5 seconds, and for conditioning to be optimum it has to be 0.5 seconds. True or False
6. Taylor's (1951) study showed that there appeared to be no difference in the rate at which anxious and nonanxious people acquired conditioned responses. True or False

Multiple choice

7. The process by which classical conditioning is purposefully eliminated is called:
   a. generalization
   b. extinction
   c. inhibition
   d. interference
8. An unconditioned reflex is:

a. an inborn response to a stimulus
b. unlearned
c. a necessary entering behavior for classical conditioning
d. all of the above

9. Parents sometimes place caustic fluids in soft-drink bottles. This is dangerous because children associate the sight of these bottles with something sweet and edible through the process of:
   a. verbal association
   b. discrimination
   c. classical conditioning
   d. habit-family hierarchy
10. Classical conditioning can be used:
    a. to reinforce an autistic child who performs the described behavior (such as says the word milk on presentation of that object)
    b. in aversion therapy with alcoholics
    c. to evaluate subject's conditionability through galvanic skin response (GSR)
    d. predominantly to teach tricks to animals
11. The basic element of a learning event is the:
    a. stimulus situation
    b. learner
    c. change in performance
    d. response
    e. all of the above
12. Most investigators of Pavlovian conditioning now believe it to be a very special kind of learning, representative of the establishment of involuntary, "anticipatory" responses. Examples of such a response are which of the following:
    1—experiencing nausea upon the sight, smell or thought of a particular food
    2—the onset of chest pain in a person with previous cardiac history who is visiting a friend in the coronary care unit
    3—the initiation of a controlled breathing pattern on perception of uterine contraction in childbirth
    4—hyperactive mobility when a bothersome relative comes to visit
    a. 1, 4
    b. 2, 3
    c. 1, 2, 3
    d. 3, 4
13. The presentation of a tone signal followed

about half a second later by an electrical shock, which leads to a change in galvanic skin response, describes the condition of:
a. repetition
b. practice
c. contiguity
d. reinforcement

Sharon, a 10-year-old child, enters the hospital and is subsequently diagnosed as having diabetes mellitus. She and her family are informed that she must receive daily insulin injections for an indefinite period of time; it is the goal of the health team that Sharon learn to give her own injections before leaving the hospital. However, she reacts to even the sight of a needle with intense anxiety and fear. A program is set up whereby the same nurse (a favorite of Sharon's) successively involves her in handling the equipment, drawing up the medication, practicing technique on inanimate objects, and ultimately administering her own injection.

14. In this situation, the sight of a needle and the anticipation of the procedure is the:
a. unconditioned stimulus
b. unconditioned response
c. conditioned stimulus
d. conditioned response
15. Sharon's extreme fear and anxiety make up the:
a. unconditioned stimulus
b. unconditioned response
c. conditioned stimulus
d. conditioned response
16. Sharon's self-administration of her insulin injections could be termed the:
a. unconditioned stimulus
b. unconditioned response
c. conditioned stimulus
d. conditioned response

Matching

Part A
_____ 17. Classical conditioning
_____ 18. Unconditioned response
_____ 19. Forgetting
_____ 20. Inhibition
_____ 21. Unconditioned stimulus
_____ 22. Stimulus generalization
_____ 23. Facilitation
_____ 24. Stimulus discrimination
_____ 25. Extinction
_____ 26. Spontaneous recovery

Part B
a. A temporary decrease in the strength of the conditioned response as a result of presentation of a second stimulus that distracts from the conditioned stimulus
b. The temporary increase in the likelihood and magnitude of the conditioned response as a result of the addition of a second stimulus not previously associated with the response
c. The ability to isolate the essential characteristics of the conditioned stimulus
d. The process whereby a neutral stimulus becomes conditioned to the point where a specific response is invariably associated with its presentation to the subject.
e. The reappearance of an extinguished conditioned response on the reappearance of the conditioned stimulus in the absence of any reinforcement
f. The extinguishing of a conditioned response because of lack of practice
g. An unlearned response invariably made by the organism when presented with stimulus
h. A stimulus having the inherent capacity to elicit a response
i. The breakdown of the conditioned response because of lack of reinforcement
j. The spread of effect (conditioned response) once a simple conditioned response is established, induced by any stimulus similar to the original conditioned stimulus

Discussion question

27. Briefly describe the difference between forgetting and extinction in classical conditioning.

TEXT
Theoretical framework

Classical conditioning is the simplest form of learning. It is often referred to also as "signal learning" or "type-1 learning." One important characteristic of classical conditioning is that the responses are general, diffuse, and emotional. The smooth muscles, rather than the skeletal muscles, are involved.

The entering behavior of the learner requires the ability to initiate involuntarily an unconditioned reflex—an inborn response to stimuli, or *unconditioned response* (UCR). The response is unconditioned in that it is unlearned.

Classical conditioning occurs when a neutral stimulus is paired with a stimulus that is adequate enough to elicit a response. When this pairing process is repeated several times, then the neutral stimulus takes on the properties of the unconditioned stimulus in eliciting the same response. It is a form of stimulus substitution. In this situation, the stimulus that has the inherent capacity to elicit a response is called the *unconditioned stimulus* (UCS).

The neutral stimulus acquires the properites of the unconditioned stimulus as a result of repeated pairing with it and is able to elicit the same response as does the unconditioned stimulus. It is now called the *conditioned stimulus* (CS). The response that is elicited as a result of the conditioned stimulus is called the *conditioned response* (CR).

A very important condition has to be maintained in pairing the conditioned stimulus with the unconditioned stimulus in order for classical conditioning to take place. The conditioned stimulus must *precede* the unconditioned stimulus by 0 to 1.5 seconds, with optimum timing being 0.5 seconds.

Pavlov's (1928) well-known conditioning experiment with the dog illustrated how classical conditioning takes place (Fig. 2-1). Pavlov discovered that when meat powder is placed in a dog's mouth, saliva flows in response (R) to the unconditioned stimulus (meat powder). This natural and relatively automatic behavior of salivation is the unconditioned response. An incidental stimulus, such as the sound of a ringing bell, does not at first result in the flow of saliva. If the bell sounds each time just before the food is presented, however, it soon comes to elicit salivation. The new response to the bell is the *conditioned response,* and the bell is the *conditioned stimulus.* An association has been made between the bell and the food so that a response resembling the one originally made to the food is now made to the bell.

Gagne (1965, 1970) referred to Pavlov's classical conditioning as "signal learning," and did research using the example of the human eyeblink. After pairing a sound ("click") with a puff of air, it was possible to demonstrate the existence of a newly learned connection, namely, the conditioned response of blinking. This was done by the click itself, *without* the puff of air, and noting that the blink response occurred. This is another example of a conditioned response.

Variables affecting classical conditioning

After experimenting with the basic elements of this study, Pavlov began to manipulate not only the nature of the stimulus, but also the time interval between the con-

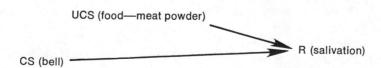

Fig. 2-1. Illustration of Pavlov's (1928) classical conditioning experiment.

ditioned stimulus and the unconditioned stimulus. He found that there are *two* requirements necessary in forming a conditioned response: (1) the conditioned stimulus must coincide in *time* with the action of the unconditioned stimulus and (2) the conditioned stimulus must *precede* the action of the unconditioned stimulus.

From Pavlov's experiment very important principles were discovered that are crucial to classical conditioning. These are events that occur in classical conditioning situations that have great importance for an understanding of this form of behavior modification, as well as of other more complex forms of learning that depend on it. The first of these phenomena is that of extinction, a kind of unlearning, that results in the disappearance of the previously learned response.

Pavlov found out that if the unconditioned stimulus (food) is omitted in a series of test trials, the conditioned response (salivation) begins to decrease and eventually fails to appear. The behavior of salivation gets extinguished. The process is called *extinction*. In classical conditioning the most dependable way to bring about extinction is by the repeated presentation, at suitable intervals, of the conditioned stimulus *without* the unconditioned stimulus.

Pavlov also noticed that after an initial period of extinction, upon presentation of the signal (the conditioned stimulus), the conditioned response may appear again after an interval. Pavlov called this *spontaneous recovery*. However, the connection is obviously weaker, and may be reextinguished in a few trials in which the conditioned stimulus is presented alone. The recurrence of the conditioned response seems to relate to two events: (1) the conditioned stimulus being presented again after a long absence and (2) the conditioned stimulus being paired with some other intense stimulus. Ultimately, however, under the extinction procedure the

newly learned connection does disappear completely.

Forgetting occurs when the learned connection is not tested over the interval concerned, that is, the stimulus or the signal is not presented. An important characteristic of classical conditioning is its great resistance to forgetting.

Stimulus generalization refers to the eliciting of the conditioned response by signals other than the one used to establish it. In other words, once a response is conditioned, a stimulus similar to the conditioned stimulus can also evoke the expected response. The closer the physical resemblance is between the other signals and the original one, the stronger the response obtained; the less similar the stimulus, the less will be the strength of the response (Bulgeski, 1964).

Discrimination is another phenomenon associated with classical conditioning. If the connection acquired to a signaling stimulus is somewhat imprecise, as the phenomenon of stimulus generalization implies, its precision may be increased and a *discrimination* established. This is accomplished by the intermittent pairing of the signal to be discriminated with the unconditioned stimulus, while the second generalized stimulus is presented alone. Through the procedure, the latter stimulus is eventually extinguished.

The limit to the fineness of discrimination that may be established by means of the contrasting-extinction procedure is determined by the sensory discrimination capacity of the organism doing the learning. The more complex the central nervous system of the organism, the greater is the degree of discrimination.

Relevant research studies

Although Pavlov's experiments were begun in 1902, the full impact of classical conditioning on American psychology was not felt until 1915, when John Watson introduced the idea in his presidential address to the American Psychological Association.

In 1920, Watson conducted the first conditioning experiment with emotions. Watson worked with an 11-months-old baby, "Albert," whose fear of loud noise was conditioned to a white rat and then to other furry objects. Watson concluded that (1) fear is conditioned or learned except to a few primitive stimuli, such as falling and loud noises; (2) reasonably permanent conditioned responses can be established through classical conditioning; (3) directly conditioned emotional responses, as well as those conditioned by transfer persist, although with a certain loss in the intensity of the reaction for a period longer than 1 month (his view being that they persist and modify personality throughout life); (4) classical conditioning can be used to establish both positive and negative emotional responses toward a neutral stimuli (DeCecco, 1968; Gagne, 1965).

Jones' (1924) study, as cited by Franks (1964), with children also showed how children's fears could be reduced or eradicated by principles of classical conditioning. Direct conditioning proved distinctly successful. To condition the child's response Jones associated with the feared object another stimulus that was capable of arousing a positive reaction (Franks, 1964). Since we learn our fears and biases by means of classical conditioning, fake fears, phobias, superstitions, and habits are all examples of conditioned responses.

Internal conditions—entering behaviors—necessary for classical conditioning to occur

What are the conditions of learning under which classical conditioning occurs? Evidently, one must deal with conditions that need to be present *within the learner* as well

as with those conditions that can be manipulated *in the learning situation*.

Referring to the internal conditions, Gagne said that for signal learning to occur there must be a natural reflex, typically a reflexive emotional response, on the part of the learner. The marked individual difference with which persons acquire signal-response learning is related to their level of anxiety. The degree of *anxiety* with which the individual typically faces life's problems and decisions has been shown to be positively correlated with ease and rapidity of conditioning (Taylor, 1951; Gagne, 1965).

Examples of typically reflexive behaviors are the eye blink, the knee jerk, the galvanic skin reflex, withdrawal from pain, the pupillary reflex, and salivation. Often the reflexive behavior is an emotional response, such as fear, startle, anger, or pleasure.

Much evidence has been accumulated that proves certain reflexes do not condition readily, such as the knee jerk and the pupillary reflex, while others, especially those involving a diffuse emotional response, have been shown to condition rather easily. Examples of these are fear and startle.

External conditions necessary for classical conditioning to take place

The conditions in the learning situation, those that can be externally controlled, are those of *contiguity* and *practice*. Contiguity refers to the proximity to each other within which the signaling stimulus and the unconditioned stimulus must be presented. These necessary time relationships have been tested in a variety of situations; it is reasonable to think that they reflect some stable characteristic of nervous-system functioning. Thus, contiguity refers to the proximity of pairing stimuli. Learning occurs dependably when the *conditioned stimulus* precedes the *unconditioned stimulus* by an interval between 0 and 1.5 seconds and most readily when the interval is about 0.5 seconds. The pairing of stimuli within this time framework fulfills the condition of contiguity.

The second condition in the learning situation is that of practice or repetition. The pairing of the unconditioned and the conditioned stimuli must be repeated. The amount of practice necessary depends on how strong the response to the unconditioned stimulus is. Signal learning is not an all-or-nothing occurrence. Rather, the connection appears to increase in strength, or dependability of occurrence, as the repetitions of paired stimuli increase in number.

A stimulus-response connection can be seen to occur in a single trial if the signal accompanies a stimulus arousing a strong emotion. This was the case, for example, when the child Albert learned to fear a rabbit when a sudden loud sound (produced by striking a metal bar) was made behind his head at the time he was reaching toward the rabbit (Watson and Rayner, 1920). Following this single event, the child showed fear whenever the rabbit was brought near him. In this case, the emotion of fear was strong enough to complete the conditioned reflex after only one pairing of stimuli.

Thus, the conditions of classical conditioning—the presence of a natural reflex within the organism, contiguity, and practice—are relatively simple to describe and rather readily controlled. In addition to the eyeblink response used in previous examples, conditioned responses have been established for many varieties of behavior in human beings, including salivation, skin-resistance changes, respiration changes, nausea, hand withdrawal, and others. It is the class of responses that are diffuse and emotional that are more easily conditioned.

A response falling in this category, for example, is the "galvanic skin reflex," which has been used frequently for the study of classical conditioning. Changes in skin resistance can be precisely measured by electrical means, and a change in galvanic skin reflex can be used to signal the acquisition of a conditioned response.

Application to nursing education and practice

On area in which nursing personnel can apply classical conditioning techniques is in assisting patients in overcoming phobias and fears of hospitalization and illness. In this case, the successive pairing of anxiety-producing situations (particularly unfamiliar environmental stimuli) with stress-reducing nursing intervention can result in the learning of a new response to these stimuli. Teaching parents principles of classical conditioning so that they can help their children to overcome inappropriate emotional responses (such as fears and phobias) would be another implication for nursing.

Teaching parents not to place caustic substances in soft-drink bottles or in food containers is another form of applying principles of classical conditioning. For example, a soft-drink bottle is an unconditioned stimulus for drinking behavior (response); the child associates the sight of the bottle with drinking. When parents place detergents in the bottle, the child may drink the caustic substance from it. When illustrated diagramatically, it looks like this:

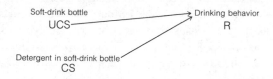

Other examples are the paired association of aspirin with the word candy, which may lead to swallowing or eating behavior.

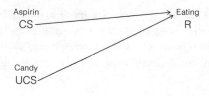

The American Cancer Society associates (pairs) "smoking" and "cancer" in their advertisements in order to produce avoidance behavior.

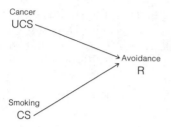

In classical conditioning, conditioned reflexes are directly related to cortical functioning; there is an excitation component and an inhibition component present. Cortical centers can at one moment be active and at the next be resting in that each time a cerebral center becomes active the brain matter around it reacts by becoming modified so as to function inversely. Excitation therefore induces inhibition, which allows the excitation to be contained and remain concentrated and not spread to the rest of the brain. Thus, only the excited focus is active, and the surrounding refractory area is functionless. Anything that reaches this refractory area is not registered by the anxiety.

Wolpe (1958, p. 70) utilized the principles of classical conditioning in psychotherapy by reciprocal inhibition. His findings led him to the following general principle:

If a response is antagonistic to anxiety evoking stimuli, so that it is accompanied by a complete or partial suppression of the anxiety responses, then the connection between stimuli and the anxiety responses will be weakened.

For example, relaxation responses are utilized for systematic desensitization.

In obstetrics, nursing has utilized the psychoprophylactic childbirth technique developed by Ferdinand Lamaze. The method entails mentally and physically conditioning the patient to suppress the pain in labor (Ulin, 1963). Conditioning techniques are used to accomplish two objectives: (1) the deconditioning of a learned attitude that fear, anxiety, and pain are intrinsic to the childbirth process; and (2) the learning of a new physiological response to uterine contractions. Both goals are accomplished by implementing principles of classical conditioning.

Both objectives are met by pairing neutral stimuli (information giving and specific respiratory responses) with the appropriate stage of childbirth preparation and actual labor and delivery to create a new association. The result is that a new response—one other than that of severe pain—is learned.

Following the view of Pavlov that the conditioned responses tend to inhibit other areas of cerebral activity, a researchable question can be raised: Would it be possible for a nurse practitioner to reeducate a patient experiencing pain by introducing new, positive conditioning whereby the patient is able to control consciously the reception of pain? In this question the *independent variable* is the introduction of new positive conditioning and the *dependent variable* is control of pain.

Conditional reflex research in psychotherapy has developed the view that, in principle, all learning is based on the formation of new temporal connections, and that psychotherapy to a great extent can be considered a process of relearning. This implies that all the applications of learning theory and the attempts to change inadequate habit patterns are fundamentally related to the conditional reflex activity. Reeducation involves extinction of pathological connections and reinforcement of more normal, adaptive behavior patterns.

Classical conditioning also serves four other functions in the area of health services: (1) diagnostic aid; (2) aversion therapy; (3) nonaversion therapy; and (4) evaluation and prediction.

Diagnostic aid. One study conducted in 1962 used classical conditioning to assist in differentiating between psychogenic and physical pain. The researcher tested subjects using the psychogalvanic skin reflex. The reflex ". . . consists of a sharply defined fall in skin resistance in response to painful stimuli, startling noises, mental challenges . . . or acutely disturbing thoughts" (Franks, 1964, p. 45). The study concluded that "the GSRs in patients suffering from physical pain were strikingly different from those suffering from psychogenic pain when spontaneous fluctuations of the skin resistance were compared with the evoked responses, especially the conditional ones" (Franks, 1964, p. 45).

Aversion therapy. Aversion therapy has been used in the past 40 years to treat numerous behavioral problems. This therapy elicits an unpleasant unconditioned response (for example, nausea) to an unconditioned stimulus (for example, emetine hydrochloride) and then attempts to condition this response to an aspect of the pathology. "This method has been most extensively applied to the treatment of alcoholism, in which alcohol is given on a number of occasions just before vomiting occurs, in the hope that eventually the alcohol will take on the properties of a CS to which the CR is intense nausea at its taste, smell or even sight" (Franks, 1964, p. 155).

Nonaversive therapy. In nonaversive therapy the subject is conditioned to a substitute stimulus that is not unpleasant or aversive in nature. One study reported success in treating constipation by associating the subject's unconditioned response of defecating to a conditioned response. The conditioned response was a specially designed belt that the subject would put on when the urge to defecate was felt. Eventually the use of the belt was enough to cause the urge to defecate (Franks, 1964, pp. 219-227).

Evaluating and predicting. One study utilizing classical conditioning in evaluation explored the relationship between subjects' alcoholic drinking patterns and the ease of galvanic skin reflex conditioning. The galvanic skin reflex changes abruptly when a loud bell rings. The bell was the unconditioned stimulus. The conditioned stimulus was a nonsense syllable. The study concluded that, "Alcoholics who reported having a steady drinking pattern more quickly established the conditioned GSR . . . than those who reported periodic drinking" (Franks, 1964, p. 97). The researcher stated that the ease of a subject's conditioning might serve as a criterion for selecting subjects for conditioned aversion therapy for alcoholism (Franks, 1964, p. 97).

Issues in classical conditioning

The phenomenon of classical conditioning has given rise to several issues. One issue regarding application of classical conditioning techniques revolves around the assumption of a general trait of conditionability within the organism. Some theorists believe it is preferable to discuss formation of conditioned responses within the context of specific conditioning situations. Others reply that if conditioning is dependent on Pavlov's central processes of excitation and inhibition, and if these processes are generalized properties of the nervous system, then a general factor of conditioning should also exist, and it should be meaningful to speak of the "conditionability" of the organism (Franks, 1964).

In other words, *the assumption that an individual has a general trait of conditionability has been questioned.* If the assumption is correct, one could speak of a person's conditionability and not speak only of how well a person conditions in a specific situation. The way a person conditions in one situation should apply to any conditioning situation. Rejection of the assumption necessitates confining one's discussion to the specific conditioning situation (Franks, 1964, p. 17).

This issue has further implications in the area of psychophysiological explorations of human behavior, where researchers have sought to find unifying concepts to explain such things as perception, intelligence, personality, and learning. The issue of internal versus external variables of conditioning becomes one of importance as one attempts to explain and duplicate learning or learning events.

A second issue is a social consideration of the ethical implications of "controlling" or "programming" another's behavior. This social issue deals with the process of conditioning, for it appears to take control of behavior out of the subject's realm of power. For example, as a psychotherapeutic technique, classical conditioning might appear far more authoritarian and directive than a more traditional psychoanalytical technique. Franks (1964) pointed out, however, that a psychoanalyst often directs the course of events in therapy on a subtle level of which the patient is probably not aware. Franks proposed that the therapist utilizing classical conditioning can at the outset be very specific about exactly what is intended and what result in the patient's behavior is expected. Thus, the patient has full knowledge of what to expect and can consent to or refuse therapy (Franks, 1964, pp. 18-19).

Researchable questions

Skinner cites various instances where a pleasant unconditioned stimulus is paired with an unpleasant stimulus. For example, in a dentist's office the client can be expected to have a favorable unconditioned response to soft music or current magazines. The unconditioned response of relaxation and comfort might be expected to carry over to the conditioned response of the therapeutic procedure (Skinner, 1953, p. 57). Pairing a pleasant unconditioned stimulus with an unpleasant conditioned stimulus might be effective

in a situation where a nurse wants to teach a diabetic patient to self-administer insulin. The nurse could have a cup of coffee with the patient while explaining the procedure of measuring and administering insulin. People by and large have favorable responses to food or a beverage, and this response could become conditioned to the less desirable stimulus of insulin injection.

In an educational institution, this pairing of stimuli could be used by instructors. An example of this could be when a nursing instructor allows students to drink coffee or eat snacks during seminars. This can be viewed as the pairing of the students' favorable unconditioned response to food and drinks with the seminar, with the hope that the pleasant unconditioned response of food will facilitate a favorable response to the conditioned stimulus of the seminar, which otherwise might have elicited fear and anxiety.

A problem arises in pairing a pleasant stimulus with an unpleasant stimulus. One cannot assume that the favorable unconditioned response will become conditioned to the unpleasant stimulus without adversely affecting the reactions to the unconditioned stimulus. It is possible that the unpleasant stimulus will elicit a response of anxiety or other undesirable emotion (response), which will then become conditioned to the more pleasant stimulus.

For example, suppose a child who has a warm, trusting relationship with mother has to have an injection in the physician's office. The physician assumes the child will respond more favorably during the procedure if the mother is present or if she is holding the child. However, the child's angry response to the injection could carry over to the mother. Therefore, the question to be asked that needs further research is, What is the effect of pairing an unpleasant stimulus to a pleasant unconditioned stimulus on the original unconditioned response of the pleasant unconditioned stimulus?

In this research question, can you identify the dependent and the independent variables? If you identified the pairing of an unpleasant stimulus to a pleasant unconditioned stimulus as the independent variable and its effect on the original unconditioned response of the pleasant unconditioned stimulus as the dependent variable, you are correct.

A second researchable question concerns the normal aging process (with central nervous system changes) and the effectiveness of classical conditioning techniques. Is there a significant relationship between aging and decrease in conditionability? The variables involved are the ease and effectiveness with which classical conditioning can be accomplished, that is, the decrease in conditionability.

ADDITIONAL LEARNING EXPERIENCES—RECOMMENDED READING LIST

DeCecco, J. *The psychology of learning and instruction: educational psychology.* (1st Ed.) Englewood Cliffs, N.J.: Prentice-Hall, Inc., 1968, pp. 241-272.

DeCecco, J., and Crawford, W. *The psychology of learning and instruction: educational psychology.* (2nd Ed.) Englewood Cliffs, N.J.: Prentice-Hall, Inc., 1974, pp. 202-204.

Gagne, R. *Conditions of learning.* (1st Ed.) New York: Holt, Rinehart and Winston, Inc., 1965, pp. 62-71.

Gagne, R. *Conditions of learning.* (2nd Ed.) New York: Holt, Rinehart and Winston, Inc., 1970, pp. 1-104.

INSTRUCTIONS TO THE LEARNER REGARDING POSTTEST

At this stage you are ready to take the posttest to determine the extent to which you have achieved the objectives. Return to the pretest of this module and take it as a posttest. Correct your own posttest utilizing the answer key that is found on this page of the module. You need to score 95% correct (26

correct points) to proceed to the next module. If your score is less than 26 correct points, correct your errors, study those aspects that you did wrong, and carefully read materials from the recommended reading list. You need to study until you achieve the 95% level.

ANSWER KEY TO PRETEST AND POSTTEST

1. True (Gagne, 1970, 37)
2. False (Gagne, 1970, p. 103)
3. True (DeCecco, 1968, p. 265)
4. False (DeCecco, 1968, p. 265)
5. False (Gagne, 1970, p. 98)
6. False (Gagne, 1970, p. 98)
7. b (Gagne, 1965, p. 100)
8. d (DeCecco, 1968, p. 265)
9. c (Text, p. 34)
10. b, c (Franks, 1964, pp. 97, 155)
11. e (Gagne, 1965, pp. 4-5)
12. c (Gagne, 1965, p. 99)
13. c (DeCecco, 1968, p. 265)
14. c (Gagne, 1965, pp. 95-97)
15. d (Gagne, 1965, pp. 95-97)
16. d (Gagne, 1965, pp. 95-97)
17. d (DeCecco, 1968, p. 265)
18. g (Gagne, 1970, pp. 95, 98)
19. f (Gagne, 1970, pp. 103-104)
20. a (Gagne, 1970, p. 101)
21. h (Gagne, 1970, pp. 95-98)
22. j (Gagne, 1970, pp. 101-102)
23. b (Franks, 1964, pp. 3-6)
24. c (Gagne, 1970, p. 103)
25. i (Gagne, 1970, p. 100)
26. e (Gagne, 1970, p. 100)
27. If there is a decrease in the learned connection following an interval of disuse, that is, if the signal is not presented, one will eventually forget the connected response. While in extinction there is an active process of trying to wipe out the response, so there is presentation of the signal alone during a number of trials, which brings about disappearance of the learned connection. (Gagne, 1970, pp. 100, 103-104)

REFERENCES

Bugelski, B. R. *The psychology of learning applied to teaching.* New York: The Bobbs-Merrill Co., Inc., 1964.

DeCecco, J. *The psychology of learning and instruction: educational psychology* (1st Ed.) Englewood Cliffs, N.J.: Prentice-Hall, Inc., 1968.

DeCecco, J., and Crawford, W. *The psychology of learning and instruction: educational psychology.* (2nd Ed.) Englewood Cliffs, N.J.: Prentice-Hall, Inc., 1974.

Franks, C. M. (Ed) *Conditioning techniques in clinical practice and research.* New York: Springer Publishing Co., Inc., 1964.

Gagne, R. *Conditions of learning.* (1st Ed.) New York: Holt, Rinehart and Winston, Inc., 1965.

Gagne, R. *The conditions of learning.* (2nd Ed.) New York: Holt, Rinehart and Winston, Inc., 1970.

Pavlov, I. P. *Lectures on conditioned responses.* New York: Liveright, 1928.

Skinner, B. F. *Science and human behavior.* New York: The Free Press, 1953.

Taylor, J. A. The relationship of anxiety to the conditioned eyelid response: *Journal of Experimental Psychology,* 1951, **41**:81-92.

Ulin, R. D. Lamaze method of antepartal conditioning prepares the patient for exhilarating moment of birth. *American Journal of Nursing,* 1963, **63**(6):60-67.

Wolpe, J. *Psychotherapy by reciprocal inhibition.* Stanford, Calif.: Stanford University Press, 1958.

MODULE 3

Operant conditioning

DESCRIPTION OF THE MODULE

The purpose of this module is to enable you to acquire knowledge about operant-conditioning theory and be able to apply the principles derived from operant-conditioning to nursing education and practice.

The content of this module is divided into five major areas: theoretical background of operant conditioning, research findings in this area, application to nursing practice and nursing education, issues in this area, and researchable questions. This module also contains behavioral objectives relevant to learning experiences, pretest and posttest, and answers to these tests to provide for immediate feedback of results.

MODULE OBJECTIVES

At the completion of this module the student will be able to perform the following objectives at the 95% mastery level:

1. Identify in writing the important facts and principles of operant conditioning theory
2. Identify in writing the differences between classical and operant conditioning, respondent and operant behaviors
3. Apply knowledge of the concept of reinforcement by differentiating in writing between examples of primary and secondary reinforcement, positive and negative reinforcement, punishment, and the conditions of reinforcement

4. Identify in writing the conditions within the learner and those in the learning situation that are necessary for operant learning
5. Identify in writing facts about extinction, generalization, and discrimination
6. Identify in writing the results of recent research specifically related to operant conditioning in the areas of punishment, avoidance, drugs, autistic children, and the control of psychiatric patients
7. Identify in writing important facts about the application of operant conditioning to nursing practice and education as related to programmed instruction, verbal behavior, chronic illness, observation and recording, psychotherapy, and strengthening and reducing the strength of behaviors
8. Identify in writing certain aspects of issues related to the application of operant conditioning to the human situation, that is, the use of behavior modification in practice as related to humanism, manipulation of human behavior, and its consequences
9. Identify in writing the independent and dependent variables of three research questions

PRETEST AND POSTTEST

Circle the correct answers. Each question is worth 1 point. For this module, 95% level of achievement is 24 points. On completion of this test, correct your answers utilizing the answer key that is found at the end of this module (pp. 55-56).

True or false

1. The major difference between operant and classical conditioning is the reinforcement procedure. True or False
2. Shaping is an example of operant conditioning. True or False
3. Negative reinforcement is the same thing as punishment. True or False
4. Operant conditioning makes it possible for an individual to perform an action by choice. True or False

Fill in the blanks

5. The process by which the learner acquires a precise response to a discriminated stimulus is called _____ .
6. The practice of reinforcing approximations of behavior that move closer to the desired behavior is known as _____ .
7. A child confronted with a new stimulus makes a response previously made to another stimulus. This behavior is called _____ .

Multiple choice

8. In operant conditioning:
   a. reinforcement follows the stimulus
   b. the stimulus must always precede the response
   c. reinforcement follows the response
   d. responses follow known stimuli
9. The strength of an operant is:
   a. proportional to its frequency of occurence
   b. a function of its stimuli
   c. dependent on the strength of the stimuli
   d. all of the above
10. An operant is:
    a. elicited by known stimuli
    b. a class of reflex behavior
    c. emitted behavior
    d. similar to a respondent
11. The following are external learning conditions necessary for operant learning to take place
    a. motivation, reinforcement, and practice

b. complexity, contiguity, and ability
   c. reinforcement, contiguity, and practice
   d. reinforcement, practice, and meaning
12. To describe the most basic condition necessary in operant conditioning, one would say:
    a. the organism must have the capability of performing the devised task
    b. the organism must want to do the devised task
13. Stimulus-response learning is more likely to be successful when reinforcement:
    a. precedes
    b. follows the devised response
14. The strongest responses are acquired through:
    a. variable schedules
    b. ratio schedules
    c. continuous schedules
    d. frequent reinforcement
15. A child who argues with peers may learn that arguing with parents is not only unsuccessful but also unacceptable. This is an example of:
    a. shaping
    b. generalization
    c. transituational responses
    d. discrimination
16. In instrumental learning, successive approximations toward a desired response are reinforced. This technique is called:
    a. fading
    b. approximation
    c. shaping
    d. selective reinforcement
17. A stimulus that is not originally a reinforcing one can become reinforcing through repeated association with one that is. This is the concept of:
    a. consequential reinforcement
    b. generalized reinforcement
    c. primary reinforcement
    d. secondary reinforcement
18. Social stereotypes result from:
    a. aversive conditioning
    b. discrimination
    c. transsitutional responses
    d. generalization
19. Research has shown that in discriminated avoidance:
    a. a neutral stimulus precedes the noxious stimulus

b. a neutral stimulus serves as a warning for the occurrence of the noxious event

c. if the subject avoids during the warning period, the noxious event fails to occur

d. all of the above

20. Tokens are which of the following:
    1—secondary reinforcers
    2—given for desirable behavior
    3—charged for undesirable behavior
    4—traded in for privileges
    a. 1 and 2
    b. 2 and 3
    c. 2, 3, and 4
    d. all are correct

21. Token-economy programs in mental health institutions and school settings, with adolescents and delinquents, represent the application of what type of learning:
    a. concept learning
    b. instrumental learning
    c. classical conditioning
    d. habit-family hierarchy

22. A nurse "accidentally" spills food on patients while feeding them. The only way the patients could prevent this situation would be to feed themselves. This is an example of:
    a. extinction
    b. punishment
    c. eliminating avoidance behavior
    d. avoidance behavior

Discussion questions

Identify the independent and dependent variables of the following questions.

23. Will patients be able to transfer conditioned responses learned under one set of circumstances to a different set of circumstances?
    a. Independent variable: _____
    b. Dependent variable: _____

24. What is the extent of continued behavioral changes over X amount of time as a result of the techniques of behavior modification as compared to the techniques of traditional psychoanalytical theory?
    a. Independent variable: _____
    b. Dependent variable: _____

25. Can nonprofessional personnel modify a patient's behavior as effectively as professional personnel?
    a. Independent variable: _____
    b. Dependent variable: _____

TEXT
Theoretical framework

Operant conditioning is also referred to as "stimulus-response learning" (S–R) by Gagne (1965), "trial-and-error learning" by Thorndike (1911), "instrumental learning" by Kimble (1961), and type-2-learning. Operant conditioning is "a kind of learning that involves making very precise movements of the skeletal muscles in response to very specific stimuli or combinations of stimuli" (Gagne, 1970, p. 38). In human beings these are voluntary behaviors or responses that can be observed. This type of learning makes it possible for the individual to perform an action by choice. Animals behave in a similar fashion.

In order to understand operant conditioning, it must be understood what is meant by "behavior." "Behavior is that part of the functioning of an organism which is engaged in acting upon or having commerce with the outside world" (Skinner, 1938, p. 6). The environment enters into a description of behavior when it can be shown that a given part of behavior may be induced at will by a modification in part of the forces affecting the organism. Such a modification of a part of the environment is called a *stimulus*, and the correlated part of the behavior is the *response* (Skinner, 1938).

In S–R, or operant, conditioning the necessary entering behavior is the availability of particular responses to the organism or the human being. In other words, the organism must be able to act or respond; for example, a rat must be able to press a bar, or a child must be able to run, smile, or perform other behaviors. These responses are called *operants* because they operate in the environment, and by doing them, the child or the organism is changing the state of the environment. The strength of an operant is proportional to its frequency of occurrence, whereas the strength of a respondent is a function of its stimuli (Hilgard, 1956). The objective of operant-conditioning procedures is simply to increase the frequency of the desirable response.

Characteristics of operant conditioning that differ from classical conditioning

The response acquired by operant conditioning is a precise, circumscribed skeletal-muscular act. In classical conditioning, or respondent learning, the response is a diffuse, generalized emotional response.

There appears to be a typical gradualness to the learning of the operant behavior. The animal or the individual does not behave correctly the first time around. Gagne (1970) cited the example of how a dog learns how to shake hands with the trainer after a series of repeated performances that are reinforced when the behavior of handshaking resembles the desired form of handshaking. The dog does not suddenly shake hands the very first time, but learns it gradually.

An example from nursing would be that a student nurse does not administer a hypodermic injection correctly prior to learning that takes place, but through practice, observation, and reinforcement, the behavior of "correct hypodermic-injection giving" gradually becomes part of the repertoire of the student nurse.

The response becomes more and more sure and precise throughout the several occasions. In other words, the response is said to undergo "shaping" through successive approximations until it becomes precise, sure, and correct. *Shaping* refers to the process of successive approximations of behavior by the use of reinforcements, until the behavior demonstrated by the organism or the individual resembles that of the desired response (criterion response). Each successive approximation toward a desired response is reinforced. By so doing, the simple is learned before proceeding to the complex. An example of this would be teaching a retarded child to use a spoon. First looking at the spoon would be reinforced, then grasping the spoon, then bringing it to the mouth. In this technique the behavior changes, but the reinforcement remains the same except it is contingent on successive behaviors.

The technique of *fading* involves initially going through a behavior with the subject and gradually fading out the teacher's participation in the behavior. Again an example of this would be with spoon feeding. Initially the experimenter's hand would hold the child's hand over the spoon as it was raised to the mouth. As the child begins to pull the spoon to the mouth, the experimentor would "fade out" by holding the wrist and eventually the elbow until the child is able to function independently.

The controlling stimulus becomes more precise. For example, when the trainer tells the dog to "shake hands," the dog responds immediately by lifting the paw, whereas at first the command of "shake hands" meant nothing to the dog. Similarly, in the case of the nursing student, the stimulus of "give a hypodermic injection to a patient" may not have produced correct administering of the injection at first; however, after several reinforced practices it produces correct behavior. It must, however, be pointed out that there are occasions with human beings that the correct response can be emitted the very first time, without any practice or shaping of behavior. For example, a person may be able to pronounce a medical term, such as hepatic, correctly the very first time it is presented.

There is a *reward,* or *reinforcement,* given *after* the correct behavior (outcome) is emitted. Some consider this point to be of utmost importance. Only correct responses are rewarded, that is, reinforcement is contingent on the animal or the human being making the correct response. The difference between operant and classical conditioning is that in operant conditioning the response determines the presentation of the reinforcer, whereas in classical conditioning the presentation of the unconditioned stimulus (food-reinforcer) determines the unconditioned response.

Gagne (1970) pointed out that the capability that has been acquired by operant-conditioning procedure implies that a particular S–R pattern is established, and at the same time other S–R patterns, equally probably at the beginning of learning, are disestablished. He illustrated this phenomena by using an arrow between S and R, as S →, rather than the line between S and R, to emphasize that a *process of discrimination* has taken place that is an integral part of operant learning. A degree of precision has been established in the response, which can be distinguished from similar but "wrong" responses. Similarly, there is precision of stimulus, which differs from other stimuli that may be present at the time the response is made.

"Any uncomplicated example of S → R learning indicates that it is motor learning"; "In S → R learning, though an important component of the *stimulus itself* is generated by muscular movements" (Gagne, 1970, p. 40). He stated that whether the behavior or the act is being established, the external stimulus (such as "shake hands" in the example of the dog) is accompanied by proprioceptive (kinesthetic) stimulation from the muscle that raised the dog's paw. Even though the behavior is fully learned, some parts of this stimulation are still present. For example, the dog raises the paw "as if voluntarily," even when no one asked the dog. Mowrer (1960) considered this portion of the total stimulation as an essential part of the capa-

bility that is learned. He presented this as

$$Ss \rightarrow R$$

where

> S = an external signal
> s = the accompanying internal proprioceptive stimulation
> R = response
> → = the precise discriminated nature of the capability

Other potential Ss → R patterns are disestablished (or estinguished) by the events of learning (Gagne, 1970, p. 40).

To conclude this portion on operant conditioning we can say that S → R learning is a more complex learning type than is classical conditioning. Gagne (1965) suggested some examples of S–R type of learning that occur in children: reaching and grasping for toys or other objects, smiling at particular people, posturing the body and limbs, and vocalizing. In adult learning, the pronunciation of unfamiliar foreign words is an example of operant conditioning. Once the correct response (operant) is made, it must be reinforced. The response and the reinforcement must be contiguous (immediate), and the response must be practiced under these conditions.

Basic conditions necessary for operant conditioning

There are two categories of conditions, or sets of variables, that are necessary for operant conditioning to take place: (1) internal conditions, which are those variables that are within the learner; and (2) external conditions, which are those variables that are in the situation—they are external to the learner and can easily be manipulated.

INTERNAL CONDITIONS—CONDITIONS WITHIN THE LEARNER

For operant learning to take place there must be a terminating *act* that provides satisfaction. This produces what Thorndike referred to as a "satisfying state of affairs." It is not necessary for the terminating act to produce innate satisfaction, that is, physical satisfaction, as long as it provides satisfaction of some kind. In order to ensure learning the learner must be able to perform such a response that terminates in reinforcement (Gagne, 1970, pp. 108-109). The operant must be part of the learner's repertoire.

EXTERNAL CONDITIONS—CONDITIONS IN THE LEARNING SITUATION

In order for operant conditioning to take place, it is essential that the external conditions of reinforcement, contiguity, and repetition be present.

Reinforcement. It was previously mentioned that the terminating behavior or response must actually result in reinforcement. That is, the terminal behavior must be satisfying to the learner. The basis of reinforcement stems from Thorndike's (1911) Law of Effect, which states:

Of the several responses made to the same situation, those which are accompanied or closely followed by satisfaction to the animal will, other things being equal, be more firmly connected to the situation, so that when it recurs, they will be more likely to recur; those which are accompanied or closely followed by discomfort to the animal will, other things being equal, have their connection weakened, so that when it recurs, they will be less likely to recur (DeCecco, 1968, pp. 250-251).

Skinner (1938, p. 62) defines the operation of reinforcement as "the presentation of a certain kind of stimulus in a temporal relation with either a stimulus or a response." He further defines a reinforcing stimulus by "its power to produce the resulting change." Some stimuli produce a change, others do not; and they are classified as reinforcing and nonreinforcing, accordingly. A stimulus may possess the power to reinforce when it is first presented, or it may acquire the power through conditioning.

In operant conditioning, an organism or an individual is presented with a reinforcing stimulus after making a desirable response. Soon, those responses that are reinforced will be repeated, and those responses that are not reinforced will be discontinued.

A brief description of the nature and the schedules of reinforcement are given as they apply to operant conditioning, Module 21 is devoted to reinforcement as a variable that influences both learning and instruction.

Nature of the reinforcer. An operant response is controlled by its consequences. An organism "acts on the environment" because of those events that immediately follow its behavior. If the events that follow a behavior increase the rate of occurrence of the behavior, the events are termed *positive reinforcers* (Whitney, 1966). A positive reinforcer then is a stimulus that when added to a situation strengthens the probability of an operant response; examples are food, water, and sexual contact (Hilgard, 1956). If the organism's behavior tends to avoid certain consequences, these consequences are termed *negative reinforcers* (Whitney, 1966). A negative reinforcer then is a stimulus that when removed from a situation strengthens the probability of an operant response; examples are, a loud noise, a very bright light, extreme heat or cold, and electrical shock. When the consequences following a behavior do not increase the probability of response, they are termed *neutral*, and the behavior preceding these neutral consequences weakens (Whitney, 1966).

Secondary reinforcement. When a stimulus that is not originally a reinforcing one is repeatedly associated with a reinforcing stimulus, it can become reinforcing (Hilgard, 1956, p. 121). A stimulus can therefore acquire the power to condition. Many secondary reinforcers accompany *primary reinfor-*

cers. Money, is a good example of secondary reinforcement because money provides access to food, shelter, and other primary reinforcers; therefore, money becomes a reinforcer for a variety of activities. Another example is the mothering individual who acquires a reinforcing value to the child by initially providing the primary reinforcers of food and warmth.

Punishment is something other than negative reinforcement as previously defined. The arrangement of the variables in punishment is opposite that in reinforcement. Punishment is: (1) the presentation of a negative reinforcer or (2) the removal of a positive reinforcer (Hilgard, 1956).

Estes (1944) found that punishment does not lead to a reduction in the total number of responses, although there is a temporary suppression of responses. Permanent weakening comes about only by nonreinforcement, and this weakening process may even be prevented by punishment because punishment suppresses the response, which must be brought to free expression before it can be redirected (Hilgard, 1956).

Schedules of reinforcement. The strength of operants depends on the schedule of reinforcement. The schedule may be one of the following types: continuous, fixed ratio, variable ratio, fixed interval, or variable interval. In a continuous schedule, reinforcement follows every response. A fixed-ratio schedule provides reinforcement for one of every so many responses, such as a reinforcement for every third response (1:3, 1:3, and so on). A fixed-interval schedule is contingent on a reinforcement every so often in terms of time; for example, a reinforcement every 4 minutes (1:4 minutes, 1:4 minutes, and so on). Variable-ratio and variable-interval schedules are based on reinforcements given without a fixed rate or time interval, such as 1:2, 1:5, 1:3, 1:7, and so on.

It has been found that a few reinforcements are sufficient to produce a constant rate of responses; for example, every 10 to 15 seconds for the lever-pressing behavior of a rat. Further reinforcement serves only to maintain the rate, not to raise it. The effect of the number of reinforcements becomes more apparent when the reinforcement is discontinued. In other words the strength of an operant may be assessed by the rate of its emission, and the probability of a response can be manipulated by the contingencies of reinforcement (Lunzer, 1968).

Behavior acquired through intermittent reinforcement is more resistant to extinction, although behavior is learned faster with continuous reinforcement. The strongest responses are produced by variable schedules. Reinforcement in the natural setting is not regular and uniform. A fisherman does not hook a fish with every cast, yet he continues to fish. In daily life reinforcement depends on many factors and is usually provided on a combined schedule with both rate and time being varied.

Contiguity. Contiguity is the second external condition necessary for operant conditioning and the establishment of an $Ss \rightarrow R$ connection. Learning occurs more quickly when reinforcement closely follows performance of the learned response (Gagne 1970). The relationship between "ease of learning" and the immediacy or delay of reinforcement has been well demonstrated in laboratory studies (Kimble, 1961, pp. 140-156).

In operant conditioning the contiguity must be maintained between the response and the reinforcing stimulus, whereas in classical conditioning the contiguity must be maintained between the conditioned and the unconditioned stimulus.

Repetition. The third external condition that must be present in the learning situation in order for operant conditioning to take place is repetition. The amount of repetition necessary to learn an $Ss \rightarrow R$ association depends on the difficulty of the discrimination involved and the degree to which the newly learned discriminated Ss → R bond conforms to responding that is either previously learned or innately determined. Repetition serves the function of selection of stimuli to be discriminated. In successive repetitions of the S → R bond certain parts of the total stimulus situation are associated with certain responses. Some responses are more successful than others in producing reinforcement, therefore the successful ones are retained while the others drop out of the picture. According to this concept, learning involves a gradual recruitment of the "bundle," or S → R connections, that lead to reinforcement (DeCecco, 1968, pp. 250-251).

• • •

The external conditions for reinforcement, contiguity, and repetition are all interrelated and they determine the ease (rapidity) with which the individual learns to discriminate the specific relevant stimulus. As Gagne (1970, p. 110) pointed out:

If suitable conditions for reinforcement both within and outside the learner, the establishment of stimulus-response learning becomes primarily a matter of arranging conditions for the desired *stimulus discrimination* to occur most readily. Anything that is done to make the selection of a correct stimulus sample easier than it would otherwise be will speed up the learning, and thereby decrease the number of repetitions required. If one is interested in *learning efficiency* for Ss → R learning, he will seek to arrange the stimulus situation so as to reduce the amount of repetition required for learning.

For example, when a mentally retarded child is learning how to hold a spoon correctly, the task of learning to hold the spoon correctly is speeded by "help" from the nurse or the therapist in positioning of hand and fingers. This association or Ss → R connection can be learned without such help, but it will require

more repetition of the situation in order for the correct set of stimuli to be selected.

Other phenomena of operant conditioning
EXTINCTION

In operant conditioning extinction occurs when the reinforcement that follows the learned response is omitted. Under these circumstances the previously learned connection gradually disappears, until it is no longer present. For example, if a rat in a cage is not reinforced with food for pressing a bar that controls the release of a pellet of food, the animal will press the bar more rapidly at first. However, each nonreinforced operant decreases the probability of the next operant. Similarly, if an infant is not reinforced by the parents' attention (picking up the infant or going to the bedroom and talking after placing the infant in the crib for a nap) for temper-tantrum behavior when placed in the crib, which controls the receiving of attention by being picked up, the infant will scream, yell, and throw a bigger tantrum at first. However, each nonreinforced tantrum (operant) decreases the probability of the next operant, until the tantrum behavior completely disappears.

GENERALIZATION

Generalization is said to have occurred when an organism or an individual is presented with a new stimulus and responds in the same manner as to a previously learned stimulus. The generalization of the learned connection to stimuli that resemble the set used in learning is another characteristic of operant conditioning, but it is similar to generalization that occurs in classical conditioning. Therefore, in generalization the conditioned response may be elicited by other stimulus situations than the one that originally established it. The closer the resemblance of the stimulus situation to the original one, the more frequently will the same response be made. For example, a diabetic patient is said to have made a generalization by reporting the result of a urine test as plus two (+2) when in actuality it was plus three (+3). In this case, the patient may not have discriminated the difference in color of the liquid in the test tube—between "yellow," "orange," or "orange with precipitation." The gradient of stimulus generalization is that range of different stimuli that resemble each other and to which the subject emits the same response to all of them.

DISCRIMINATION

Operant conditioning involves the establishment of discrimination. The occurrence of learning involves the selection of stimuli that are successful in bringing about reinforcement and the rejection of those that are not. Therefore differential reinforcement is necessary for establishing the discrimination of stimuli. An example of this would be related to the lever-pressing experiment cited previously. When the lever is pressed in the presence of a light, a pellet of food is delivered to the rat. When the light (discriminated stimulus) is absent, the pellet of food is withheld. The rat learns only to respond in the presence of the light, however the light does not elicit the response; it creates the occasion for a response (Hilgard, 1956, p. 125).

Another example would be when the previously mentioned diabetic patient would say the result of a urine test is plus three (+3) when the color of the liquid (test) in the test tube is deep orange and say it is plus four (+4) when it is deep orange and has precipitation. The extent to which the patient has learned to pick the correct stimulus and respond correctly is the extent to which the patient has learned to discriminate.

In the literature, discrimination learning has been designated S^D and S^Δ. The discriminative stimulus S^D is the occasion on which a behavior is reinforced. The response is not reinforced in the S^Δ situation (De-Cecco, 1968).

RETENTION

Type-2 learning, or operant conditioning, appears to be quite resistant to forgetting and extinction, especially when intermittent schedules of reinforcement are used in the learning stages. Skinner (1950) demonstrated retention of pecking behavior in his pigeons after 4 years. Some authors (Leavitt and Schlosberg, 1944) have suggested that complex motor skills are extremely resistant to forgetting as compared to verbal association, because complex motor skills are relatively isolated acts, having few activities to exhibit *interferences* with them, as opposed to verbal associations, which have many interferences. Interference is the main cause of forgetting.

Relevant research studies

Ss → R learning has been extensively studied in animals like white rats, pigeons, monkeys, and others. Large amounts of objective data have been published concerning the effects of variations in the basic conditions of Ss → R learning on the rapidity of the learning event. For example, Ferster and Skinner (1957) compiled a large amount of evidence on the effect of different schedules of reinforcement on learning and execution of Ss → R connections. Even though many of the experiments have been conducted on animals, cautious extrapolations of the findings can be made to human learning and performance. Important principles of operant conditioning have also been applied and investigated in clinical situations involving human beings.

The application of operant concepts of behavioral events outside the laboratory has taken place, for the most part, during the past 40 years. In this interval a great deal of relevant empirical research has accumulated.

The following discussion merely highlights some of the research that has taken place, for it is beyond the scope of this module to deal comprehensively with the research that has been accumulated in the area of operant conditioning.

Honig (1966) and Franks (1966) conducted numerous studies concerning the application of principles of both operant and classical conditioning to clinical situations with humans.

Ferster (1964) demonstrated the effect of positive reinforcement on behavioral deficits of autistic children. He pointed out that much of the performance of the autistic child is a result of operant conditioning, that is, it is controlled by its consequences on the environment. For example, the autistic child produces stimuli or situations such as tantrums and other self-destructive behaviors that are aversive enough so that the relevant audience will escape or avoid the aversive stimulus, often by providing a reinforcer. The child who throws a tantrum for candy will sooner or later get the candy.

In another study Ayllon and Michael (1964) applied the principles of operant conditioning in controlling the disruptive behaviors of psychiatric patients. Disruptive behaviors, such as failure to engage in normal and necessary activities or persistent participation in activities that are harmful, may be considered the result of events occurring in the patient's immediate or historical environment rather than the manifestation of mental disorder. Therefore the environmental variables must be manipulated in order to modify the problem behavior. In order to control the problem, however, one must first know what the naturally occurring reinforcement is, what the duration and frequency of the problem behavior is, and what the possibilities are of controlling the reinforcement. In this research each patient was observed every 30 minutes for 1 to 3 minutes to determine the frequency of the behavior. It was found that what maintained the undesirable behavior in most cases was the attention or social approval of the nurses toward that behavior. The nurses therefore switched to giving or withholding social reinforcement contingent on a desired class of behavior. Undesirable behavior was extinguished because it was ignored.

A research study by Ayllon and Haughton (1962) involved patients who refused to eat. Coaxing and persuading the patients to eat was not effective; furthermore, this approach conditioned the patients to eat only with assistance. When the attention that was given for "refusal to eat" was withdrawn, the patients started eating unassisted.

Boren (1966) conducted a study to describe how operant conditioning principles could be applied when the organism was under the influence of different types of drugs. The independent variable in all of these studies was always the administration of a chemical agent. The dependent variable was any biological effect, such as modification of the behavior. The object was to give graded doses of a drug and then observe the graded effect on the system under study. For example; a pigeon was given pentobarbital to see how it affected the pigeon's pecking rate above or below an already established baseline. Rate-increasing drugs could then be called stimulants and rate-decreasing drugs could be called depressants. This and other studies with animals have shown that behavior controlled by a fixed-interval schedule of reinforcement is more sensitive to drugs than behavior controlled by fixed-ratio schedules.

Azrin and Holtz (1966) studied the effects of punishment on behavior. Results of this study showed the following: (1) punishment simply reduces the frequency of the punished response, it does not eliminate it; (2) sudden intense introduction of punishment is better than a gradual increase in intensity; (3) punishment should be delivered immediately after the response that is to be punished; (4) the greater the intensity of the punishing stimulus, the greater the reduction of the punished response; (5) continuous punishment is superior to intermittent punishment; (6) if a response is punished but not reinforced in some manner, it will extinguish through the absence of reinforcement; (7) if punishment is associated with the delivery of reinforcement, the punishing stimulus may acquire conditioned reinforcing properties; (8) mild punishment as compared to intense punishment allows a characteristic recovery from punishment; (9) an alternative response should be available that will produce the same or greater reinforcement as the punished response; (10) a reduction of positive reinforcement may be used as punishment when the use of physical punishment is not possible.

It was found by Azrin and Holtz (1966) that aversive stimuli in general and punishment in particular produce disruptive and undesirable emotional states. The primary disadvantage of punishment has been found to be the resulting social disruption. To the extent that punishment eliminates or disrupts social interaction, it can be expected to make the individual incapable of living in society. The following three sources of disruption have been found to result from punishment: (1) escape from a situation in which punishment is delivered, (2) expression of operant aggression where the punished tries to destroy the individual who is delivering the punishing stimulus, (3) expression of elicited aggression where the aggression or attack is against a nearby individual, even though that individual did not deliver the punishment.

Hoffman (1966) studied the analysis of *discriminated avoidance*, using the following strategy: a neutral stimulus was scheduled to precede, and in this sense served as a warning for, each occurrence of a noxious event. If the subject emitted an appropriate operant during the warning period, the noxious event failed to occur. When the subject failed to avoid, however, both the warning signal and the noxious event remained until an escape response occurred, whereupon both were terminated.

Application to nursing education and practice

The principles of operant conditioning have several implications for nusing education and practice. The following section deals with an overview of some of the ways in which operant theory has been applied.

Operant conditioning in chronic illness

Operant conditioning techniques are being applied to chronically ill patients in order to help these patients extinguish "sick" behaviors. Traditionally, nurses give attention to patients who make the most noise. Many patients prefer this negative attention to having very little attention. It has been found that patients can learn to walk faster if unwarranted complaints about dizziness, or some other complaint, are tended to but ignored socially while attempts to ambulate are reinforced socially. Operant techniques are also helpful in assuring proper fluid intake. Instead of paying attention to when the patient does not drink—for example, by nagging—the nurse ignores nondrinking behavior and reinforces drinking behavior. In a similar situation a graph was made by the patient and was used to reinforce back-brace wearing. Non–back-brace wearing was ignored where previously it warranted nagging, which was attention (Fowler, Fordyce, and Bernie, 1969).

Operant approach to observation and recording

Peterson (1967) devised a way to apply operant principles to observation and recording in the hospital or clinical setting. Such an approach helps nursing students learn how to assess and intervene with patients who lack expected behavior skills or who demonstrate inappropriate behaviors. The students are helped to identify discriminitive stimuli that set off behaviors in their patients through the use of a special recording form. This form has also proved useful as an assessment of the students' effectiveness in either building independent skills in their patients or reducing inappropriate behaviors.

Only observable interactions are recorded. The emphasis is placed on those events that immediately precede and follow a behavior of interest. Observation of consequent events gives the nurse cues as to what conditions may maintain or increase a particular behavior. The recording form is set up as follows:

	Antecedent	Patient	Consequent
Time	events	behavior	events

Behavior modification with tokens

Eighteen withdrawn patients were studied to determine first of all what they liked to do (preferred behavior) and what things they needed to do (desired behavior). Fixed amounts of *tokens* (poker chips) were given to the patients for desired behaviors, such as making the bed and getting dressed. Tokens were exchangeable for preferred behaviors, such as weekend passes and use of the dayroom. Two methods of implementing the token system were studied—the deprivation method and the nondeprivation method. Each patient was assigned at random to a deprivation or nondeprivation group. In the nondeprivation group the patients were allowed a baseline amount of preferred behaviors and, as they earned tokens, were

given even more. In the deprivation group the patients were not allowed any preferred behaviors unless they had earned tokens to exchange for such opportunities. Through this study it was shown that the nondeprivation method was easier to administer and more humane, which allowed the nursing staff to establish close meaningful realtionships with the patients (Beal, and others, 1969)

A subsequent study by Burley and Steiger (1972) has also shown the success with which tokens can be used to modify the behavior of psychiatric inpatients. Tokens were paid for desirable behavior, and unacceptable behavior was ignored. If ignoring the undesirable behavior did not extinguish it, tokens were then charged for the undesirable behavior. Behavior was shaped by increasing the requirements for which tokens would be awarded. Tokens were then used for food, dayroom privileges, pass privileges, and buying things like cigarettes. Burley and Steiger found that after behavior modification was instituted the staff became more enthusiastic; there was increased social awareness among the patients, less "crazy" talk, a decrease in disturbing behaviors, an improvement in personal hygiene, and less fighting; there were fewer physical complaints; and the patients required less medicine, believed they were being treated fairly, and asked for more privileges.

Increasing and reducing the strength of behaviors

Whitney (1966) studied the application of operant theory to increase and reduce the strength of certain behaviors. The following are examples of methods that have been used to modify behavior.

Shaping new behavioral repertoires. The shaping of self-feeding of a severely retarded child who had to be tube fed because he had never been known to raise his arms or respond in any way was studied. A milk-sugar solution was presented to the retardate as a reinforcement that was contingent on some approximation of hand or arm movement. At first mere eye blinking was reinforced, then progressively more was demanded before the milk was received.

Increasing low rates of behavior. Allen and Johnson increased the rate of a child's interaction with other children by selectively giving teacher attention as a reinforcer whenever the child engaged in interaction with other children (Whitney, 1966).

Reinstating behavioral repertoires. Sherman (1963) employed shaping procedures to reinstate verbal behavior for a psychotic who had been institutionalized for 30 years and had been mute for 27 years. Initially the experimenter reinforced head nodding with pennies in response to questioning; then he informed the patient that pennies would not be given unless the patient responded to the questioning with "huh-uh" or "no." After sixteen sessions the psychotic patient was able to converse with simple statements (Whitney, 1966).

Eliminating avoidance behavior. Bentler (1962) reported an instance of a child who exhibited avoidance behavior to bath water. The technique used was to place the child's toys in such a way that in order to play with them she had to first approach an empty bathtub, then a sink filled with water, and so forth until the behavior of bathing in a bathtub was reestablished (Whitney, 1966).

Escape and avoidance of aversive stimuli. Ayllon and Michael (1964) used escape and avoidance of an aversive stimulus (food spilling) to strengthen self-feeding behavior. The nurse "accidentally" spilled food on the patients while feeding them. The only way the patients could avoid having food spilled on them and still receive food was to feed themselves (Whitney, 1966).

Extinction. Williams programmed extinction for bedtime tantrum behavior. Under normal circumstances when the child cried at night the parents would remain in the bedroom until he had fallen asleep. During the extinction period, the parents were instructed to put the child to bed and leave the room. If the child cried, they were not to reenter the room and reinforce the tantrums. The child's rate of tantrum throwing soon became zero (Whitney, 1966).

• • •

In conclusion, it can be seen that facilitating social recovery—that is, a patient's ability to function in society—is one of the primary responsibilities of nursing. Nursing intervention that can promote such social recovery by eliminating ineffective behaviors is a true contribution. Changing patient behaviors has other implications in addition to preparing patients to function in society. Many patients may never be able to leave the hospital, but a better adjustment within the hospital may be an attainable goal. Such advances not only benefit the patient but also lighten the work of the nursing staff, leaving the staff with more time to spend in constructive activities with the patients. Another attribute of this technique is that it can be employed by nonprofessionals as well as professionals, and the guidance of a psychologist is not required. In addition, the use of behavior therapy does not necessitate the allocation, the use of behavior therapy does not necessitate the allocation of more money and staff; it only requires an interest in rehabilitating patients (Layton, 1966).

The principles of operant conditioning have also been applied in preparing programmed instruction and in modifying verbal behaviors.

Programmed instruction

In 1954, Skinner undertook a series of investigations and related inventions designed to increase the effectiveness of teaching academic subjects like reading, spelling, and arithmetic. A "machine" is used, and the child punches the answer; if the answer is correct, "reinforcement" occurs by the machine moving to the next problem. Skinner believes that no teacher can be as skilled a reinforcer as the machine, since the teacher cannot be with every student at once, commending proper responses and correcting erroneous ones. Skinner's teaching devices have come to be known as "teaching machines," and the materials that become the basis for instruction are called "programs," some of which appear in programmed books. The use of operant conditioning techniques in education shows that what has been learned through the study of laboratory animals can be generalized (Hilgard, 1956).

Verbal behavior

Operant conditioning theory has been extrapolated to verbal learning. Speech sounds are emitted—and reinforced—as are any other behaviors. Some speech utterances known as "mands" make demands on the hearer and get reinforced as the hearer complies. A second function, the "tact" function, is concerned mostly with naming, and its reinforcement by the hearer is more general than is mand reinforcement. A third term introduced by Skinner is "autolytic" behavior, referring to verbal behavior that is dependent on other verbal behavior, such as "I was about to say. . . ." It can be seen that our verbal behavior is "shaped" by the reinforcement contingencies of the verbal communities in which we live.

Issues in operant conditioning
The experimental situation versus the human situation

In many ways operant conditioning has come to typify an experimental, objective approach to human behavior. As such it has been the prime critical target for those psychologists who are concerned that an adequate understanding of human behavior must involve more than the experimental methods of physical science. The following are offered by Hall and Lindzey (1957, pp. 461-462) as reasons for this criticism.

1. In operant theory the majority of the investigations have been concerned with simple rather than complex behavior and have been carried out with animal species far removed from the human organism.

2. Most of the positive features of operant theory—its careful definitions, explicitness, and wealth of research—exist only when the theory is applied to animal behavior. As soon as the theory is generalized to complex human behavior, concepts that were crystal clear become ambiguous, and definitions that were tight become flaccid.

3. The terms stimulus and response operate quite well with a limited organism in a restricted environment, but with the adult human organism, operating in a natural environment, specification of the stimulus can only come after there is a relatively complete understanding of the behavioral event in question. It can be argued that if the psychologist can define the stimulus, the task is at an end; therefore, it is implied that the necessary definitions for operant theory can only be provided after the fact. Therefore, if the theory operates on a post-hoc basis, its generality and predictive efficiency is impaired. (Hall and Lindzey, 1957, p. 461.)

4. Another criticism of operant theory points to its simplicity and molecularity. It has been believed that "this theory is the very essence of a segmented, fragmented, and atomistic approach to behavior. There is no appreciation of the importance of the whole." (Hall and Lindzey, 1957, p. 462.)

5. Some critics point to operant theory as "nothing more than a refinement of common sense. For the ordinary individual it is easy to view behavior as determined by a series of relationships between stimuli on one hand and responses on the other." (Hall and Lindsey, 1957, p. 462.)

Dehumanization versus humanization

Roos (1970) asserted that rather than having "dehumanizing" consequences, conditioning procedures are designed to foster the development of human qualities. While reinforcement contingencies can be established without the subject's knowledge, this approach is not desirable. Conversely, other strategies aimed at "treatment" can be equally manipulative if the subject is kept unaware of the contingencies; for example posthypnotic suggestion and other procedures. Those who criticize conditioning on the basis that it is "mechanistic" or "dehumanizing" fail to grasp its basic purpose, for conditioning approaches if successfully applied should maximize interaction with social and physical environments.

Free versus controlled behavior

Schoenfeld (1969) directed his attention to an issue between humanists and scientists working on the experimental analysis of behavior. Humanism regards the human being as a thinking and feeling organism, as the discoverer or inventor of morality, as having a philosophical mind, as being creative, as possessing a will and choice of action, and as being "free." Humans are not a machine and cannot be controlled like a machine. Science argues that behavioral control is inevitable. Science sees itself as no threat to anyone, but rather as seeking knowledge only, and knowledge cannot be bad. Control is only consequential to knowledge. Schoenfeld asserted that humanism needs no defense because we are all humanists; however, behavioral science must deal with the following question if it is to have peace with humanism: will science be able to salvage the human and the unique humanity that humanism defends?

Psychoanalytical theory versus behaviorism

Perhaps the most crucial area of all as far as the patient is concerned—apart from the question of remission—is that of symptom substitution. According to psychoanalytical theory, symptoms are the result of the conflict between impulses struggling to express themselves and the controlling defensive forces. Hence according to the analyst, treating the symptom and leaving the conflict unresolved may result in substitution of symptoms that are more harmful than those they replaced. Therefore, the resolution of the original conflict situation may be a necessary component of the effective treatment of behavioral pathology (Franks, 1966).

Another problem yet unresolved is that of the tendency to relapse following an initial response to treatment. Two possible ways of coping with this problem have been looked at: (1) to develop "booster" follow-up conditioning sessions and (2) to develop initial conditioning techniques that minimize relapse, such as the use of intermittent reinforcement schedules (Gardner, 1968).

Researchable questions

Results of research studies concerned with the application of techniques of operant conditioning have clearly demonstrated that behavior modification is an effective therapeutic tool. There remain however numerous unanswered questions concerning the utility and the applicability of operant conditioning techniques in modifying maladaptive human behaviors. This is one area where research is needed. Here are a few researchable questions that need investigation.

A descriptive (exploratory) study, stage one

1. What are the reinforcers that health care personnel (nurses, physicians, and others) unconsciously give to patients that foster maladaptive dependency behaviors in patients?
   a. Independent variable: is the type of reinforcers health-care personnel unknowingly give

b. Dependent variable: dependency behavior

An experimental study—follow-up of the first one—stage two

1. What is the effect of withholding reinforcement (that was made contingent on dependency behavior) on dependency behavior?

   a. Independent variable: withholding reinforcement

   b. Dependent variable: dependency behavior

2. What is the effect of delivery of positive reinforcement (that is made contingent on behaviors of independence) on behaviors of independence?

   a. Independent variable: delivery of positive reinforcement

   b. Dependent variable: behaviors of independence

3. Will psychiatric patients be able to transfer operants (such as self-feeding, self-dressing) learned under one set of circumstances (institutional setting) to a different set of circumstances (home)?

   a. Independent variable: changes in circumstance

   b. Dependent variable: transfer of learned responses

4. Can nonprofessional personnel (such as paranursing personnel or family members) modify a patient's behaviors as effectively as professional personnel? In most institutions this is a necessity because of staff limitations and also for follow-up behavior modification therapy at home.

   a. Independent variable: professional versus nonprofessional personnel

   b. Dependent variable: effectiveness of behavior modification

Conclusion

It can be seen that knowledge of the principles and techniques of operant conditioning can be very useful in our daily personal and professional lives. The relative simplicity of the techniques involved allows the implementation of programs without the need for professional psychiatric guidance or additional staff. The end result of the effective use of these techniques could, as Skinner has said, "lead to the creation of the type of world we want to live in." An inspiring thought!

ADDITIONAL LEARNING EXPERIENCES—RECOMMENDED READING LIST

DeCecco, J. *The psychology of learning and instruction: educational psychology.* (1st Ed.) Englewood Cliffs, N. J.: Prentice-Hall, Inc. 1968, pp. 243-272.

Gagne, R. *The conditions of learning.* (2nd Ed.) New York: Holt, Rinehart and Winston, Inc., 1970, pp. 38-42, 104-122.

Hilgard, E. R. *Theories of learning.* New York: Appleton-Century-Crofts, 1956, pp. 107-145.

Hilgard, E. R., and Bower, G. H. *Theories of learning.* New York: Appleton-Century-Crofts, 1966, pp. 107-145.

Honig, W. K. *Operant behavior: areas of research and application.* New York: Appleton-Century-Crofts, 1966.

INSTRUCTIONS TO THE LEARNER REGARDING POSTTEST

You are now ready to take the posttest to determine the extent to which you have achieved the objectives of this module. Return to the pretest and take it again as a posttest. Correct your answers utilizing the answer key that begins at the bottom of this page. You need to score 24 correct points (95% level) to proceed to the next module. If your score is less than 24 correct points, correct your errors, study those parts that you did incorrectly, and carefully read some of the articles in the recommended reading list. You need to study until you achieve the 95% level.

ANSWER KEY FOR PRETEST AND POSTTEST

1. True (DeCecco, 1968, p. 271)
2. True (Gagne, 1970, pp. 104-105)

3. False (Hilgard and Bower, 1966, pp. 113, 138)
4. True (Gagne, 1970, p. 38)
5. operant or S–R learning (Gagne, 1970, p. 63)
6. shaping (Gagne, 1970, p. 110)
7. generalization (DeCecco, 1968, p. 259)
8. c (Skinner, 1938, p. 21)
9. a (Hilgard 1956, p. 108)
10. c (Hilgard, 1956, p. 108)
11. c (DeCecco, 1968, p. 266)
12. a (DeCecco, 1968, p. 166)
13. b (Gagne, 1970, pp. 120-121)
14. a (Layton, 1966, p. 41)
15. d (DeCecco, 1968, p. 260)
16. c (Whitney, 1966, p. 230)
17. d (Whitney, 1966, p. 230)
18. d (DeCecco, 1968, p. 259)
19. d (Hoffman, 1966, pp. 499-500)
20. d (Burley and Steiger, 1972, pp. 9-15)
21. b (Burley and Steiger, 1972, pp. 9-15)
22. d (Whitney, 1966, p. 231-232)
23. a. changes in circumstance
    b. transfer of conditioned response
24. a. behavior modification technique versus psychoanalytical technique
    b. extent of continued behavior change over a period of time X
25. a. professional versus nonprofessional personnel
    b. effectiveness of behavior modification

REFERENCES

Ayllon, T. and Haughton, E. Control of the behavior of schizophrenic patients by foods. *Journal of the Experimental Analysis of Behavior*, 1962, **5**(3):343-352.

Ayllon, T. and Michael, J. Control of disrupting behaviors of psychiatric patients. In C. M. Franks (Ed.), *Conditioning techniques*. New York: Springer Publishing Co., Inc., 1964.

Azrin, N. H., and Holtz, W. C. Punishment. In W. K. Honig (Ed), *Operant behavior: areas of research and application*. New York: Appleton-Century-Crofts, 1966.

Beal, E., Sletten, I. W., Ogn Janov, V., and Hughes, D. Nursing care approaches for operant reinforcement with psychiatric patients. *Journal of Psychiatric Nursing and Mental Health Services*, 1969, **7**(4):157-159.

Bentler, P. M. An infant's phobia treated with reciprocal inhibition therapy. *Journal of Child Psychology and Psychiatry*, 1962, 3:185-189.

Boren, J. J. The study of drugs with operant techniques. In W. K. Honig (Ed.), *Operant behavior: areas of research and application*. New York: Appleton-Century-Crofts, 1966.

Burley, E. J., and Steiger, T. B. Behavior modification: two nurses tell it like it is. *Journal of Psychiatric Nursing and Mental Health Services*, 1972, **10**(1):9-15.

DeCecco, J. *The psychology of learning and instruction: educational psychology*. (1st Ed.) Englewood Cliffs, N.J.: Prentice-Hall, Inc., 1968.

DeCecco, J. *The psychology of learning and instruction: educational psychology*. (2nd Ed.) Englewood Cliffs, N.J.: Prentice-Hall, Inc., 1974.

Estes, W. K. An experimental study of punishment. *Psychological Monograph*, 1944, **57**(263):124-137.

Ferster, C. B. Positive reinforcement and behavioral deficits of autistic children. In C. M. Franks (Ed.), *Conditioning techniques*. New York: Springer Publishing Co., Inc., 1964.

Ferster, C. B., and Skinner, B. F. *Schedules of reinforcement*. New York: Appleton-Century-Crofts, 1957.

Fowler, R. S., Fordyce, W. E., Bernie, R. Operant conditioning in chronic illness. *American Journal of Nursing*, 1969, **69**(6):1226-1228.

Franks, C. M. Clinical application of conditioning and other behavioral techniques. *Conditioned Reflex*, 1966, 1(1):36-50.

Gagne, R. *The conditions of learning*. (2nd Ed.) New York: Holt, Rinehart and Winston, Inc., 1970.

Gardner, J. M. Issue at point. *Mental Retardation*, 1968, **6**(4):54-55.

Hall, C. S., and Lindzey, G. *Theories of Personality*. New York: John Wiley & Sons, Inc., 1957.

Hilgard, E. R. *Theories of learning*. New York: Appleton-Century-Crofts, 1956.

Hilgard, E. R., and Bower, G. H. *Theories of learning*. New York: Appleton-Century-Crofts, 1966.

Hoffman, H. S. The analysis of discriminated avoidance. In W. K. Werner Honig (Ed.), *Operant behavior: areas of research and application*. New York: Appleton-Century-Crofts, 1966.

Honig, W. K. (Ed.) *Operant behavior: areas of research and application*. New York: Appleton-Century-Crofts, 1966.

Kimble, G. A. Hilgard and Marquis' *Conditioning and learning*. New York: Appleton-Century-Crofts, 1961.

Layton, Sister Mary Michele. Behavior therapy and its implications for psychiatric nursing. *Perspectives in Psychiatric Care*, 1966, 4(2):38-51.

Leavitt, H. J., and Scholosberg, H. The retention of verbal and of motor skills. *Journal of Experimental Psychology*, 1944, 37:247-249.

Lunzer, E. A. *The regulation of behaviour.* New York: American Elsevier Publishing Co., Inc., 1968.

Mowner, O. H. *Learning theory and behavior,* New York: John Wiley & Sons, Inc., 1960.

Peterson, L. W. Operant approach to observation and recording. *Nursing Outlook,* 1967, **15**(3):28-32.

Roos, P. Normalization, de-humanization, and conditioning—conflict or harmony? *Mental Retardation,* Aug. 1970.

Schoenfeld, W. N. Humanism and the science of behavior. *Conditioned Reflex,* 1969, 4(3):139-144.

Sherman, J. A. Reinstatement of verbal behavior in a psychotic by reinforcement methods. *Journal of Speech and Hearing Disorder,* 1963, **28**:398-401.

Skinner, B. F. *Behavior of the organism.* New York: The Macmillan Co., 1938.

Skinner, B. F. Are theories of learning necessary? *Psychological Review,* 1950, **57**:193-216.

Thorndike, E. L. *Animal intelligence,* New York: The Macmillan Co., 1911.

Whitney, L. R. Operant learning theory: a framework deserving nursing investigation. *Nursing Research,* 1966, **15**:(3):229-235.

Williams, C. D. The elimination of tantrum behavior by extinction procedure. *Journal of Abnormal Social Psychology,* 1959, **59**:269.

MODULE 4

Chaining

DESCRIPTION OF THE MODULE

This module is concerned with "skill learning," also known as "chaining." It is the third condition of learning, following classical and operant conditioning. The text of the module is organized to cover five relevant areas— theoretical framework, research studies, application to nursing education and practice, issues, and researchable questions.

In addition, this module contains learner objectives, and pre- and posttests to measure the degree of learning or knowledge that has been acquired. It also contains an answer key to the pre- and posttests to enable the learner to receive immediate feedback on the tests.

MODULE OBJECTIVES

At the completion of this module—having studied each part of it very carefully, including the recommended reading list—the student will be able to:
1. Define what "chaining" or "skill learning" is
2. Describe how skill learning takes place— theoretical background
3. Describe the characteristics of a chain
4. Describe the external and internal conditions necessary for chain learning to take place
5. Describe and give an example of the phenomena associated with chaining— extinction, generalization, discrimination, and forgetting

6. Teach correctly two chains (nursing procedures) and identify *all* areas, using the checklist in the module
7. Apply the principles of chaining to other nursing-education and nursing-practice situations
8. Identify at least one issue in chaining
9. Raise one researchable question and identify both the independent and dependent variables

PRETEST AND POSTTEST

Circle the correct answers. Each question is worth 1 point. For this test 95% level of achievement is 19 points. On completion of this test correct your answers utilizing the answer key that is found at the end of this module (p. 93).

True or false

1. An important point in chaining is that the person receives some kinesthetic feedback from the immediate response before going on to the next link in the chain. True or False
2. It is not necessary to learn the particular links of a chain in sequence in order to accomplish chain learning effectively. True or False
3. Contiguity refers to the timing of a chain. True or False

Multiple choice

4. The occurrence of _____ appears to be extremely essential to the establishment of chains.

58

a. conditioned stimulus

b. terminal satisfaction

c. external cues

5. Chaining, or skill learning, refers primarily to:

a. motor responses

b. the sequence of S–R units

c. both of the above

d. none of these

6. In a chain each S–R (stimulus—response) units acts as the stimulus for:

a. the antecedant S–R unit

b. the following S–R unit

c. the preceding S–R unit

d. the next series of S–R units

7. A skill or chain has three characteristics. A chain does *not* include which of the following as a characteristic:

a. a series of motor responses

b. eye-hand coordination

c. the organization of small chains into complex response patterns

d. contiguity

8. When performing a chain, an individal receives internal feedback by

a. kinesthetic senses

b. chemical reactions

c. cognitive processes

d. reflex responses

9. Which of the following is *not* a phase of learning?

a. cognitive

b. fixation

c. reinforcement

d. autonomous

10. During the cognitive phase, the student _____ the skill.

a. practices

b. intellectualizes

c. understands

d. uses

11. In the fixation phase, the student:

a. practices until speed is tops

b. practices the chain in sections

c. practices until becoming an expert

d. practices until there are zero errors

12. Practice provides many benefits. Which of the following does *not* refer to practice?

a. helps strengthen each S–R segment

b. helps prevent extinction and forgetting

c. helps learn proper timing.

d. helps learning in the cognitive phase

e. helps during the fixation and autonomous phases

13. Feedback is an important part of learning a chain. Feedback refers to which of these?

a. knowledge of results

b. reinforcement

c. punishment

d. generalization

14. There are four phenomena of chaining: extinction, generalization, forgetting, and discrimination. Which of these refers to the unlearning of a chain?

a. forgetting

b. generalization

c. discrimination

d. extinction

15. Which phenomenon refers to the discreteness of each S–R unit?

a. forgetting

b. generalization

c. discrimination

d. extinction

16. Which phenomenon refers to applying a chain to learning another similar chain?

a. forgetting

b. generalization

c. discrimination

d. extinction

17. The cause of forgetting is:

a. massed practice

b. discrimination

c. deletion of practice

d. lack of feedback

18. The function of verbal instruction in chain learning (such as in performing a catheterization procedure) is to:

a. ensure that the student does not make a mistake

b. enable the student to perform creatively

c. provide external cues for selection of correct links

d. to reinforce the student's response

19. In teaching the diabetic patient or student the procedure of testing urine for sugar, the teacher must be aware of and provide which of the following types of external conditions:

a. repetition and reinforcement

b. contiguity and reinforcement
c. reinstatement of procedures in proper order
d. discrimination
e. contiguity

Discussion question

20. Define "chaining."

TEXT
Theoretical framework

Chaining, or skill learning, refers primarily to motor responses, that is, muscular movements. Each movement is viewed as an individual stimulus—response (S–R) association. *A chain or skill is a sequence of stimulus–response (S–R) units which the preceding S–R unit acts as a stimulus for the next S–R unit.* The example of eating illustrates this definition:

S (food on plate)—R (pick up fork)
S (fill fork with food)—R (place fork in mouth)
S (food in mouth)—R (fork withdrawn)
S (food in mouth without fork)—R (chewing begins)

For the acquisition of sequences that are nonverbal the word *chaining* is usually used. However, in the acquisition of sequences that involve a subvariety of verbal behaviors, the term *verbal chains*, or *verbal associates*, is used.

The principles of chaining are important for the nurse-educator to understand because so much of nursing involves the teaching and learning of chains. In nursing, a good use of chaining is illustrated in the procedure in which a nurse learns how to cope with and implement the management of cardiac arrest and other emergency procedures. Other examples are the learning of skills of sterile technique, the wearing of gloves, and the performing of sterile procedures (for example, catheterization or surgical procedures).

In chaining, the important thing is the *correct sequencing* of appropriate responses. In chain learning, a chain cannot be learned unless the learner is capable of performing the individual links. For example, in the wearing of sterile gloves, the nurse must be able to perform each of the S–R links prior to putting it together with proper sequencing. During the process of chain learning, at times, it is necessary to guide the chaining through verbal instruction ("how-to-do" explanations). The function of this instruction is to provide *external cues* for the selection of exactly the right links for the chain. This process might appear in the following form:

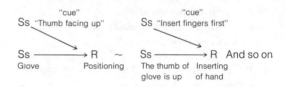

In this example, let us assume that the student nurse or the patient is to learn the procedure of putting on gloves. The sight of the glove (Ss) elicits the response (R) of positioning the glove in such a way that the thumb of the glove is facing upward. If the learner fails to respond in this way, the nurse-teacher can give verbal instruction (cue) to have the thumb of the glove facing upward. After the learner correctly positions the glove, the sight of it will be the second stimulus (Ss) to produce the response of inserting the hand (R). If the learner fails to insert the hand, then the teacher can again provide the external verbal cue of "insert fingers first," which in turn will produce the correct response of "inserting the hand" from the learner. In this way the entire procedure of donning the glove can be performed. It should be stressed that the last link in the procedure should be reinforced positively. The last act (S–R link, the wearing of the gloves) constitutes a consummatory act that provides reinforcement for the first link and also for the entire chain.

Verbal instruction (cue) may be self-administered. After the skill is learned, the cueing may not be necessary. In learning nursing skills and procedures, it may help the students to verbally repeat what they are doing and what the next step will be. This acts as self-administered cueing.

With young children, when one cannot use verbal cues, it is possible to teach chaining by using other means of cueing; for example, the additional stimuli of pictures and gestures. Again, these additional cues may not be necessary once the chain has been learned.

A skill or chain has three characteristics:

1. It is a chain of motor responses (S–R units)
2. It involves eye-hand coordination
3. It includes the organization of chains into complex response patterns

The first characteristic involves a chain of *motor responses*. In a motor response, the stimulus for each S–R link or unit is partly kinesthetic. In other words, the stimulus comes from an internal muscular feeling that one has learned is correct. When one picks up a fork, one knows that it is being held correctly without thinking about it because of the way it feels. This feeling is called *kinesthetic feedback*. Therefore, in a motor response the kind of feedback that helps the learner to know by feeling if a performance is correct is kinesthetic feedback.

When a skill is first learned external feedback (outside the body) is required, such as someone saying the performance is adequate. In the example of eating, mother uses external feedback by showing and telling how to hold a fork and by correcting errors. During the process of learning a skill or chain, reliance on internal cues, such as kinesthetic feedback, increases while the use of external feedback decreases.

The second characteristic of a chain involves *eye-hand coordination*. Skill learning requires varying degrees of eye-hand coordination. Placing a fork in the mouth utilizes the perception of where hand and mouth are and the coordinating of muscular movement so the two meet in a desired fashion. This type of activity is very basic eye-hand coordination. A more complex example is that of a pilot coordinating what is seen on the instrument panel with the pushing of appropriate buttons and levers.

The third characteristic of a chain is that *it includes the organization of chains into complex response patterns*. Chains are often part of a larger response pattern. The chain or skill of giving an injection is part of the overall chain of dispensing medications. The chains that make up the total response patterns are thought to be hierarchically organized. Each smaller chain must be individually learned, in sequence, before the whole response pattern is learned.

An example from nursing is about giving an injection. The student has to learn sequentially several small chains, or subtasks, such as how to use a syringe, how to use a vial or ampule, how to draw the desired amount, how to locate the correct anatomical site, and so on, before the final or overall response pattern can be performed smoothly.

Another example from nursing would be teaching a student to do a tube feeding. Which of the following subtasks or smaller chains would have to be taught and in what order?

1. Clamping and unclamping nasogastric tubing
2. Handling a 50-ml syringe
3. Pouring the desired amount of feeding
4. Checking for feeding temperature
5. Checking the tube for proper placement in the stomach
6. Administering the feeding to the patient
7. Cleaning the equipment

The correct sequence of the S–R chains is 4, 3, 5, 1, 2, 6, 7.

Three phases of chain learning have been identified by Fitts (1962, pp. 186-189) as (1) cognitive, (2) fixation, (3) autonomous. *In the cognitive* phase a new skill is just being learned. During this phase, the student tries to intellectualize the skill. This intellectualization process constitutes the cognitive phase of skill learning. In this phase, as the instructor explains the skill, the student assimilates the information and mentally visualizes how to perform the skill.

The second phase of skill learning is *fixation.* During the fixation phase the correct behavior is practiced until the error rate is zero. When this occurs the chain is said to be fixed. The length of the fixation phase varies with the learner and the complexity of the chain. When the student first attempts the chain, all energy is directed toward connecting the units of the chain together in proper sequence. With practice, the student then tries to organize the chains into an overall pattern.

The final state of skill learning is the *autonomous stage.* During this phase, the student increases the speed and efficiency of the chain while maintaining a zero error rate. At this stage the skill becomes involuntary, or automatic, and inflexible.

Conditions of chain learning

There are *two categories of conditions* necessary for chaining to occur: conditions within the learner, internal, and conditions within the situation; external.

INTERNAL CONDITIONS

The first condition necessary for chaining to occur is that the *student must have the physical and intellectual capabilities necessary to perform the chain.* We would not expect a 2-year-old child to be capable of learning a complex chain, such as giving an injection; a 2-year-old has both insufficient dexter-ity (physical) and retention (intellectual). It is therefore important to assess a learner's physical and intellectual capabilities as they pertain to the learning of a specific chain prior to teaching it.

The second condition within the learner necessary for chain learning is that *each S–R connection must be previously learned.* Before the next link, or S–R unit, can be learned, the preceding link must be mastered. One could not expect a student who has not fully learned how to fill the syringe to give an injection. Each S–R link acts as a stimulus for the next S–R unit. If one S–R unit is not fully learned, there is no stimulus, or there is an incorrect stimulus, for the next one.

EXTERNAL CONDITIONS

In order for chaining to occur, four conditions must be present in the *situation:* (1) contiguity, (2) practice, (3) feedback, and (4) sequencing.

The first condition, *contiguity,* refers to the timing involved in presenting and executing a chain. The individual S–R units of a chain must be performed in close time succession if the chain is to be learned. Since each S–R unit acts as a stimulus for the next, no pauses should be present when learning a chain. When practicing a chain to improve performance, rest periods are necessary. Learning and performance are not the same. Learning requires contiguity.

The second external condition necessary for chaining is *practice.* Practice is important for four reasons:

1. To strengthen each S–R segment
2. To help the student learn the S–R segments in proper sequence and with proper timing
3. To help prevent extinction (loss of the chain) and forgetting
4. To strengthen both the fixation and autonomous phases of skill learning

The third external condition for chaining is

feedback and reinforcement. Feedback refers to *knowledge of results.* Two types of feedback exist: intrinsic and extrinsic. Intrinsic feedback is synonomous with internal or kinesthetic feedback. Extrinsic, or external, feedback comes from the situation or the teacher. Feedback also acts as a reinforcing agent. Praise from the teacher reinforces the student to duplicate the chain. Feeling (kinesthetic feedback) the correct performance helps the learner continue in the same way. The satisfaction a student receives from completing a chain is also reinforcing (internal feedback). *Reinforcement* of the terminal link is therefore an essential aspect of the chain or skill learning. The terminal link must lead to a satisfying state of affairs; for example the positive feeling that a procedure is completed correctly, as when the urine has come out in a catheterization procedure or the glove is put on in a glove-donning procedure. The occurrence of some terminal satisfaction appears to be essential to the establishment of chains. If the reinforcement is omitted, extinction of the final link occurs, and the chain as a whole disappears. It has been found that the reinforcement needs to be immediate in order for chain learning to occur most readily. If reinforcement is delayed, learning is delayed (Gagne, 1965).

The final external condition necessary for chain learning is *sequencing*. Sequencing refers to the presentation of the parts of a chain in proper order so that the student can reinstate them correctly. There are two methods for presenting a chain: (1) beginning to end or (2) end to beginning (backward chaining). The first method is logical and obvious. The second method was developed by Thomas Gilbert (1962) and is also called *mathetics*. Gilbert taught riflery beginning with firing a shot and working toward the beginning. An example from nursing can be in the catheterization procedure, where the student can work backwards in collecting the equipment necessary to perform the catheterization procedure. For example, in order for the urine to come out of the patient's bladder, what things are needed? A catheter. In order to put the catheter into the patient's bladder, what things are needed? Lubricating jelly, gloves, and syringe. The question is asked to the beginning of the procedure.

Phenomena associated with chain learning

Four *phenomena* of conditioning also apply to chaining: (1) extinction, (2) generalization, (3) forgetting, and (4) discrimination.

Extinction, the first phenomenon, is the unlearning of a chain that occurs when feedback or reinforcement is withdrawn. If a student no longer receives satisfying reinforcement at the completion of a chain or no longer gets feedback, or if the last link is forgotten, the chain will be extinguished.

The second phenomenon of chaining is *generalization.* It occurs when the learning of a particular chain or part of it can be applied to other similar situations. For example, the learning of aseptic technique in the changing of dressings can also be applied with some modification to the handling of sterile equipment.

The third phenomenon of chaining is *forgetting.* Forgetting occurs when practice is deleted. Any part or all of a chain may be forgotten. It is known, however, that in some cases reinstatement of one part of a chain will elicit the entire chain; for example, in trying to ride a bicycle after many years without practice, the stimulus of sitting in the seat and peddling elicits remembrance of the entire chain.

The final phenomenon associated with chaining is *discrimination.* Each S–R segment is a discrete unit. In teaching or learning a chain the discreteness of each unit must be preserved or confusion will occur. The need for discrimination places a responsibility on the teacher to make sure the student sees the discreteness of each S–R unit.

Relevant research studies
Phases of skill learning

William Bryan and Noble Harter (1897, 1899) were among the first researchers to notice a pattern of skill learning. When they observed students learning the Morse code, they found beginning students had to identify each letter and correspond with dots or dashes. As the students progressed, they seemed to respond to whole words, phrases, and even sentences at once.

A similar experience was observed by William Book (1908) as he regarded typing students. The novice had to identify the letter to be typed, locate the letter on the keyboard mentally, place a finger on the proper key, and finally, say and strike the key simultaneously. As students progressed, they were able to identify groups of letters or syllables, use mental spelling, and strike the keys. Experts are able to read words and phrases ahead, striking the correct keys.

Miller, Gallanter, and Pribam (1960) identified the difference between the beginner's and the expert's approaches to learning a chain. Beginner and expert both have a plan, or approach, to the skill. The beginner's plan is voluntary, flexible, and communicable. The expert's version of the plan is involuntary, inflexible, and not easily communicated; often the expert is unable to explain how to execute the skill.

Sequencing

Thomas Gilbert (1962) studied presentation, or ordering, of S–R units. He developed a method of reverse contiguity, called mathetics. The students in Gilbert's study were taught riflery. They began with the final step, or shooting the rifle, and then went backwards until all the steps were covered. The theory behind this is that completing the final step acts as a reinforcing or motivating agent.

Cox and Boren (1965) compared Gilbert's method with a traditional method and found both to be equally effective.

Part versus whole method of teaching

The research question involved in this section is whether the student should perform the entire skill at once (whole method) or first practice the parts of the skill (part method).

McGuigan and MacCaslin (1955) compared the two methods in teaching riflery to army recruits. One group was taught each S–R segment and then allowed to practice before going on to the next segment. The whole-method group was given a demonstration of firing a rifle. Next, they were given instruction and practice time on all aspects of firing a rifle. The researchers found that the whole method was superior to the part method.

Further research was summarized by James Naylor (1962), who concluded that for skills that are not highly organized nor difficult, the part method is best. For skills that are moderately or highly difficult and very organized, the whole method is best.

Massed versus distributed practice

The research issue of this section deals with the benefits of massed versus distributed practice. Massed practice does not provide time for rest. Distributed practice allows for rest periods.

Irving Lorge (1930) performed a classical experiment on this topic. Three groups of students were assigned a task to draw a figure using only a mirror image. The first group was given twenty trials without any rest (massed practice). The second group had twenty trials with 1-minute rest periods between each trial. The third group had 1-day rest periods between each trial. The length of time to complete the task decreased after about four trials for groups 2 and 3. The first group's performance stayed the same. Distributed practice proved beneficial.

Mary Kientzle (1946) experimented to see

what amount of rest time was optimal. The task was printing the alphabet upside down. Rest periods varied from none to 7 days. Forty-five seconds proved to be the optimal rest period. Periods less than 45 seconds proved detrimental to performance. Periods longer than 45 seconds proved to be ineffective in increasing performance.

Carl Duncan (1951) studied further the effects of rest and practice. Two groups were given a task to complete. Group 1 received no rest periods but three times as much time for practice. Group 2 received periodic rest periods. When the groups were compared, group 2 had better performance despite the fact that group 1 had practiced three times longer. Both groups were then given a rest period, but group 2's performance still remained superior.

Feedback

J. L. Elwell and G. C. Grindley (1938) studied the effects of withholding feedback. Students were taught to beam a light on the bull's-eye of a target. This required coordination of both the left and right hands. The students received kinesthetic feedback as well as external feedback when the light hit the bull's-eye. At one point, the feedback was withdrawn (Fig. 4-1) and performance plummeted. Motivation was also affected. Students complained of boredom and displeasure and arrived late for successive meetings.

Lorge and Thorndike (1935) studied the effects of delaying feedback. Students were to learn to toss two wooden balls over their shoulders at an unseen target. The groups were treated as listed:

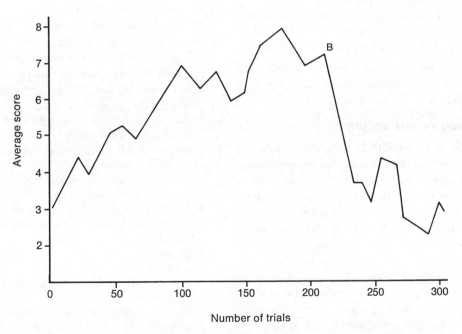

Fig. 4-1. Average performance of 10 subjects. Feedback removed at B (After Elwell and Grindley, 1938, p. 45; DeCecco and Crawford, 1974, p. 261.)

Group 1—received money (motivation) and feedback (information regarding accuracy)
Group 2—received no feedback
Group 3—received immediate feedback
Group 4—received feedback after 1 second
Group 5—received feedback after 2 seconds
Group 6—received feedback after 3 seconds
Group 7—received feedback after 4 or 6 seconds
Group 8—received feedback after the next-to-previous throw

Group 2 (no feedback) and group 8 (intervening toss before feedback) were the only groups showing no improvement. Also less improvement was demonstrated in group 7 than in groups 3, 4, 5, and 6.

A similar experiment was done by Greenspoon and Foreman (1946). They assigned specific length lines to be drawn by five groups of blindfolded students. The treatments were as follows:

Group 1—received immediate feedback
Group 2—received no feedback
Group 3—received feedback after 10 seconds
Group 4—received feedback after 20 seconds
Group 5—received feedback after 30 seconds

Increasing the delay of feedback decreased the rate of learning. This is illustrated in Fig. 4-2.

Speed versus accuracy

William Solley (1952) performed an experiment to test which was more important, speed or accuracy. He found that in skills in which speed is the primary focus, speed should be emphasized right from the beginning. In skills in which both speed and accuracy are important, emphasis should be placed on both speed and accuracy.

Robb (1966) discovered in studying the effects of slow practice—in which the student slowly goes through each step—that this method hindered the student's learning of a simple skill. If timing is an important factor in learning a skill, slow practice is not useful.

Application to nursing education and practice—identification of an issue

This section deals with teaching a skill. First, principles involved in chain learning will be identified. This will be followed by an example of a task in which the principles will be applied to the teaching of a specific skill.

The first principle is *analysis of the skill,* that is, the breakdown of the chain into S–R units. This step is not as easy as it may appear. The teacher must be careful to discriminate clearly each S–R unit to prevent student confusion. The teacher must also begin to think about internal feedback and external feedback. It probably will be necessary to explain how the student should "feel" (kinesthetic feedback) when performing. Also, the teacher needs to look at what cues from the environment (external feedback) will help the student discriminate. These cues can be either verbal or pictorial or in actual demonstration form.

To implement the principle of analysis of the skill more explicitly let us use the example of drawing 1 ml of solution from an ampule into a 3-ml syringe, aseptically. The teacher must be able to identify each of the following S–R units:

S (take an alcohol sponge in right hand)–R (pick up ampule in left hand)
S (ampule in left hand)–R (place sponge around top of ampule)
S (sponge in place)–R (snap off top)
S (top off)—R (discard top and sponge)
S (top discarded)–R (place ampule on counter)
S (ampule on counter)–R (pick up syringe in right hand)
S (syringe in right hand)–R (unsheath needle with left hand)
S (unsheathed needle)–R (place needle cover on counter)
S (needle cover on counter)–R (place needle in ampule)
S (needle to bottom of ampule)–R (withdraw 1 ml of solution)

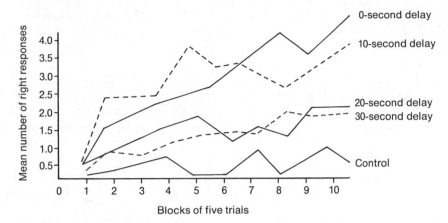

Fig. 4-2. Mean number of correct responses of the control and experimental groups for successive blocks of five trials. (After Greenspoon and Foreman, 1946, 227; DeCecco and Crawford, 1974, p. 262.)

S (solution withdrawn)–R (check amount)

S (amount checked)–R (replace needle protector)

The second step in skill analysis is *assessing the complexity of the skill*. The teacher must look at the skill to see what physical and intellectual requirements will be needed, and later must ascertain if the student posesses them. For example, assessing the complexity of skill for the above example includes:

1. Physical requirements
   a. Good eyesight
   b. Good eye-hand coordination
   c. Good dexterity
2. Intellectual requirements
   a. Ability to understand the principles of sterility
   b. Ability to concentrate for at least 10 minutes
   c. Ability to retain information

The third step in analyzing a chain is *assessing component skills*. The teacher must determine if there are other chains necessary to know before this skill can be learned. An example is that students need to know how to

read a bath thermometer before learning how to give an enema. In the previous example, the students must know how to operate the syringe. Not only does the teacher need to analyze necessary preexisting skills but also the hierarchy of the S–R units within the chain, in other words, how to organize the S–R units.

The fourth step in teaching a chain is to assess the *entering behavior of the student*. The teacher has already analyzed what is necessary for the student to do to achieve. Now, it is necessary to determine if the student is capable of achieving. The teacher will want to know two sets of information:

1. Does the student possess both the physical and intellectual capabilities to achieve?

2. Does the student have the necessary prerequisite skills? One way in which the teacher can determine this is by means of testing. The teacher also can do the following:

   a. Observe the student's ability to operate a syringe, which also checks dexterity
   b. Check medical records for the report of

student's eye examination or ask the student about eyesight

c. Test the student on knowledge of aseptic technique

The next step in teaching a chain is to *prepare the approach*. The teacher must have some strategy for presenting the chain. Research findings dictate some of the strategy. Most important is that the teacher needs to provide the following *four basic conditions for learning:*

1. *Contiguity* means that the teacher must make sure the chain is presented without pause, so that each S–R unit will act as a stimulus for the next; for example, presenting the students with the entire chain of withdrawing 1 ml of solution into a 3-ml syringe, aseptically, without interruption.

2. *Feedback and reinforcement* serve a similar purpose. Feedback means the teacher provides knowledge of results. This is one of the most important parts of teaching. The teacher not only tells the students when the task is being performed correctly, but also prompts and cues them as they proceed. The teacher has to make environmental cues clear. To teach students to manipulate a syringe, the teacher might demonstrate cues, such as the feel of the syringe, the placement of the plunger when the syringe is filled at different levels, and so on.

Feedback is a form of reinforcement. Praising students who are succeeding helps them and motivates them to continue.

3. *Practice* involves deciding how much practice is needed, how often rest periods are needed, and what kind of practice is needed. The teacher's role in practice is again prompting and providing feedback, including correction of errors. Determination of the amount of practice and rest is dependent on the complexity of the chain and the aptitude of the students. It is different for each student. Types of practice vary. Mental practice has been shown to be helpful, while practice in a simulated situation is more helpful. The best practice is obtained from actual performance, and this method is recommended whenever feasible.

One of the great issues in nursing education is in the area of determination of the amount of practice the students need in learning nursing procedures. What amount of practice is necessary to master and overlearn a task has been a hot issue in nursing for several decades. One school of thought views the need for practice in, for example, "learning how to give a bed bath to a patient" as "if you know how to give a bath to yourself, then that's all the practice you need to give a bed bath to the patient." The other extreme stresses practice to the point of overlearning, where the gain from additional practice is not worth the time invested in practicing.

4. *Sequencing* must be provided for; it can be forward or reverse chaining. Forward chaining is preferrable in some situations, as in the "bed bath" example; however, whichever is chosen, it must reflect a logical pattern, based on component S–R units.

The next step in teaching a chain includes the actual implementation of the teaching. In so doing the teacher must do the following: (1) provide the four conditions of learning as explained before and (2) assist the students in the three phases of learning—cognitive, fixation, autonomous. During the cognitive phase when the student is intellectualizing the chain, a clear explanation and demonstration is needed. Audiovisual aids can help. The teacher must make sure that each S–R unit is discrete. During the fixation stage, the students require more demonstration, prompting, feedback, and practice. When they no longer make errors, the students are ready for the autonomous stage, during which they practice in order to increase speed.

Examples of important S–R chains in a procedure	Pass	Not pass
1. Followed principles of asepsis		
2. Broke ampule using an alcohol sponge		
3. Unsheathed needle without contamination		
4. Placed needle properly in ampule		
5. Withdrew correct amount of solution		
6. Checked correct amount of solution		
7. Resheathed needle		
8. Finished in 5 minutes		

Fig. 4-3. Observation checklist.

The final step in teaching a chain is *evaluation*. At this time, the teacher must test to determine the student's grasp of the chain. The teacher can use a procedure checklist based on a chain. For example, the observation checklist may look like the one presented in Fig. 4-3. It can be checked on a "pass" – "not pass" basis.

In summary, in teaching a specific skill one can start by analyzing the skill, then decide how to assess the entering behavior, how to implement and provide the four basic conditions for learning, and how to evaluate the student's performance.

Researchable questions

There are many research questions that need to be answered concerning chaining. A couple are listed below.

1. Of the two types of cueing or prompting procedures (verbal versus pictorial), which one is more effective in teaching chain learning to student nurses?
   a. Independent variable: verbal versus pictorial cueing or prompting procedures

   b. Dependent variable: effectiveness of teaching chain learning
2. What is the effect of teacher-administrated versus student- (self-) administered verbal cueing on the ease of chain learning?
   a. Independent variable: teacher- versus student- (self-) administered verbal cueing.
   b. Dependent variable: ease of chain learning

Conclusion

Chain learning is something that all of us experience from the time we are little children throughout our lives. In nursing, especially, where emphasis is placed on learning technical skills, chain learning and teaching are of paramount importance. Daily, nurses are expected to teach patients, families, and staff and community members various skills. The teaching of skills is universal to all types of nurses. It seems, therefore, that the teaching of chains based on a sound theoretical background is important for all nurses to know. For what is nursing but action based on knowledge and reason.

ADDITIONAL LEARNING EXPERIENCES—RECOMMENDED READING LIST

Gagne, R. *The conditions of learning.* (1st Ed.) New York: Holt, Rinehart and Winston, Inc., 1965.

Gagne, R., *The conditions of learning.* (2nd Ed.) New York: Holt, Rinehart and Winston, Inc., 1970, pp. 42-45, 123-134.

DeCecco, J. *The psychology of learning and instruction: educational psychology.* Englewood Cliffs, N.J.: Prentice-Hall, Inc., 1968, pp. 273-321.

INSTRUCTIONS TO THE LEARNER REGARDING POSTTEST

You are now ready to take the posttest to determine the degree of achievement of the module objectives. Go back to the pretest and take the same test as a posttest. Correct your own answers utilizing the answer key given on this page. You need to score at least 95% correct (19 correct points) to proceed to the next module. If you score less than 19 points, correct your errors and study the text and the recommended reading list. Study until you achieve the 95% correct level.

ANSWER KEY TO PRETEST AND POSTTEST

1. True (Gagne, 1965, p. 129)
2. False (Gagne, 1965, p. 129, DeCecco, 1968, p. 48)
3. True (DeCecco, 1968, pp. 285; Gagne, 1970, p. 130)
4. b (Gagne, 1970, p. 131)
5. c (Gagne, 1970, p. 123)
6. b (DeCecco, 1968, p. 277)
7. d (DeCecco, 1968, pp. 277-278)
8. a (DeCecco, 1968, p. 290)
9. c (DeCecco, 1968, pp. 282-283)
10. b (DeCecco, 1968, p. 282)
11. d. (DeCecco, 1968, pp. 282-283)
12. d (DeCecco, 1968, pp. 286-290, 314-317)
13. a and b (DeCecco, 1968, pp. 290-295)
14. d (Gagne, 1970, p. 131)
15. c (Gagne, 170, p. 132)
16. b (Gagne, 1970, p. 132)
17. c (DeCecco, 1968, pp. 314-319)

18. c (Gagne, 1965, p. 89)
19. a, c, and e (Gagne, 1965, pp. 93-94)
20. "Chaining" is defined as the connection of a set of motor Ss → R units in a sequence. These sequences are made up of motor responses. If learning has occurred, the sequence not only will be repeated, but will be repeated without error. (Gagne, 1965, pp. 123-124)

REFERENCES

Book, W. F. *The psychology of skill.* Missoula, Mont.: University of Montana Publications in Psychology, 1908.

Bryan, W. L. and Harter, N. Studies in physiology and psychology of the telegraphic language. *Psychological Review*, 1897, **4**:27-53.

Bryan, W. L. and Harter, N. Studies on the telegraphic language: the acquisition of a hierarchy of habits. *Psychological Review*, 1899, **6**:345-375.

Cox, J. and Boren, L. M. "A study of backward chaining. *Journal of Educational Psychology.* 1956, **56**:270-274.

DeCecco, J. *The psychology of learning and instruction: educational psychology.* (1st Ed.) Englewood Cliffs. N. J.: Prentice-Hall, Inc., 1968.

DeCecco, J., and Crawford, W. *The psychology of learning and instruction: educational psychology.* (2nd Ed.) Englewood Cliffs, N. J.: Prentice-Hall, Inc., 1974.

Duncan, C. P. The effect of unequal amounts of practice on motor learning before and after practice. *Journal of Experimental Psychology*, 1951, **42**:257-264.

Ebel, R. *Measuring educational achievement.* Englewood Cliffs, N.J. Prentice-Hall, Inc., 1965.

Elwell, J. L., and Grindley, G. C. The effect of knowledge of results on learning and performance. I.: A coordinated movement of the two hands. *British Journal of Psychology*, 1938, **29**:39-53.

Fitts, P. Factors in complex skill training. In R. Glaser (Ed.), *Training research and education.* Pittsburgh: University of Pittsburgh Press, 1962, pp. 177-197.

Gagne, R. *Conditions of learning.* (1st Ed.) New York: Holt, Rinehart and Winston, Inc., 1965.

Gagne, R. *Conditions of learning.* (2nd Ed.) New York: Holt, Rinehart and Winston, Inc., 1970.

Gilbert, T. Mathetics: the technology of education. *Journal of Mathetics*, 1962, **7**:73.

Greenspoon, J., and Foreman, S. Effect of delay of knowledge of results on learning a motor test. *Journal of Experimental Psychology*, 1956, **36**:187-211.

Kientzle, M. J. Properties of learning curves under varied distribution of practice. *Journal of Experimental Psychology*, 1946, **36**:187-211.

Lorge, I. *Influence of regularly interpolated time intervals upon subsequent learning.* Teachers College Contributions to Education, No. 438, New York: Teachers College Press, 1930.

Lorge, I., and Thorndike, E. The influence of delay in the after-effect of a connection. *Journal of Experimental Psychology,* 1935, **18**:186-194.

McGuigan, F., and MacCaslin, E. Whole and part methods in learning a perceptual motor skill. *American Journal of Psychology,* 1955, **68**:658-61.

Miller, G., Galanter, E., and Pribram, K. *Plans and the structure of behavior.* New York: Holt, Rinehart and Winston, Inc., 1960.

Naylor, J. Parameters affecting the efficiency of part and whole training methods: a review of the literature. In *NAUTRADEVGEN Technical Report,* U.S. Training Devices Center, Port Washington, N. Y., 1962.

Robb, M. Feedback *Quest,* Monograph VI, 1966, pp. 38-43.

Solley, W. The effects of verbal instructions of speed and accuracy upon the learning of a motor skill. *Research Quarterly,* 1952, **23**:231-240.

Verbal learning—verbal associates

DESCRIPTION OF THE MODULE

This is a self-contained module on the process and implications of verbal learning. It is necessary for the student to have mastery of the concepts of classical and operant conditioning and be aware of the basic concepts of the chaining process prior to studying this module.

The content presented in this module is an integrated form. The essential areas that are presented and discussed are: theoretical framework of verbal learning, research studies, application to nursing education and practice, issues, and researchable questions.

MODULE OBJECTIVES

The student, on successful completion of the learning tasks contained in this module and studying the recommended reading list on verbal learning, will be able to:
1. Demonstrate an understanding of the theoretical framework of verbal learning by:
   a. Listing the necessary entering behaviors for successful verbal learning
   b. Properly classifying the internal and external conditions for verbal learning
   c. Defining by example the types of verbal learning
   d. Defining the types of and appropriately using verbal mediators
   e. Stating the principles of interference

and extinction and correctly applying these to the internal and external learning conditions
   f. Identifying five methods of measurement of verbal learning
2. Demonstrate in oral or written form knowledge of how to incorporate the principles of verbal learning in teaching educational programs (units, procedures, and the like) to nursing students
3. Discuss how the process of verbal learning can be used in the promotion of professional status (individually and/or collectively)
4. Indicate ways in which verbal learning can be a contributing factor to the discovery and collection of nursing research
5. Discuss how the principles of verbal learning can be utilized effectively in assisting the nursing profession to solve, identify, such as or assess any of the poignant issues in which it is currently involved, such as legislation, career ladder, and curriculum

PRETEST AND POSTTEST

Circle the correct answers. Each question is worth 1 point. The 95% level of mastery equals 21 correct points. On completion of this test correct your answers utilizing the answer key that is found at the end of this module (p. 83).

Multiple choice

1. The activity of naming an object involves:
   - 1—the response enabling the child to identify properly the object seen
   - 2—an emotional response
   - 3—an internal stimulus enabling the child to say the proper name
   - 4—learning different response for stimuli that might be confused
   - a. 1, 3
   - b. 3, 4
   - c. 1, 2, 3, 4
   - d. 2, 3

2. In verbal association, the length of the chain to be learned as a single entity is:
   - a. unlimited
   - b. determined by the kinds of words involved
   - c. limited to a range of five to nine words
   - d. determined by previous experience

3. The length of the chain that may be learned is:
   - a. unlimited
   - b. determined by the content of the chain
   - c. limited to five to nine chains
   - d. determined by previous experience

4. Interference that affects knowledge to be learned in the future is called:
   - a. retroactive
   - b. proactive
   - c. subsequent
   - d. mediation

5. The two internal conditions (entering behaviors) necessary for verbal learning are:
   - a. meaningfulness
   - b. practice
   - c. verbal mediation
   - d. instruction

6. Meaningfulness in verbal learning is determined by:
   - a. the number of different associations elicited by a verbal unit
   - b. word frequency and familiarity
   - c. frequency with which words have been experienced
   - d. habit family hierarchy
   - e. originality of the concept

7. Which of the following are *not* types of mediators? (Choose the correct answer.)
   - 1—visual pictures
   - 2—spoken words
   - 3—written words
   - 4—conceptual images
   - a. all of the above
   - b. none of the above
   - c. 3 and 4
   - d. 2 and 4

Labeling

8. Label the following process   A   B   C   D

   when learning of A (what is learned earlier) interferes with the rentention of B, C, and D (what is learned later).

9. Label the following process   A   B   C   D

   when learning of D interferes with the retention of previously learned A, B, and C.

Matching

Match the internal and external conditions of verbal learning:

Part A
_____ 10. Massed/distributed practice
_____ 11. Overlearning
_____ 12. Mediating
_____ 13. Prior discrimination
_____ 14. Part-whole practice

Part B
a. External
b. Internal

Match the definition with the appropriate term:

Part A
_____ 15. Recognition
_____ 16. Anticipation
_____ 17. Savings
_____ 18. Reproduction
_____ 19. Reconstruction

Part B
a. Correlating dates and events
b. Taking multiple choice examinations
c. Arranging scrambled items
d. Recollecting step B, given step A
e. Learning a set of materials to mastery, then relearning it at a future time

Discussion questions

20. Discuss how the principles of interference can be used to enhance the acceptance of the new roles of nurses, such as nurse practitioner, by professional colleagues and the general public.
21. List principles to be included in creating a lesson plan teaching nursing students the principles of safe medication administration.
22. Discuss how the process of verbal chaining, paired associates, and the previously learned cognitive structure could lead to the discovery of problems for nursing research.
23. Outline a sequence of instruction, using the principles of verbal learning that could be used to assist a career-ladder nurse in grasping a new role concept.

TEXT
Theoretical framework

As a child you began to learn about yourself and the world around you by seeing and touching. Pretty soon people began putting names (or sounds as you probably perceived them then) to the things you were observing and touching. At the point when you began to label these things, the process of verbal learning had begun for you.

Almost simultaneously you began another learning process, that of chaining. You simply connected or linked two entities, that is, the sound (the name) with the object. The more frequently you repeated this sequence correctly and were praised for it (by parents) the easier it became. Soon, even without the praise, you could identify the object at any time.

What you actually were doing was developing a system of response integration and associative "hook-ups." You repeated the word frequently until you could pronounce it fairly accurately and with ease. That is the response integration. Henceforth, whenever you saw a ball or a chair you could quickly associate the response (name) with the object. This is the associative hookup. This process is also called paired-associate learning and is frequently used with learning a foreign language.

Therefore, verbal learning is the process of forming verbal associations; it is attaching a name (label) to an object. According to Gagne (1965), verbal learning is like skill learning in that it involves a chain of at least two links: (1) the presentation of object (stimulus, S; for example, catheter) and the observing of the object (response, R); (2) the observing response results in certain internal stimuli (Si) that give rise to the verbal response, as in the following diagram:

$$Ss \longrightarrow R \sim s \longrightarrow R$$

(Presentation of object "catheter")   Observing   Observing R Si   Verbal response "catheter"

Research in verbal learning is mostly done in terms of nonsense syllables, paired associates, and serial learning (Gagne, 1970, pp. 134-137; DeCecco, 1968, pp. 326-328; Ellis, 1969, pp. 78-80).

Development of verbal behavior

Jensen (1966a, b) has proposed a theory for the development of verbal behavior in children. These verbal behaviors can be used as a means of assessing any cognitive disturbances in children and as evaluation of cognitive development.

Age 1 year: S_v–R learning. At 1 year of age children respond to words about four times faster than they respond to other sounds in their environment. The symbol S_v refers to a verbal stimulus, which can be a syllable, a word, a phrase, or others. The R refers to the physical movement the child makes in response to the verbal stimulus. The movement may be touching, grasping, or other motions; for example, S_v may be the child crawling or walking toward the doll and "holding the doll" or "bringing the doll" (DeCecco, 1968, p. 329).

Ages 2 to 3 years: S–R$_v$ learnings. The child begins to utter the word (R$_4$) "ball" or "doll" on seeing (S) the ball or the doll. The child learns to discriminate between various objects. It almost appears as if the child is attempting to catalogue the environment. The child discriminates sounds and associates these sounds with certain objects. Such verbal labeling behavior may be lacking in the development of disadvantaged children.

Ages 3 to 4 years:

R$_v$–R and V–R learning. The child's movement comes under the control of the child's own verbal behavior. R$_v$–R learning consists of making an overt response (R) to one's own spoken response (R$_v$); for example, saying "bite" (R$_v$) and indeed biting (R). V–R learning consists of making an overt response (R) to one's own thoughts (V); for example, thinking "bite" (V) and then proceeding to bite (R). Thus, with the ability to say and think various words the child has the capacity to self-direct behavior. These movements however are not entirely divorced from the environment.

S–V–R learning. To show the relationship among environment, verbal response, and movement, Jensen (1966a) described the V–R level as S–V–R learning where:

S = environmental stimuli (such as, child sees a ball)
V = verbal response (that the child says to self, such as, "will run")
R = physical movement that finally results (for example, runs)

S–V–R–V$_c$ learning. The addition of V$_c$ does not indicate another learning type, but simply another aspect of S–V–R (or V–R). The V$_c$ refers to verbal confirming response or feedback, as where the child:

S = sees a ball that is soft
V = thinks about biting the ball
V$_c$ = says, "yum, yum"

S–V–V–R learning. Words may become linked to other words in ways that facilitate the association of the stimulus and response. The notation S–V–V–R indicates such connections between verbal responses as well as connections between environmental stimuli and verbal responses; for example, (De-Cecco, 1968, pp. 329-331), where a child:

S = sees a ball
V = decides to touch the ball (first V)
V = which in turn suggests biting the ball (second V)
R = bites the ball

Conditions of verbal learning — internal and external
INTERNAL CONDITIONS—ENTERING BEHAVIOR

Before continuing, the basic principles of entering behavior should be delineated. They are relatively simple but could easily be taken for granted. If they are overlooked and in fact are not present, the teaching or evaluating of verbal learning would be useless.

It was stated that as a child you saw or felt objects. This implies the *possession of some sensory powers.* The next step was to connect the object and sound, which was defined as the *ability to chain.* As you repeatedly identified the object correctly as a chair and not a ball, you were in fact making a *discriminatory remark.* These three elements plus another, *mediation,* are the necessary entering behaviors for verbal learning (Gagne, 1970, pp. 136-137; DeCecco, 1968, pp. 328-332).

Mediation. In nursing education students are exposed to a myriad of new information as they learn anatomy and physiology, pathophysiology, nursing procedures, and other information. One thing that is learned is that most of the information is somewhat related. Often, the problem is in learning always to connect information A with nursing procedure B. It is most likely that this goal is accomplished through the process of mediation. Mediation has been defined as "talking to yourself in relevant terms when faced with a problem to be solved or something to be learned." Of course, this talking is usually silent and many times is subconscious. The types of mediators people use are as varied as the people. There are single-step (or link) and multiple-step mediators.

Single-step mediators include items such as rhyming words, similar sounds, and similar meanings and letters of words. Disadvantaged children have difficulty in utilizing verbal mediation because of a lack of reference (verbal or pictorial reservoir) (DeCecco, 1968, pp. 339-340, 341-344).

Another frequent form of a mediator is a *pictorial image*, or even a *conceptual image*. Having once actually seen a gangrenous limb, or a photograph of one, or heard a vivid description of it, the connection between that and the importance of good circulation will never be forgotten. This image is a mediating link and is now a part of the memory system.

It has been established that verbal learning is primarily a process of chaining with the appropriate use of mediators of some sort. The question logically arises, "How long of a verbal chain can be learned at one time with or without mediators?" Research (Deese, 1958) has generally proved that chains of seven links plus or minus two are the maximum that can be retained in the immediate memory span (DeCecco, 1968, p. 356; Gagne, 1970, pp. 136-140).

Meaningfulness. Meaningfulness is an aspect of both the materials the student attempts to learn and previous experience with those materials.

Meaningfulness is the variety of associations the student makes with a verbal unit. It refers to the frequency of use or familiarity with the words (DeCecco, 1968, p. 339).

The *spew hypothesis* proposes that "the frequency with which words have been experienced determines their availability as re-

sponses in new associative connections. Meaningfulness influences both learning and retention. The higher the meaningfulness, the more rapid the learning and the longer the materials are retained" (DeCecco, 1968, p. 339).

Therefore, based on the previous definition of meaningfulness and the spew hypothesis, the abstract concept of "meaning" can be evaluated in concrete terms. Thus, if a response or association is frequently used, it becomes more familiar through the process of response integration. This response, once familiar, is then readily available as a response to new associations. Hence, the increase of knowledge through meaningfulness occurs.

For instance, once the concept of the blood pressure has been learned, the concepts of shock, blood volume, and circulation could be easily associated to blood pressure—a previously learned, meaningful response.

In the previous paragraph, the word "concept" was used instead of listing specific information. This is an important inclusion. Research has proved that meaningful ideas or concepts are retained much better than mechanical or verbatim chains or associations (Gagne, 1970, pp. 147-150; DeCecco, 1968, pp. 333-339).

In this module, most of the concepts presented have been related to some aspect of nursing. It is hoped that this is of more value and significance than relating the examples of biophysics or politics. If it in fact has helped in the understanding of concepts, then this device has demonstrated the important principle of verbal learning—that of meaningfulness. The greater the meaningfulness of the material to be learned, the more rapid is the learning. And, contrary to popular belief, the more rapid the learning, the slower is the forgetting. Conversely, slow learning results in rapid forgetting. Meaningfulness has the greatest influence on the rapidity of learning.

Thus, when a nurse is teaching a student or a patient about a procedure, disease, diagnostic test, or other area, it is necessary to use information and concepts that are pertinent and meaningful to that person at that particular time.

• • •

To summarize the internal conditions (conditions within the learner) for verbal learning, it would now be useful to delineate the conditions that must be present for any type of verbal learning to occur. As discussed previously, the learner must have some sensory perception and must possess the ability to disciminate and chain. The learner must also have completed the response integration of mediators and must have previous experience with meaningful material (Gagne, 1970, p. 141; DeCecco, 1968, p. 338).

EXTERNAL CONDITIONS

There are five external conditions that are present within the learning situation that affect verbal learning and can be manipulated by the teacher: (1) instruction to learn, (2) practice conditions, (3) reinforcement, (4) interference factors, and (5) method of measurement.

Instruction to learn (set to learn). The supplying of instruction varies from the situation where the teacher provides no information (guideline) before learning begins to the situation where specific instructions are given—incidental learning versus intentional learning.

In an *incidental learning* situation the teacher does not provide instructions to prepare students for a test on the materials they are to learn, or the teacher directs students to learn one task and then tests them on another task.

Intentional learning provides for the prior announcement of the test and the learning task and objectives. For instance, at one time during nursing education students are probably instructed to learn the specific psychosocial theories of behavior. They are also probably given a list of objectives on which they are to be tested. The learning that occurs as a result of this teaching strategy is called intentional learning. It is also very possible that while students are studying these theories, they also learn something about their own behavior. The latter is an example of incidental learning.

The difference between intentional and incidental learning is only quantitative. Because individuals can and do supply their own direction and motivation when these are not provided externally, in the strict sense there may not be such a phenomenon as incidental learning (DeCecco, 1968, p. 346).

In an experiment on incidental versus intentional learning with six groups of undergraduate students who were given different instructions to learn, Postman and Senders (1946) found that: (1) intentional learners obtained higher test scores than incidental learners; also, the direction varied highly in effectiveness; (2) the students who were told that they would be tested for details of content also did better on test items on general comprehension; and (3) students who were given directions to learn specific materials did better than students in the incidental-learning situations who received no directions to learn (DeCecco, 1968, p. 345).

Practice conditions. Practice is the second external condition for verbal learning. Since practice is the condition that describes the amount of work output, there is strong empirical support for the common-sense observation that the longer a person practices at learning the more that will be learned (Underwood, 1964; DeCecco, 1968, p. 349). How to get students to increase the vim and vigor of their efforts is the problem of motivation, but the beneficial effects of that effort, once it is invested, are beyond questioning.

It is not practice itself, but the conditions of practice that pose problems for the experimenter and the teacher. There are three types of practice conditions: massed versus distributed, overlearning, and part versus whole.

Massed versus distributed practice. Massed practice refers to the practice condition in which the learner does not take a rest period. Cramming for state borad examinations is an example of massed practice. Distributed practice refers to the practice condition in which the learner takes a rest after a period of study. For example, studying anatomy for 2 hours each evening is distributed practice.

Evidence indicates that intervals for distributed practice must be shorter when the material is difficult and the probability of erroneous responses is high (Underwood, 1961, 1964). Theoretically, distributed practice is beneficial because the intervals allow time for unwanted or erroneous responses to drop out or to become extinguished (Underwood, 1961; DeCecco, 1968, pp. 347-349).

If the likelihood of the forgetting response is very high, massed practice should replace distributed practice. Massed practice is better for retention (Underwood, 1964). This principle can apply both to skill learning and verbal learning.

Overlearning. For students to acquire or secure mastery of materials and verbal skills, overlearning can be employed; that is, learning beyond original mastery. However, overlearning can reach a point of diminishing returns (Kreuger, 1929). At this point, additional practice increases retention so slightly that the effort surpasses the gain. Research has proved that practice over 50% of initial mastery is virtually useless (DeCecco, 1968, pp. 347-348).

Part versus whole practice. The choice of the part or the whole method of practice must depend on the internal organization of the learning material. Some materials divide into parts and recombine into wholes much more easily than others. The part method can be used effectively with such materials (De-Cecco, 1968, p. 349).

In their study Deese and Hulse (1967) gave the subjects two types of lists and tested the speed with which the lists were learned under part versus whole practice conditions. The lists consisted of the following words:

List A   north, man, red, spring, woman, east, autumn, yellow, summer, boy, blue, west, winter, girl, green, south

List B   north, east, south, west
spring, summer, autumn, winter
red, yellow, green, blue
man, woman, boy, girl

The result was that list B was learned faster in part form; however, if list A was split, students learned less well. Therefore, part versus whole learning depends on internal organization of the content to be learned.

Reinforcement. Another external condition of verbal learning is the reinforcement of correct responses. Such reinforcement is often called *confirmation.* The student's correct responses are confirmed. It is a form of feedback or knowledge of results. This confirmation of results or correct responses can be done either by the teacher or by the learner after checking the answers with the criteria.

According to Underwood (1959), most of the verbal learning observed in the laboratory is not dependent on immediate reward. Only the informational feedback on the correctness of responses remains (DeCecco, 1968, p. 350).

Interference factors. Interference is the competition of old and new responses, which results in forgetting.

In *retroactive inhibition,* what is learned later in time interferes with the retention of what was learned earlier; for example:

The learning of D inhibits and interferes with what was learned earlier, A or B or C.

In *proactive inhibition,* what was learned earlier in time interferes with the retention of what is learned later; for example:

A B C D

A represents past learned material that interferes and inhibits the learning of B, C, and D, things learned later in time.

From the standpoint of entering behavior, proactive inhibition is the major cause of forgetting. This conclusion is at odds with the traditional belief that what was learned subsequently (retroactive inhibition) rather than what was learned previously (proactive inhibition) is the chief source of forgetting (Underwood, 1964).

Present evidence also suggests that *extinction* is the process underlying interference.

Serial-position effect describes the tendency to remember the material in the beginning and the end and to forget the material in the middle of a list. This is because the middle links are subjected to both proactive and retroactive inhibitions (DeCecco, 1968, pp. 350-354; Gagne, 1970, pp. 143-145). For example, in a long chain of a procedure that is composed of ten links, as is illustrated in Figure 5-1, the center links of D, E, and F are adversely affected by both proactive and retroactive inhibition. Therefore, the chance of these links being learned and remembered is slim unless additional practice is provided to strengthen these links and other cueing techniques (mediational procedures and linking codes) are provided to ensure their being learned.

For example, let us assume that at the beginning of the semester students studied and learned the signs, symptoms, and pathological process of diabetes mellitus; 5 weeks later in their medical-surgical nursing class they had to study and learn the signs, symptoms, and pathological process of diabetes insipidus. If they start having difficulty remembering and retaining what they are studying now (diabetes insipidus) and seem to be mixing up the signs and symptoms of the two types of diabetes, the type of interference or inhibition that is taking place in proactive inhibition. If, on the other hand, the studying of diabetes insipidus made them forget some of the signs and symptoms of diabetes mellitus that they had learned earlier, the type of inhibition that is taking place is retroactive.

The methods that should be used to reduce these interferences are verbal or pictorial mediation to enable the learners to discrimi-

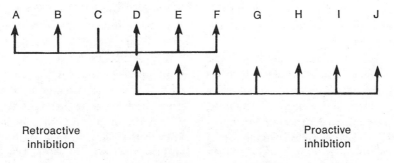

Fig. 5-1. Serial position effect.

nate between the two diabetes and the more opportunities for practice.

Method of measurement. The way in which retention of verbal learning is measured affects what is retained. As with all types of learning, there must be some satisfactory or behaviorally measurable methods of evaluating the extent of verbal learning. There are five such methods of measurements:

1. *Reproduction*, or the recall method, requires that the student reproduce the material that has been learned; for example essay exams, descriptions, and definition exams employ this method.

2. *Recognition* requires the student to select from a series of items those which are the responses that have been learned. For example, multiple choice questions in which the student selects the correct choice from several others are primarily an exercise in discrimination. Recognition method of measurement produces the highest score.

3. *Reconstruction* requires the student to unscramble a set of scrambled items (De-Cecco, 1968, p. 358). For example, from a set of givens, the learner is asked to rearrange the items in the proper order, either chronologically or sequentially.

4. *Anticipation* requires the student to recall the next step or item in a series or in a previously learned sequence given only cues or clues. An example would be for the instructor to start a nursing procedure such as the wearing of sterile gloves by opening the sterile package and then asking the student, "What is the next step?"

5. *Savings* is the measurement of the amount of time necessary to relearn a previously mastered set of materials. In other words, the savings, or relearning, method requires the student to learn a set of materials to mastery (errorless performance) and then to relearn the materials. Using a fairly simple calculation, the teacher determines how much less time was required for relearning than for original learning. It was surprising to find that relearning takes less time when the subject does not recognize the materials as familiar.

After 1 or 2 days of learning, the amount of retention is greatest for the recognition method and diminishes as one moves through the reconstruction, reproduction, relearning, and anticipation methods. The most demanding or sensitive measures of retention are the relearning (or savings) and the anticipation methods (DeCecco, 1968, pp. 358-359).

Other phenomena associated with verbal learning
EXTINCTION

The phenomenon of extinction is closely related to interference. Gagne (1970) states that the important event underlying interference is extinction of previously learned connections; that is, forgetting, as it occurs in verbal chains is a matter of interference, and this is often thought of as extinction. For example, when an error is made in attempting to reinstate a link in a verbal chain, the student to some degree extinguishes the correct response. When a correct link suffers extinction, new learning must take place again if the verbal chain is to be reestablished.

GENERALIZATION AND DISCRIMINATION

Stimulus generalization that was explained in operant conditioning can also occur within any of the links in a verbal chain. For example, if one patient's physician orders, "atropine 1 gt OS b.i.d.," and if another patient's physician orders, "atropine 2 gtt O.D. t.i.d.," there will be a generalizing tendency from the first set of orders to the second one. The two sets of units are physically similar, both in their appearance and in their sounds, and the response appropriate to the first unit will tend to be connected by generalization to the stimulus of the second chain. As a consequence, the requirements for discrimination of each link will be severe. The second chain (or the second physician's order), accordingly, is harder to learn or carry out than the first because it tends to give rise to "generalization errors." These in turn have the typical consequences for interference that have already been discussed. Generalization in such instances has the effect of making the learning of verbal sequences more difficult by increasing the difficulty of discrimination of the individual links (Gagne, 1970, p. 147).

Sometimes, however, generalization facilitates the learning of a second task rather than making it more difficult; for example, the generalizing tendencies of *mediating* links.

Application to nursing education and practice

DeCecco (1968) presents instructional implications as a series of teaching steps that conform to the basic teaching model. There are seven steps that facilitate verbal learning in students. These are as follows:

1. *Describe for the student what is to be learned.* In other words, state the objectives of what the students should accomplish by the end of instruction. This principle is derived from the research study of Postman and Senders (1946) on incidental versus intentional learning that showed that intentional learners obtained higher test scores than did incidental learners.

2. *Examine the instructional test and materials for meaningfulness.* Meaningfulness was defined as word frequency and word familiarity. In teaching groups of students or patients, the teacher must find out what the students' entering behaviors are with regard to important words and concepts and make a list of words or concepts that will occur in the materials the teacher will use and for which there will not be explicit instruction. These

are words or concepts the teacher assumes will be in a student's entering behavior. If a student's entering behavior lacks this specific vocabulary, then it is both the teacher's as well as the learner's responsibility to learn them and to raise the level of entering behavior (DeCecco, 1968, pp. 362-363).

3. *Assess entering behavior for the availability of meaningful responses and verbal mediators.* In assessing the availability of meaningful responses, the teacher is attempting to make relatively meaningless materials meaningful and unfamiliar materials familiar. This the teacher does by:

a. Assessing the student's entering behavior to discover not only which responses are available but also their relative availability and to present the new material in terms of meaningful responses now available to the student

b. Using instruction to bridge the old and the new meanings

The methods of assessing the entering behavior for availability of verbal mediators are as follows:

a. Determining which verbal and pictorial mediators may be useful for the instructional task

b. Assessing entering behavior to determine which of these may be available

c. Supplying mediators that may be useful in the learning of the task

4. *Provide the appropriate practice conditions.* As was explained before under "external" conditions of verbal learning, the teacher must:

a. Provide opportunities for the student to make the necessary responses

b. Schedule practice on a massed or a distributed basis

c. Determine the degree of mastery the student must attain

d. Provide either part or whole practice.

5. *Provide knowledge of correct responses through reinforcement.* The teacher must

provide prompting or confirmation of correct responses. The student must have some way of discovering the correct answers and have the opportunity to compare answers. In prompting, the teacher provides the correct answer before the student responds. In confirming, the teacher provides the correct answer after the student responds.

6. *Provide conditions that reduce interference.* Factors that influence and cause interference and forgetting should be reduced. This is done by:

a. Doing a task analysis to reduce the major task into a series of component tasks that are properly sequenced from the simple to the complex

b. After the task analysis, presenting the subtasks to the student in such a way as to avoid both proactive and retroactive interference

c. Finding those points in the material that are frequently sources of interference or confusion to students

d. Introducing dissimilarity into potentially confusing materials through the use of various devices such as color, symbols, and drawings

e. Knowing what the student has previously learned (entering behavior) and planning instruction accordingly to reduce proactive inhibition, since it is the major cause of forgetting (DeCecco, 1968, pp. 367-368).

7. *Use suitable methods of measurement.* It is important to decide which method of measurement to use. The basis for this decision should be the standard of acceptability specified in the statement of objectives. If the objective states that the student will recognize the correct response, or reconstruct a list by unscrambling, or be able to recall, then the teacher should use only those methods of measurement (DeCecco, 1968, p. 368).

Researchable questions

Two areas of research that need investigating are:

1. What is the effect of the use of mediators (teacher-initiated versus student-initiated) on the retention of learned material?

a. Independent variable: use of mediators (teacher-initiated versus student-initated)

b. Dependent variable: retention of learned material

2. What is the effect of verbal versus pictorial mediators on retention of materials learned?

a. Independent variable: verbal versus pictorial mediators

b. Dependent variable: retention of materials learned

ADDITIONAL LEARNING EXPERIENCES—RECOMMENDED READING LIST

DeCecco, J. *The psychology of learning and instruction: educational psychology.* (1st Ed.) Englewood Cliffs, N.J.: Prentice-Hall, Inc., 1968, pp. 322-384.

Gagne, R. *The conditions of learning.* (2nd Ed.) New York: Holt, Rinehart and Winston, Inc., 1970, pp. 134-154.

INSTRUCTIONS TO THE LEARNER REGARDING POSTTEST

At this stage you are ready to take the posttest to determine the extent to which you have achieved the objectives of this module. Return to the pretest of this module and take it as a posttest. Correct your own answers using the answer key found at the end of this module (p. 83). You need to score 21 correct points to achieve a 95% level of mastery. If you score less than 14 correct points, correct your errors, study the text again, and read some of the materials from the recommended reading list. Then take the posttest again. You need to study until you achieve at least a 95% level of mastery.

ANSWER KEY TO PRETEST AND POSTTEST

1. a (DeCecco, 1968, p. 48)
2. c (DeCecco, 1968, p. 354; Gagne, 1970, p. 142)
3. a (DeCecco, 1968, p. 354; Gagne, 1970, p. 142)
4. b (Gagne, 1970, p. 143)
5. a and c (DeCecco, 1968, p. 333)
6. a, b, and c (DeCecco, 1968, p. 338)
7. b (DeCecco, 1968, p. 337; Gagne, 1970, pp. 147-148)
8. proactive inhibition (DeCecco, 1968, p. 356)
9. retroactive inhibition (DeCecco, 1968, p. 356)
10. a (Gagne, 1970, p. 141; DeCecco, 1968, pp. 346-349)
11. a (Gagne, 1970, p. 141; DeCecco, 1968, pp. 346-349)
12. b (Gagne, 1970, p. 141; DeCecco, 1968, pp. 346-349)
13. b (Gagne, 1970, p. 141; DeCecco, 1968, pp. 346-349)
14. a (Gagne, 1970, p. 141; DeCecco, 1968, pp. 346-349)
15. b (DeCecco, 1968, pp. 356-358)
16. d (DeCecco, 1968, pp. 356-358)
17. e (DeCecco, 1968, pp. 356-358)
18. a (DeCecco, 1968, pp. 356-358)
19. c (DeCecco, 1968, pp. 356-358)
20. Answer must include: (a) definition of retroactive interference, (b) definition of extinction, (c) definition of nurse practitioner, (d) conceptual image as a possible mediator
21. Answer must include information that shows the student's understanding of the (a) effectiveness of using short chains; (b) use of mediators; (c) problem of interference and importance of learning correctly the first time; (d) necessity of sequencing, feedback, and reinforcement; (e) concept of meaningfulness in material learned and cues used
22. Answer must include: (a) definition of verbal chaining, (b) definition of paired associates,

(c) definition of origin of cognitive structure, (d) proper sequencing of these components.
23. Answer must include: (a) principles of extinction, (b) use of a role model (real or conceptual) as a mediator, (c) use of meaningful concepts instead of items.

REFERENCES

DeCecco, J. *Psychology of learning and instruction: educational psychology.* (1st Ed.) Englewood Cliffs, N.J.: Prentice-Hall, Inc., 1968.

DeCecco, J., and Crawford, W. *The psychology of learning and instruction: educational psychology.* (2nd Ed.) Englewood Cliffs, N.J.: Prentice Hall, Inc., 1974.

Deese, J., *The Psychology of Learning,* (2nd Ed.), N.Y.: McGraw-Hill Book Co., 1958.

Deese, J., and Hulse, S. H. *The psychology of learning.* (3rd Ed.) New York: McGraw-Hill Book Co., 1967.

Ellis, H. *The transfer of learning.* New York: The Macmillan Co., 1969.

Gagne, R. *The conditions of learning.* New York: Holt, Rinehart and Winston, Inc., 1970.

Jensen, A. Individual differences in concept learning. In H. J. Klausmeier and W. Harris (Eds.), *Analysis of Concept Learning.* New York: Academic Press, Inc., pp. 139-154, 1966a.

Jensen, A., Verbal mediation and educational potential. *Psychology in the schools,* 1966b, 3:99-109.

Kreuger, W. C. F. The effect of over-learning on retention. *Journal of Experimental Psychology,* 1929, 12:71-78.

Postman, L., and Senders, V. L. Incidental learning and generality of set. *Journal of Experimental Psychology,* 1946, pp. 36, 153-165.

Underwood, B. J. Verbal learning in the educative process. *Harvard Education Review,* 1959, 29:107-117.

Underwood, B. J. Ten years of massed practice on distributed practice. *Psychological Review,* 1961, pp. 68, 229-247.

Underwood, B. J. Laboratory studies of verbal learning. In E. R. Hilgard (Ed.), *Theories of Learning and Instruction.* Part I of the 63rd Yearbook of the National Society for the Study of Education (NSSE). Chicago: University of Chicago Press, 1964, pp. 133-152.

MODULE 6

Discrimination learning

DESCRIPTION OF THE MODULE

This module on discrimination learning is a self-directed and self-contained independent unit of instruction. It is the fifth type of learning according to Gagne's (1970) hierarchy of conditions of learning. The major intent of this module is to provide the learner with the basic theoretical content of discrimination learning and its application to nursing practice and education. Included herein are the following: behavioral objectives, pre- and posttest, and the text on discrimination learning. The text covers five specific areas: theoretical framework, research studies in the field, application to nursing education and practice, issues, and two researchable questions. An additional recommended reading list is also provided that is essential for the student's learning experience.

As prerequisite skills (entering behavior), the student must have knowledge about the first four conditions of learning—classical conditioning, operant conditioning, chaining, and verbal associates.

MODULE OBJECTIVES

At the completion of this independent learning module on discrimination learning and after studying the recommended reading material on this subject, the student will be able to:

1. Define and explain orally or in writing what discrimination is and how it takes place—the process of discrimination learning
2. Describe the theoretical framework of discrimination learning
3. Identify the conditions within the learner that are necessary for discrimination learning to take place
4. Identify the external conditions of discrimination and multiple discrimination learning and give one example in each category
5. State or describe orally or in writing some of the relevant research studies that have been conducted in the area of discrimination learning
6. Apply the major principles of discrimination learning to a specific patient-teaching or student–teaching situation and implement all the external conditions that are necessary for discrimination learning
7. Identify one issue in teaching discrimination learning
8. Raise one researchable question beyond the ones that are mentioned in this module, and identify both the independent and dependent variables

PRETEST AND POSTTEST

Circle the correct answers. Each question is worth 1 point. You should achieve 100% level of achievement for this test, which is 10 correct points. Correct your answers using the answer key found at the end of this module (p. 93).

True or false

1. Multiple discrimination has the same potential for interference as does single discrimination. True or False
2. Once the multiple discriminations are learned, whether they have been difficult or easy, they are subsequently remembered just about equally well. True or False
3. Increasing the similarity of the set of stimulus objects involved in multiple discrimination learning decreases the difficulty of learning. True or False

Multiple choice

4. Forgetting of chains in multiple discrimination learning is:
   a. not related to interference
   b. not too likely to occur once learned
   c. lessened by repetition
   d. all of the above
5. The amount of repetition required in discrimination learning is:
   a. directly proportional to the number of chains to be discriminated
   b. inversely proportional to the number of chains to be discriminated
   c. is not affected by the number of chains to be discriminated
6. An important aspect of discrimination learning is:
   a. symbolization
   b. class stimuli
   c. distinctive features
7. Interference in discrimination learning can be overcome by:
   a. chaining
   b. generalization
   c. repetition
8. In teaching students to discriminate between insulin shock and insulin coma, the instructor should provide which combination of the following conditions
   1—repetition
   2—reduction of interference
   3—presentation of each chain or concept one by one
   4—generalization
   5—reduction of similarity
   6—confirmation of correct response
   7—availability of links
   a. all of the above
   b. all except 4 and 7
   c. 2, 3, 5, and 7
   d. 1 and 7
9. The process by which an individual learns to make different responses to two or more stimuli is called _____.
10. In multiple-discrimination learning there must be a condition that provides for confirmation, which some learning theorists call _____.

TEXT
Theoretical framework

In identifying and defining discrimination learning it should be noted that the process involves not only differentiating between two or more stimuli, but also delivering the appropriate response to the discriminated stimulus or stimulus pattern (Deese and Hulse, 1967, p. 170). The discrimination model, or paradigm, involves learning to make a response (R) in the presence of a discriminative stimulus (S^D) but not in the presence of another stimulus (S^Δ). On first-learning trials, response may occur with either S^D or S^Δ, but as training and learning progress and reinforcement is given only for S^D–R and not for S^Δ–R; the response will be elicited only in the presence of the S^D. When this occurs in a criterion number of trials, discrimination has occurred and to some extent behavior has come under the control of the environment (DeCecco, 1968, p. 261).

The discrimination model just described accounts for the instrumental conditioned discrimination in which it was necessary to differentiate between two stimuli and associate a response with the relevant stimulus (S^D). However, the same learning task also applies to stimulus patterns in which multiple discrimination learning tasks must be accomplished (Hilgard, 1956, p. 52).

Perceptual learning and discrimination learning are related to each other. Gibson (1968) described the relevance of "perceptual learning" as a matter of increasing differentiation of parts of the environment in the learning of a child during the early years. Discrimination learning leads to perceptual differentiation in five media: objects, space, events, representations, and symbols. Perception and differentiation of objects and space are developed first in a child, followed by discrimination of events, when the child learns to manipulate objects and can move about. Still later, during the early school years, the learning of discrimination of representations (pictures) and the learning of symbols are developed (Gagne, 1970, p. 157).

Discrimination learning is facilitated by the use of *distinctive features*. Distinctive features are those characteristics of an object, event, or picture that enable the person to distinguish them from one another. Thus, an individual learns to respond differentially to these characteristics.

In multiple-discrimination learning the individual acquires a number of different chains. A set of discriminations may be represented as follows:

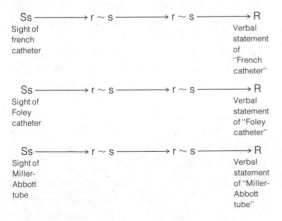

The middle s ~ r in each chain represents

the coding link. The others may be thought of as stimulus link and response link respectively. For example, let us assume that a student nurse is given a set of three catheters, one for each different purpose or use. Initially, the catheters all look alike. Soon the student can distinguish them by the number of holes there are at the end of the catheters, the color, the thickness of the lumens, and whether they are single or double lumened. In this kind of learning, the student nurse who becomes capable of making different responses (correctly labelling each of the catheters) to the different collection of catheters is said to have learned how to make discrimination or multiple discriminations.

The learning of each object (catheter) by itself can readily be understood and learned as a simple chaining process. But what happens, as far as learning is concerned, when the student nurse must acquire all the chains at once rather than only one? First, the task of discriminating the stimuli, one (catheter) from the other, increases the *difficulty of the learning*. When the "French catheter" is presented alone, the discrimination task is easy, not demanding. But when "French catheter" is presented along with the "Foley catheter," the chance of confusion as a result of a lack of discrimination is increased. The chance of confusion in the appearance of a "French catheter" and a "Foley catheter" and a "Miller-Abbott tube," chest tubes, and all the other tubes is even greater. As a set of stimulus associates for multiple discrimination, these catheters need to be well discriminated, so that they can generate very different mediating responses. A teaching technique that can be used is *to magnify the differences* among the catheters when they are initially being learned; for example, by emphasizing the distinctive feature of each catheter—such as the French catheter is a simple long tube with one or two holes at the tip, the Foley catheter on the other hand has two holes on one end and also an air pocket that can be filled either with air or water. Also at the other end of the Foley catheter there is a Y-shaped bifurcation. One of the bifurcations is used for injecting water or air; the other one is used for urine to come out. The Miller-Abbott tube has a double lumen and is a very long tube that is placed nasogastrically. Another coding link to keep in mind with regard to the Miller-Abbott tube is its "double name" as "Miller and Abbott." Thus, it can be associated with double-lumened catheter. If the student can generate these mediating links or codes, the student will remember them longer and be better able to discriminate the catheters. Otherwise, the teacher can provide such helpful mediating links to ease the task of discrimination learning by students. Another teaching technique that is designed to make stimulus differences more permanent is to have the student nurses feel or manipulate the catheters, thus providing additional tactual and kinesthetic cues to their differences.

The second major difficulty that exists in learning multiple discriminations as opposed to single discrimination is that a great potential for *interference* exists, which causes forgetting in the individual. No sooner has the student learned the proper responses (names) for French and Foley catheters than the names of other nasogastric tubes, chest tubes, and so on must be learned. When the student attempts to recall any of these, interference occurs and reduces the probability of recall.

Keeping in mind these two sources of difficulty in discrimination learning, the following steps must be taken in the teaching of associates:

1. The sight of the stimulus object (catheter) must be identified distinctively, that is, the learner must be able to match one French catheter with another one
2. The student must be able to make a dis-

tinctive response (label as "French catheter") to the sight of the French catheter
3. A coding response must be available to the learner; this varies from one learner to another, and also some associates may generate more readily available mediating links or codes than others

When all these prerequisite learnings have occurred, the student learns the individual chains first by having the teacher use the "prompting" procedure. For example, the teacher may demonstrate the catheter and label it as "French catheter," or cue the student. The student may repeat the name later. Therefore, for each single associate the learner is then able to reinstate the entire chain alone when a picture of a catheter or an actual catheter is presented.

As can be seen, it is quite difficult for the learner to retain learning in a set of multiple discriminations. One method used is to learn each associate, then *repeat* them in somewhat different order. It has not been established yet how many single associates must be learned before initiating recall and repetition.

Other approaches listed in the literature are "progressive-part" learning (McGeoch and Irion, 1952) and initial exaggeration of the differences in the stimuli with gradual reduction in these differences to those that are normal. Possibly the most efficient technique for the learning of multiple discrimination is a combination of these approaches (Gagne, 1970, pp. 161-162).

Gibson's (1942) study with multiple discrimination supports Gagne's concept of the process of multiple-discrimination learning. Gibson found that a set of multiple discriminations containing highly similar stimuli required 19.8 repetitions to learn, whereas the set with stimuli low in similarity needed only 8.9 repetitions. Increasing the similarity of the set of stimulus objects involved in multiple-discrimination learning has the definite effect of increasing the difficulty of learning. The interference that takes place during the learning session is greater when there is more stimulus generalization. Therefore, in order to overcome the forgetting that occurs when an entire set of chains must be learned at once, it is necessary to increase repetition (Gagne, 1970, p. 164).

It is of interest to note that once the multiple discriminations are learned, whether they have been difficult or easy, they are remembered equally well. Gibson's study also confirmed this finding. In other words, as Gagne (1970, p. 165) stated it, "Once the multiple discriminations have been fully established, retention is no longer affected by interference *within* the set. It may be, of course, and undoubtedly is, affected by interference from other sources, such as the learning of still other verbal chains."

Conditions of discriminations learning
INTERNAL CONDITIONS

"In order for optimum learning to take place, the learner must have previously acquired, *in isolation,* each of the chains that is to be learned." "The initial stimulus links must have been previously discriminated from each other, and the response links must also have been previously learned as discriminated Ss → R connections" (Gagne, 1970 p. 165). For example, in the example of student nurses learning to discriminate between the different types of catheters, the student nurses acquire this type of learning faster if:

1. They can identify each catheter by itself
2. They are able to name the catheters when they see them
3. They have available a mediating link

Availability of links varies with individuals. Evidence suggests that those people who possess more mediating links acquire a set of chains more rapidly than those who have fewer available links (Deese, 1967).

EXTERNAL CONDITIONS

"The entire set of stimuli that are to be associated in different chains must be presented to the learner one by one so that he is able to reinstate the chain for each." Also, an external cue or prompt should be utilized to elicit the desired response (Gagne, 1970, p. 166).

Repetition is required in order for the links of various chains to be discriminated. The amount of repetition needed will vary according to the similarity of the Ss → R links and the number of chains to be discriminated. With the presentation of similar stimuli, interference occurs, and generalizations may take place. Generalization can be reduced if the learner has already acquired discrimination learning of the links of various chains. The arrangement of repetition to accomplish learning of the entire set of discriminations best is unknown. Whether one should learn two or three or ten chains before repeating those previously learned is not known. However, it is known that repetition in multiple-discrimination learning does not appear to have the function of strengthening individual connections. What repetition does is overcome the effects of forgetting brought about by interference (Gagne, 1970, pp. 166-167).

As in the case of single-chain learning, there must be a condition in multiple-discrimination learning that provides for *confirmation* of the correct response. When the learner reinstates a chain, the learner must have a way of knowing that it contains a correct terminal response (Gagne, 1970, p. 167).

Other phenomena associated with multiple-discrimination learning

Generalization. Stimulus generalization occurs among (1) the stimuli being differentiated and (2) among the stimuli of other links in each chain, including the response link. The greater the similarity of the elements that are to be discriminated within the chain, the greater is the generalization and the more difficult is discrimination learning (Gagne, 1970, p. 170).

Discrimination. The need for discrimination learning (Ss → R) of each link of each chain is created because of the generalization tendencies among the stimuli of each chain. When single-chain discrimination occurs as a prerequisite to multiple discrimination, the latter occurs most rapidly.

Extinction. Extinction of any particular chain (single or multiple) in the set occurs when confirmation or positive reinforcement of the correct response is omitted. Extinction is important in the unlearning of incorrect responses by omitting the reinforcement. However, occurrence of errors also fosters extinction of correct responses so that they cannot be recalled and, therefore, must be relearned. Interference is the main cause of the extinction that is characteristic of multiple-discrimination learning (Gagne, 1970, p. 170).

Forgetting. Forgetting of individual chains results because of interference generated by learning other chains that make up the total set. Repetition aids retention of chains for longer periods of time. The curve of forgetting for multiple discriminations is similar to that described by Ebbinghaus for chains: retention falls off rapidly at first, then more slowly over a period of days and weeks. In order to overcome the phenomenon of forgetting, properly spaced repetitions, reviews, or practices are used to maintain retention at a high level (Gagne, 1970, p. 170-171).

Issues and relevant research studies in discrimination learning

Discrimination learning has given rise to two major positions that separate cognitive theorists from behaviorists. The behaviorist position, or continuity theory, attributes discrimination learning to the accumulation of positive habit strength, which occurs over a series of reinforced trials in which reinforcement only follows S^D–R. "Continuity theory

accounts for present learning in terms of past associative learning" (Hilgard, 1956, p. 435). Cognitive theorists, however, explain such learning in terms of insight and problem solving, which implies some mediation process. This theory describes an organism as shifting from one response to another until the correct or rewarded behavior is found. Such theory predicts sharp breaks in learning curves as insight or problem solving is achieved (Hilgard, 1956, p. 435). In this way "noncontinuity" theories explain how the correct response to a discrimination task can be learned on the basis of one trial.

Another theory relevant to this issue of continuity is Harlow's "learning set." This theory postulates that as a number of successive discrimination problems of the same type are learned, a gradual improvement occurs in the ability to solve the task until at some point a task is solved immediately (Deese and Hulse, 1967, p. 202). On the basis of this, Harlow believes that an organism (animal or human) learns about the nature of the task or develops a set used in solving the next similar task.

The second major issue over which the two groups of theorists disagree is in regard to the stimulus characteristics that facilitate discrimination. The behaviorist position tends to hypothesize that only the absolute characteristics of the stimulus are important, while the cognitive position contends that relationships between stimuli are important to discrimination learning. One phenomenon of discrimination learning that is related to this relative versus absolute issue is that of transposition. Transposition is the ability to learn discriminations based on the relationship or similarity between two stimuli rather than on the basis of reinforcement alone. A transposition effect is not obtained when the stimuli are very dissimilar. Cognitive theorists use this to support their position that discrimination is based on relational qualities, while behaviorists explain the effect as caused by the generalization that occurs in a gradient according to the degree of similarity between any two stimuli.

Other issues surrounding the learning problem pertain to how attention to cues is selected and to what degree learning relevant discrimination cues facilitates transfer of learning in one problem to that of another problem. Research in human learning has revealed some knowledge about attention and discrimination learning. Pasnak (1971) reported that in complex discrimination learning, attention is given to a characteristic of a complex contour rather than to the entire contour. The opposite is true in learning simple discrimination tasks. Pasnak hypothesized that in complex learning one attends to those features that in past experience have consistently marked differences in stimuli. Ellis (1965) reported that observation of simple shapes was enough to facilitate discrimination of such shapes, whereas verbal labeling along with observation of more complex shapes was necessary in learning more complex tasks. Ellis labels such verbal association as acquired distinctiveness and notes that such distinctiveness facilitates transfer of learning to new situations.

Studies have also been undertaken to discover how the presentation of stimuli affects the discrimination task. One such study reported by Croll, Knauss, and Knauss (1970) indicates that children learn discrimination tasks faster when the stimuli are presented in sequence rather than simultaneously. The same study indicates that for children the number of irrelevant dimensions of the stimuli presented affected rate of learning. In this case learning occurred more readily when irrelevant dimensional cues were kept to a minimum.

The relationship of learning set and discrimination has also been studied by DiVesta and Blake (1959). In this study three groups of students were asked to learn a discrimination task with only one of the three being instructed that some principle was operating as the basis for the discrimination. Of the three groups, the instructed group, learned the task more rapidly. The study also indicates the importance of reinforcement and learning in that only one of the two uninstructed groups was consistently reinforced for correct responses. As could be expected, this group learned at a more rapid rate than did the third group, which was not consistently rewarded for correct responses. In summarizing this review some additional conditions for learning discrimination tasks might also be offered in addition to those already outlined. These would include sequential presentation of stimuli rather than simultaneous presentation; drawing of attention to stimulus distinctiveness by pointing out distinguishing characteristics; decreasing irrelevant stimuli, especially when the task is complex; and providing relevant cues along as many dimensions as possible to facilitate discrimination of one stimulus from another.

Application to nursing education and practice

Discrimination learning is of great importance to nursing education and practice in that nurses are constantly faced with distinguishing one class of conditions from another by learning and employing a system of signs and symptoms. Nursing intervention is also based on the assessment of patients, which involves the process of discriminating normal or expected conditions from abnormal ones.

A multitude of relevant and specific problems could be raised for discussion in terms of discrimination learning, but one example will be presented for discussion and that will be the task of learning to discriminate abnormal electrocardiogram patterns from normal ones, and then learning to differentiate among the various abnormalities. The nurse-learner is faced first with the task of identifying what pattern and sequence of waves constitutes the cardiac cycle and secondly with associating each wave of the sequence with the corresponding cardiac action and letter classification (verbal associate). Having discriminated the cardiac sequence or chain and each link of that chain, the nurse must then learn to discriminate the variations that occur within the link and chain and associate them with their physiological correlate and respond to them with the appropriate intervention.

One approach to this learning problem that greatly utilizes discrimination learning theory is that of programmed instruction. In this method of instruction, learning the stimulus-response connections can be accomplished on an individual and isolated basis before links are associated in relevant and discriminated chains. Because of the high degree of similarity among the stimulus waves, repetition and reinforcement are extremely important in learning to discriminate both individual waves and patterns of waves. Programmed instruction allows for the amount of repetition necessary to the individual learner, facilitating learning and retention and also providing immediate reinforcement and feedback for correct responses, which facilitates stimulus-response connections both in links and chains. Verbal associates are used in distinguishing stimulus-response connections as well as observation, thus employing at least two stimulus dimensions. Verbal associates and cues also provide assistance in learning the mediating factors necessary to discrimination of a complex task.

Another area of application of the principles of discrimination learning to nursing is in situations where there is a similarity of manifestations of diseases, such as with diabetes mellitus and diabetes incipidus, insulin coma and diabetic coma, and rubella and rubeola. The instructor who is aware of the role and effect of similarity of stimuli on retention of facts and its function in interference will make a special effort to make salient the differences in similar materials, will emphasize the distinctive features, and will provide the students with mediating links or help them to generate their own mediating links. For example, in the case of rubella and rubeola, even the names sound so much alike that confusion (interference factors) is very real. They are both childhood disorders called measles, but they are different types. Both have incubation periods, and, in both, children suffer from fever, rash, and malaise. When the student is presented with a 2-year-old child with measles (S) in a public health visit, the student can reach the conclusion that it is rubeola (R) because of the presence of (1) a fever of 101° to 104° F (s–r), (2) a sore throat, (3) nasal discharge, (4) a dry "barking" cough, (5) conjunctivitis, (6) Koplik's spots inside the mouth, and (7) a rash all over the body. The student rules out rubella because the child does not have (1) a mild fever, (2) a faint, flat rash on face, neck, and upper trunk only, or (3) increased tenderness behind the ears. The intervention is important here because of the discrimination in diagnosis. The mother of this child is pregnant, but the unborn child is not in danger since it is not rubella that her 2-year-old has now. However, nursing invervention is essential to the child in order to prevent meningitis. Detailed instruction must be given to the mother to watch the child's temperature, and if a stiff neck develops to take the child to the hospital.

The instructor who has made salient the differences in the above diseases by (1) making the distinctive features (differences in symptoms) very obvious by the use of magnification of spots, showing slides of the rashes, and pointing out the differences; (2) utilizing other methods of attracting the students' attention to the differences between the diseases; (3) providing the students with repetition of the learning task, and (4) confirming correct responses (that is, correct identification of differences between the two diseases) will enable the students to discriminate between these two similar diseases and will help them to retain the material longer.

Another example where nursing students seem to have tremendous difficulty is in differentiating which nerve fiber carries the sensory impulse to the brain (central nervous system) and which one brings it back to the sensory organ (motor). The task to be discriminated is between the afferent nerve and the efferent nerve. The teacher can utilize the above mentioned four teaching strategies to reduce the similarity of these two anatomical features and in addition may provide the students with a mediating link; for example, the word SAME can be used in making the distinction. Each letter of the word SAME given in this sequence can be used in helping the students keep in mind which nerve fiber carries which impulse: *s*ensory—*a*fferent, *m*otor—*e*fferent. In other words, the *se*nsory impulse (touching a hot object) is carried by the *a*fferent nerve fibers to the central nervous system, and the *m*otor impulse comes from central nervous system through the *e*fferent nerve fibers to the sensory organ (hand) and commands the hand to be pulled back, as occurs in any reflex system. In this example, the word SAME is a "linking code," or a "mediating link," that enables the student to associate Ss → R; it is the small s → R in the following situation:

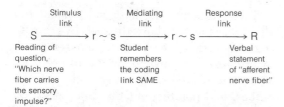

Stimulus link	Mediating link	Response link
S ⟶ r ~ s	⟶ r ~ s	⟶ R
Reading of question, "Which nerve fiber carries the sensory impulse?"	Student remembers the coding link SAME	Verbal statement of "afferent nerve fiber"

Other coding links could also be used and might consist of nonsense syllables, rhymes, or whatever else aids the student in remembering necessary information.

Discrimination theory could also be utilized in identifying and operationalizing problems in nursing research. Much is being said in nursing today about the process of assessment of patients in terms of a nursing model, with the hope that common nursing problems can be described and classified in terms of appropriate intervention. Use of a model itself probably can be seen as analogous to the theory of learning set in that once problems among relationships within the model framework are learned, similar discrimination problems among reality situations can be more easily recognized. However, it might also be interesting to approach the assessment of nursing problems from another view. It must be assumed that nurses in practice do discriminate normal from abnormal even though many or most are unaware of the basis on which they make their "discrimination" and response or intervention. Nursing research might address itself to the study of those cues that are most relevent to the nurse in the identification of a specific problem in practice. If this were accomplished, nursing education not only could address itself to problem identification set, but also could focus concentration on learning those cues that are most relevent to the identification. Such a focus might also assist the nursing profession in developing a more specific and universal language, which would facilitate professional communication.

In conclusion, therefore, principles from discrimination learning are useful in nursing education and practice. The important points to keep in mind in teaching patients and students any discrimination tasks are:

1. Discrimination learning is difficult when materials to be learned are similar, so the teacher's task is to reduce similarity between tasks
2. Chains must be presented to the learners one by one
3. Repetition is needed to overcome forgetting
4. Measures must be taken to reduce in-

terference by making stimuli more distinctive and by providing "coding links"

5. Correct responses must be confirmed or positively reinforced

Researchable questions

1. What is the effect of different types of mediators (pictures versus words versus symbols) on reducing the interference factors in a multiple-discrimination learning situation?

   a. Independent variables: the types of mediators—pictures versus words versus symbols

   b. Dependent variable: reduction of interference

2. What is the effect of confirmation that is self-administered versus teacher delivered on the rapidity of discrimination learning?

   a. Independent variable: confirmation (reinforcement) that is self-administered versus that which is teacher delivered

   b. Dependent variable: the rapidity of discrimination learning

ADDITIONAL LEARNING EXPERIENCES—RECOMMENDED READING LIST

DeCecco, J. *The psychology of learning and instruction: educational psychology.* Englewood Cliffs, N.J.: Prentice-Hall, Inc., 1968, pp. 260-264.

Gagne, R. *The conditions of learning.* New York: Holt, Rinehart and Winston, Inc., 1970, pp. 47-51, 155-171.

INSTRUCTIONS TO THE LEARNER REGARDING POSTTEST

Having completed the studying of this module, you are now ready to take the posttest to determine the level of achievement of the objectives. Return to the pretest of this module and take it over again as the posttest. Correct your answers, using the answer key found on this page of the module. You need to score 10 correct points for achievement at the 100% mastery level before proceeding to the next module. If your score is less than 10 correct points, correct your errors, study

the text over again, and read some of the articles in the recommended reading list. Take the posttest again. It is necessary to study until you achieve 100% mastery.

ANSWER KEY TO PRETEST AND POSTTEST

1. False (Gagne, 1970, p. 160)
2. True (Gagne, 1970, p. 164)
3. False (Gagne, 1970, p. 164)
4. c (Gagne, 1970, p. 170)
5. a (Gagne, 1970, p. 166)
6. c (Gagne, 1970, p. 157)
7. c (Gagne, 1970, p. 169)
8. b (Gagne, 1970, pp. 160-163)
9. discrimination (Ellis, 1965, p. 33)
10. reinforcement (Gagne, 1970, p. 168)

REFERENCES

Croll, W., Knauss, D., and Knauss, M. Sequential contiguity and short term memory in children's discrimination learning. *Journal of Experimental Child Psychology,* 1970, **10**:337-343.

DeCecco, J. *The psychology of learning and instruction: educational psychology.* Englewood Cliffs, N.J.: Prentice-Hall, Inc., 1968.

Deese, J. From the isolated verbal unit to connected discourse. In C. N. Cofer (Ed.), *Verbal learning and verbal behavior.* New York: McGraw-Hill Book Co., 1961.

Deese, J., and Hulse, S. *The psychology of learning.* (3rd Ed.) New York: McGraw-Hill Book Co., 1967.

DiVesta, F. J., and Blake, K. The effects of instructional "sets" on learning and transfer. *American Journal of Psychology,* 1959, **72**:57-67.

Ellis, H. *The transfer of learning,* New York: The Macmillan Co., 1965.

Gagne, R. *The Conditions of Learning.* New York: Holt, Rinehart and Winston, Inc., 1970.

Gibson, J. A. Intra-list generalization as a factor in verbal learning. *Journal of Experimental Psychology,* 1942, **30**:185-200.

Gibson, E. J. Perceptual learning. In Gagne, R., and Gephart, W. R. (Eds.), *Learning research and school subjects.* Itasca, Ill.: F. E. Peacock Publishers, Inc., 1968.

Hilgard, E. R. *Theories of learning.* New York: Appleton-Century-Crofts, 1956.

McGeoch, J. A., and Irion, A. L. *The psychology of human learning.* New York: David McKay Co., Inc., 1952.

Pasnak, R. Pattern complexity and response to distinctive features. *American Journal of Psychology,* 1971, **84**:235-244.

MODULE 7

Concept learning

DESCRIPTION OF THE MODULE

Concept learning is the sixth condition of learning. This module presents the bases of concept learning. The five major areas that are presented in integrated form are: the theoretical framework, relevant research studies to support the different view points, issues that are still unresolved, application to nursing education and practice and to education in general. Researchable questions are also raised. Since this module is a self-contained learning kit, it also contains information about the module objectives and the pretest and posttest to determine the extent to which students know the content prior to learning it and at completion. The content of the module is presented in sequential order.

MODULE OBJECTIVES

On completion of this module, having studied it very carefully and having studied the content in the recommended reading list, the learner will be able to perform the following objectives at the 95% level or better. The student will be able to:

1. Describe in writing or orally the different theoretical frameworks of concept learning that are presented by:
   a. Piaget's (cognitive) description of concept formation
   b. The computer model of concept formation
   c. The behavioristic view of concept formation and learning, specifically as

presented by Gagne and by DeCecco
2. Evaluate each of these theories according to preestablished criteria
3. State the internal and external conditions that are necessary for concept learning to take place
4. Differentiate and describe the different types of concepts and their characteristics
5. Identify at least one issue in the area of concept learning
6. Provide evidence (research studies) to support the principles of concept learning
7. Apply the principles of concept learning as proposed by DeCecco in teaching of a specific nursing concept to a patient or a student
8. Raise one researchable question and identify both the dependent and independent variables

PRETEST AND POSTTEST

Circle the correct answers. Each question is worth 1 point. The 95% level of achievement for this test is 24 correct points. Correct your answers using the answer key that is found at the end of this module (p. 110).

True or false

1. The emotional aspect of our concepts may be a product of early classical conditioning and consistent reinforcement and therefore may be difficult to extinguish. True or False
2. The concept of health can be classified as a concrete concept. True or False

94

3. A student answers a test question correctly to the effect that muscle tissue is made up of striated fibers. This shows that the student definitely has acquired the concept of striated muscle. True or False

4. Unlike some other learning types, concept learning does not involve any learned chains. True or False

5. A concept can be one stimulus or a class of stimuli. True or False

Multiple choice

6. The attributes of concepts are:
   a. the distinguishing characteristics of the concepts
   b. of equal number in different concepts
   c. varying in dominance according to the importance of the concepts
   d. all of the above

7. The role of a verbal associate in concept learning is to:
   a. serve to reinforce the abstract idea represented by the concept
   b. function as an external stimulus to recall
   c. eliminate the need for chaining

8. It can be determined that concept learning has occurred by having:
   a. the learner demonstrate that the concept can be generalized to specific instances
   b. the learner indicate component parts of the concept
   c. the learner recognize the verbal cue that stimulates recall

9. In learning to convert milliliters (ml) to teaspoons, a student is dealing with what type of concepts?
   a. concrete
   b. conjunctive
   c. attribute
   d. disjunctive
   e. relational

10. The "test" for the presence of concepts is itself a matter of demonstrating that:
    a. the learner can discriminate between stimuli
    b. the learner can verbally repeat the definition
    c. generalization can occur
    d. problems can be solved

11. A student nurse is attempting to find out what the concept of sodium retention means. Which response by an instructor would provide the greatest possibility for remembering?
    a. Sit down and think of the alternatives.
    b. Tell me what you think, and I'll give you feedback.
    c. Can you recall any of the functions of sodium in the body?

12. When teaching a nursing student the concept of cyanosis, the instructor may show pictures of normal patients and pictures of patients who are cyanotic. By what processes does the student learn that concept?
    a. generalization and discrimination
    b. repetition and reinforcement
    c. discrimination and reinforcement

13. Which of the following is true?
    a. As the number of attributes of a concept increases, the complexity of the concept increases.
    b. As the number of attributes of a concept increases, the process of learning the concept gets easier.
    c. Variations in the attributes of a concept does not affect the rate at which the concept is learned.

14. Which of the following items are correct for concept learning?
    a. Reinforcement and contiguity are essential
    b. Reinforcement and contiguity help but are not vital
    c. Concept learning allows the learner to generalize to stimuli in other classes
    d. Concept learning allows the learner to generalize to other stimuli in the same class

15. The attributes and values of a conjunctive concept are:
    a. unrelated
    b. diminutive
    c. additive
    d. nonspecific

Matching

Part A

_____ 16. Relational concepts
_____ 17. Conjunctive concepts
_____ 18. Disjunctive concepts

_____ 19. Concept by observation
_____ 20. Concept by definition
_____ 21. Attribute

Part B
a. Clean, white sheet
b. One white bedspread and/or one yellow bed-spread
c. All linen carts have more towels than wash-cloths
d. Urine
e. Specific gravity
f. Dosage
g. Distinctive feature of a concept

Discussion questions

22. Describe how you would teach a diabetic child (age 7 years) the concept of carbohydrate foods.
23. List two ways individuals respond to a collection of things.
24. Distinguish between concept by observation and concept by definition.
25. A nursing instructor is teaching students about different types of wounds. How might knowledge about concept learning be utilized in teaching the students the concept "laceration"?

TEXT
Theoretical framework
Introduction

The purpose of this module is to present several theories or models of concept formation or learning and to evaluate them in terms of the criteria set forth by this writer.

There are three major schools of thought in explaining the process of concept formation. These are: first, the cognitive theorists (Ausubel, Bruner, and Piaget); second, the behaviorists (Skinner, Osgood, Staats, Kendler, Wittrock, Gagne, and DeCecco); and third, those who favor the computer model of cognitive functioning (Newell, Shaw, Simon, and Hovland). Within each school, the form of explanation of concept formation ranges from an extreme view point to a moderate;

for example, Ausubel (1966) tried to explain concept formation in terms of "meaningful learning." Piaget and his followers asserted that the child does not acquire important concepts, such as the notion of number, just from teaching, but on the contrary, to a remarkable degree, develops them independently and spontaneously. Furthermore, cognitive theorists rule out a role for "external reinforcement," asserting that the development of important cognitive processes is primarily a method of inner organization and coordination (Anderson, 1966, p. 396).

Bruner and Oliver (1963) believed that concepts are formed in a process in which "transformations" are imposed on data by the organism and that a person's cognitive structure does reflect a specific history of learning. In general, "for cognitive theorists, *information* is the key to concept formation: information is available from stimuli in varying amounts, information is assimilated, and information is processed with strategies that are more or less parsimonious and efficient" (Anderson, 1966, p. 395). They stressed the importance of events within the organism.

The behaviorists' point of view ranges from a strict stimulus-response (S–R) approach (Skinner) to the mediational (S–r–s–R) approach (Osgood, Staats, Kendler, Wittrock, Gagne, and DeCecco). In behavioral terms, "concept" refers to the contingency in which a common response (R) is evoked by a class of stimuli (S). A concept is acquired when response emitted in the presence of the discriminative stimulus is differentially reinforced (Anderson, 1966, p. 395).

The computer model of cognitive functioning is one of the more eclectic positions. It cannot be identified with either the neobehavioristic or with the cognitive viewpoint. However, it is more like the behavioristic viewpoint because it deals with input-output relationships.

Criteria for selecting a model, or theory, of concept learning and instruction

A model, or theory, of concept learning or instruction must be able to:

1. Explain the problem under study
2. Identify the conditions of learning and transfer that are important areas for basic research in school learning
3. Predict outcomes
4. Initiate further research
5. Help build findings of empirical studies into a systematic body of knowledge
6. Transfer and communicate results of empirical and conceptual work
7. Have practical value and significance and be easily implemented
8. Handle individual differences
9. Help to program material
10. Have heuristic value

Presentation of selected models

Three theoretical frameworks of concept formation will be presented, and each fulfills most of the previously mentioned criteria. These are: (1) Piaget's theory of concept formation (cognitive approach), (2) the computer model of cognitive functioning and concept formation, and (3) behavioristic theory (stimulus-response and mediational approaches), including the behaviorists' view of concept learning in general and Gagne's and DeCecco's view of concept learning.

To fully understand what is involved in concept learning, it is necessary to know what a concept is. There are many definitions of a concept. DeCecco defines a concept as "a class of stimuli which have a common characteristic" (DeCecco, 1968, p. 388). Kendler (1964) defined concept learning as "an acquisition of a common response to dissimilar stimuli . . . that concepts are associations and that they function as cues or mediators of learned behavior. Carroll (1964)

defined a concept as an abstraction from a series of experiences which defines a class of objects or events" (Klausmeir and Harris, 1966, p. 83).

According to Gagne, these definitions have the following properties in common:

1. A concept is an inferred mental process.
2. The learning of a concept requires discrimination of stimulus objects (distinguishing "positive" and "negative" instances)
3. The performance that shows that a concept has been learned consists of the learner being able to place an object in a class (Klausmeir and Harris, 1966, p. 83).

An important point to remember in teaching concepts is that a concept is a class of stimuli and not a particular stimuli. For example, a "patient" is a concept. There may be a sick boy or girl or a sick man or woman, or a sick adult or child, but they all fall under the classification of "patient."

PIAGET'S THEORY

As mentioned in the introductory section, Piaget (1965, p. 406) stated that, "It is a mistake to suppose that a child acquires the notion of number or other mathematical concepts just from teaching." But, he said, "The child develops them himself independently and spontaneously." Furthermore, he said that the child's comprehension of mathematical concepts comes only as a function of age and mental growth. Also, he asserted that the development of important cognitive processes is primarily a matter of "inner organization and coordination."

Several of Piaget's studies on number concepts (1965, p. 407) with 5-year-old or younger children have shown that children must grasp the principal of conservation of quantity before they can develop the concept of number. He also concluded from these studies that the formation and conservation of concepts of number, space, and geometry are all stage-bound, and each has certain sequences. This is also how Piaget explained the phenomenon of transfer. He stated that a child cannot transfer or conserve without having learned the prerequisites for the specific task (concept) and without being mentally and physically ready (age-wise). In his words " . . . children do not appreciate the principle of conservation of length or surface until somewhere around the age of seven. They discover the reversibility that shows the original quantity has remained the same (e.g., the realignment of equal length blocks the removal of the wall, and so on). Thus, the discovery of logical relationships is a prerequisite to the construction of geometrical concepts, as it is the formation of the concept of number" (Piaget, 1966, p. 411).

Piaget has been criticized by many U.S. psychologists. There are two issues that are paramount in regard to Piaget's delineation of stages of intellectual development and concept formation. The first issue concerns the empirical validity of these stages and his unsystematic and "unscientific" methods of conducting his research and reporting his findings. He seems to be indifferent to such considerations as sampling, reliability, intersituational generality, statistical significance, and experimental control. The second issue concerns the theoretical criteria that any designated stage of development must meet, irrespective of its empirical status. Piaget's critics contend that a genuine stage of development does not exist if it arises gradually rather than abruptly, reflects environmental as well as endogenous influences, fluctuates over time, and manifests variability over subject matter (Ausubel, 1966, pp. 13-14).

Even though Piaget has been criticized widely, his ideas are closely tied to observation of behavior, and this makes them the sort of psychology that moves science forward because it is testable by reference to the facts of behavior.

Flavell (1963, pp. 405-433) furthermore pointed out some of Piaget's contributions as they pertain to concept development and developmental psychology in general. Here are some of them:

1. Piaget has shed new light and emphasis on the cognitive aspect of child development.

2. His intricate theory, which is mostly based upon observational type of research (mostly of his children), opened a new area of research. Most U.S. psychologists are trying to test part of his theory, thus adding to the body of developmental and educational psychology.

3. His conservation experiments of surface area (the cow and the meadow) and volume (fluid content in different beakers) are being standardized and used as measures of intelligence to assess individual child's intellectual development and scholastic aptitude and readiness for various kinds of instruction.

4. Planning curricula in the context of Piaget's developmental findings. Two forms: (a) Grade placement of instructional content, i.e., what courses to teach at what grade level. (b) How to make use of Piaget's data on developmental sequences to anticipate and guard against subtle, non-obvious "misacquisitions" which he has shown the child is likely to fall prey to in trying to master a new area.

5. His theory offers an explanation about the cognizing organism and the process by which external unknowns become known internals. It might tell something about the most favorable conditions for learning and thus the way we should go about teaching.

COMPUTER MODELS

The information approach based on a computer model of cognitive organization and functioning has been one of the most eclectic positions in recent years. The general idea of this approach is behavioristic, since it deals mechanistically with input-output relations. But, instead of a reflexive model of symbolic processes, it uses a more substantive view of the nature of information as well as the cybernetic principle of a control system that is both (1) sensitive to feedback that indicates behavioral error and (2) differentially responsive to such feedback in ways that correct the existing error or discrepancy (Ausubel, 1966, p. 11).

The computer model of human thinking proposed by Newell, Simon, and Shaw (1966) involves a receptor mechanism capable of interpreting coded information, plus a control system, consisting of a large store of memories and a variety of processes for operating on the information in these memories, and rules for combining the processes into complex strategies or programs, which in turn can be selectively activated by the input information. This type of research has led Miller, Galanter, and Pribram (1960) to propose a new cybernetic or discrepancy-testing unit of analysis to replace the stimulus-response paradigm.

The theoretical and heuristic value of the computer model depends on the tenability of theories to account for human cognitive functioning. Computer programs are capable of generating cognitive operations that are performed by humans, such as generalizing, abstracting, and logical decision-making. The crucial question is whether they are genuinely comparable to the processes that are performed by humans. Hovland (1966) stated that the computer can be used merely as a simulator of human cognitive processes rather than as a cybernetic model. It is theoretically possible to program a computer in accordance with the hypothesized properties of human cognitive functioning, but the fidelity of the simulation might be open to question.

A computer can be used either to test predictions made by different theoretical models or to obtain additional information about cognitive functioning that is too complex to permit prediction or experimental investigation (Hovland, 1966).

The other advantages of using a computer model are: the computer can be used as subjects and variables and controls can be introduced that would be impossible to control with human subjects. Computer models place great emphasis on developing theories that have both descriptive and predictive power. Finally, programmed material can be developed and written.

There are limitations to computer models. The following are some of the reasons why a computer at this stage of development cannot perfectly simulate human brain functioning and thinking. (1) They simulate only those behaviors that are rule-bound. All human behaviors are not rule-bound. (2) If the system is to simulate human thinking processes, it lacks the elements of forgetting and fatigue that are so much a part of human thinking and brain functioning. (3) With computers, one can know the initial level or the amount of memory storage that exists at a specific time, but with humans, one cannot specifically state the level at which knowledge starts or the previous history of knowledge is. (4) Simulation methods have been successful where it is possible to define performance of a task as an outcome of a succession of single steps. Much more difficult are those processes where a number of stages are going on simultaneously, in parallel fashion, and it appears that much of our perceptual and thought processes operate in this fashion. (5) To date, most simulation has been of the performance of one individual. For simulation to be maximally effective it should be able to predict machine solutions not only of one individual under specific conditions, but also the effects for different individuals under different environmental conditions, after various amounts of experience (Hovland, 1966).

BEHAVIORISTIC POINT OF VIEW

This includes the stimulus-response theorists and the neobehaviorists, or mediation theorists.

Behavioristic view of concept learning in general. As mentioned in the introductory section, for behaviorists, the word "concept" refers to "the contingencies in which a common response is evoked by a class of stimuli" (Anderson, 1966, p. 395). A concept is acquired when a response emitted in the presences of the S[D] is differentially reinforced.

Behaviorists are currently producing increasingly powerful analyses of concept formation based on the role of mediating responses, particularly verbal or symbolic mediators. Hull (1920) originally proposed that concepts are developed by *abstracting the common stimulus elements* in a series of stimulus objects. Osgood (1953, pp. 667-668) however, believed that Hull's consideration of a concept formation would not distinguish the process from any other learning. He stated that ". . . the only essential condition for concept formation is the learning of a common mediating response (which is the meaning of the concept) for a group of objects or situations, identical elements and common perceptual relations merely facilitating the establishment of such mediators." Osgood, while rejecting the notion that concepts are based on identical stimulus elements, did not adequately specify how the objects come to elicit a common response or what the common response is.

Kendler and D'Amato (1955) have considered concept formation to be the acquisition of a common implicit response to different stimuli. In addition, Kendler and Karasik (1958, p. 278) have extended this to verbal concept formation, which they assume occurs "when subject learns to respond to a set of different works with the same implicit response."

Staats (1966) regarded concepts as a verbal habit-family hierarchy formed on the basis of a class of stimulus objects having identical elements; for example, the "animal" concept. The individual words in the concept gain their meaning through classical conditioning, where the word is paired with the appropriate stimulus object.

Using a conception of meaning, that is, an implicit mediating response, Mowrer (1954) suggested that a sentence is a conditioning device, and that communication takes place when the meaning response that has been elicited by a predicate is conditioned to the subject of the sentence.

On the basis of verbal habit families and language conditioning and generalization, learning that is originally derived from experience with a relatively small class of objects, usually having identical elements, may be transferred to many new situations and tasks. It has been suggested by Staats (1966) that these are the processes that underlie the progression from concrete to abstract thinking that have frequently been said to occur in child development and are involved in "understanding a concept."

Thus, the process of concept formation is seen as one that involves complicated principles of learning, communication, and mediated generalizations. In an unpublished paper, Wittrock (1966) stated that the mediated generalization approach leads one to study problems of transfer often given little attention by researchers adopting the one-step stimulus-response model. These important problems include verbally mediated transfer and secondary or acquired generalizations and discriminations. This approach also uses reinforcement and contiguity in the learning of verbal mediators (p. 22).

Mediated generalization approach has been used to study transfer to concepts. Two types of research have been conducted on child learning. The first is by Kendler (1964), who has emphasized the age development for use of verbal mediators and has also exemplified how the concepts of practice, contiguity, and reinforcement are applied to hypothetical mediating stimuli and responses to make useful predictions about transfer. Second, Wittrock and others at the University of California in Los Angeles have studied conditions for teaching verbal mediators, especially hierarchically ordered sets of verbal mediators (Wittrock, 1966).

The type of research that has been produced by behaviorists, as such, has been more in the area of testing the effects of variables that influence concept formation. There has been very little research on the process or the acquisition of concept formation. Mediation theorists have contributed some, but they have been too busy trying to defend their own hypothesis. The areas of study have been very broad and rather vague.

Gagne's and DeCecco's view of concept learning. Both Gagne (1970) and DeCecco (1968) viewed the process of concept learning as being when an individual can learn to respond to collections of things by distinguishing among them and also by putting things (objects or events) into a class and responding to the class as a whole. In order to state that an individual is using a concept, one must be able to demonstrate that the performance is impossible on the basis of simple forms of learning.

There are several meanings to the term "concept." The most fundamental meaning of the term "concept" that is exhibited in individual behavior is the response to a class of observable objects or object qualities, such as those implied by the names "color," "shape," "size," "heaviness," and so on, or by common objects, such as "cat," "chair," "house," or "human." These are generally referred to as *concrete concepts*, or *concepts by observation*, since these are observable items.

Abstract concepts and those that involve relations are referred to as *concepts by definition*; for example, "temperature," "volume," "feelings," and mathematical concepts, such as "square root," "ratio," and so on.

The process of concept learning is the same both in children and adults. An example of the process is a student nurse who is studying basic concepts in nursing and must learn the concepts of "asepsis" and "sterile field." In such a case one assumes that the basic learning of 'the words has already been accomplished. But the verbal chains must be established that connect several instances of observed procedure of aseptic technique and a field that is free from any live bacteria to the response "sterile field" and "asepsis." Furthermore, a number of multiple discriminations must be acquired. The student nurse must distinguish "sterile field" from "clean field" from "contaminated field" and also sterile field in different situations, such as in the operating room while conducting surgery, in a treatment room while doing a thoracentesis or a catheterization. Once these have been mastered, the basic instructional conditions can be carried out for concept learning, that is, various instances of "asepsis" and "sterile field" are shown at one time or in quick succession and are identified by the student, who is then ready to classify a new example of "sterile field" or "asepsis" as a member of the concept class.

Gagne (1970) pointed out that the learning of a concept is not always or necessarily a verbal matter, since concepts can be learned by animals as well as human beings. However, using verbal cues (words), which are external stimuli that help the student recall the concept, provided the student has already learned the chains in which the word occurs, makes it relatively easy to structure the situation so that concept learning takes place.

Characteristics of concepts. Concepts are distinguished by their attributes and values of their attributes. An *attribute* is a distinctive feature of a concept, and it varies from one concept to another, such as red, round pill, which has two attributes: color and form (shape).

Values of an attribute. The values of an attribute are the various forms it may take (DeCecco, 1968, p. 389). For example, color as an attribute has values, such as red, sanguine, serosanguineous, pink, and so on. Form has values, such as round, rectangular, square and others. Some concepts have attributes with very few values; for example, a human being or a patient (concept) has a series of two values—man or woman, dead or alive, child or adult, married or single—whereas a color as an attribute may have several values ranging from pale color to very dark.

Number of attributes. The number of attributes varies from one concept to another; for example "red, round pill" has two attributes: color and shape; "small, red, round pill" has three attributes: size, color, and shape. As the number of attributes increases, the difficulty of learning the concept increases. Scanning the values of several attributes is a strenuous and a time-consuming affair. Bruner, Goodnow, and Austin (1956) suggest that under ordinary time pressures, individuals tend to reduce the number of attributes to which they attend (DeCecco, 1968, p. 389).

Dominance of the attribute. Dominance refers to the fact that some attributes are more obvious than others. Dominance refers to both the concept and to its attributes. Concepts with a few obvious attributes are easier to learn than concepts with several obscured ones. As a teacher, one must determine the relative dominance of the attributes of the concepts to be taught and must use this information in the planning of instruction. Important attributes that lack dominance must be given special emphasis; for example, the teacher can resort to underscoring, diagramming, drawing, using hand and arm gesticulation and vocal inflections, magnifying the obscure attribute, and other techniques. Large numbers of attributes can be reduced by ignoring some and focusing attention on others or by combining the attributes into a smaller number of patterns (DeCecco, 1968, p. 390).

Types of concepts. Attributes combine in three different ways to produce three types of concepts.

Conjunctive concepts. In a conjunctive concept certain values of several attributes occur simultaneously (DeCecco, 1968, p. 391). For example, two red, round pills is a conjunctive concept, because it has three attributes (number, color, and form) each attribute has a value (two, red, round), and these specific attributes are jointly present. Other examples are "bird machine" (respirator) or curved emesis basin. Both of these concepts have attributes of color, size, shape, function, and weight, and each attribute has values; for example, the bird machine may be yellow in color; large, medium or small in size; come in several different shapes; function in helping the patient breath, and vary in weight. Similarly, the curved emesis basin has several attributes, and each attribute has several values.

Conjunctive concepts are often the easiest to learn and to teach because of the additive quality of their attributes and values. Students need to learn a list of attributes and appropriate values in learning concepts.

Disjunctive concepts. In disjunctive concepts the appropriate values of one attribute or of another or of both are present. In disjunctive concepts the attributes and the values are substituted for one another. An example is "two squares and/or two circles" as a disjunctive concept. The concept is disjunctive because the value of the form can change—it can be a circle, a square, or both. Another example of a disjunctive concept from nursing is "shock" (lowered blood pressure). It can occur as a result of excessive loss of blood and/or anaphylaxis (such as with a drug that dilates the blood vessels, thus lowering the blood pressure).

Disjunctive concepts are difficult to learn

because of the arbitrary equivalence of their attributes. Disjunctive concepts are rules that the student must learn to apply to equivalent stimulus situations (DeCecco, 1968, p. 392).

Relational concepts. Relational concepts possess specifiable relationships between attributes. An example is that all children between the ages of 3 to 7 years can take so many ounces of milk. Specific dosages of medicine—for example, children between the ages of 3 to 5 years should take so many mg of drug X every 6 hours—are relational concepts. The age ranges and the quantity of drug or milk are the attributes of the above-mentioned relational concepts. The statement of the relationship of these attributes describes the concepts. "Distance" and "direction" are examples of relational concepts because both have as their attributes points in space and time. Carroll (1964) discussed several relational concepts that are difficult for students to learn: time, many, few, average, longitude, mass, weight, and others.

The effect of intellectual development on concept learning: limits imposed by developmental periods. According to Piaget (1965), the child's stage of development determines the level of thought of which the child is capable. The learning of concepts and principles requires the student to engage in abstract thought. Piaget classifies the intellectual development of the child into three major stages:

Preoperational stage (ages 1 to 7 years). The preoperational stage includes the sensorimotor stages in the subclassification that occurs from birth to 2 years of age. In the preoperational stage the child uses and describes words in terms of function, such as the concept of fruit (apple) is described as something to bite or eat. At this stage the child learns concepts from experience, and since this experience is limited, the child learns them incompletely. Gagne (1965) suggested that a child entering kindergarten may know the concepts of above, below, on top of, underneath, next to, the middle one, start, stop, go, come, sit, stand, and so on. but may not know such concepts as the one before, the next one, double, like, unlike, grapheme-phoneme correspondences, and number names for quantities. In the case of disadvantaged children, Gagne suggested that teachers must be very careful to avoid unwarranted assumptions about what they have and have not learned.

Period of concrete operations (ages 7 to 11 years). During the period of concrete operations, the child's thinking is oriented toward concrete objects in the immediate environment. The child relinquishes the physical attributes of objects one by one, and each grouping remains an isolated organization. In this stage the child can learn concepts that require the classification of concrete objects and events and in acquiring new concepts can employ rudimentary concepts of time, space, number, and logic. Intellectual operations or groupings of this period show the characteristics of closure, associativity, reversibility, and identity (DeCecco, 1968, p. 395).

Formal operations stage (ages 12 years and up). Development of abstract and relational concepts occurs during the formal operations stage. The child's thoughts concern the possible as well as the real. The capability for hypotheticodeductive and propositional thinking develops.

The conditions of concept learning

Internal conditions. Prerequisite to the learning of a concept the individual should have as entering behavior the capabilities that have previously been established by multiple discrimination. These include "a set of verbal (or other) chains that have been acquired previously to *representative* stimulus situations, that exhibit the characteristics of the class that describes the concept, and that distinguish these stimuli from others not included in the class. Of course, the acquisition of multiple discrimination is in turn dependent upon other prerequiste learnings the individual chains, and the stimulus-response connections that compose them" (Gagne, 1970, p. 180).

External conditions. In human learners, the situational conditions for concept learning are largely embodied in a set of *verbal instructions*.

1. "The specific *stimulus objects*, to which chains that include a common final link have been previously learned are *presented simultaneously* or in *close time succession*" (Gagne, 1970, p. 181).

2. *Instructions* should elicit a common link to a stimulus situation belonging to the proper class but to which the learner has not previously responded; for example, instructions asking "What is this?" to a new stimulus situation including a "sterile field" or "asepsis" or asking "Where is the sterile field?"

3. "Once these events have occurred, the new capability may be verified by asking for the identification of several additional instances of the class, again using stimuli to which the learner has not acquired verbal chains" (Gagne, 1970, p. 181).

4. *Immediate reinforcement* needs to be given when the concept is learned. Confirmation has to be immediate, that is, contiguity of reinforcement is important. Also, contiguity is important in presentation of the instances (in the first external condition). The absence of contiguity may be a factor in the slowness of concept learning.

Repetition, or *practice*, does not seem to be necessary when all the other conditions are optimal.

Generalization as a phenomenon associated with concept learning. The possession of the capability generated in the learner by the learning of a concept is the characteristic of generalization. For example, having acquired the concept of "asepsis," the student nurse is able to generalize this concept to other stimulus situations that were not part of the learning and can immediately identify a sterile field.

The effect of concept learning is to free the individual from control of specific stimuli. Generalization of concepts is very important to most kinds of intellectual activity done by the humans. It is used in reading, communicating and thinking. As Gagne (1970, p. 182) pointed out, "It is not surprising that the 'test' for the presence of concepts is itself a matter of demonstrating that generalizing can occur." The generalizing capability provided by concept learning goes beyond the *stimulus generalization* that is the fundamental property of stimulus–response learning. It is not limited by physical resemblances only.

Uses of concepts and principles

Concepts reduce the complexity of the environment. The fact that we can group events into classes is an important source of mastery over the environment. Archer (1966, p. 46) suggested that reducing the complexity of the world takes on the character of motivation and striving. The individual attempts not only to reduce the complexity of the chaotic environment but also "to seek and search out peculiarities and differences in the elements in its environment in order to optimize its environmental complexity."

The learning of concepts and principles enables one to grasp, in an array of environmental stimuli, similarities and differences with which one would otherwise have difficulty coping.

Concepts help identify objects of the world. Identification involves the placing or classifying of objects into a class; therefore, it reduces the complexity of the environment. The use of concepts to identify objects points out to the teacher the importance of having concepts as entering behaviors. Gagne (1970) stated that concepts and principles may be related to the world and to each other in hierarchical form. If a child does not learn the subordinate concepts and principles, the learning of higher ones will be very difficult or impossible.

Concepts and principles provide direction for instrumental activity. Concepts and principles enable one to know in advance the actions that can be taken. Placing objects or persons in the right class, which is very important in problem-solving behaviors, enables one to make important decisions.

Concepts and principles make instruction possible. The steps described for the teaching of concepts and principles are largely embodied in a set of verbal instructions. It would not be possible to instruct a student about these strategies if the student had not already learned some concepts and principles. Concepts and principles can become an obstacle to instruction when the student has an inadequate grasp of them and does not know their relationship to the concrete environment (DeCecco, 1968, p. 399).

Concepts can be stereotypes. McDonald (1965) defined a stereotype as a rigid or inaccurate concept, impervious to experience. The teacher must sometimes provide corrective experiences for an additional use of concepts. As concepts, stereotypes can sometimes be changed when the student is provided with a wider array of positive and negative examples than those previously experienced. The emotional aspects of concepts may be a product of early classical conditioning and consistent reinforcement, as in the case of fears and appetites; therefore, they may be difficult to extinguish (DeCecco, 1968, p. 400).

Strategy of teaching concepts. The principles that are put forth by DeCecco (1968) to facilitate the acquisition of concepts by the learner apply to any teaching situation—education in general or nursing education in particular. With proper adaptation of these principles, the strategies can also apply to teaching of concepts to any age level, provided that the teacher adapts it to the level and capabilities of the learner.

DeCecco has proposed nine steps that are involved in teaching concepts to the learner. Some of these proposed steps have been scientifically tested, and some still await testing. In the following section, these nine steps are presented with their research findings.

1. *The teacher informs the student of what performance will be expected after the concept is learned.* The expected performance is the correct identification of new examples of the concept—not the definition alone. In other words, the student should be told what the objectives are. Describing the terminal behavior has two purposes: first, it provides the teacher with a means of assessing the adequacy of the student's performance and of determining the areas that need further instruction; second, it provides the student with a way of assessing personal performance and of determining when the objective has been achieved. The student's self-evaluation and knowledge of results has positive reinforcement value, because it confirms the degree of achievement.

2. *The teacher reduces the number of attributes to be learned in complex concepts and makes the important attributes dominant.* This step requires that the teacher analyze the concept to be taught prior to the actual teaching to determine the values and the number of attributes, the dominant and conspicuous attributes, and the relevant and irrelevant values and attributes and to determine which of these are more important than others. This is done to know which are the important attributes to stress in the actual teaching situation. Two general procedures are suggested by DeCecco (1968) to reduce the number of attributes of complex concepts:

   a. Ignore some of the attributes of complex concepts that are not relevant in learning the concept
   b. Focus on those attributes that are important or code the attributes into fewer patterns; for example the study by

Carroll (1964) of teaching of the complex concept of *"tort"* (a legal concept) illustrates the validity of this procedure

3. *The teacher provides the student with useful verbal mediators.* The teacher needs to find out if the student possesses the entering behaviors of verbal associations before undertaking the teaching of concepts. A series of experiments conducted by Wittrock, Keislar, and Stern (1963, 1964, 1965) indicate that certain names or labels (verbal mediators) facilitate the student's learning of concepts. For example, in the study by Stern (1965), students were tested to determine their ability to identify new examples of a concept, new concepts of the same type, and a new category of concepts. It was found that those students who were given class labels as a verbal mediator did better than those students who were given the name of an example of the concept.

In another study, Wittrock, Keislar, and Stern (1964) utilized kindergarten children to test the role of different types of verbal mediators on concept learning. Four types of mediators were given: classification of French words. These were four groups:

Group 1—*no mediator:* were told, "Something you have learned in the past will help you"

Group 2—*general mediator:* were told, "Recalling the articles "le" and "la" would help you find the right answer"

Group 3—*class mediator:* were told, "The top picture is a *la (le)* word; find a *la (le)* picture on the bottom that goes with it"

Group 4—*specific mediator:* were told, "The name of the top picture is (French word)"

The class mediator (group 3) represented an intermediate amount of instructional guidance—more guidance than provided by the general mediator (group 2) and less guidance than provided by the specific mediator (group 4).

Results showed that the children who received the class mediator (intermediate guidance) retained the concept longer and recog-

nized more new examples of the concepts. However, in a later study (Wittrock and Keislar, 1965), the class mediator and the specific mediator were equally effective in teaching concepts. These studies refuted the popular myth that young children can learn concepts best with little or no instructional guidance, a position that was upheld by "developmental stage" theorists.

4. *The teacher provides the student with positive and negative examples of the concept.* A "positive example" of a concept is one that contains the attributes of the concept. A "negative example" is one that does not contain the attributes of a concept. For example, positive examples of *respirators* are the bird machine and iron-lung machine. Negative examples are tongue depressor or tracheostomy tube. Research studies have indicated that provision of positive and negative examples is a major condition of concept learning. In a study done by Huttenlocker (1962), students were taught a concept with positive examples only, negative examples only, or a mixture of both. It was found that students learned the concept better when both positive and negative examples were used. The students had the most difficulty in learning a concept when only negative examples were used.

As for the number of positive examples that the teacher should provide, there should be enough to represent the range of attributes and attribute values of the concept. In the case of negative examples, the teacher should present enough of these to eliminate irrelevant attributes that students are likely to include as part of the concept. All negative examples of the attribute that usually confuse students should be presented and, if necessary, explained (Gagne, 1965). Finally, a direct experience or realistic examples are not necessarily preferable to simplified presentations of the concept, such as line drawings, diagrams, cartoons, and charts. These presentations help simplify the learning of concepts by focusing on the major attributes (DeCecco, 1968, pp. 407-412).

5. *The teacher presents the examples in succession or simultaneously.* The major concern of this step is the order with which positive and negative examples are presented to the students. The external learning condition of contiguity is essential in this step, that is, the almost simultaneous presentation of examples of the concept. The study by Kates and Yudin (1964) indicated that *simultaneous presentation* (keeping all examples in view at the same time) was superior and more effective in teaching a concept than *successive presentation* (in which one example at a time is shown and removed after 20 seconds) or the *focus condition* (in which two examples—the focus example, which is always positive, and the new example, which is positive or negative—are presented together). The simultaneous presentation is superior because the student does not have to rely on memory for previous examples. It also helps the student to make discriminations among examples.

6. *The teacher presents a new positive example of the concept and asks the student to identify it.* In this step the teacher provides both contiguity and reinforcement. In the previous steps the teacher emphasizes discrimination or distinction between positive and negative examples. In this step, however, the teacher emphasizes generalization, or the ability of the student to make the conceptual response to a new but similar pattern of stimuli.

7. *The teacher verifies the student's learning of the concept.* The teacher verifies the student's learning by presenting several new positive and negative examples of the concept and asking the student to select only the positive ones. The available evidence does not indicate whether this step is essential for concept learning; however, it provides the teacher with a means of assessing whether the student has understood the concept. It also provides the student with additional opportunities to make responses and obtain reinforcement from teacher, self, or both (DeCecco, 1968, p. 413).

8. *The teacher requires the student to define the concept.* Much of concept learning is prelingual (before the child learns the language) or alingual (without the use of language). In the experiment by Johnson and O'Reilly (1964) there were three groups of students. Group 1 (pictorial group) had to classify pictures of two types of birds by their attributes. Group 2 (verbal group) had to classify verbal phrases that described birds with the same attributes as those in the pictures. Group 3 (pictorial-definition group) had to classify the same pictures used by the first group, but they were also asked after every five cards, "How do you tell a gunkle bird?" The first and second groups were asked this question after they had completed their examination.

The researchers found that the pictorial-definitions group (group 3) gave twice as many good definitions as did the pictorial group (group 1). The classification task was learned fastest by the verbal group (group 2). The researchers concluded that small amounts of practice with the definition improves the quality of the definition. They also argue that if concept learning includes the ability to use concepts in communication, special attention should be given to the learning of definitions. Of course, the teacher cannot assume that the student who is able to define a concept is also capable of identifying the concept. It is also true that some concepts in science and mathematics are difficult to define or describe in words. It is therefore necessary for the teacher to provide special training for concept definition when it is difficult to formulate (DeCecco, 1968, p. 414).

9. *The teacher provides occasions for student responses and for reinforcement of these responses.* The purpose of reinforcement is to

provide feedback on the student's correctness of response. Since feedback is crucial in concept learning, or any other type of learning, any inconsistency, delay, or failure to provide feedback will impair student learning. The research studies of Rhine and Silun (1958), Carpenter (1954), and Sax (1960) support the conditions of reinforcement as a factor in the efficient learning of concepts.

The mode of response should not be shifted, at least during the early stages of concept learning. The study of Wilder and Green (1963) showed that the shift from spoken to written responses is less inhibiting than the shift from drawing to writing or writing to drawing. Various mechanical or electronic devices may maintain consistency of response mode and informational feedback better than what can now be done under ordinary classroom conditions (DeCecco, 1968, p. 415-416).

Concluding comments of different theoretical frameworks of concept learning. There is no ultimate answer to the question of which kind of theory—behaviorist, cognitive, or some other—gives the best account of concept formation. The choice between approaches must be made on more general grounds, such as comprehensiveness, simplicity, and usefulness. The type of research that behaviorists have conducted has been more fruitful and on the whole has been more tightly designed and executed.

Attitudes toward cognitive psychology have improved greatly in recent years because of such factors as high visibility and the readability of cognitive theorists like Bruner and the increased believability of the information-processing model accompanying the rise of computer technology. Scholars from other disciplines, such as mathematics and hard sciences, have given a boost to cognitive psychology because they have been involved in school curriculum reform and have

attempted to rationalize innovations with an appeal to psychology.

APPLICATION TO NURSING EDUCATION AND PRACTICE

Whether teaching a student or a patient, the nurse needs to be aware of the nature of the material. Are concepts being taught? If they are, then the terminal behavior of the student or patient will be when the learner is able to identify an object class. Demonstration may not be necessary—only correct identification of new examples of the concept. This expected behavior must also be communicated to the learner. For example, with the concept of proper body alignment, can the student identify a patient in proper body alignment or not in proper body alignment?

Also, because concept learning requires verbal chains and discriminations as a prerequisite, the teacher needs to be aware of the entering level of the learner. For example, in discussing foods high in sodium with a patient, the nurse must assess whether the patient understands what sodium is? Does the patient connect it with salt? Can the patient tell the difference between salty and sweet foods?

As a teacher, the nurse also needs to be aware of the type of concepts being taught. If the material is concepts by observation, then it will be necessary to provide concrete examples of the concept. Learning experiences should provide a class of concrete situations because in order to be accurate tools for thinking about and dealing with the real world concepts must be referable to actual stimulus reactions. Not only should the teacher provide positive examples of the concept, but also negative examples of the concept. In the example of body alignment, the instructor might show the students several examples of proper body alignment in patients in different positions (sitting, bending, lying), then show them examples of improper body alignment. To test if the students understand the concept, the teacher then might ask them to point out a patient who is in proper body alignment.

If the nurse, as a teacher, is teaching concepts by definition, then the method of teaching might differ. A carefully constructed sequence of instruction involving verbal communication would be used. However, testing for evidence of learning would be the same—correct identification of new examples of the concept. For example, the concept of arrest, whether cardiac or respiratory, would be similar. The attributes are cessation of breathing, heart beat, or both. Concrete examples might be hard to provide here, but simulated experiences could be provided with other students playing roles. Again, identification of the concept is required.

If the concept is very complex with many attributes to be learned, the nurse, as a teacher, might reduce the number of attributes to be learned and make important attributes dominant. For example, in teaching about arrhythmias, the teacher could stress the most common disturbances and could group them according to similar causes, similar characteristics, or common effects on the heartbeat.

As a teacher, the nurse must also decide whether to teach for initial learning of a few responses or for retention and transfer. This will effect the teaching methodology employed (that is, rule and example versus guided discovery). If guided discovery is chosen, then the instructor must decide on useful verbal mediators relevant to the material with which to provide the student.

The nurse who is teaching children must also keep in mind that the learning of concepts is related to the intellectual development of the child (that is, concrete thinking versus hypotheticodeductive and propositional thinking).

RESEARCHABLE QUESTIONS

1. What is the effect of self-generated versus teacher-generated examples (positive or negative) on (1) the speed of learning of concepts, (2) the retention of concepts, and (3) the transfer of concepts?
   a. Independent variable: self-generated versus teacher-generated examples (positive or negative)
   b. Dependent variables: the speed of concept learning, the retention of learned concepts, and the transfer of concepts
2. What is the effect of verbal versus pictorial cues (mediators) on (1) the speed of concept learning, (2) the retention of concepts, and (3) the transfer of concepts?
   a. Independent variable: verbal versus: pictorial cues (mediators)
   b. Dependent variables: the speed of concept learning, the retention of learned concepts, and the transfer of concepts

ADDITIONAL LEARNING EXPERIENCES—RECOMMENDED READING LIST

DeCecco, J. *The psychology of learning and instruction: educational psychology.* (1st Ed.) Englewood Cliffs, N.J.: Prentice-Hall, Inc., 1968.

DeCecco, J., and Crawford, W. *The psychology of learning and instruction: educational psychology.* (2nd Ed.) Englewood Cliffs, N.J.: Prentice-Hall, Inc., 1974, pp. 385-427.

Gagne, R. The learning of principles. In H. J. Klausmeier and C. W. Harris (Eds.), *Analyses of concept learning.* New York: Academic Press, Inc., 1966.

Gagne, R. *The conditions of learning.* (2nd Ed.) New York: Holt, Rinehart and Winston, Inc., 1970, pp. 51-65, 171-194.

Gagne, R., and Brown, L. T. Some factors in programming of conceptual learning. *Journal of Experimental Psychology,* 1961, 4:355-365.

Hilgard, E. R., Irvine, R. P., and Whipple J. E. Rote memorization, understanding and transfer: an extension of Katona's card-ticket experiments. *Journal of Experimental Psychology,* 1953, 46:288-292.

Hunt, E. B. *Concept learning: an information processing problem.* New York: John Wiley & Sons, Inc., 1966.

Klausmeier, H. J., and Harris, C. W. *Analyses of concept learning.* New York: Academic Press, Inc., 1966.

Osler, S. F., and Trottmen, G. E. Concept attainment: II. Effect of stimulus complexity upon concept attainment at two levels of intelligence. *Journal of Experimental Psychology,* 1961, **62**:9-13.

Shulman, L. S., and Keislar, E. R. (Eds.) *Learning by discovery: a critical appraisal.* Chicago: Rand McNally & Co., 1966.

Wittrock, M. C., Verbal stimuli in concept formation: learning by discovery. *Journal of Educational Psychology,* 1963, **54**(4):183-190.

Wittrock, M. C. The learning by discovery hypothesis. In L. S. Shulman and E. R. Keislar (Eds.), *Learning by discovery: a critical appraisal.* Chicago: Rand McNally & Co., 1966.

Wittrock, M. C., Keislar, E. R., and Stern, C. Verbal cues in concept identification. *Journal of Educational Psychology,* 1964, **55**(4):195-200.

INSTRUCTIONS TO THE LEARNER REGARDING POSTTEST

At this stage you are ready to take the posttest to determine the extent to which you have achieved the objectives. Return to the pretest and take the same test again as the posttest. Correct your answers using the answer key found on this page. You need to achieve 24 correct points (95% level) to proceed to the next module. If your score is less than 24 correct points, study the text again and correct your errors. Also, read some of the articles found in the recommended reading list. You need to study this module until you achieve a 95% level of mastery or better.

ANSWER KEY TO PRETEST AND POSTTEST

1. True (DeCecco, 1968, p. 400)
2. False (Gagne, 1970, p. 172)
3. False (Gagne, 1970, pp. 172, 187)
4. False (Gagne, 1970, p. 180)
5. False (DeCecco, 1968, p. 388)
6. a (DeCecco, 1968, p. 388)
7. b (Gagne, 1970, p. 177)
8. a (Gagne, 1970, p. 183)
9. e (DeCecco, 1968, p. 390)
10. c (Gagne, 1970, p. 182)
11. c (Wittrock, Keislar, and Stern, 1964, pp. 195-200)
12. a (DeCecco, 1968, p. 408)
13. a (DeCecco, 1968, p. 389)
14. a and d (Gagne, 1970, pp. 181, 182)
15. c (DeCecco, 1968, p. 392)
16. c and f (DeCecco, 1968, pp. 391-392)
17. a and d (DeCecco, 1968, pp. 391-392)
18. b (DeCecco, 1968, pp. 391-392)
19. a and d (Gagne, 1970, p. 172)
20. e (Gagne, 1970, p. 172)
21. g (DeCecco, 1968, p. 389)
22. First, tell the child that he will be expected to name and identify carbohydrate foods. Define which attributes of carbohydrates that you want learned, such as sweet, breadlike, and others. Make sure that the child understands the meaning of the words chosen to represent the attributes. Show the child in pictures or actuality foods that are carbohydrates and those that are not. Present the examples in close succession. Show the child a different example and ask for it to be named. Then show a variety of foods, some positive and some negative examples of carbohydrates and ask that the carbohydrates be identified. Have the child define in words the concept of carbohydrates. Set up practice situations for choosing foods to reinforce the knowledge. (DeCecco, 1968, pp. 402-415; Gagne, 1970, pp. 171-172)
23. a. By distinguishing among them
    b. By putting things into a class and responding to the class as a whole (Gagne, 1970, pp. 171-172)
24. An individual responding to a class of observable objects or qualities that can be named or observed—color, shape, size, cat, girl, and so on—is referring to concepts by observation. An individual describing the relationship between two concepts is referring to concept by definition (abstraction); examples are physical concepts such as mass and temperature, language concepts of subject, and mathematical concepts such as square root and prime numbers (Gagne, 1970, p. 172).
25. a. Tells the students what performance is expected of them after they learn the concept

(to be able to identify a laceration from other types of wounds)

b. Identifies two important attributes of a laceration: (1) a wound (2) made by tearing

c. Gives students useful verbal mediators to help them pick out lacerations from other wounds (cues like "jagged," "ripped," or others)

d. Gives students positive and negative examples of the concept; laceration examples plus any other kinds of wounds that may confuse the student must be presented and explained

e. Presents examples of lacerations and other wounds simultaneously or in succession

f. Asks students to identify a new positive example of a laceration—to provide contiguity and reinforcement

g. Verifies students' learning by giving both positive and negative examples of lacerations for students to identify only the positive examples

h. Has students define a laceration

i. Provides actual clinical experience in identifying lacerations as opposed to other wounds and gives more reinforcement (such as emergency room experience) (DeCecco, 1968, pp. 402-415)

REFERENCES

Anderson, R. C. Introduction. In R. C. Anderson and D. P. Ausubel (Eds.), *Readings in the psychology of cognition.* New York: Holt, Rinehart and Winston, Inc. 1966, pp. 395-405.

Archer, J. E. The psychological nature of concepts. In H. J. Klausmeier and C. W. Harris (Eds.), *Analyses of Concept Learning.* New York: Academic Press, Inc., 1966, pp. 37-49.

Ausubel, D. P. Introduction. In R. C. Anderson and D. P. Ausubel (Eds.), *Readings in the psychology of cognition.* New York: Holt, Rinehart and Winston, Inc. 1966, pp. 3-17.

Bruner, J. S., Goodnow, J. J., and Austin, G. A. *A study of thinking.* New York: John Wiley & Sons, Inc., 1956.

Bruner, J. S., and Olver, R. R. *Development of equivalence transformation in children.* Monograph of the Society for Research in Child Development, 1963, **28**(whole #86):125-141.

Carpenter, F. Conceptualization as a function of differential reinforcement. *Science Education,* 1954, **38**: 284-294.

Carroll, J. B. Words, meanings and concepts. *Harvard Educational Review,* 1964, **34**:178-202.

DeCecco, J. P. *The psychology of learning and instruction: educational psychology.* (1st Ed.) Englewood Cliffs, N. J.: Prentice-Hall, Inc., 1968.

DeCecco, J., and Crawford, W. *The psychology of learning and instruction: educational psychology.* (2nd Ed.) Englewood Cliffs, N.J.: Prentice-Hall, Inc., 1974.

Flavell, J. H. *The developmental theory of Jean Piaget.* New York: Van Nostrand Reinhold Co., 1963.

Gagne, R. *The conditions of learning.* (2nd Ed.) New York: Holt, Rinehart and Winston, Inc., 1970.

Hovland, C. I. Computer simulation of thinking. In R. C. Anderson and D. P. Ausubel (Eds.), *Readings in the psychology of cognition.* New York: Holt, Rinehart and Winston, Inc. 1966, pp. 158-172.

Hull, C. L. Quantitative aspects of the evolution of concepts. *Psychological Monograph,* 1920, **28**(1): 1-86.

Huttenlocker, J. Some effects of negative instances on the formation of simple concepts. *Psychological Reports,* 1962, **11**:pp. 35-42.

Johnson, D. M., and O'Reilly, C. A. Concept attainment in children: classifying and defining. *Journal of Educational Psychology,* 1964 **55**:71-74.

Kates, S. L., and Yudin, L. Concept attainment and memory. *Journal of Educational Psychology,* 1964, **55**:103-109.

Kendler, H. H. The concept of the concept. In A. W. Melton (Ed.), *Categories of Human Learning.* New York: Academic Press, Inc., 1964, pp. 211-236.

Kendler, H. H., and D'Amato, M. F. A comparison of reversal shifts in human concept formation. *Journal of Experimental Psychology,* 1955, **4**:165-174.

Kendler, H. H., and Karasik, A. D. Concept formation as a function of competition between response-produced cues. *Journal of Experimental Psychology,* 1958, **55**:278-283.

Klausmeier, J. H., and Harris, C. W. *Analyses of concept learning.* New York: Academic Press, Inc., 1966.

McDonald, F. J. *Educational psychology.* (2nd Ed.) Belmont, Calif.: Wadsworth Publishing Co., Inc., 1965.

Miller, G. A., Gallanter, E. H., and Pribram, K. H. *Plans and the structure of behavior.* New York: Holt, Rinehart and Winston, Inc., 1960.

Mowrer, O. H. The psychologist looks at language. *American Journal of Psychology,* 1954, **9**:660-694.

Newell, A., Simon, H. A., and Shaw, J. C. Elements of a theory of human problem solving. In R. C. Anderson and D. P. Ausubel (Eds.), *Readings in the Psychology of Cognition,* New York: Holt, Rinehart and Winston, Inc., 1966, pp. 133-157.

Osgood, C. E. *Method and theory in experimental psychology.* New York: Oxford University Press, 1953.

Piaget, J. How children form mathematical concepts. In R. C. Anderson and D. P. Ausubel (Eds.), *Readings in the Psychology of Cognition.* New York: Holt, Rinehart and Winston, Inc., 1966, pp. 406-414.

Rhine, R. J., and Silun B. A. Acquisition and change of a concept attitude as a function of consistency of reinforcement. *Journal of Experimental Psychology,* 1958, **55**:524-529.

Sax, G. Concept acquisition as a function of differing schedules and delays of reinforcement. *Journal of Educational Psychology,* 1960, **51**:32-36.

Staats, A. W. Verbal habit-families, concepts, and the operant conditioning of word classes. In R. C. Anderson and D. P. Ausubel (Eds.), *Readings in the Psychology of Cognition,* New York: Holt, Rinehart and Winston, Inc., 1966, pp. 18-40.

Stern, C. Labeling and variety in concept identification with young children. *Journal of Educational Psychology,* 1965, **56**:235-240.

Wilder, N., and Green, D. R. Expressions of concepts through writing and drawing and effects of shifting medium. *Journal of Experimental Psychology,* 1963, **54**:202-207.

Wittrock, M. C. Verbal stimuli in concept formation: learning by discovery. *Journal of Educational Psychology,* 1963, **64**:183-190.

Wittrock, M. C. Three conceptual approaches to research on transfer of training. Unpublished article. University of California, Los Angeles, Oct. 1966.

Wittrock, M. C., and Keislar, E. Verbal cues in the transfer of concepts. *Journal of Educational Psychology,* 1965, **56**:16-21.

Wittrock, M. C., Keislar, E., and Stern, C. Verbal cues in concept identification. *Journal of Educational Psychology,* 1964, **55**:195-200.

Principle learning

DESCRIPTION OF MODULE

Principle learning is the seventh condition of learning. The content of this module on principle learning is presented in sequential order and in an integrated form. The five essential areas that are discussed are: theoretical framework, relevant research studies conducted in the field, issues, application to nursing education and practice, and researchable questions. The module also contains a set of behavioral objectives to be accomplished by the learner and a pre- and posttest to measure the degree of accomplishment of the objectives. The answer key to the pretest and posttest is also provided.

MODULE OBJECTIVES

At the completion of this module, and having read and studied the required reading materials, the student should be able to accomplish the following objectives at the 95% level of achievement:

1. Define verbally or in written form what principle learning is
2. Differentiate between concrete concept, abstract concept, and defined or relational concepts
3. Describe the theoretical framework of principle learning as described by Gagne and DeCecco

4. Identify the internal conditions of principle learning
5. Identify the external conditions of principle learning
6. Identify and implement the essential steps of teaching principle learning to a specific nursing situation
7. Identify at least one issue in principle learning and state its good and bad aspects
8. Apply the principles of rule learning to nursing education and nursing practice
9. Formulate a researchable hypothesis in the area of principle learning and identify both the dependent and independent variables
10. Identify the hierarchy of concepts and principles when given specific nursing concepts or principles within a course, such as sterile technique, carbohydrate diet, and so on.

PRETEST AND POSTTEST

Circle the correct answers. Each question is worth 1 point except the last two. Question 11 is worth 2 points and question 12 is worth 8 points. The 95% level of mastery equals 19 points for this test. On completion of the test correct your answers using the answer key found at the end of this module (p. 122).

True or false

1. Principle learning is affected by interference to the same degree as other types of learning. True or False
2. Simpler kinds of learning (verbal chains and multiple discriminations) are retained for longer periods of time than are the more complex types of learning (concepts and rules). True or False

Multiple choice

3. In order to determine whether an individual has acquired a principle, the individual should:
   a. only verbally state the definition of the principle
   b. be asked to apply the principle
   c. practice the principle consistently
   d. supply an instance of the principle, that is, give a positive example
   e. all of the above
4. Rule learning is:
   a. similar to simple forms of Ss → R chaining
   b. chaining of concepts
   c. concerned with several concrete concepts
   d. exemplified by the word "catheter"
5. Which of the following are relational concepts?
   a. a patient
   b. health
   c. diagonal
   d. hospital
6. The internal condition for principle learning is:
   a. to be able to discriminate between simple chaining and more complex chaining forms
   b. to have as entering behavior knowledge of component concepts that formulate the rule
   c. to have knowledge of at least one of the key concepts that constitutes the rule
   d. to be able to classify stimuli into a class
7. Practice conditions for learning of principles are:
   a. not essential because rule learning is a higher form of learning
   b. essential with all types of learning, including rule learning

c. useful when the learning of one principle interferes with the retention of another
   d. dependent on the learner's capabilities
8. The role of reinforcement in principle learning:
   a. is not as essential as in simpler forms of learning
   b. should be given when the learner is trying to recall the individual component concepts
   c. should be given when the learner demonstrates the principle in its complete form
   d. should only be self-generated when matching the terminal act with the set criteria
9. The teaching of abstract concepts:
   a. should be given to children 7 years old and up
   b. should be reserved for those children who have reached the formal operations stage of development
   c. cannot be used with children in the concrete operational stage of development
10. Identify the proper sequencing hierarchy of principles involved in the scientific method, which is also referred to the problem-solving process:
    1—assessment
    2—intervention, or testing of hypothesis
    3—evaluation, or verification of hypothesis
    4—collection of data
    5—implementation of changes
    6—diagnosis of the problem, or formulation of hypothesis
    a. 1, 2, 3, 4, 5, 6
    b. 6, 5, 4, 3, 2, 1
    c. 4, 1, 6, 2, 3, 5
    d. 1, 4, 6, 3, 2, 5
11. "If digitalis 0.25 mg is to be administered to an adult patient, then pulse rate of the patient should be above 60 pulses per minute." In this example of a principle, identify the component concepts that the student nurse should have as entering behavior, that is, as internal conditions.
12. If you were a nursing instructor, what is the principle to be taught in question 11 and how would you teach it to a freshman nursing student? To narrow the learning task let us assume that you first will teach how to take a

pulse and count it correctly. Identify each essential step of teaching any principle and apply them to the above situation.

TEXT
Theoretical framework
Introduction

A *principle* is defined as the relationship between two or more concepts (DeCecco 1968, p. 393). Gagne (1970, p. 191) defines it as "an inferred capability that enables the individual to respond to a class of stimulus situations with a class of performances."

Principles are also called *rules*. When students are able to apply a rule, their behavior is said to be rule governed, and they are said to have learned the rule because they respond regularly to a large class of specific situations, that is they *apply* the rule. Principles are the primary organizing factors of intellectual functioning. Rules guide the individual's behavior in meeting a variety of particular situations and in solving problems. This means that most observed human behaviors are principle governed. This enables people to be subjected to a tremendous amount and variety of sensory input and still function effectively.

Since a rule is composed of several concepts, in order to be able to learn the rule an individual must have as entering behavior the capability of identifying the component concepts that are to be chained and of demonstrating that these concepts relate to one another in a particular manner. Therefore, knowledge of the individual concepts within a principle is prerequisite to learning a principle. It should be emphasized that rule learning is a *chaining of concepts*, not the more simplistic Ss → R chaining of Gagne's third condition, or type, of learning.

There are many types of principles, depending on their content. Rules may be composed of *defined concepts*, which serve "the purpose of distinguishing among different ideas, and they may be capabilities that enable the individual to respond to specific situations by applying classes of relations" (Gagne, 1970, p. 193). A "defined" concept is operationally defined as the type of concept that is not concrete, cannot be observed. It is an abstract concept and is learned by *definition*. In other words, in defined concepts, the individual uses a rule in order to *identify* something that itself embodies a relation. For example, the concepts of health, fatigue, and worry are defined concepts. Defined concepts may also be called relational concepts because they do relate two or more simpler concepts; for example the concept of health represents a relation between concepts of "absence of illness" and "feelings of being well." In nursing science, the student learns many rules having the form of defined concepts, like those of adaptation, insufficiency, dominance, assessment, and many others that relate these concepts. Rules, therefore, may vary in such properties as abstractness and complexity, although the dimensions of these characteristics have not been made specific.

A principle can be explained in the form, "if A, then B" where A and B are previously learned concepts, and a correct sequence is learned. This kind of learning is most broadly used in formal education. To be considered educated, humans must learn many *ideas* (principles), such as "gases expand when heated." Gagne uses the word idea to show that this is not rote memorization. It is important to remember this distinction between Gagne's fourth step (verbal association) and the seventh step (principle learning). Through verbal chaining (step 4), the statement ("gases expand when heated") could be learned. However, if this is the type of learning that has taken place, then the learner's performance would be limited. The learner would only be able to answer a true or false statement about what happens when gases are heated or to complete the statement, "When gases are heated_____." To learn the principle involved, the student must already know certain concepts about gases, molecules, and heat. Understanding the principle means being able to *demonstrate* this knowledge by knowing why not to throw aerosol cans into fires or why it is important to know where the oxygen shut-off is in case of a fire. This ability to give examples and apply the rules differentiates between the student who has learned a principle and one who is using verbal chaining only. Verbal statements are usually part of the process of principle learning, but principle learning is not required for verbal association to take place.

Principle learning cannot be accomplished by simply ignoring all other types of learning. This kind of learning is possible only because it has been preceded by the acquisition of learning sets from the most simple classical conditioning through concept learning.

Conditions of principle learning
INTERNAL CONDITIONS

The learner must have as entering behavior knowledge of the component concepts that constitute the principle. In other words, the prerequisite for learning rules that are made up of chains of concepts is knowing the concepts. For example "gases expand when heated" can be learned as a rule when the learner has already learned all three concepts—gases, expansion, and heat. If the learner knows only two of these concepts, then the rule learning and its application will be inadequate.

As Gagne (1970, p. 200) points out, "knowing the concepts means being able to identify any member of the class by name. It is only when such prerequisite concepts have been mastered that a rule can be learned with full adequacy. Otherwise there is

danger that the conceptual chain, or some parts of it, will become merely a verbal chain, without the full meaning that inheres in a well-established rule."

EXTERNAL CONDITIONS

Verbal instructions constitute the major external conditions of principle learning. DeCecco (1968) referred to these external conditions as strategies in teaching principles and cited eight steps. He considers all of them to be crucial.*

1. Specify the general nature of the performance that is expected when learning is completed. This step allows the learners to monitor their own performance and to generate their own reinforcement. This step is like a statement of learner objectives; for example, the completion of instruction the student will apply the principle of "gases expand when heated."

2. Decide and indicate which concepts and principles the student must recall in learning the new principle. The teacher must analyze the principle to determine what the component concepts of the principle are and must assess the stduent's entering behavior to determine if these concepts have been mastered. Kendler and Vineberg's (1954) study supported this recommendation that knowing the component concepts is essential in learning the principle. Results of this study showed that the group that knew all of the component concepts required twenty three trials to learn the test concept, whereas the second group that knew only one of the two component concepts required twice as many trials as the first group to learn the test concept. The third group that did not know either of the two concepts required four times as many trials as the first group.

Gagne recommends that the teacher ask

---

*Gagne (1970) considers the external conditions only to be those mentioned in steps 1, 3, 4, 5, and 8.

the following in order to determine the pre-requisites for any given question: "What does the student have to know in order to be instructed in the principle?" It is important that teachers do task analysis before presenting a principle to students. In the case of the component concepts, the teacher must determine which concepts the students should know before teaching them the principle. Similarly, in the case of higher-order principles the teacher must determine which lower-order principles the student must recall. The teacher can do this task analysis by asking the above-mentioned question. In the previous example, the student should know the component concepts of gases, expansion, and heat. Other related concepts and lower-order principles that the student should know are, molecules, the behavior of molecules when heated, types of gases that are volatile, and so on.

3. **Assist the student in the recall of component concepts.** In other words, verbal instructions continue by *invoking recall of the component concepts.* The teacher needs to provide contiguity by having the student simultaneously recall the component concepts. For example, the teacher may say "Do you remember what gases are? . . . Do you remember what heat does? . . . Do you remember how molecules act when heated?" In most cases, the recall of component concepts can be done by verbal means. Pictures also can be used to help the student recall the important concepts.

4. **Use verbal statements (cues) that will help the learner combine the concepts in proper order (as a chain of concepts) to formulate the rule.** This step requires that verbal instruction provide contiguity of concepts and for the proper relationship of the concepts. The student will need guidance (cueing) in putting the relevant concepts in proper order to formulate the rule. It is not enough to instruct "order the concepts prop-

erly." For example, the teacher may say, "Now tell me why we do not throw aerosol cans, such as hair spray cans, into the fire?" The student should respond, "Because the left-over pressured gas may expand when heated and explode." The teacher should then reinforce the student enthusiastically by saying, "That's correct."

5. **Ask the student to demonstrate the principle fully.** Both Gagne and DeCecco emphasize the importance of having the student demonstrate a grasp of the principle to the teacher. One way this can be done is by asking the student to give positive and negative examples of the application of the principles. For example, the teacher may give the names of ten different molecules of gases and metals and ask the student to indicate which of these molecules are gases and which should not be heated.

6. **Ask the learner to give a full statement of the principle.** Gagne points out that this step is not essential for rule learning itself, but it is useful for later instruction. The teacher can use verbal mediators to elicit the definition; for example, the teacher may ask, "What happens when gases are heated?" The student should respond, "Gases expand when heated."

7. **Verify the student's learning of the principle.** In order to ensure that the student has not given the teacher the "rote definition" of the rule, the teacher needs to ask the student to apply the rule to new situations; for example, as mentioned in step 5, the student may be asked to identify the positive examples when given a list of both positive and negative examples of the rule. The verification process provides an opportunity for the teacher to assess how well the new capability has been established.

8. **Provide for contiguity, reinforcement, and practice.** *Contiguity* is an important condition applicable to the time interval between the recall of component concepts and

the verbal cueing of the rules with these parts properly sequenced.

Reinforcement is provided when the principle is demonstrated in its complete form. Reinforcement may be given either by the instructor, as "That's correct," when the student demonstrates the correct application of the principle, or the student can generate self-reinforcement by matching the terminal act with the set criteria (objective) or with a form remembered from initial instruction (step 1).

Repetition, or practice, has not been found to be essential for principle learning or retention (Gagne and Bassler, 1963); however, the possible need for reinforced practice of a principle is crucial when the learning of one principle interferes with the retention of other. The study conducted by Entwisle and Huggins (1964) found that beginning engineering students who studied voltage principles first and the corresponding current principles immediately following retained less of what they had learned than when they studied the principles of voltage alone. These researchers also found that learning several principles of electrical circuits interfered with retention of the rules and caused forgetting. Based on these findings DeCecco (1968) point out the need for both proper sequencing of the subject matter and reinforced practice of potentially confusing principles.

Other characteristics of principle learning
HIERARCHIES OF RULES

Rules are not learned in isolation, except by very young children. Adults learn related sets of rules pertaining to a large topic. What they learn is an *organized set of intellectual skills.* The rules that compose the set may be related to one another in a logical sense. They are also related psychologically, referring to the learning of some rules as prerequisites to the learning of others (Gagne 1970).

The psychological organization of intellectual skills may be represented as a *learning hierarchy,* often composed of large set of rules. Two or more concepts may compose a rule, therefore, they are prerequisite conditions (subordinate levels of knowledge) that the individual should have in learning that single principle. Similarly, two or more rules may join together to formulate a higher-order rule, therefore, the subordinate rules are prerequisite for learning the higher-order rule. The entire set of rules, organized in this way, forms a learning hierarchy that describes and generally determines the efficient route to attainment of an organized set of intellectual skills that represent understanding of a topic (Gagne, 1970, p. 206). It also determines the sequence of learning tasks ranging from the simple (subordinate level of knowledge) to the complex (superordinate level of knowledge and rules).

Evidence for the hierarchical nature of learning was provided by Gagne and Associates (1965). They tested to see what happens when learners actually undertake to acquire a set of rules that appear to have a hierarchial structure and if mastery of one set actually affects the learning of the next "higher" set, as would be expected. These expectations were listed with sixth graders who were asked to learn nonmetric geometry definitions from a booklet that was prepared as a self-instructional program. The material was carefully sequenced so that the concepts were prepared and ranged from levels one to four, depending on their complexity. Students were asked to learn the concepts at the bottom of the hierarchy first, then the second, third, and fourth, until the final task was given as a terminal exercise. Results showed that the learning of higher-level rules was dependent on the mastery of prerequisite lower-level rules in a highly predictable fashion.

The learning of organized intellectual skills, according to these results, seems to be predictable from the *pattern of prerequisite rules* that make up the hierarchy of skills to be acquired (Gagne, 1970, p. 207). These findings have also been verified by several other studies (Gagne and Paradise, 1961; Gagne and Bassler, 1963).

Determining the prerequisites for any given rule may be accomplished by asking the following question, "What would the student have to know how to do in order to be instructed in this rule?"

Gagne (1970, p. 208) also posed the question, "If all the prerequisite rules are known, does this mean that the higher-order rule is immediately known also?" The answer is no, because, just knowing the prerequisite rules is not enough, and the rule has to be learned. Knowledge of subordinate categories of knowledge fulfills the criteria that the student possesses the entering behaviors, that is the conditions within the learner are satisfied but not the conditions of the learning situation. There must be appropriate *instruction* that (1) informs the learner about the expected performance—the objectives, (2) encourages recall, and (3) cues the proper sequence of acts, as described in previous sections.

RETENTION OF RULES OR PRINCIPLES

There is a marked difference between forgetting the simpler forms of learned capabilities, such as chains and multiple discriminations, and forgetting of the more complex capabilities, such as concepts and rules. Concepts and principles have shown marked resistance to forgetting and are frequently remembered with little loss over periods of months and years (Gagne, 1970).

Katona's (1940) study has shown that subjects who learned just the verbal statement of the principles forgot most of them within a month. Those subjects who learned the rules and were able to demonstrate them retained almost all of the rules after the same interval.

Briggs and Reed's (1943) study also showed

that retention of factual details in prose passages was poorer than retention of ideas, that is, rules. Furthermore, many other studies of rules and organized sets of rules that occur in school learning have shown marked resistance to forgetting over periods of months (Ausubel, 1968, pp. 111-115).

Of course the interference factor that produces forgetting in other forms of learning also causes forgetting of rules. However, according to Gagne (1970) the organized nature of rules appears to resist the effects of interference and to maintain retention at high levels. However, research conducted by Entwisle and Huggins (1964) found that confusing principles learned by engineering students on voltages and electrical circuits interfered with retention of the principles. The major practical implication that is pointed out by Gagne is that in general, learning of rules produces understanding and establishes a capability that is retained over a long period of time.

DEVELOPMENTAL DETERMINATION—LIMITS IMPOSED BY INTELLECTUAL DEVELOPMENT

The learning of principles requires the student to engage in *abstract thought* process. According to Piaget, the stage of development determines the level of thought of which a child is capable. For example, children from the ages of 7 to 11 years are classified as being in the period of *concrete operations*. During this period, children's thinking is oriented toward concrete objects in the immediate environment. They relinquish the physical attributes of objects one by one, and each grouping remains an isolated organization.

During the period of *formal operations* (ages 12 years and up), children's thought processes can handle the possible as well as the real. They are capable of hypotheticodeductive and propositional thinking. Children in this age group can handle principles as well as concepts since principles are a form of if-then statements and are a form of propositional and hypotheticodeductive thinking. During the period of formal operations, students are capable of thinking in terms of possible combinations of concepts in an orderly and systematic way.

It would appear therefore that the younger child in the period of concrete operations is not capable of engaging in abstract thought process, but the older child in the period of formal operations is. Even though teaching can contribute to the development of abstract thought in both periods of development, the rigors of abstract thought process should be reserved for older children (De Cecco, 1968).

Use of principles

DeCecco (1968, pp. 398-399) cite three major uses of principles:

1. *Principles reduce the necessity of constant learning.* In school settings the learning of principles enables students to progress through a discipline, acquiring increasing amounts of knowledge.

2. *Principles provide direction for instrumental activity.* By using concepts and principles, we know in advance the actions to be taken, which enables us to solve problems.

3. *Principles make instruction possible.* The steps described for teaching principles are largely embodied in a set of verbal instructions. It would not be possible to instruct a student who had not already acquired some concepts and principles.

Application to nursing education and practice

Each of the eight steps that were described and illustrated as external conditions of principle learning are teaching strategies that should be applied in the teaching of principles to students and patients. Any teaching to patients or students should stress the underlying principles that are involved in the learning task, since principles are retained longer than any factual information. It is especially important to find out what the entering behavior of the patient or student is, that is, what level of knowledge is possessed prior to instruction.

Once the entering behavior of the student is determined then the following teaching steps or strategies can be applied to ensure that the student or patient "understands" the concepts and the principles of the learning task—whether it is determination of "what categories of foods are allowed in a diabetic diet," "how to maintain good circulation in the leg," or "how to transfer ounces to milliliters."

The essential steps that DeCecco and Gagne recommend in teaching principles that can be applied to any learning situations are:

1. Describe the performance expected of the student or patient, that is, state the objective

2. Decide and indicate which concepts or principles the student or patient must recall in learning the new principle. (This the teacher can do by asking Gagne's basic question, "What does the learner have to know in order to be instructed in this principle?" By utilizing this questioning tool, the instructor can determine the sequence of the content and principles to be taught to the patient or student, remembering that "lower-order" principles must be learned before "higher-order" principles can be taught.)

3. Assist the student or patient in the recall of the component concepts by means of cueing and the use of mediators.

4. Help the student or patient combine the concepts in the proper order by the aid of cues and mediators

5. Require the student or patient to demonstrate the principle fully by applying the principle to new but similar situations

6. Require the student or patient to state the principle fully, that is, to define it verbally

7. Verify the student's learning of con-

cepts by asking the learner to apply the principle to other situations

8. Provide for contiguity, practice of principles, and reinforcement of correct responses

The application of Gagne's basic question in determining which principles are of lower level and which are superordinate is extremely applicable to nursing education, especially in determining the proper sequencing of contents and courses within the curriculum. The same strategy also applies in sequencing a course or a lesson plan. This basic question is also a valid tool in assessing the entering behavior of students or patients in learning a specific task.

It is almost impossible to enumerate the implications of the important principle of rule learning in teaching of concepts and principles to patients and students. Every teacher can and should apply the basic points that are illustrated in this module.

Issues in principle learning

One of the major issues in teaching of principles is the method of instruction, that is, what is the best way to accomplish *principle learning*? One group says that the principles need to be discovered by the individual student. Gagne believes that, provided students have learned the required concepts, telling them the principle is much quicker and perhaps as effective.

The second issue deals with whether to limit the teaching of principles to the formal operational stage of development or also to teach him to younger age groups. Piaget (1966) and his followers argue that intellectual development is age related. Until the children reach the age of formal operations (12 years and up) they are not capable of abstract thinking. The other school of thought, however, insists that it is possible to teach abstract concepts and principles to younger children, if the content matter can be brought down to their level. For example,

the study conducted by Wittrock (1963) showed that younger children were able to learn the molecular nuclear theory. Also the study by Gelman (1967) demonstrated the learning of relational concepts and conservation of volume by younger children.

Researchable questions

1. An exploratory study might be to determine the hierarchy of basic principles of nursing taught in baccalaureate nursing programs.

2. What is the effect of the use of mediators—cues (teacher-delivered versus self-generated)—on the recall of the component concepts of a principle?

   a. Independent variable: the use of mediators (cues)—teacher delivered or self-generated

   b. Dependent variable: recall of the component concepts of a principle

3. What is the effect of inductive versus deductive teaching strategy on the speed of learning and retention of principles?

   a. Independent variables: inductive versus deductive teaching strategy

   b. Dependent variables: speed of learning and retention of principles

ADDITIONAL LEARNING EXPERIENCES—RECOMMENDED READING LIST

DeCecco, J. *The psychology of learning and instruction: educational psychology.* (1st Ed.) Englewood Cliffs, N.J.: Prentice-Hall, Inc. 1968, pp. 385-427.

DeCecco J., and Crawford, W. *The psychology of learning and instruction: educational psychology.* (2nd Ed.) Englewood Cliffs, N.J.: Prentice-Hall, Inc., 1974, pp. 287-323.

Gagne, R. *The conditions of learning.* N.Y.: Holt, Rinehart and Winston, Inc., 1970, pp. 56-59, 189-213.

INSTRUCTIONS TO THE LEARNER REGARDING POSTTEST

Having completed studying this module, you are now ready to take the posttest to determine the extent to which you have

Essential steps of teaching principles	Application to specific situation
1. Describe the performance expected of the student after the principles have been learned	1. At the completion of instruction, the freshman nursing student will be able to locate correctly sites where the pulse of the patient can be felt and count it correctly for 1 minute.
2. Decide and indicate which concepts or principles the student must recall in learning the new principle.	2. As entering behavior, the student must have the concepts of: a. Pulse—anatomy and physiology b. Time: 1 minute = 60 seconds c. Ability to hear, feel, and see correctly
3. Assist the student in the recall of the component concepts	3. To help students recall the component concepts, the teacher may: a. Make statements such as: "You know what the heart does." "You know which blood vessels carry the blood to the parts of the body." "You know where arteries are located that are superficial and can be felt." b. Show pictures of the circulatory system
4. Help the student combine the concepts in the proper order	4. The teacher provides contiguity of concepts and for the proper relationship of concepts; it is not enough to ask the student to order the concepts properly—teacher's questioning should guide the ordering. For example, the teacher may say, "Now I want you to tell me under what anatomical conditions can a pulse be felt?" and the student should respond, "Whenever arteries come to the surface, such as just under the skin so that one can feel them—or one can listen to the heart (apical pulse) directly." The teacher should then enthusiastically give feedback to the student by saying, "Correct." Next, the teacher may say, "Where do you expect the arteries to run more superficially—you may use the picture of circulatory system if you wish." The student should respond, "Near temporal area, brachial area, carotid area, dorsalis pedis, and others." The teacher should then reinforce the student by saying, "That is very good, it is correct," and so on.
5. Require the student to demonstrate the principle fully	5. The teacher may ask the student, "Show me where you can take the pulse and count the pulse rate for 1 minute."
6. Require the student to give a full statement of the principle	6. The teacher may use verbal mediators to elicit the definition, such as, "Where would you feel pulses?" The student may reply, "Pulses are felt when the artery runs superficially—close to the skin, such as the temporal area, carotid, and others." The teacher may also ask, "Could you define a pulse rate?" The student may answer, "A pulse is the number of heart beats per minute." The teacher says, "That's correct."
7. Verify the student's learning of the principle	7. The teacher may ask for the student to take the pulses of different patients utilizing different pulsation sites.
8. Provide for practice of the principle and for reinforcement of student responses	8. The student is provided with additional learning experiences of taking pulses of children, adults, normal individuals, patients with circulatory problems to the lower extremities, and others.

achieved the objectives. Return to the pretest of this module and take it again as a posttest. Correct your own posttest utilizing the answer key that is found on this page. You must score 95% correct (19 correct points) to proceed to the next module. If your score is less than 19 points, correct your errors, study those aspects you did incorrectly, and carefully read some of the articles in the recommended reading list. Study until you achieve the 95% correct level.

ANSWER KEY TO PRETEST AND POSTTEST

1. False (Gagne, 1970 p. 210)
2. False (Gagne, 1970 pp. 209-210)
3. b and d (Shulman and Keislar, p. 144; DeCecco, 1968, pp. 418-425)
4. b (Gagne, 1970 p. 193)
5. b and c (Gagne, 1970 p. 193)
6. b (Gagne, 1970 p. 200)
7. c (DeCecco, 1968, p. 424) (Gagne, 1970 p. 202)
8. c (Gagne, 1970 p. 202)
9. c (DeCecco, 1968, pp. 394-395)
10. c (Gagne, 1970 pp. 203-209)
11. Digitalis:
    a. Indications—effect of medicine
    b. Dosage—calculation of dosage
    c. Route of administration
    d. Precautuions
    Adult versus child patient
    Pulse:
    a. Anatomy and physiology of pulse and heart beat
    b. Ability to count pulses correctly
    Knowledge of time—one minute is 60 seconds, etc.
12. The principle to be taught is that if the adult patient's pulse is to be counted correctly, then correct identification of the site of pulse taking should take place and the pulse should be correctly counted. (DeCecco, 1968, pp. 418-425)
    (See boxed material opposite page.)

REFERENCES

Ausubel, D. P. *Educational psychology: a cognitive view.* New York: Holt, Rinehart and Winston, Inc. 1968.

Briggs, L. J., and Reid, H. B. The curve of retention for substance material. *Journal of Experimental Psychology*, 1943, **32**:513-517.

DeCecco, J. *The psychology of learning and instruction: educational psychology.* (1st Ed.) Englewood Cliffs, N.J.: Prentice-Hall, Inc., 1968.

DeCecco, J., and Crawford, W. *The psychology of learning and instruction: educational psychology.* (2nd Ed.) Englewood Cliffs, N. J.: Prentice-Hall, Inc., 1974.

Entwisle, D., and Huggins, W. H. Interference in meaningful learning. *Journal of Educational Psychology*, 1964, **55**:75-78.

Gagne, R. The acquisition of knowledge. *Psychological Review*, 1962, **69**:355-365.

Gagne, R. M. *The conditions of learning.* (2nd Ed.) New York: Holt, Rinehart and Winston, Inc. 1970.

Gagne, R., and Bassler, O. C. Study of retention of some topics of elementary non-metric geometry. *Journal of Educational Psychology*, 1963, **54**:123-131

Gagne, R., and Paradise, N. E. Abilities and learning sets in knowledge acquisition. *Psychological Monograph*, 1961, **75**(14):(whole No. 518).

Gagne, R., and staff, University of Maryland Mathematics Project. Some factors in learning non-metric geometry. *Monograph of Social Research Child Development*, 1965, **30**(1):42-49.

Gelman, R. S. *Conservation, attention and discrimination.* Doctoral dissertation. University of California, Los Angeles, 1967.

Katona, G. *Organizing and memorizing.* New York: Columbia University Press, 1940.

Kendler, H. H., and Vineberg, R. The acquisition of compound concepts as a function of previous training. *Journal of Experimental Psychology*, 1954, **48**:252-258.

Piaget, J. How children form mathematical concepts. In R. C. Anderson and D. P. Ausubel (Ed.) *Readings in the Psychology of Cognition.* New York: Holt, Rinehart and Winston, Inc. 1966, pp. 406-414.

Shulman, L. and Keislar, E. K. (Eds.) *Learning by discovery: a critical appraisal.* Chicago: Rand McNally and Co., 1966.

Wittrock, M. C. Response made in the programing of kinetic molecular theory concepts. *Journal of Educational Psychology*, 1963, **54**:89-93.

Problem solving

DESCRIPTION OF MODULE

Problem solving is the eighth condition of learning and the most complex one within the hierarchy of learning. This self-contained independent unit of instruction on problem solving describes the content of problem solving in an integrated form. The five major areas that are presented in a synthesized form are: theoretical framework, relevant research studies that have been conducted in the field, issues, application and extrapolation to nursing education and practice, and researchable questions.

In addition to the content presented on problem solving, this module has necessary information in the form of guidelines that the learner needs to follow in order to understand the material. The content of the module is properly sequenced. In addition to the above mentioned items, the module contains module objectives, pretest, posttest, and an answer key to the tests for feedback purposes.

MODULE OBJECTIVES

At the completion of this module on problem solving and after having studied the content of the recommended reading list, the student should be able to accomplish the following objectives at the 95% level of achievement. The student will be able to:

1. Define the process of problem solving

2. Explain in writing or orally the differences between the four basic approaches to problem solving
3. Describe Gagne's (1970) and DeCecco's (1968) model and theoretical framework of problem solving
4. Identify the internal and external conditions of problem solving
5. Describe the areas within which individuals differ in exhibiting problem-solving behavior
6. Support statements with regard to the theoretical framework with relevant research studies
7. Apply the principles of problem solving to patient teaching and student learning
8. Describe the relationship between problem solving and discovery learning and between problem solving and creativity
9. Identify the issues in problem solving and discuss the positive and negative aspects of each
10. Raise at least one researchable question and identify both the independent and dependent variables

PRETEST AND POSTTEST

Circle the correct answers. Each question is worth 1 point. The 95% level of mastery for this test is 13 correct points. Correct your answers using the answer key that is found at the end of this module (p. 140).

True or false

1. Presenting the solution of the problem, that is, showing the learner how to solve the problem, aids in more effective problem solving. True or False
2. Problem solving and rule learning differ only in the number of component concepts the individual may have to recall. True or False
3. Cues that verbally state the solution are a vital part of learning problem solving. True or False
4. Convergent thinking is characteristic of high creativity. True or False
5. Once the problem solution is achieved, learning appears to be unaffected by repetition. True or False

Multiple choice

6. According to Maltzman's theory of habit-family hierarchy, mediated generalizations occur:
   a. when stimuli become associated with more than one response
   b. correct responses gain strength because of reinforcement
   c. some stimuli rise in importance in the hierarchy because of familiarity
   d. some responses are elicited for more than one stimulus
7. A divergent mechanism according to Maltzman's theory of problem solving is the:
   a. hierarchy of responses that are made to a given stimulus; correct response low in the hierarchy
   b. hierarchy of responses that are made to a given stimulus; correct response high in the hierarchy
   c. hierarchy in which various stimuli exhibit the same response; correct stimuli high in the hierarchy
   d. hierarchy in which various stimuli exhibit the same response; correct stimuli high in the hierarchy
8. Factors essential for problem solving include all except:
   a. contiguity of rules
   b. repetition
   c. guidance provided by verbal instruction
   d. recall of relevant rules
9. Problem solving is:

a. the process by which the learner discovers a combination of previously learned rules that can be applied to achieve a solution for a novel problem situation
b. the process by which the learner applies previously learned rules to achieve a goal
c. the process by which concepts and principles are combined in a hierarchy leading to resolution of any problem learned in the process

10. Problem solving:
    1—is an act of learning
    2—is a change in human performance and capability
    3—has inherent generalizability
    4—produces a generalizable rule that is novel to the individual
    5—is in need of repetition
    a. all of the above
    b. 1, 2, 4
    c. 1, 2, 3, 4
    d. 3, 4, 5

11. Individual differences in problem solving depend on:
    1—retaining the solution model
    2—guidance of thinking
    3—recalling previously learned rules
    4—amount of information stored
    5—making cues distinctive
    a. all of the above
    b. 1, 3, 5
    c. 1, 3, 4
    d. 2, 3, 5

12. The following diagram represents:

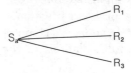

a. learning by discovery
b. habit-family hierarchy
c. generalization
d. convergent thinking
e. divergent thinking

13. The following diagram represents:

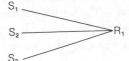

a. learning by discovery
b. habit-family hierarchy
c. generalization
d. convergent thinking
e. divergent thinking

Discussion question

14. Define "inductive leap."

TEXT
Theoretical framework
Introduction

Problem solving is the most complex kind of human learning. The process of problem solving may be viewed as a form of principle learning in which the learner discovers a combination of previously learned lower-level rules and applies them in the learning of higher-order rules, thus achieving a solution for a novel problem situation. Successful problem solving results in the acquisition of new knowledge just as does successful learning of concepts and principles.

The process of problem solving has been consistently viewed as similar to the scientific method. The sequence of events involved in problem solving are:

1. *Presentation of the problem.* Gagne suggests that the problem presented by means of verbal statement or another mode

2. *Definition of the problem.* The learner identifies and distinguishes the essential features of the problem situation.

3. *Formulation of a hypothesis.* Hypotheses may be possible solutions to the problem.

4. *Verification of the hypothesis.* The learner tests the different hypotheses until the problem is solved.

As can be seen from these four steps, only the first step is externally determined. The other three steps or events are internal to the problem solver and deal with the utilization of previously learned rules. These rules have to be present in the learner's entering be-

havior. Therefore, problem solving depends on rules and on a particular type of rule that governs the individual's own thinking behavior—this is called a *strategy* (Gagne, 1970).

Two very famous experiments, which are classics in implementing and illustrating the principles of problem solving, are those of Katona's (1940) matchsticks problem and Maier's (1930) pendulum problem.

Katona (1940) presented the students with a set of square figures made from an arrangement of matches. Instructions for changing the shapes of the forms with limited maneuvers by the students were given. Results of this study showed that:

1. The least effective method was to demonstrate to the student the specific matches to be removed or rearranged in order to solve the problem and for the learner to recall the correct moves.

2. The method in which the learner was instructed through a set of *verbal propositions* was more effective in leading to problem-solving. The two different propositions were in the form of instructions given to the learner. One was called "arithmetic proposition," which stated that the matches that have double functions should be changed to have single functions. The second one was called "structural proposition," which instructed the learner to proceed making holes and disassembling the figures. These two propositions were equally effective.

3. The best results were obtained by the method that informed the students to proceed a step at a time to illustrate the changes that would be brought about by using a rule but without actually stating the rule. Several examples were given to students by utilizing the rule, but not stating the rule; for example, some of the squares were shaded to create holes in the original figure. Gagne referred to this type of help as "learning by help" or "guided discovery" method of teach-

ing problem solving. The students were able to discover the rule after the presentation of these examples.

This experiment points out that when a problem is solved, a higher-order rule is acquired, which in turn may be generalized to other new problem situations. The presentation of the solution was not effective in teaching students how to solve problems, because it did not initiate acquisition of new knowledge in the form of higher-order rules. The solution was learned in the form of a simple chain. The most dependable way to teach problem solving was to stimulate the student to discover the rule.

Maier's (1930) pendulum experiment also illustrated the basics of problem solving. The learners were placed in a room 18 feet by 20 feet in size, containing only a work table. They were also provided with a set of poles, lengths of wire, chalk, and several clamps. The problem was to construct two pendulums so designed that each would make a chalk mark on the floor at the designated place when swung over it. The correct solution to the problem was to clamp two poles together, wedging them vertically against another pole that they pressed horizontally against the ceiling. It made a T-shape frame. From the two ends of the T they suspended two wires weighted at their lower ends with clamps that held the chalk. When the pendulum was swung, the chalk made marks at the correct spots on the floor.

Maier used different sets of instructions with different subjects. For example, he used additional sets of instructions that helped the subjects to recall certain previously learned rules, for example, (1) instructions on how to make a plumb line by using a clamp, a pencil, and string; (2) how to make a long pole by clamping two short ones together; (3) how to hold up an object against a wall with two poles, by wedging them together tightly. With another group of subjects he also gave the added instructions of how simple the problem solution would be if he "could just hang the pendulums from a nail in the ceiling."

Results of this study showed that those subjects who obtained added instruction that helped them to recall relevant principles solved the problem faster than those who were just told the problem. The added instruction, which Maier called *direction*, improved the probabilities of solution even more. The proportion of college students who were able to solve this problem under the three conditions were 0:15 for group 1, which received only the statement of the problem; 1:18 for group 2, which received added instruction; and 4:10 for group 3, which received instruction plus direction.

Gagne pointed out that in Maier's experiments the verbal instructions served several functions:

1. They informed the learners about the nature of the solution or the performance expected, that is, they defined the goal
2. They enabled the recall of relevant subordinate rules
3. They guided the students' thinking

Different approaches to the explanation of problem solving

The process of problem solving is viewed from different prospectives. There are several theories of problem solving. Forehand (1966) separates the theories into four basic contemporary approaches to problem solving.

Gestalt psychology. The first and oldest contemporary approach to problem solving has developed from classical Gestalt psychology. These psychologists, such as Kohler (1925) and Wertheimer (1945), viewed problem solving as an internal cognitive process or function where the learner integrates previously learned responses. Problem solving occurs as an insightful, or "aha," experience.

Psychometric approach. The psychometric approach is concerned with understanding the nature of intelligence and the traits of the individual. Its characteristic method has been the attempt to discover and interpret additive components of mental activity. The factors defined are the theoretical constructs derived from statistical relationships among the end results of problem-solving activity. The major concern in this approach is with traits of the individual. It has little to say about processes or conditions of problem solving. Guilford (1961) and Green (1964) have done research in this area.

Information-processing approach. Information processing deals with the programming of computers to solve complex problems. Often it is referred to as "artificial intelligence." Forehand (1966) described an information-processing approach to problem solving in which computer programs might supplement human cognitive processes and provide theoretical models and complex theories. Newell, Simon, and Shaw (1958) pioneered this approach in studies where subjects proceeded through the problem from start to finish without passing through stages. The student is given a set of operations in the initial situation and is then expected to produce a given result. Computer models have a built-in "sufficiency test" of specifications. Its processing system includes: coding, storage, retrieval, and transformation.

Like behaviorism this approach is elementalistic as opposed to holistic, and is insistent on discipline and detail in theory statement. Like Gestalt psychology it accepts the validity of complex internal events and eschews the assumption that such processes obey the laws of classical and operant conditioning.

The behavioristic approach. Learning theory never denied the reality or the importance of the phenomena of problem solving and conceptualization, but instead maintained that the phenomena can be accounted

for most efficiently by means of a simple relationship between stimuli and responses and that the premature invention of nonoperational concepts is a hindrance rather than help to the development of the desired explanation. Internal processes have been expressed cautiously in terms of mediating $Ss \rightarrow R$ processes.

Foremost among the proponents of behavioristic approach is Maltzman. Maltzman (1955) proposed a theory of problem solving that deals with the stimulus-response hierarchies. According to Maltzman, convergent and divergent mechanisms combine to produce habit-family hierarchies, which in turn determine the process of problem solving.

A stimulus-response hierarchy is shown in Fig. 9-1. S is a stimulus; R_1, R_2, and R_3 are three responses to this stimulus. This figure indicates that R_1 is stronger (higher in hierarchy) than R_2 and R_3. A stronger response is one that is more likely to occur in the presence of a stimulus. Maltzman gives the example that if the word table represents S_1, the three responses in order of strength might be chair (R_1), legs (R_2), and floor (R_3). The chair is the most dominant response, and, therefore, occupies the highest level of the hierarchy. However, it is possible that in a given situation floor is the correct response. Maltzman refers to this situation, where the correct response is low in the hierarchy, as the *divergent mechanism.*

An example of divergent mechanism in a

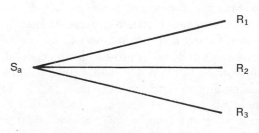

Fig. 9-1. Divergent mechanism.

nursing situation would be as follows: S is the stimulus: sight of a red, enlarged tonsil; the responses may be: R_1, surgery; R_2, give ice chips; R_3, give antibiotics. Often the response to an enlarged, red tonsil is that it has to be removed, or surgery. However, it is possible that the correct response may be the R_3 (give antibiotics) or some other response that may be even less dominant (R_5 or R_6). A person who can respond and give the less dominant answer, which may be the correct one, is said to be thinking in divergent ways.

In a *convergent mechanism* (Fig. 9-2) different stimuli within a hierarchy elicit the same response to varying degrees.

An example that is cited by DeCecco is that the words book (S_1), pen (S_2), and future (S_3) can all elicit the same response: student (R). But S_1 (book) has the strongest tendency to elicit this response and, therefore, it occupies the highest position in the hierarchy.

An example in nursing that illustrates the convergent mechanism is that the words pa-

tient (S_1), therapist (S_2), and medical-social worker (S_3) can all elicit the same response: hospital (R). The S_1 (patient) has the strongest tendency to elicit the response of hospital; therefore, it occupies the highest position in the hierarchy.

Convergent and divergent mechanisms combine to produce what Maltzman calls habit-family hierarchies as illustrated in Fig. 9-3.

S_a is an external stimulus that produces three different responses by means of the divergent mechanism, each response varying in strength. These responses in turn are connected with three stimuli that have varying tendencies to elicit a given response by means of the convergent mechanism. The R_{Ga} is the solution to the problem. In Maltzman's theory then, habit-family hierarchies combine to produce compound habit-family hierarchies. He believes that problem solving is accomplished by choosing habit-family hierarchies as well as specific responses within a hierarchy.

The role of *mediated generalization* is very important in solving problems utilizing Maltzman's theory of habit-family hierarchy. According to Maltzman, the strength of a correct response within a hierarchy must be increased in order for the individual to be able to solve the problem, especially when the correct response or the correct habit-family hierarchy is low in a compound hierarchy.

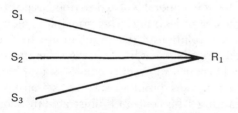

Fig. 9-2. Convergent mechanism.

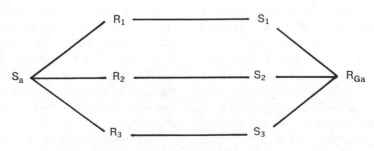

Fig. 9-3. Habit-family hierarchy.

The originally dominant but incorrect response or hierarchy will be extinguished gradually since it does not solve the problem. In the meantime, through the process of mediated generalization, the strength of the correct response, which has been low in the hierarchy, is increased. In mediated generalization effects on one member of a hierarchy also influence other members and finally increase the strength of the initially weak but correct member. The effects of mediated generalization are the result of reinforcement. Through mediated generalization, when one member of a hierarchy gets reinforcement, all other individual members of that hierarchy receive added strength.

The studies of Judson, Cofer, and Gelfand (1956) and Staats (1957) support the findings on the positive effects of mediated generalization on problem-solving behavior. Mediated generalization through the use of verbal mediators is affected by the factor of age. Kendler, Kendler, and Learnard's (1962) study on reversal and nonreversal shifts found that age differences affect the use of mediation. Very young children, under 4 years of age, do not appear to use verbal mediation. In the study these children had great difficulty solving problems with reversal shifts and were relatively more successful with problems of nonreversal shifts. These three experiments that dealt with mediated generalization in the solution of problems show that it is a form of verbal mediation.

In describing problem-solving behavior, Maltzman distinguishes between *productive* and *reproductive* thinking. In reproductive thinking, the student is presented with a succession of problems belonging to the same class. The solution to a series of algebraic problems that require essentially the same operations as in calculating dosages of medicine is an example of reproductive thinking. The solution involves reproductive thinking because it elicits various responses of the same habit-family hierarchy.

In *productive thinking* (also called *creative thinking*) the habit-family hierarchy that is low in dominance must gain strength in the compound hierarchy, and the dominant but incorrect hierarchy must be extinguished in order for the problem to be solved. As in the case of Katona's (1940) matchstick problem, the initial incorrect responses must be extinguished, and the less dominant correct responses must gain strength (for example, double functions for sticks, and disassembling the figure by making figures) by reinforcement of their individual response members. Productive thinking is more complex and more difficult than reproductive thinking. Reproductive thinking involves primarily the response members of a single hierarchy. Productive thinking involves competition among several hierarchies. The divergent mechanism is similar to productive thinking; the convergent mechanism is similar to reproductive thinking. However, both of these types of thinking are forms of learning (DeCecco, 1968, pp. 438-439).

DeCecco (1968) pointed out that problem solving in general is also described as positive transfer of learning. The principles relevant to the solution of the problem are transferred. In other words, if we consider the second task in a series of two tasks as a problem, we can view problem solving as transfer of learning. This concept is illustrated by Schulz (1960) as follows in Fig. 9-4.

In this design, if either the experimental (E) or the control group performs reliably better on task B (which represents the problem and the solution), transfer of learning has taken place. Transfer is positive if the performance of the experimental group is superior, and negative if the performance of the control group is superior. Zero transfer has occurred when both groups perform at the same level.

The transfer view of problem solving "underscores an important characteristic of this type of learning: successful problem solving

	Task A	Task B
Experimental group	X	X
			Reliable difference
Control group		X

Fig. 9-4. Operations for defining transfer. (From Schultz, R. W. *Problem solving behavior and transfer*. Harvard Educational Review **30**:61-77. Copyright 1960 by President and Fellows of Harvard College.

results in learning of high generalizability and transferability—in learning of higher-order principles of wide applicability" (De-Cecco, 1968, p. 476).

Conditions of problem solving
INTERNAL CONDITIONS

The major internal condition that the learner should possess in order to problem solve is the ability to *recall the relevant rules* that have been learned previously. For example, in the pendulum problem, the subject must recall the rules of weighting a length of wire, clamping, wedging poles, and so on. For the matchstick problem one has to recall rules governing the construction of multiple patterns of squares either in "arithmetic" or "structural" terms. Similarly, a nurse who is going to solve a problem in drugs and solutions, such as withdrawing 8 mg of morphine from a vial that contains 10 mg/ml, has to know and recall the previously learned rules of transformation in terms of ratios and rules of addition, subtraction, multiplication, and division. Problem solution always depends on previous experiences of the learner and the recall of previously learned rules.

EXTERNAL CONDITIONS

Contiguity of rules. There should be contiguity of rules that are to be put together in order to solve the problem and the stimulus situation that sets the problem. That is, the component principles must be kept in mind

all at once or be recalled or reactivated at will in close succession (Gagne, 1970, p. 222). The required contiguity may be made more probable if the relevant rules can be recalled quickly. One function of instruction can be to *stimulate such a recall by asking questions.*

Verbal instructions. Verbal instructions that are provided externally can *"guide"* or *"channel" thinking in certain directions.* This guidance can be self-generated. Guidance can be minimal when it takes the form of informing the learner of the goal of the activity and of the general form of the solution. Gagne thinks that this amount of guidance appears to be required if learning is to occur at all. Greater amounts of guidance may function to limit the range of hypotheses to be entertained by the learner in achieving the solution.

When these external conditions are present, the learner is able to solve the problem, although the time required to solve the problem varies with the amount of guidance that is provided and also with the individual differences variable, that is the varying abilities of learners.

Individual differences variable in problem-solving behavior

Gagne (1970) pointed out several areas in which individual differences may occur in solving problems.

Store of rules. It appears that a problem is more likely to be solved rapidly if the individual has a store of rules available. Individuals who have greater numbers of relevant rules available to them arrive at the solution to a problem faster than those who have few.

Ease of recall. Individuals differ in their ease of recall of relevant rules.

Distinctiveness of concept. Some individuals are able to distinguish and sort out the relevant aspects of the stimulus situation faster than others; thus they are able to "define the problem" more readily than others.

Fluency of hypothesis. The ability to formulate a hypothesis differs in individuals. Some people are more fluent than others on the basis of the facility with which rules are combined into hypotheses. Factors of intellectual fluency have been emphasized by in-

vestigators of creativity (Taylor, Berry, and Block, 1958; Getzels and Jackson, 1962; Guilford, 1967).

Matching of specific instances to a general class. Individuals may differ in the ability to match specific instances to generalizations. It is an operation performed by the problem solver in verifying the solution (Gagne, 1970, pp. 222-223).

• • •

Regardless of individual differences, the external conditions of contiguity of rules, recall of relevant rules, and guidance provided by verbal instruction are essential for problem solving. Once problem solution is achieved, what is learned is highly resistant to forgetting.

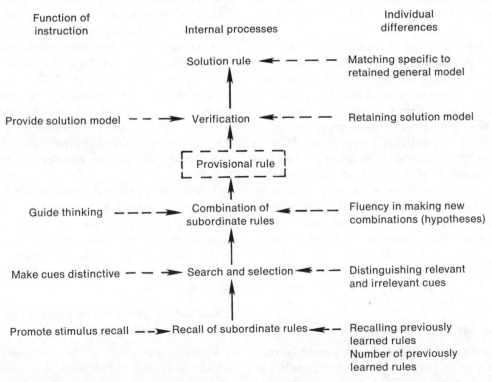

Fig. 9-5. Factors in problem solving, according to Gagne. (After Gagne, R. M. Human problem-solving: internal and external events. In B. Kleinmuntz (Ed.), *Problem-solving: research method and theory.* New York: John Wiley & Sons, 1966, p. 139.)

Gagne (1970) also pointed out that the capability that is established by problem solving is one that generalizes immediately and without repetition to an entire class of problems. That is, the individual has acquired a *higher-order rule* that can be generalized in a wide variety of stimulus situations belonging to a given class.

Gagne's (1966) model for problem solving includes four additional components or phenomena. The first of these is *sequential action*, which connotes that successful completion of any stage of problem solving depends on the existence of a capability in the preceding stage. The *threshold phenomena* is the second component of Gagne's model, and it indicates that certain stages must be reached before progression occurs in problem solving. The third component is *nongraded responses*, which indicates that action resulting from some preceding event is positive and nongraded, that is, it either takes place or does not take place, such as a cue is either discriminated or not or a hypothesis is either formed or not. This is also known as the "all or none law." Lastly, the model includes *multiple connections*, wherein any event can contribute to a number of subsequent events, or any number of events can be required to produce just one subsequent event; for example, a hypothesis may require a combination of rules. The factors that Gagne (1966, 1970) considered to be involved in problem-solving situations are illustrated in Fig. 9-5.

Learning of strategies in problem solving

As mentioned previously, the role of verbal instruction in providing guidance of thinking in the problem-solving process is of utmost importance as one of the external conditions. These instructions can be given either by the teacher, a book, or another external source; or they can be by *self-instruction*. A learner needs to know how to use self-instruction in solving problems. Such a capability is composed of higher-order rules, which are usually called strategies. Strategies may not be part of the goal of learning, but they are learned. *Study skills* are a form of strategies. Rothkopf (1968) defined a class of *mathemagenic behaviors* that are used by the student as capabilities for learning and remembering. Skinner (1957) emphasized the importance of *self-management behaviors*, which guide the individual in learning. Strategies in discovery and problem solving are described by Bruner (1961).

Rothkopf (1968) found that questions interspersed at intervals during the reading of passages of material to be learned improve retention of the information in the text, as compared to straight reading without questions. On the basis of such evidence, Rothkopf hypothesized that the effect of questions is to establish certain kinds of "inspection behaviors," a class of "mathemagenic behaviors" that facilitate learning and retention of information obtained from the study of printed texts. These facilitative effects are a form of strategy. These findings emphasize that a considerable variety of strategies need to be taken into account in describing conditions of learning. There must be strategies of: attending, coding, storage and retrieval, hypothesis forming, and other strategies that are particularly relevant to solving problems. All such strategies constitute a special class of rules, and they become a very useful portion of the repertoire of intellectual skills available to a sophisticated learner.

However, as Gagne (1970) points out, knowing a set of strategies is not all that is required for thinking; it is not even considered to be a substantial part of what is needed. To be an effective problem solver, the individual should have acquired masses of structurally organized knowledge and intellectual skills. Such knowledge is made up of content principles and not heuristic ones. Strategies deal with heuristic rules.

Instructions for problem solving

DeCecco cites five steps for teaching effectively for problem solving. These steps are based on Gagne's external conditions. These five steps can be utilized in teaching problem solving at any level—elementary to graduate school—in any subject matter where problem solving takes place, whether it is an elementary school arithmetic class or in nursing-school patient-care problems.

1. *Describe for the learner the terminal performance that constitutes the solution of the problem.* The description of the student's terminal performance fulfills two learning conditions: the student's attention is directed to those aspects of the materials that will lead to a particular solution, and the learner will know when the solution has been achieved and thereby can generate self-reinforcement. For example, the teacher may say to the student nurse, "You have a vial of morphine that contains 10 mg/ml, and you want to withdraw only 8 mg. What is the proportion of 8 to 10?"

2. *Assess the student's entering behavior for the concepts and principles that will be required in solving the problem.* This step fulfills the requirements of the second component of the basic teaching model. Here the teacher analyzes the problem to determine the lower-order principles necessary to solve this problem; in the previous example, principles dealing with ratio, multiplication, subtraction, division, and addition. The nurse-teacher next tries to find out if the student nurse knows how to multiply subtract, divide, add, and construct equal ratios.

3. *Invoke the recall of all relevant concepts and principles.* The teacher should provide for contiguity of relevant rules. The student must recall these principles in the presence of the problem and discover the relationship between them, that is, generate

the higher-order principle, which will result in the problem's solution. By asking questions and demonstrating relevant subordinate rules, the teacher can help the student nurse recall the relevant principles and recognize the relationship between these subordinate rules. Ausubel (1960) suggested the use of *advance* organizers in invoking recall of relevant principles. Advance organizers are a particular form of verbal mediation. They are concepts or principles introduced before the presentation of the main body of instructional material. They are chosen for their usefulness in explaining and organizing that material.

For the previous example the nurse-teacher can read or have the student read about the concept of ratio and how to use ratios in planning amounts of fluid the patient is to drink every hour in order to have the patient drink a predetermined amount of liquid in a particular number of hours. After reading and solving such a problem, the student may then be asked to solve the problem of withdrawing 8 mg morphine from a vial that contains 10 mg/ml. The first reading assignment should act as an advance organizer and help the student nurse solve the second problem.

4. *Provide verbal direction to the students' thinking without giving the solution to the problem.* Verbal direction can be in the form of directing the student's attention and channeling thinking for problem solving. The teacher may say, "You may want to formulate equal ratios, or you may have to divide some numbers in order to solve the morphine problem." Both Maier's (1930) and Katona's (1940) experiments showed that added direction enhanced problem solving.

5. *Verify the student's learning by requiring full demonstration of the problem solution (using other problems of the same class.)* As mentioned previously, problem solving has high transferability. Once higher-order principles are learned, the student should be able to transfer and immediately solve new

problems to which the principle applies. This step is very important in assessing the adequacy of the instruction and the student's learning. For example, the teacher may give a different problem to the student, but the problem is of the same category or hierarchy. The student who has understood the principles involved in the previous problem situation should be able to apply that higher-order principle and solve a new problem immediately.

Relationship between problem solving and discovery learning

Gagne (1970, p. 224) pointed out that, basically, the capability learned by means of problem solving is no different from that which is learned by combining lower-level rules in the manner described by principle learning. Both learning types result in the establishment of higher-order principles. Problem solving and principle learning appear to differ only in the *nature* and the *amount of guidance* given by means of verbal instruction. In principle learning the instructions include a sentence or a question that verbally cues the solution. In problem solving they do not.

In problem solving, the learner is asked to *discover* the higher-order principle without any specific help. The study by Worthen (1968) compared instructional methods of discovery to expository. He taught fifth and sixth graders mathematical concepts and problems over a 6-week period. Results showed that the expository method produced superior recall of rules learned when measured immediately following the learning period. The presentation of problems by means of the discovery method produced greater amount of transfer of rules acquired. This finding seems to have important implications to education, if one assumes that the main purpose of education is to produce transfer of learning. However, as Ausubel

(1963) pointed out, the evidence of experimental studies does not demonstrate that higher-order principles *must* be learned by discovery. Problem solving, or discovery, is only the final step in a sequence of learning that extends back through much prerequisite learning.

The issue of whether problem solving should be done by means of discovery as opposed to expository method is still unresolved. In general, however, as Gagne pointed out, the key to achievement of a higher-order rule does not lie solely in the discovery method. However, evidence strongly suggests that achievement of a higher-order principle by means of problem solving produces a new capability that is effective, generalizable, and retained over a long period of time.

There is further argument about whether learning by discovery refers to a method of teaching, a method of learning, or something one learns (Wittrock, 1966). Also, as Cronbach (1966) pointed out, even when there is agreement that it is something learned, it is not clear whether this something is a specific principle, the problem solution, the ability to solve problems by applying a single principle, the structure of knowledge in a given discipline, the techniques of discovery, or simply interest in the satisfaction of the creative urge.

DeCecco (1968) viewed discovery learning as occurring when the student has little or no direction from the teacher yet reaches the instructional goal. The main characteristic of discovery learning is the degree of guidance provided. Wittrock (1963) classified the degree of guidance provided in solving problems into four categories. In the first the teacher may give both the rule and the example, that is, the solution to the problem—"ruleg." This is often referred to as expository type of teaching. In the second, the rule is given, but an example or solution is not given. In the third category the solution is given, but the rule is not given. Neither the rule nor the solution is given in the fourth type. The second and the third conditions are referred to as "guided discovery." The fourth situation is "complete discovery," or "unguided discovery."

Suchman (1960) developed another strategy that he called "inquiry training." This is a method to teach both strategy and tactics of scientific inquiry. This method does not define the terminal behavior expected of the student. Inquiry is "motivated by the desire to obtain a new level of relatedness between and among separate aspects of one's consciousness" (Suchman, 1966, p. 178). Suchman's major emphasis is the teaching of means of acquiring knowledge, whatever it is, and not substantive knowledge itself. His teaching method neither provides the principle nor the problem solution, and it does not view application of the principle and the discovery of solutions as its major goals.

The procedure of problem solving that is proposed by Gagne (1970) and by DeCecco (1968) differs from inquiry training in three ways:

1. The major instructional objective is the acquisition of a higher-order rule as represented in the problem solution rather than the learning of techniques of inquiry.

2. The teacher gives direct assistance to the learner in recalling relevant principles in order to arrive at a problem solution

3. The student is required to demonstrate fully a newly learned capability by solving new and similar problems

These differences result between problem solving as viewed by Gagne and De-Cecco and inquiry training as viewed by Suchman because of the different emphasis that is placed on the instructional objectives—substantive knowledge versus inquiry training.

In concluding the debate on the different techniques of teaching problem solving, De-Cecco (1968, p. 474) made the following comment that stresses the major points that one ought to take into consideration before deciding which technique to employ to produce what type of learning.

Intrinsic to our concept of teaching is the assumption that the selection of teaching procedures must be based on prior statements of instructional objectives and a description and assessment of the prerequisite entering behavior. The complex inter-relationship among objectives, students, and procedures should make all a priori claims about the universal suitability of particular instructional procedures for all objectives and all students immediately questionable.

Relationship between problem solving and creativity

As Gagne pointed out, a great deal of scientific discovery and a great work of art have resulted from problem-solving activity. The act of discovery, even in every-day learning situations, involves a "sudden insight" that changes the problem situation into a solution situation. It, too, requires the individual to possess previous knowledge of the principles involved in the solution. Major discoveries or acts of creation occur rarely, and they involve a feat of generalizing that goes far beyond what may be expected in the usual learning situation. Gagne referred to this as an "inductive leap," where "there is a combining of ideas that come from widely separated knowledge systems, a bold use of analogy that transcends what is usually meant by generalizing within a class of problem situations" (Gagne, 1970, p. 228).

Gagne asked what learning has to do with creative discovery. He answered by saying that great discoveries of great social importance have been made by people who have acquired many kinds of hierarchies of principles. They have been deeply involved for long periods of time, and they have been consistently asking or trying to find relationships that exist between what appear on the surface to be remotely related disciplines.

Gagne further pointed out that these people learned to relate principles, as did anybody else, by combining sets of subordinate rules, partly with the aid of verbal instructions, partly by making "small" discoveries that may be involved in the acquiring of the higher-order principles of any particular knowledge system.

The use of discovery as a method of learning principles leads to development of capabilities that are very effective from the standpoint of transferability, generalizability, applicability, and retention. This method of learning generates new knowledge in the learner. Also, because it has tremendous positive reinforcement value, this method of learning also creates in the individual love of learning and "thirst for knowledge."

Of course, different authors view the nature of creativity from different perspectives. Ausubel believes that creativity refers to a "rare and unique talent in a particular field of endeavor," also that "creative achievement . . . reflects a capacity for developing insights, sensitivities, and appreciations in a circumscribed content area of intellectual or artistic activity" (Ausubel, 1963, pp. 99-100). He also stated that such an individual is uncommon, much rarer than the intelligent person.

Guilford (1962) maintained that creative abilities are somewhat general and can be applied to a variety of tasks and are not associated with a particular subject matter or discipline. He stated that a distinctive aspect of creative thinking is divergent thinking, which is characterized by flexibility, originality, and fluency. *Flexibility* refers the divergent responses made to a given word and is tested by Guilford's Unusual Uses Test. *Originality* is tested by Guilford's Plot Title Test. It also taps for unusual and uncommon

responses. *Fluency* refers to the quantity of output, that is, the number of unusual answers produced to a given word in a given time. The more output, the more fluent the person is said to be.

According to Getzels and Jackson (1962), divergent thinking tends to be stimulus free, while convergent thinking is stimulus bound.

Maltzman (1958, 1960) preferred the term originality to creativity because he could define originality in terms of unusual or uncommon verbal responses without engaging in the debate of whether it was creative or not. He performed a very successful experiment where he demonstrated that originality was a learning activity in that he could train the individual to give original responses. He had three groups. Group 1 was given a training test of words five times, and were asked to give different responses each time. Group 2 was given five new tests of common words and were asked to respond to each word as quickly as possible. Group 3 received five tests of low frequency (uncommon words) and were asked to respond as quickly as possible. Results showed that the first group gave the greatest number of uncommon responses to the words in the list. The third group did the next best. On the basis of this study, one can conclude that asking students to produce different responses to the same stimulus does increase originality.

Torrance and associates (1960) defined creative thinking as the process of recognizing incomplete or missing components, then forming and testing hypotheses about them and expressing conclusions, making necessary modifications, and retesting.

INSTRUCTIONS FOR CREATIVITY

DeCecco (1968) proposed methods by which to foster creative ability in learners in the form of flexibility, fluency, and originality solutions to problems.

Classify the kinds of problems. Getzels

(1964) distinguished between presented problems and discovered problems. Getzels believed that creative thinking begins with situations in which the problem is presented to the students, but the solution is not. The less that is known about the problem situation, the more the student will create. In his view, the type of problem-solving situation in which the problem and the solution are known requires the least or the lowest level of creativity. When the situation is based on complete discovery technique, the student requires considerable amount of assistance, even though the exact nature of assistance may not be clear. In any case, the teacher can use Getzel's scheme in classifying the problems students are expected to solve.

Provide for the development and use of problem-solving skills. One popular method of problem solving is by means of *brainstorming* (Osborne, 1957). This is a form of free association. It generates new and unusual types of solutions to problems.

An extensive study on brainstorming was conducted by Parnes and Meadow (1959). Their findings indicated that: (1) training in brainstorming increases creative problem solving, (2) brainstorming produces more solutions than do methods that penalize bad ideas in some way, (3) more good ideas are produced by brainstorming than by traditional methods, (4) extended efforts to produce ideas (latter part of brainstorming) lead to an increased number of ideas and an increased proportion of good ideas, and (5) students in creative problem-solving courses (which include brainstorming) obtain higher scores on Guilford's test of creative abilities than those students who have not had these courses.

Contrary evidence to the positive effects of brainstorming is provided by the studies of Taylor, Berry, and Block (1958). They found that individuals who worked in groups using brainstorming technique produced ideas that were both inferior in quality and quantity to those produced by people who worked alone. Torrance (1961) also found that directions that emphasized quantity of output (responses) without regard to quality resulted in fewer responses than did directions that emphasized interesting, clever, and unusual ideas.

Teach research skills. Another technique to foster creativity is teaching certain basic research skills. This technique is consistent with Torrance's (1960) definition of creative thinking as forming and testing hypotheses. The research of Torrance and Myers (1963) supports this proposal.

Promote creative reading. Creative reading is another useful approach to fostering creativity and problem-solving skill. The study of Torrance and Harmon (1961) supports this proposal. They had two groups of subjects. Group 1 was asked to read the articles critically and look for the following factors:

1. Defects in the statement of the problem and its importance
2. Underlying assumption of the hypotheses
3. Procedures for collecting and analyzing data
4. Conclusions and interpretation of data
5. Critical appraisal of the worth of research

The creative group (group 2) was asked to think in terms of:

1. New possibilities suggested by the statement of the problem
2. Other possible hypotheses related to the problem and its solution
3. Improvements that could have been made in the collection of the data
4. Other possible conclusions and interpretation of the findings
5. Appraisal of the possibilities stemming from the findings

Students in both groups were then asked to perform a research study of their own. Results showed that the creative group was judged to have more new and creative ideas than the critical group. One important implication of this finding for teachers is that the teacher should emphasize the creative function rather than asking students to read critically. The teacher may ask for both types of reading—creative and critical.

Reward creative achievements. Torrance (1960, 1965) listed five ways in which the teacher can positively reinforce creative achievements:

1. Treat unusual questions with respect
2. Treat unusual ideas and solutions with respect
3. Show students that their ideas have value
4. Provide opportunities and give credit for self-initiated learning
5. Provide chances for students to learn, think, and discover without threat of immediate evaluation.

Application to nursing education and practice

The external conditions for problem solving are variables in the form of verbal instructions that could be manipulated by the nurse or the nursing instructor in teaching patients or students problem-solving techniques. Important items among the external conditions are for the teacher to: (1) provide contiguity of rules, (2) help the student to recall relevant principles, and (3) guide or channel the student's thinking.

The teacher also can and should utilize the important steps that DeCecco has suggested in teaching problem solving. He suggested a very practical approach:

1. State the objective to the student, that is, the terminal behavior expected of the student. In other words, state the problem and the nature of the solution required, not the solution itself.

2. Assess the student's entering behavior either by means of pretest or by informal questioning to determine if the student or the patient has or knows all the necessary rules in order to solve the problem.

3. Help the student recall the rules either by cueing or by verbal means.

4. Guide the student's or the patient's thinking; for example, by saying, "What does this concept remind you of?" or "Look here first." or "Focus on this issue first."

5. After the student solves the problem, verify the solution by asking the student to apply the higher-order rule discovered in solving that specific problem to another similar but new problem situation.

The discussion on the relationship of problem solving to discovery learning and creativity provided several practical means of initiating creativity in learners. Also, it was pointed out that the subject matter, the objectives of the lesson plan, and the student's entering behavior determine whether the teacher should use complete discovery, guided discovery, or expository type of teaching in initiating problem-solving behavior in learners.

Researchable questions

1. What is the affect of teaching problem solving by means of a complete discovery as opposed to a guided discovery method of instruction on the affective behavior of learners?
   a. Independent variable: complete discovery versus guided discovery technique of instruction
   b. Dependent variable: affective behavior of learners

2. What is the effect of a self-instructional strategy of solving problems versus a teacher-generated strategy of solving problems on the transfer of problem-solving behavior?
   a. Independent variable: self-generated versus teacher-generated strategies for problem solving
   b. Dependent variable: transfer of problem-solving behavior

ADDITIONAL LEARNING EXPERIENCES—RECOMMENDED READING LIST

DeCecco, J. *The psychology of learning and instruction: educational psychology.* (1st Ed.) Englewood Cliffs, N.J.: Prentice-Hall, Inc., 1968, pp. 428-479.

DeCecco, J., and Crawford, W. *The psychology of learning and instruction: educational psychology.* (2nd Ed.) Englewood Cliffs, N.J.: Prentice-Hall, Inc., 1974.

de Tornyay, R. Measuring problem-solving skills by means of the simulated clinical nursing problem test. *Journal of Nursing Education*, 1968a, 7(3):3-35.

de Tornyay, R. The effect of an experimental teaching strategy on problem solving abilities of sophomore nursing students. *Nursing Research*, 1968b, 17:108-113.

Gagne, R. *The conditions of learning.* (2nd Ed.) New York: Holt, Rinehart and Winston, Inc., 1970, pp. 59-62, 214-236.

Gagne, R., and Smith, E. C., Jr. A study of the effects of verbalization on problem solving. *Journal of Experimental Psychology*, 1962, **63**:12-18.

Kleinmuntz, B. *Problem-solving: research method and theory.* New York: John Wiley & Sons, Inc., 1966.

Kramer, M., Tegan, E., and Knauber, J. The effect of the presets on creative problem solving. *Nursing Research*, 1970, **19**:303-310.

Maltzman, I. On the training of originality, in R. C. Anderson and D. P. Ausubel (Eds.), *Readings in the psychology of cognition.* New York: Holt, Rinehart and Winston, Inc. 1966, pp. 657-680.

Mednick, S. A. The associative basis of the creative process. *Psychological Review*, 1962, **69**:220-232.

Newell, A., Shaw, J. C., and Simon, H. A. Elements of a theory of human problem solving. *Psychological Review*, 1958, **65**:151-166.

Sorenson, G. An honors program in nursing. *Nursing Outlook*, 1968, 16(5):59-61.

Wittrock, M. C. Teaching problem-solving to young children. *UCLA Educator*, 1966, 8(3):4-6.

Wittrock, M. C. Replacement and non-replacement strategies in children's problem solving. *Journal of Educational Psychology*, 1967, 58(2):69-74.

INSTRUCTIONS TO THE LEARNER REGARDING POSTTEST

At this stage you are ready to take the posttest to determine the extent to which you have achieved the objectives of this module. Return to the pretest and take it again as the posttest. Correct your answers using the answer key that is found on this page. You must score 13 correct points to proceed to the next module. If your score is less than 13 points, correct your errors, study the text over again, and read some of the articles in the recommended reading list. You need to study until you score at least 13 correct points, which is 95% level of mastery or better.

ANSWER KEY TO PRETEST AND POSTTEST

1. False (DeCecco, 1968, pp. 443-448; Gagne, 1970, pp. 218-219)
2. False (Gagne, 1970, p. 224)
3. False (Gagne, 1970, p. 226)
4. False (DeCecco, 1968, p. 455)
5. True (Gagne, 1970, p. 224)
6. b (DeCecco, 1968, pp. 435-436)
7. a (DeCecco, 1968, pp. 433-434)
8. b (Gagne, 1970, p. 224)
9. a (Gagne, 1970, p. 214)
10. c (Gagne, 1966, pp. 3-18)
11. c (Gagne, 1966, pp. 3-18)
12. e (DeCecco, 1968, p. 428)
13. d (DeCecco, 1968, p. 428)
14. A major discovery involving a feat of generalizing that goes far beyond what may be expected in the usual learning situation; a combining of ideas that have come from widely separated knowledge systems; a bold use of analogy that transcends what is usually meant by generalizing within a class of problem situations. (Gagne, 1970, p. 228)

REFERENCES

Ausubel, D. P. Use of advance organizers in the learning and retention of meaningful verbal material. *Journal of Educational Psychology*, 1960, **51**:267-272.

Ausubel, D. P. *The psychology of meaningful verbal learning: an introduction to school learning.* New York: Grune & Stratton, Inc., 1963.

Brunner, J. S. The act of discovery. *Harvard Educational Review*, 1961, **31**:21-32.

Cronbach, L. J. The logic of experiments on discovery. In L. S. Shulman and E. R. Keislar (Eds.), *Learning by discovery.* Chicago: Rand McNally & Co., 1966, pp. 72-92.

DeCecco, J. *The psychology of learning and instruction: educational psychology.* (Ed. 1) Englewood Cliffs, N.J.: Prentice-Hall, Inc., 1968.

Forehand, G. D. Epilogue: constructs and strategies for problem-solving research. In B. Kleinmuntz (Ed.), *Problem-solving: research method and theory.* New York: John Wiley & Sons, Inc., 1966, pp. 355-383.

Gagne, R. Human problem solving: internal and external events. In B. Kleinmuntz (Ed.), *Problem solving: research, method and theory.* New York: John Wiley & Sons, Inc., 1966, pp. 3-18.

Gagne, R. *The conditions of learning.* (2nd Ed.) New York: Holt, Rinehart and Winston, Inc., 1970.

Getzels, J. W. Creative thinking, problem solving and instruction. In E. R. Hilgard (Ed.), *Theories of learning and instruction,* the 63 Yearbook of NSSE. Chicago: University of Chicago Press, 1964.

Getzels, J. W., and Jackson, P. W. *Creativity and Intelligence.* New York: John Wiley & Sons, Inc., 1962.

Green, B. F. Intelligence and computer simulation. *Transaction of the New York Academy of Science,* 1964, **11**(27):55-63.

Guilford, J. P. Factorial angles to psychology. *Psychological Review,* 1961, **68**:1-20.

Guilford, J. P. Factors that aid and hinder creativity. *Teachers College Record,* 1962, **63**:380-392.

Guilford, J. D. *The nature of human intelligence.* New York: McGraw-Hill Book Co., 1967.

Judson, A., Cofer, C., and Gelfand, S. Reasoning as an associative process: II. Direction in problem solving as a function of prior reinforcement. *Psychological Reports,* 1956, **2**:501-507.

Katona, G. *Organizing and memorizing.* New York: Columbia University Press, 1940.

Kendler, T. S., Kendler, H. H., and Learnard, B. Mediated responses to size and brightness as a function of age. *Journal of Comparative and Physiological Psychology,* 1962, **53**:80-87.

Kohler, N. *The mentality of apes.* New York: Harcourt Brace, 1925.

Maier, N. R. F. Reasoning in humans: I. On direction. *Journal of Comparative Psychology,* 1930, **10**:115-143.

Maltzman, I. Thinking: from a behavioristic point of view. *Psychological Review,* 1955, **62**:275-286.

Maltzman, I. On the training of originality. *Psychological Review,* 1960, **67**:229-242.

Maltzman, I., Bogartz, W., and Breger, L. A procedure for increasing word association originality and its transfer effects. *Journal of Experimental Psychology,* 1958, **56**:392-398.

Newell, A., Simon, H. A., and Shaw, J. C. Elements of a theory of human problem solving. *Psychological Review,* 1958, **65**:151-166.

Osborne, A. *Applied imagination.* New York: Charles Scribner's Sons, 1957.

Parnes, S. J., and Meadow, A. Effects of brainstorming instructions on creative problem solving by trained and untrained subjects. *Journal of Educational Psychology,* 1959, **50**:171-176.

Rothkopf, E. Z. Two scientific approaches to the management of instruction. In R. Gagne and W. R. Gephart (Eds.), *Learning research and school subjects.* Itasca, Ill.: F. E. Peacock Publishers, Inc., 1968.

Schulz, R. W. Problem solving behavior and transfer. *Harvard Educational Review,* 1960, **30**:61-77.

Skinner, B. F. *Verbal behavior.* New York: Appleton-Century-Crofts, 1957.

Staats, A. W. Verbal and instrumental response-hierarchies and their relationship to problem solving. *American Journal of Psychology,* 1957, **70**:442-447.

Suchman, R. J. Inquiry training in elementary school. *Science Teacher,* 1960, **27**:42-47.

Suchman, R. J. A model for analysis of inquiry. In H. J. Klausmeier and C. W. Harris (Eds.), *Analyses of concept learning.* New York: Academic Press, Inc., 1966.

Taylor, D. W., Berry, P. C., and Block, C. H. Does group participation when using brainstorming facilitate or inhibit creative thinking? *Administrative Science Quarterly,* 1958, **3**:23-47.

Torrance, E. P. Creative thinking through the language arts. *Educational Leadership,* 1960, **18**:13-18.

Torrance, E. P. Priming creative thinking in the primary grades. *Elementary School Journal,* 1961, **42**:34-41.

Torrance, E. P. *Gifted Children in the Classroom.* New York: The Macmillan Co., 1965.

Torrance, E. P., and Harmon, J. A. Effects of memory evaluative, and creative reading sets on test performance. *Journal of Educational Psychology,* 1961, **52**:207-214.

Torrance, E. P., and Myers, R. E. Teaching gifted elementary pupils research concepts and skills. *Gifted Child Quarterly,* 1963, **6**:1-6.

Torrance, E. P., Yamamoto, K., Schentzki, K., Palamutlu, N., and Luther, B. *Assessing the creative thinking abilities of children.* Minneapolis Bureau of Educational Research, University of Minnesota, Minneapolis, Minn., 1960.

Wertheimer, M. *Productive thinking.* New York: Harper & Row, Publishers, 1945.

Wittrock, M. C. Verbal stimuli in concept formation: learning by discovery. *Journal of Educational Psychology,* 1963, **64**:183-190.

Wittrock, M. C. The learning by discovery hypothesis. In L. S. Shulman and E. R. Keisler (Eds.), *Learning by discovery.* Chicago: Rand McNally & Co., 1966, pp. 33-76.

Worthen, B. R. Discovery and expository task presentation in elementary mathematics. *Journal of Educational Psychological Monograph Supplement,* 1968, **59**(1), Part 2.

MODULE 10

Social learning

DESCRIPTION OF THE MODULE

This module teaches the ninth type of learning—social learning. It encompasses most of the previous eight conditions of learning. Social learning is not as complex as problem-solving behavior; however, aspects of it utilize the problem-solving conditions.

This independent unit of instruction presents the major theoretical approaches to social learning. Social learning, which is also referred to as observational learning, is concerned with the acquisition of behavior by means of modeling. The content is presented in sequential order, and the five major areas are presented in integrated form. They include: theoretical background, relevant research, issues, application to nursing education and practice, and researchable questions.

The module also contains behavioral objectives that are implemented within the text and a pre- and posttest to determine the degree to which these objectives have been accomplished.

MODULE OBJECTIVES

At the completion of this module, having read and studied the content and utilized a variety of available instructional materials, the student will be able to accomplish the following set of objectives at the 95% level of accomplishment. On completion of this module, the student will be able to:

1. State, discuss and compare three theorists' views of social learning
2. Identify and discuss four fundamental factors of learning
3. List three instances wherein imitation can hasten independent learning
4. Distinguish between same behavior, copying, and matched-dependent behavior and give examples of each
5. Identify the four categories of people that children are most likely to imitate
6. Discuss generalization and discrimination in reference to social learning
7. Discuss reinforcement and secondary rewards (social rewards) as variables of social behavior
8. Describe the three types of effects models can have on a subject
9. Identify the antecedent social-stimulus events necessary to the development of all forms of social behavior
10. State and explain an effect punishment has on imitative learning responses
11. Describe at least two recent research findings relevant to social learning
12. Draw some extrapolations to nursing from the readings; illustrate how social-learning theory can be applied to nursing education and practice
13. Discuss at least two current issues that have a basis in social-learning theory; give supporting findings
14. Propose at least two researchable ques-

tions on the subject of social learning as related to nursing, stating the hypothesis and the independent and dependent variables for one of them

PRETEST AND POSTTEST

Circle the correct answers. Each question is worth 1 point except questions 25 (worth 4 points), 26 (worth 5 points), and 27 (worth 5 points). The 95% level of mastery for this test is 36 points. Correct your answers using the answer key found at the end of this module (p. 164).

True or false

1. The greater the amount of affection and nurturance existing between a model (such as a parent) and an imitator (such as a child), the greater will be the reproduction of the behavior of the model by the imitator. True or False
2. Imitation behavior of a superordinate individual or role model occurs only on a conscious level. True or False
3. Imitative behavior is more likely to be elicited by those children who have developed strong dependency habits, rather than in children whose dependency responses have been weakly established. True or False
4. The greater the degree of competency and prestige held by the model, the less the amount of modeling behavior in the learner. True or False
5. Social behavior patterns are most rapidly acquired through either the influence of the model or differential reinforcement. True or False
6. It has been found by Bandura, Ross, and Ross (1963) that film-mediated models, including television, are less effective than real-life models in eliciting and transmitting aggressive responses in children. True or False
7. The Bandura, Ross, and Ross (1963) study also demonstrated that children readily imitate behavior exhibited by an adult model in a new situation in the absence of the model. True or False

Matching

Part A

____ 8. Copying
____ 9. Same behavior
____10. Matched-dependent behavior
____11. Modeling effect
____12. Inhibitory and disinhibitory effects
____13. Eliciting effect

Part B

a. Imitation that occurs through an intricate routine of watching and imitating that is dependent on relevant cues
b. When one person learns to model behavior on that of another with the individual being aware that the behavior is the same as that of the model
c. Learning that occurs when two persons perform the same act in response to individual stimulation by the same cue in which each learns to make the same response
d. The acquisition by the observer of new responses that were not previously part of the behavior repertory and that through observation are substantially produced.
e. The strengthening or weakening of response patterns that are already a part of the observer's repertory, but that by observation of a model take on a new pattern
f. The elicitation of previously learned matching responses of the model and the observer through the observation of the model by the observer

Multiple choice

14. When children are punished by being hit, they not only learn not to do the behavior for which they are being punished, but they also learn another means of aggression toward others. They learn this by:
    a. intentional learning
    b. incidental learning
    c. chaining
15. A child is more likely to model the behavior of another individual if:
    a. the child has dependent feelings toward that individual causing the child to want that individual's approval
    b. the child feels independent of the indi-

vidual and does not care about approval from that person

c. the model is not an aggressor

16. When a model (for imitation) is used as a teaching strategy, learning can be produced using:
    1—direct techniques (face to face)
    2—symbolic techniques (words)
    3—mathematical techniques
    4—pictorial techniques (films, television)
    a. 1 and 2
    b. all of the above
    c. 1, 2, and 3
    d. 1, 2, and 4

17. Mowrer refers to imitation learning in children as empathetic learning. Which of the following best explains his rationale?
    a. The child observes that the model gains satisfaction from the behavior and so expects to gain the same satisfaction.
    b. The child intends to please the model through imitation.
    c. The child engages in similar behavior in an attempt to become emotionally close to the model.

18. In a study that compared the aggressive behaviors portrayed by cartoon models versus human models versus film-mediated models, Bandura, Ross, and Ross (1963) found out that:
    a. the cartoon models elicited imitation of aggressive behavior in children that was equivalent to that elicited by human models
    b. the children were not as attentive to the cartoons as to the human models
    c. the boys were more attentive to the cartoon models than the girls

19. Social restrictions, or the suppression of responses, can be enforced by which of the following techniques?
    a. nonreward
    b. punishment
    c. inhibition
    d. a, b, and c
    e. none of the above

20. Antecedent social-stimulus events necessary to the development of all forms of social behavior include:

a. reinforcement contingencies of the child's learning history

b. methods of training that have been used to develop and modify social behavior

c. the behavior characteristics of the social models to which a child has been exposed

d. all of the above

21. Behavior is dependent on the following fundamental factors of learning *except:*
    a. drive
    b. copying
    c. rewards
    d. cues
    e. responses

22. Imitation that occurs through an intricate routine of watching and imitating that is dependent on relevant cues is an example of
    a. copying
    b. matched-dependent behavior
    c. same behavior
    d. social inhibition
    e. none of the above

23. B. F. Skinner proposes the use of which of the following as a basis for social learning?
    a. modeling
    b. continuous reinforcement
    c. punishment
    d. differential reinforcement
    e. restrictions

24. Conditions under which imitation can hasten independent learning include all *except:*
    a. the model must be correct
    b. there must exist a dependency relationship between the model and the subject doing the imitating
    c. the cue response connections producing the units of matched behavior must be present
    d. the subject must generalize from the situation in which the model's cue is present to a situation in which it is absent

Discussion questions

25. List the four classes of persons who are most often imitated by others.
    a. _____
    b. _____
    c. _____
    d. _____

26. Briefly discuss the following situations in terms of their relevance to social-learning theory.
    a. A clinical nursing instructor is about to teach a student nurse the procedure for administering an intramuscular injection. Relate this situation to concepts of modeling.
    b. A 5-year-old child is admitted to the hospital where you are employed. The child has second- and third-degree burns over the lower portion of her body. It is a suspected case of battering. Briefly discuss this situation as it relates to social learning.

TEXT
Introduction

Social learning is a theory in which people learn to fit in with the manners and customs of the family, neighbors, community, and society in which they live (Watson, 1967, p. 75). In the last 50 years it has become important in the development and modification of human behavior and also in the understanding of social and antisocial behavior. Originally, social learning meant how humans as biological organisms became behaviorally acceptable through the process of socialization; the emphasis was on learning-theory approaches to personality development, and most learning was based on cognitive, intelligent selection of responses to explain social learning. However, no explanation was given for unconscious, unintelligent behavior. Thorndike's (1932) studies seem to indicate that most social learning was of the direct, unconscious kind (Dollard, 1950, p. 44). Today the theory seems to aim in the direction that social learning is a form of observational learning and can occur without a stimulus-response being elicited from the observer and also without reinforcement (Miller, 1961, p. 12).

Social learning is a process of learning new behaviors, modifying undesirable behavior, or changing behavior through a process of imitation, or role-taking. According to Bandura and Walters (1963, p. 47), "Imitation plays an important role in the acquisition of deviant, as well as conforming, behaviors. New responses may be learned, or the characteristics of existing response hierarchies may be changed as a function of observing the behavior of others and the response consequences without the observer performing any overt responses or receiving any direct reinforcement during the acquisition period. In some cases the amount of learning acquired by the observer can, in fact, be as great as that acquired by the performer" (McBrearty, 1961, p. 425).

Miller and Dollard (1941, p. 1) pointed out that:

> To understand thoroughly any item of human behavior—either in the social group or in the individual life—one must know the psychological principles involved in its learning and the social conditions under which this learning took place. It is not enough to know either principles or conditions of learning; in order to predict behavior both must be known.

Gagne (1970, p. 352) pointed out that "children readily learn by imitation such behaviors as aggressiveness, dependency, ways of reacting to frustration, reactions to the opposite sex, self-control, and many particular kinds of moral behavior." Therefore, it is extremely important for them to have models from which to learn desirable social behavior.

Historical background

The historical background of social learning probably began with Aristotle, who has been translated as saying that "man is the most imitative of living creatures, and through imitation learns his earliest lessons; and no less universal is the pleasure felt in things imitated" (Miller and Dollard, 1941, p. 311). Some social-learning theorists, as it appears does Aristotle, tend to stress imitative tendencies as innate. Walter Bagehot was one of the theorists who believed that imitativeness is an inate part of human nature. While Bagehot (1873) was concerned primarily with groups and how some customs are fixed and broken down, his theoretical considerations in 1873 did much in laying the foundations for the reinforcement theory of learning. He is quoted in Millard and Dollard (1941) as saying, "The truth is that the propensity of man to imitate what is before him is one of the strongest parts of his nature" (p. 291).

"The concept of imitation has roots in psychological theory with a long history dating back to Morgan (1896), Tarde (1903), and McDougall (1908), who regarded imitativeness as inate or instinctive. As the doctrine of instinct fell into disrepute, a number of psychologists, notably Humphrey (1921) and Allport (1924), attempted to account for imitative behavior in terms of Pavlovian conditioning principles. In dealing with language learning, for example, Allport suggested that a child makes the first approximations to human speech in the course of babbling and that these approximations elicit from adults, who perceive the child's utterances as socially significant, the word-sound to which the child's vocalization has approximated, together (on some occasions at least) with a demonstration of the act or object to which this word refers. As a result, the child is classically conditioned to produce the word whenever the adult produces it or whenever the object or event with which it is associated appears in the environment" (Bandura and Walters, 1963, pp. 52-53).

In keeping with the view that classical conditioning accounts for imitative tendencies in humans, Holt (1931) also worked with language development in the small child, and he offered an analysis of observational learning similar in many respects to Allport's. Holt noted that "when an adult copies a movement made by a child, the latter tends to repeat this movement, and that this sequence may

be continued time after time with the child's imitative responses becoming increasingly spontaneous" (Bandura and Walters, 1963, p. 53). One main weakness of classical-conditioning theories of imitation, however, is "their failure to account satisfactorily for the emergence of *novel* responses during the model-observer sequence" (Bandura and Walters, 1963, p. 53).

Still other social-learning theorists believe that imitative behavior is learned and takes place in response to rewards and punishments. E. L. Thorndike purported that imitative habits are generated by instinct, exercise, and effect. He placed major importance on the influence of the family and social structure in setting up conditions for modeling and imitative behavior. He failed, however, to detail the conditions under which imitation is rewarded or punished (Miller and Dollard, 1941, p. 307).

La Piere and Farnsworth presented concepts that suggest the term "imitation" be abandoned in favor of the term "model," and like Gagne refer to the process of learning by the human model, or human example. They suggest that this type of learning reduces the chance of learning by trial and error and increases the chance of a successful and lasting response (Miller and Dollard, 1941, p. 314).

According to Mowrer's social-learning theory, the focus is on proprioceptive feedback as a mediator in imitative learning. As such he regards imitative learning as parallel to habit formation, differing only in the origin of the response-correlated stimuli. The model produces the stimuli in imitative learning, and the learner produces the stimuli in habit formation. The feedback in both cases is associated through classical conditioning (Bandura and Walters, 1963, p. 56.)

Piaget (1948) suggested that modeling is a method of socialization. He conceived of it as a circular process or sequence of alternating imitations (Kramer, 1972, p. 50).

B. F. Skinner proposed the use of differential reinforcement (strict operant conditioning), rather than modeling, as the basis for social learning (Kramer, 1972, p. 50). In keeping with this idea, Rheingold, Gerwitz, and Ross (1959) found that reinforcement of vocalizations in 3-month-old infants did increase their frequency of vocalizations.

Theories of social learning

Social learning is often referred to as observational learning. The main causal factor of social learning is by means of imitation or modeling. Social learning is similar to learning by means of modeling. There are many theories of social learning proposed by different theorists and experimenters. Three major theories of social learning are presented in the following pages; namely, (1) the social-learning theory of Miller and Dollard (1941), (2) the behavioristic theory of social learning, and (3) the sociobehavioristic theory of social learning (Bandura and Walters, 1963). The theoretical issues and relevant research studies to support each school of thought are also presented and discussed.

Miller and Dollard's theory of social learning

"Although imitation received considerable attention during the earlier part of the twentieth century, it was not until the publication of *Social Learning and Imitation* by Miller and Dollard (1941) that the concept was fully integrated into a behavior-theory framework, and the phenomenon of imitative behavior was presented as a major problem confronting learning theorists" (Bandura and Walters, 1963, p. 54).

Imitation is defined by Miller and Dollard (1941, p. 10) as "a process by which 'matched,' or similar acts are evoked in two people and connected to appropriate cues." They refer to their theory of imitation as a "reinforcement theory of social learning" (p. 91). According to this theory, the necessary conditions for learning through imitation include a *motivated subject*, who is positively reinforced for matching the correct responses of a model during a series of initially random, trial-and-error responses. According to this social-learning theory, behavior is dependent on four fundamental factors of learning:

1. Drive—a strong stimulus that impels action (either primary—inate—or secondary—learned, or acquired), the strength of which is in direct proportion to the stimulus
2. Response—the observable behavior that occurs as a result of the drive
3. Cues—the stimuli that elicit and are elicited by the response distinctive to the drive
4. Rewards—the reinforcement received as a result of the response (Miller and Dollard, 1941, p. 18-35)

Mechanisms that account for the learning of imitative behavior within this theoretical framework are:

1. *Same behavior.* Learning that occurs when two persons perform in the same way in response to individual stimulation by the same cue in which each learns individually to make that response; for example two students with the same career goals choosing the same university.

2. *Copying.* Learning that occurs when one person learns to model behavior on that of another, with the copier aware that the behavior is the same as that of the model. The essential learning centers around this knowledge and, in the end, the copier must be able to respond independently to the cues of sameness and difference. Copying units are established early in the history of each individual and appear to play a considerable role in all fundamental social learning. Copying is learned only when the appropriate conditions of reward for learning it are present.

3. *Matched dependent behavior.* Learning that occurs when one person is older, shrewder, or more skilled than another. Imi-

tation occurs through an intricate routine of watching and imitating that is dependent on relevant cues. The behavior of the imitator is dependent on the discriminating ability of the leader to determine appropriate behavior in response to specific cues that evoke the desired terminal reward or drive satisfaction; for example, children matching the behavior of parents, social climbers, and nursing students to instructors. In other words, in matched-dependent behavior, the leader is able to read the relevant environmental cues, but the follower is not. The latter must depend on the leader for the signal as to what act is to be performed, and where and when; the follower does not need to be keenly aware that the act is matched (Miller and Dollard, 1941, pp. 91-92).

The essential difference between copying and matched-dependent behavior is that in matched-dependent behavior the imitator responds only to the cue from the leader; while in copying, the imitator responds also to the cues of sameness and difference produced by stimulation from personal responses as well as the model's. In copying, the cues of difference acquire anxiety value, and the cues of sameness acquire reward value. The theorists' suggest a continuum with pure matched-dependent behavior at the lower level and copying at the other end (Miller and Dollard, 1941, pp. 159-160).

Miller and Dollard also purported that imitation of a given response will be learned if rewarded and that when learned in one situation, it will generalize to somewhat similar but new situations (Miller and Dollard, 1941, p. 131). For example, using imitative learning (watching) of the nurse's feeding behavior while in the nursery to teach a new mother the skills of feeding a premature infant should generalize to the mother's actual feeding of the baby in the nursery, and if rewarded (with praise) would be expected to generalize

to home feeding of the infant when discharged.

The conceptualization of secondary rewards (social rewards) is also very important in social learning because it is quite clear that a great deal of social learning depends on this type of gratification rather than the direct gratification of primary drives; for example, delaying immediate satisfaction of a behavioral goal because of social pressure, such as praise, prestige, and the like, and thus establishing an imitative response pattern. However, the primary drives (direct and biological, such as food, shelter, and protection) must be met if the secondary drives are to have any goal value. An example is a child who has not been well cared for by the mother will not place as much reward value on being near her as will a child who had previously been nurtured by the mother (Miller and Dollard, 1941).

The social conditions under which imitative behavior is most likely to occur seem to Miller and Dollard to be associated with hierarchical status with regard to specific skills and social status. They feel there are at least four classes of persons who are imitated by others. They are: "(1) superiors in age-grade hierarchy, (2) superiors in a hierarchy of social status, (3) superiors in an intelligence ranking system, and (4) superior technicians in any field" (Miller and Dollard, 1941, p. 183).

Based on their theory and the research studies, Miller and Dollard (1941, pp. 210-211) suggested three conditions under which imitation hastens the process of learning independent responses.

1. The cue-response connections producing the units of matched behavior must be present if example is to be useful. One of the purposes of education is to supply proper units of behavior. The individual must have these copying units—be they fundamental dance steps, steps in a nursing procedure,

phonemes of a new language, or medical terminology—before being able to use copying as a shortcut to further learning.

2. The model must be correct. If a model is wrong and the person has a tendency to imitate, this tendency must be extinguished before a correct, rewarded response can occur.

3. The subject must generalize from the situation in which the model's cue is present to the situation in which it is absent. The probability of this occurring is greater when the environmental stimulus is a distinctive component of the total stimulus pattern. If responding to the cues from the model directs the dependent subject's sense organs and attention toward the proper environmental cue, this may enhance the distinctiveness of the stimulus. If, on the other hand, responding to the cues from the model directs the dependent subject's sense organs and attention away from the proper environmental cue, the subject may not be exposed to the stimulus at all. In this case, no generalization will occur, and there will be no benefit from imitation.

Miller and Dollard's theory of imitation has been criticized by Bandura and Walters (1963, p. 55), who view the theory and the experiments conducted by Miller and Dollard to demonstrate learning by imitation as "special cases of discrimination place learning in which the behavior of others provides discriminative stimuli for responses that already exist in the subject's behavioral repertoire." Bandura and Walters state that "the theory of Miller and Dollard may account adequately for learning of this kind, but that it does not account for the occurrence of imitative behavior in which the observer does not perform the model's responses during the acquisition process and for which reinforcers are not delivered either to the models or the observers. Moreover, the theory presents imitative learning as being contingent on the observer's performing a close approximation

to the matching response before being able to acquire it imitatively and thus places a severe limitation on the behavioral changes that can be attributed to the influence of a model." Also, the experiments on which Dollard and Miller (1950) based their theory included no instances of novel responses in the absence of rewards to the observers for imitative behavior, so it is perhaps not surprising that they viewed observational learning as a special case of instrumental conditioning.

By the following example Miller and Dollard (1941) concluded that imitation cannot be used to produce a novel response unless the component cue-response matchings have already been learned. A small boy was taken to the snake house in the zoo. He saw a big colored snake behind the glass. He seemed fascinated and asked what it was. He was told, that it was a snake. After hearing this, he repeated, "nake, nake," and was rewarded by being lifted up to get a better view. Afterward, he asked to go back and see the "nake." In this case, the connection between the cue of hearing someone else pronounce an initial "s" before a consonant and make the response of pronouncing the initial "s" himself was not present. Independent evidence for this conclusion comes from the fact that the little boy was mispronouncing all words beginning with "s" before a consonant (for example, saying "mells" instead of "smells.") Because the matching of the unit had not already been learned the response elicited imitatively was, inevitably, imperfect. Thus the response elicited by generalization to the cue of the object alone, in the absence of the mother's pronunciations of the word "snake" was also imperfect. Although imitation did not produce the independent learning of a perfectly correct response, it nevertheless speeded learning by immediately eliciting a closer approximation than would be expected after thousands of purely random responses.

According to Miller and Dollard, the imperfections of the child's speech in this example emphasize the point that imitation cannot be used to produce either a sound or a novel combination of sounds in a new situation unless the component cue-response matchings have already been learned. This also demonstrates that there is no general unlearned capacity to imitate, a fact that is painfully obvious to a person trying to learn the phonetic elements of a foreign language.

In contrast to the previous experiment conducted by Miller and Dollard, Bandura and Huston (1961) conducted an experiment to demonstrate the acquisition of novel behavior through imitation. In this experiment one group of nursery-school children experienced a highly nurturant and rewarding interaction with a female model, whereas for a second group of children the same model behaved in a distant, nonrewarding manner. Following the social interaction sessions, the model played a game with each child. The object of the game was to guess which of the two boxes contained a picture sticker. In executing each trial, the model exhibited relatively novel verbal, motor, and aggressive responses that were totally irrelevant to the game. A measure was obtained of the number of imitative responses the child reproduced while performing the trials. Except for aggressive responses, which were readily imitated regardless of the nurturant quality of the model, children who experienced the rewarding interaction with the model imitated her behavior to a substantially greater extent than did children with whom the same model had reacted in a distant and nonrewarding way. Moreover, the children in the model-rewarding condition displayed more behavior that was only partially imitative of the model's social responses. This study indicates that exposure to a model possessing rewarding qualitites not only facilitates precise imitation but also increases the probability of the occurrence of responses falling within the same class as those made by the model but that the model does not in fact emit.

Behavioristic theory of social learning
MOWRER'S THEORY OF IMITATION

"Mowrer (1960) described two forms of imitative learning that differ from the matched-dependent learning of Miller and Dollard. In one case, organism A makes a response and at the same time rewards organism B. As a result, A's response takes on secondary reward value for B; consequently, B attempts to reproduce A's response at times when it is not being made by A. An analogous process is assumed in the account given by Whiting and Child (1953) of the development of *identification*" (Bandura and Walters, 1963, p. 55).

Mowrer (1960, p. 115) also described another form of imitation, which may be called *empathic learning*. Bandura and Walters (1963, p. 55) viewed this case as: "A both provides the model and experiences the reinforcement. B, in turn, both experiences some of the same sensory consequences of A's behavior as A experiences it and also *intuits* A's satisfactions or dissatisfactions."

Mowrer's theory focuses primarily on positively valenced proprioceptive feedback as the crucial process mediating imitative learning. According to Mowrer, as perceived by Bandura and Walters (1963), "imitation occurs only when the observer is directly or vicariously rewarded by the sensory consequences of the model's instrumental responses. Consequently, the observer regards imitative learning as precisely parallel to habit formation, and views the two forms of response acquisition as differing only in respect to the origin of the response-correlated stimuli that sustain the learned responses." Bandura and Walters (1963, p. 56) also pointed out: "In the case of habit formation these stimuli are produced by the acts of the learner; in the case of imitation, by the acts of the model; nevertheless, in both cases they take the form of rewarding (motivational or emotional) proprioceptive feedback associated through classical conditioning with the learner's execution of the acts performed. It is evident, however, that proprioceptive feedback can account only in the part for the acquisition, facilitation, and inhibition of responses that are attributable to the influence of a model. Therefore it is also necessary to take account of external stimulus elements, which probably play the role of key discriminative cues."

"Moreover, behavior is influenced by models even when there are no response-generated cues that have positive or negative valence. Indeed, Mowrer himself at times emphasized the role of conditioned sensations, or images that provide sensorimotor linkage between cognitive and emotional responses. In most cases of observational learning such perceptual responses may be the only important mediating processes" (Bandura and Walters, 1963, p. 56).

SHEFFIELD'S THEORY OF IMITATION

"In a recent study of programmed learning from filmed demonstrations, Sheffield (1961) focused on the role of mediating perceptual and symbolic responses possessing cue properties that are capable of eliciting, sometime after a demonstration, overt responses corresponding to those that were demonstrated. Sheffield's theory of imitative learning is consistent with Mowrer's in several important respects. From both points of view, learning of this kind is based on the principle of contiguity and is mediated, at least in part, by essential similar cues, producing cognitive responses. Sheffield, however, makes no assumptions concerning the role of mediating conditioned emotional reactions or proprioceptive feedback. This may be because Sheffield has addressed himself mainly to "the learning of perceptual-motor tasks from filmed demonstrations that do not contain strong positive or aversive stimuli essential for the classical conditioning of emotional responses. Mowrer's theory may be primarily relevant to cases in which the model's responses incur social reward or punishments" (Bandura and Walters 1963, pp. 56-57).

An experiment conducted by Bandura (1962b), as cited by Bandura and Walters (1963, p. 57) strongly suggested that "the *acquisition* of imitative responses results primarily from the contiguity of sensory events, whereas response consequences to the model or to the observer have a major influence only on the *performance* of imitatively learned responses. Three groups of children observed a film-mediated model who exhibited four novel aggressive responses accompanied by distinctive verbalizations. In one condition of the experiment, the model was severely punished; in a second, the model was generously rewarded with approval and food; while in the third condition no response-consequences were presented to the model. During the acquisition period, the children neither performed any overt responses nor received any direct reinforcement; therefore, any learning that occurred was purely on an observational or vicarious basis. The results of a postexposure test of imitative behavior revealed that the differential, vicarious reinforcement had produced differential amounts of imitative behavior. The children who were in the model-punished condition performed significantly fewer imitative responses than children in both the model-rewarded and the no-consequences groups. Moreover, boys reproduced more imitative responses than girls, and the differences were more marked in the model-punished condition." When the experiment was extended one step further by offering attractive incentives contingent on reproducing the model's responses, results showed that "the introduction of positive incentives completely wiped out the previously observed performance differences, revealing an equal amount of learning among the children in the model-rewarded, model-punished, and no response-consequences conditions. Similarly, the sex difference was substantially reduced. The fact that some of the children failed to reproduce all the model's responses indicates that factors other than sensory stimulation undoubtedly influence response acquisition" (Bandura and Walters, 1963, pp. 58-59).

The process of imitation is receiving increasing attention from learning theorists, but it is still usually treated as a form of instrumental conditioning, as conceptualized by Miller and Dollard. There is considerable evidence, however, that learning may occur through observation of the behavior of others even when the observer does not reproduce the model's responses during acquisition and therefore receives no reinforcement (Bandura, 1962).

Bandura and Walters (1963) believed that the learning principles set out by Hull (1943) and Skinner (1938, 1953) should be "revised and extended in order to account adequately for observational learning. Moreover, these principles deal only with the role of direct reinforcement. Since the eliciting and maintaining of imitative behavior are highly dependent on the response consequences to the model, an adequate social-learning theory must also take account of the role of *vicarious reinforcement*, through which the behavior of an observer is modified on account of the reinforcement administered to a model" (p. 4).

Bandura and Walters' sociobehavioristic theory of social learning

The sociobehavioristic approach to social learning, as purported by Bandura and Walters (1963), is especially useful since its primary emphasis is on accounting for the acquisition and modification of human behavior via the social-learning process in a group situation. They believe that social behavioral patterns are learned fastest and are most lasting through the combined influence of social models and differential reinforcement (operant conditioning). Since it is impossible for any learning to take place in a vacuum, it seems feasible that this would hold true not only for operant conditioning but also for the other forms of learning.

The conceptualization of *schedules of reinforcement*, such as fixed-ratio, fixed-interval, variable-ratio, and variable-interval, is an important part of Bandura and Walter's social-learning theory. However they contend that social reinforcers are usually dispensed on a *combined schedule*, with both the number of reinforced responses and the time interval between reinforcements continually changing (Bandura and Walters, 1963, p. 7). Because the social situation and social demands continually change, this aspect holds many implications for nursing practice and education. Unless the nurse can successfully control the patient's social situation completely (which is doubtful), this notion must be dealt with if nursing interventions are to be successful. This seems particularly true when interventions are aimed at child-rearing practices.

Generalization and *discrimination* are other conceptualizations of the social-learning theory, as purported by Bandura and Walters, that must be present in order for social learning to take place. "Learned patterns of response tend to generalize to situations other than those in which they were learned, the extent of generalization being a function of the degree of similarity between the original learning situation and the novel sets of cues" (Bandura and Walters, 1963, p. 8). When responses overgeneralize or generalize on the basis of irrelevant cues, maladaptive behavior may occur. For instance, the study done by Watson and Raynor (1920) with "Albert" and "the white rat" in which a 1-year-old child was conditioned by classical learning to fear white rats (by the pairing of loud noise with the presentation of a white rat). The irrational fear and overgeneralization to all fluffy objects that occurred in Albert is an example of this conceptualization.

A study done by Bandura, Ross, and Ross (1961) with preschool children attempted to show that imitative learning involves the generalization of imitative response patterns. The study dealt with the imitative behavior of children when exposed to models with aggressive behaviors. The study showed significantly that in the absence of the model the subjects imitated not only the discriminated responses but also the behaviors performed by the models (Bandura, Ross, and Ross, 1961).

When discussing social learning, one must always include aspects of the extinctability of undesirable behavior. Bandura and Walters focus on punishment, inhibition, and nonreward as means of producing socially approved patterns of behavior. However, within the framework of social-learning theory, the effect of any type of reward is highly dependent on both external cues, especially as associated with the presence of the socializing agent, and individual internal cues, which together contribute to the response pattern (Bandura and Walters, 1963, p. 13).

As an attempt to explain the development of all forms of social behavior, Bandura and Walters found it to be of theoretical significance to classify behaviors in terms of: (1) antecedent social-stimulus events; for example, the behavioral characteristics of the social models to which a child has been exposed; (2) reinforcement contingencies of the learning history; and (3) methods of training that have been used to develop and modify social behavior (Bandura and Walters, 1963, p. 44).

They also noted that ". . . the provision of

models not only serves to accelerate the learning process but also, in cases where errors are dangerous or costly, becomes an essential means of transmitting behavior patterns" (p. 52). These models may be *observational* or *symbolic*, in which the model is presented to the learner either verbally, pictorially, or in combination. It is often said that such models play a major role in shaping behavior. Another research study by Bandura, Ross, and Ross (1963) attempted to determine the extent to which film-mediated aggressive models served as a source of imitative behavior. The research revealed that the observation of models portraying aggression on film substantially increases the probability of aggressive reactions to subsequent frustrations being displayed by the subjects. The subjects were nursery-school children, and although it was not studied by the researchers, they did observe that the children did not, as a rule, perform indiscriminately the behavior of the filmed characters. They explained this by saying that the aggressive behavior is possibly either a function of negative reinforcement patterns in the methods of the child's rearing or as a result of the probability that proprioceptive feedback alone (the filmed model's behavior) is not sufficient to account for response inhibition or demonstration. Finally, the model may be *exemplary*, in which case the model is already known to the subject, and any reference elicits a response pattern, either negative or positive; for example, the "hero-worship" phase in children.

In an attempt to explain the observer's matching-response (imitative) behavioral patterns, Bandura and Walters (1963, p. 60) listed three effects of the observation of models:

1. Modeling effect—the acquisition by the observer of new responses that were not previously part of the repertory and that, through observation, the

observer is substantially able to reproduce

2. Inhibitory and disinhibitory effects—the strengthening or weakening of response patterns that are already a part of the observer's repertory, but that, as a result of observation of a model, take on a new pattern

3. Eliciting effect—the eliciting of previously learned matching responses of the model and the observer through the observation of the model by the observer

Bandura and Walters supported each of the three effects of the models by experimental means. During recent years, a number of investigators have conducted laboratory-experimental studies in which subjects have been exposed to aggressive real-life or fantasy models. These investigators have varied considerably in their choice of stimulus conditions and of dependent variables. The results of these studies suggest that observation of the behavior of models has three rather different effects, each of which may be reflected in an increase in the number, range, and intensity of the observer's matching responses.

TRANSMISSION OF NOVEL RESPONSES BY MEANS OF MODELING EFFECT

The observer may acquire new responses that did not previously exist in the repertory. In order to demonstrate this *modeling effect* the model must exhibit highly novel responses, and the observer must reproduce them in a substantially similar form.

"In a study designed to test for delayed imitation of deviant models in the absence of the models, Bandura, Ross, and Ross (1961) exposed one group of nursery-school children to aggressive adult models and a second group to models who displayed inhibited and nonaggressive behavior. Half of the children in each of these conditions observed models of the same sex as themselves, while the remaining children in each group were exposed

to models of the opposite sex. For the aggressive-model group, the model exhibited unusual forms of physical and verbal aggression toward a large inflated plastic doll. In contrast, the nonaggressive-model group observed an adult who sat very quietly, totally ignoring the doll and the instruments of aggression that had been placed in the room" (Bandura and Walters, 1963, p. 61). Results showed that, in the absence of the model, children imitated not only the discriminated responses, but also behaviors performed by the models. They also produced new types of aggressive behavior that fell within the same category of aggressive behavior but that the model did not exhibit. For example, if the model hit the Bobo doll by hand, the children who observed the model's aggressive behavior not only hit the doll but also kicked it with their feet.

Later, Bandura, Ross, and Ross (1963), as cited by Bandura and Walters (1963, p. 61), "compared the effects of real-life models, human-film aggression, and cartoon-film aggression on the aggressive behavior of preschool children. Subjects in the human-film–aggression condition saw a movie that showed the adults who had served as the male and female models in the real-life conditions portraying aggression toward the inflated doll. Children in the cartoon-aggression condition observed a cartoon character make the same aggressive responses as the human models did in the other two conditions. After exposure to the models, all children were mildly frustrated, and measures were than obtained of the amount of imitative and nonimitative aggression they exhibited in a new setting with the model absent." Results of this experiment showed that "the children who observed the aggressive models displayed a great number of precisely imitative aggressive responses, whereas such responses rarely occurred in either the nonaggressive-model group or the control group. Moreover, children in the nonagressive-model group displayed the inhibited behavior characteristic of their model to a greater extent than did the control children. In addition, the results indicated that film-mediated models are as effective as real-life models in transmitting deviant patterns of behavior." (Bandura and Walters, 1963, p. 61.)

"Experimental demonstrations of modeling effects have so far employed only aggressive behavior as the dependent variable. Anthropological and field-study data suggest that other classes of responses may be acquired through the observation of social models; for example, Bandura (1960) compared the behavior patterns of parents of highly aggressive children with those of parents of children who displayed generalized inhibition of social behavior and found that the parents of inhibited children were generally more inhibited and controlled in their behavior than were the relatively expressive and sometimes impulsive parents of the aggressive children. . . . A somewhat similar modeling effect is reflected in the findings of Levin and Baldwin (1959) that indicated that parents who were socially retiring had children who were shy and inhibited when required to perform in public." (Bandura and Walters, 1963, p. 64.)

INHIBITORY AND DISINHIBITORY EFFECTS

"Observation of models may strengthen or weaken inhibitory responses; these *inhibitory* and *disinhibitory* effects are apparent in studies in which the responses evoked already exist in the subject's repertory." Of course these responses may not precisely match those made by the model (Bandura and Walters, 1963, p. 60).

An experiment was conducted by Lovaas (1961) in which he permitted children to play with either of two toys, each of which could be operated by depressing a lever. In one case the lever operated a hitting doll; in the other case it caused a ball to rise within a cagelike structure. Children who had watched an aggressive cartoon gave a greater proportion of responses to the lever that operated the hitting doll than the children who had watched the nonaggressive movie. In this case the model appears to have had a disinhibitory effect. Furthermore, the author suggests that there are times when the presentation of aggressive material may serve as a discriminative cue signaling an occasion on which aggressive behavior is unlikely to meet with punishment.

"Inhibitory effects are more likely to be produced through the observation of painful consequences resulting from a model's behavior or of fearful reactions by the model that the observer has already learned to recognize as danger signals" (Bandura and Walters, 1963, p. 79).

ELICITING EFFECT

"It is possible that observation of a model sometimes elicits previously learned matching responses in the observer simply because the perceiving of acts of a certain kind serves as a 'releaser' for responses of that same class. This *eliciting effect* can be distinguished from disinhibition if we know the past history of the subjects. However, since the classification of a response as deviant implies social censure and since children are generally taught not to make socially censured responses, it is probably safe to assume that the eliciting of previously learned deviant responses through exposure to a deviant model usually, if not always, reflects a disinhibitory process" (Bandura and Walters, 1963, p. 60)

Independent variables that influence the effect of modeling in the acquisition of behavior
Culture

According to Bandura and Walters (1963, p. 47), it is evident from informal observation that models are utilized in all cultures to promote the acquisition of socially sanctioned behavior patterns, the cultural importance of observational learning is especially apparent in accounts given by anthropologists of the process of socialization in societies other than our own." In many languages "the word for 'teach' is the same as for 'show' and the synonymity is literal" (Reichard, 1938, p. 471).

A study by Nash (1958) of the social training of children in a Cantalense subculture of Guatemala pointed out the manner in which complex adult role behavior can be acquired almost entirely through imitation. "The young Cantalense girl is provided with a water jar, a broom, and a grinding stone, which are miniature versions of those used by her mother. Through constantly observing and imitating the domestic activities of the mother, who provides little or no direct tuition, the child readily acquired a repertory of appropriate sex-role responses. Similarly, small Cantalense boys accompany their fathers while the latter are engaged in occupational activities and reproduce their father's actions with the aid of smaller versions of adult implements" (Bandura and Walters, 1963, p. 48).

North American parents also provide their children with miniature functioning replicas of the complex appliances that are customarily found in their households. "While playing with these toys that stimulate imitation of adults, children frequently reproduce not only the appropriate adult role-behavior patterns, but also characteristic or idiosyncratic parental patterns of response, including attitudes, mannerisms, gestures, and even voice inflections, which the parents have certainly never attempted directly to teach." (Bandura and Walters, 1963, p. 48.)

In many cultures, "children do not do what adults tell them to do, but rather what they see other adults do" (Reichard, 1938, p. 471). "While it is evident that much learning in North American society is still fostered through the presentation of real-life models, with advances in technology and written and audiovisual means of communication, increasing reliance is placed on the use of the symbolic models" (Bandura and Walters, 1963, p. 49).

Symbolic models may be presented "through oral or written instructions, pictorially, or through a combination of verbal and pictorial devices. Verbal instructions that describe the correct responses and their sequencing constitute one widely prevalent means of providing symbolic models. Indeed, without the guidance of manuals and directives, members of technologically advanced societies would be forced to engage in exceedingly tedious and often haphazard trial-and-error experimentation." (Bandura and Walters, 1963, p. 48.)

"Pictorially presented models are provided in films, television, and other audiovisual displays, often without the accompaniment of any direct instructions to the observer. In fact, audiovisual mass media are, at the present time, extremely influential sources of social behavior patterns . . . Such models play a major part in shaping behavior and in modifying social norms and thus exert a strong influence on the behavior of children and adolescents. Consequently, parents are in danger of becoming relatively less influential as role models and often are greatly concerned with the problem of regulating their children's television viewing." (Bandura and Walters, 1963, p. 49.)

"Rate and level of learning may vary as a function of mode of model presentation, since an actual performance is apt to provide substantially more relevant cues with greater clarity than is conveyed by a verbal description" (Bandura and Walters, 1963, p. 50).

In the child-training literature a good deal of attention has been given to parental use of *exemplary models*, which may be presented to the child through verbal description, pictorially, or, if the behavior of the model is already known to the child, simply by reference to the model and one or more of the model's characteristics. Exemplary modeling may be positive, as when parents point to some child or adult as an example of how to behave; in contrast, in negative exemplary modeling, the parents select some person as demonstrating undesirable behavior, attitudes, or attributes, often pointing out their consequences for the model and exhorting the child not to follow in those footsteps. The problem with negative modeling is that, "in attempting to deter their children from socially undesirable activities, the parents are forced to focus, and sometimes to elaborate, on deviant behavior which otherwise may have received little attention from the children. Exemplary models often reflect *social norms* and are thus a means of describing or displaying in varying degrees of detail the appropriate conduct for given stimulus situations." (Bandura and Walters, 1963, p. 50.)

Characteristics of the model – prestige and sex

Experiments conducted by Miller and Dollard on the prestige of models and their effect on imitation have confirmed the deduction from learning theory that an individual can learn to discriminate between leaders as good and bad models. They learn to copy the leader they are rewarded for copying and not to copy the leader they are not rewarded for copying. Once such learning occurs, it generalizes to new leaders, so that there is a tendency to copy the new leaders who are similar to those whom the individual has been rewarded for copying and to "noncopy" the new leaders who are similar to others whom the individual has been rewarded for "noncopy." A leader who has acquired prestige as a good model for several responses is likely to be copied in other new responses, and one who has acquired "negative prestige" as a bad model for several responses is likely not to be copied in new responses. Miller and Dollard stated that a similar analysis could be applied to other forms of prestige,

such as that involved in compliance with suggestions and obedience to commands (Miller and Dollard, 1941, pp. 181-182).

Differences between the sex of a model and the sex of a child also influence the extent to which imitative behavior is elicited, thus channeling social responses in the direction of sex-role behavior (Bandura, Ross, and Ross, 1963). Moreover, reinforcement procedures are more effective when the agent of reward is a high-prestige person than when the reinforcers are dispensed by a person of low prestige (Prince, 1962, p. 378.)

Influence of response consequences to the model

"The influence that the behavior of a model will exert on an observer is partly contingent on the response consequences to the model. Children who observe an aggressive-model rewarded display more imitative aggression than children who see a model punished for aggression. Similarly, rewarding and punishing consequences to a model who violated a prohibition influence the extent to which his transgression will be imitated. In addition, models who are rewarding, prestigious, or competent, who possess high status, and who have control over rewarding resources are imitated more readily than are models who lack these qualities. Such factors also determine in part which models will be selected as major sources of exemplary social-behavior patterns. While immediate or inferred response consequences to the model have an important influence on the observer's *performance* of imitative responses, the *acquisition* of these responses appears to result primarily from contiguous sensory stimulation" (Bandura and Walters, 1963, p. 107).

Characteristics of the subjects – observer characteristics

Characteristics of the observers, deriving from their previous reinforcement histories, also influence the extent to which imitative behavior occurs. Persons who have received insufficient rewards, such as those who are lacking in self-esteem or who are incompetent, and those who have been previously rewarded for displaying matching responses are especially prone to imitate a successful model; so too are highly dependent individuals who are probably also persons who have frequently been rewarded for conforming behavior. Moreover, observers who believe themselves to be similar to models in some attributes are more likely to match other classes of responses of the models than are observers who believe themselves to be dissimilar. Also, "susceptibility to the social influence of model is increased by temporary or transient states of the observer, such as emotional arousal of a moderate degree of intensity or the intensified dependency that can be induced through hypnotic procedures" (Bandura and Walters, 1963, p. 108).

Summary and conclusion

In conclusion, imitative behavior is often rewarded by the model and, in addition, brings rewarding consequences, provided the model exhibits socially effective behavior; consequently, most children develop a generalized habit of matching the responses of successful models. Indeed, social behavior patterns are most rapidly acquired through the combined influence of models and differential reinforcement. While the principles of successive approximation and imitation are crucial for understanding the acquisition of social-behavior patterns, maintenance of these patterns over a long period of time is best explained in terms of principles derived from studies of the effects of the scheduling of reinforcement (Bandura and Walters, 1963).

Application to nursing education and practice

An important aspect of behavior in the educational process is imitative behavior. The stress that communities place on having teachers of fine character partly stems from the concept that the commendable attributes may rub off on the pupils by some kind of imitative process. In addition, a considerable part of what the teacher does in the classroom is a process of demonstrating in such a way that the pupils can effectively imitate the performance. The importance of imitation varies with the subject matter. The teaching of surgery, for example, would be hardly feasible if it did not lean heavily on an imitative process. On the other hand, work in creative writing should avoid any imitative process, for it would clearly defeat the purposes of the course. (This is not to say that a course in creative writing does not depend on certain language skills, some of which have been learned by an imitative process.)

There is another aspect of imitative behavior that is of immediate practical importance to the beginning teacher; this is the tendency for pupils to imitate the general characteristics of the teacher. Anybody who has spent time visiting schools probably noted that in the quiet rooms the teachers are typically quiet people who rarely if ever raise their voice. On the other hand, noisy classrooms are typically run by noisy teachers, who talk loudly and who commonly raise their voice to recover control. Some systematic studies support this common observation. In the studies conducted by Anderson and his associates (1945 to 1946) at Michigan State University, the findings showed that aggressive teachers had many pupils manifesting aggressive behavior. Low aggression on the part of the teacher was accompanied by little aggression among pupils (Travers, 1967, p. 378).

Role of matched-dependent and copying behaviors in the school setting

Matched-dependent behavior is well illustrated by the tendency for pupils to reflect many of the aspects of the behavior of the teachers. It is not that the pupils intentionally copy the behavior of the teachers, for they do not. Without being aware of what they are doing, they nevertheless manage to reflect aspects of the teacher's behavior; but they are not particularly concerned about the fact that some of their behaviors do not match very well. This tendency to match behavior is typically found in situations in which persons have to relate to figures of prestige, such as the pupils relating to the prestigious figure of the teacher.

An important aspect of matched-dependent behavior, when it has occurred over a long period, is the phenomenon known as *identification.* Much evidence indicates that matched-dependent behavior and its consequences— identification— represent major elements in the development of personality; and it is particularly effective as a generator of attitude. For this reason, the attitudes of children tend to show a considerable resemblance to those of their parents. Children tend to vote the same way their parents do, and they also tend to show a considerable resemblance to them in their religious attitudes. Furthermore, identification with the parents must necessarily play a greater role in the molding of personality than does contacts with teachers (Travers, 1967, p. 376).

Matched-dependent behavior and identification also represent major elements in the development of a role. Much has been written (both by nurses and by social scientists) about the nursing role, especially as it is practiced in the bureaucracy of the hospital. Nursing educators have spent so much time trying to define nursing's role that they have not given much attention to the *process* of transmitting this role to students. Hadley (1967) touched on this issue in her presentation of the dynamic interactionist concept of role. She established that role behavior emerges out of interaction between the self and another. The "other" she focuses on is

the patient and the patient's role. While this is indeed significant, it is far less crucial in terms of social learning than the relationship between the student and the teacher or staff nurse, or between the neophyte and the head nurse.

In 1968, Kramer identified role models of new graduate nurses and noted how these models changed over time with employment. It is noteworthy that as a nurse's models changed, so did role conception and values. Much of the socialization of the nursing student is done by direct teaching. Kramer's study indicates that the significance of modeling should not be minimized.

Nursing educators themselves should act as good nursing role models, and the attitude of "do as I say, but don't do as I do" should be abolished. A teacher who is also a nurse has a strong influence on the students' responses in the role taking of "nurse," for they will imitate both the good and bad patterns of behavior picked up from cues provided by the role model. The outcome of the students' affiliation with each instructor will shape their ultimate nursing role.

In contrast to matched-dependent behavior, copying behavior is a much more complex process. For example, in teaching the student nurse the procedure of withdrawing 1 ml of vitamin B complex from a vial and inject it intramuscularly (I.M.) to a patient, the nursing instructor carefully demonstrates and illustrates with pictures each of the steps of the procedure. The student nurse then makes an attempt to copy and demonstrate the steps. During this learning phase (acquisition phase), if the student realizes that the position of the vial or the angle of the needle to the site of injection is not correct, that is, not similar to the model presented, then the student begins again, paying greater attention to the proper handling of the vial and correct angle of the needle to the site of injection. What the student nurse is doing in this instance is *discriminating* between the model and his or her own efforts to reproduce the model. The student recognizes similarities and differences and takes action to correct the differences.

Miller and Dollard (1941) showed that copying behavior may have disadvantages as well as advantages in the learning process. Through copying a person may learn to perform certain essential acts related to the solution of a particular problem, but may not have the ability to solve the problem. A student nurse may be baffled by a transformational problem about drugs and solutions but may eventually complete it to the teacher's satisfaction by copying the procedure from the paper of another. This copying behavior does nothing to help the student solve future transformational problems in drugs and solutions because it does not include the copying of certain internal behaviors that form an essential part of the process. Copying behavior, if it is to be effective must permit the learner to copy most of the essential processes of the skill to be learned. When imitation is incomplete, learning is generally ineffective.

Another example of this phenomenon is when students learn to do mathematics by formula without understanding the basic principles underlying the formulas. For example, a student nurse who learns by rote the formula for transforming fahrenheit (F) to centigrade (C) by memorizing

$$(F - 32)^5/_9 = C$$

may be able to produce right answers, but only as long as all the problems remain in exactly the same format. Give the problem a new twist, such as changing centigrade to fahrenheit, and the student is completely lost. Incomplete imitation creates a situation in which there is little transfer of learning.

Role of imitation and independent learning–language learning

Imitation can greatly hasten the process of independent learning by enabling the subject

(such as an autistic child) to perform the first correct response sooner than usual. Imitation is particularly important when the occurrence of the correct response would otherwise be exceedingly improbable (such as in cases involving combinations of a number of different units, such as the syllables of a long word). In order for imitation to elicit the first correct response, the essential units of coying or matched-dependent behavior must already have been learned (Miller and Dollard, 1941, p. 217)

When one is copying or learning to say a word for the first time, the crucial cues for producing the correct response are the syllables that are heard from the model. At the same time, part of the stimulus pattern is just having heard and felt oneself say the preceding syllable. Thus, by generalization there is a tendency on subsequent trials to respond appropriately, not only to the stimulus of hearing the model's syllable (cue) but also to the stimulus of hearing the preceding syllable being said and, in the case of the initial syllable, to the stimulus of the situation, the name of the word, or the thought of the name of the word. Because responses are weaker in situations to which they generalize than in the original situation in which they were rewarded, it is easier for the subject to say the word, such as milk or orange, on the second trial with the aid of hearing the model than it is if the model does not continue to say the word or cue the child. As soon as the generalized tendencies become strong enough so that the correct response occurs in the absence of the model, this generalized response can be rewarded, and the subject is learning independently (Miller and Dollard, 1941, p. 204).

It may take approximately three to five repetitions before a normal child will say the word milk, for example. However, in an autistic child, the first utterance of the word may not take place until the model (therapist) has made several hundred repetitions of the word. Often the model may have to clasp the lips of the autistic child together and force the sound of "m" to come out. Through the process of shaping the behavior, the therapist can eventually get the child to say the word correctly.

"If a child has no opportunity to hear speech, as in the case of deaf persons (Keller, 1927), and no opportunity to match the mouth and laryngeal muscular responses of a verbalizing model, it would probably be impossible to teach that child the kind of verbal responses that constitute a language. In such cases where some other stimulus is known to be capable of arousing an approximation to the desired behavior, the process of acquisition can be considerably shortened by imitation and the provision of social models" (Bandura and Walters, 1963, p. 3).

Other implications

The role of vicarious reinforcement is very important in social learning. Bandura and Walters (1967) demonstrated that learned behavior can occur when "the learner merely views and does not reproduce the response for reward during the learning process" (p. 12). Positive reinforcement would not be present by the model during the observational learning sequence. Maintaining and eliciting this behavior, however, is highly dependent on vicarious reinforcement, or the observation of the reward the model receives for this behavior. An example could be the young child who watches an older brother prepare to go to the hospital. If the brother were given special attention and gifts then indeed the younger child learns that hospitalization is not a threat. A meaningful and socially successful model in the learning situation, such as the brother's experience, heightens the reinforcement level of the younger child.

The human being is continually being molded and oriented to society by extinction, counterconditioning, positive reinforcement, social imitation, and discrimination. The child who continually throws tantrums in order to control the parents' behavior will reduce this tendency if there is no response by the parents. Nonresponse must be continually reinforced or the tantrum behavior will not be extinguished.

Counterconditioning of a child—such as that the syringe and white uniform do not signify fear—may be approached by playing "water guns" with the nurse. Incompatible responses of fun—water-gun syringes—are paired with receipt of intramuscular medication to reduce fear responses in the patient.

Positive reinforcement by fixed-interval, fixed-ratio, and continuous reinforcement are inherent in our society. Fixed-interval time schedules tend to regulate our daily lives. Why do we eat three meals at 7, 12, and 6 o'clock? Fixed-interval time and fixed-rate ratio are often combined to produce a tenacious and inflexible responding rate. The patient who leans on the buzzer may be conditioned by the nursing personnel to give loud and frequent complaints before they will appear. A busy mother may have more time to spend with her child at specific times and, therefore, only responds to much louder cries at other times. In both instances, the model can vary the intensity of both rate and time by rewarding quieter less-frequent demands. Frequent contact with patients in response to low reasonable requests also builds a trust and rapport needed in meaningful communication.

These learned social patterns of behavior tend to generalize into similar overlapping areas. Using internal and external cues as guides, Kahn (1960) noted two interesting generalizations encouraged by lower- and middle-class mothers: the lower-class mother regarded her child as being good only when obedient and respectful, and the middle-class mother positively reinforced curiosity, self-control, and happiness in the child. Dependency, which is reinforced in the lower-class child's formative years, when combined with low school achievement, because of unfamiliar teaching models, will very likely be reinforced in the ghetto scene. The effects of meaningful education and social-class reinforcement are a wide-open area for research (Bandura and Walters, 1963).

For social learning to be effective, it must also provide discrimination. Socially inappropriate behavior is reduced by punishment, inhibition, and nonreward. Mowrer (1960) defined the progressive modeling of behavior to avoid punishment as "response inhibition." The noncommunicative, self-stimulating child—the autistic child—whose behavior is gradually modeled to avoid a shock stimulus used in learning, would be an example of this principle. *Place-avoidance* learning teaches the individual to substitute appropriate behavior for inappropriate behavior.

From infancy on, people are continually developing internal and external cues that guide behavior. From early childhood, the development of these cues is combined into a framework that culminates in adult cognitive morality at about 12 years of age. Piaget postulated that through authority and punishment the child's concept of morality develops into the cognitive mediating processes of reciprocity and cooperation.

Huckabay (1971) found that this cognitive moral judgment was positively associated moral behavior and cooperation at the 6- to 8-year-old age level. Awareness of the consequences of behavior with their effects on the self and others was part of this mature morality. This study also found that the negative social behaviors of cheating, lying, lack of resistance to temptation, and aggression decrease as the child grows older, and that these negative social behaviors are positively related to one another. Also, they are not inversely related to positive social behaviors of empathy, cognitive moral judgment, and generosity. The latter finding indicates that a child is capable of performing both negative and positive social behaviors at the same time; for example, cheating in one situation and being generous and empathetic in another.

Personality development is an integral part of socially learned behavior. Dependency and physical comfort form the basis of the habit hierarchies that are learned as very young children. As people grew older, they learn to communicate, and are positively reinforced by verbal-cognitive processes. These more elemental hierarchy levels of attention seeking, dependency, and physical comfort, however, are reverted to when stress or illness strikes. Social learning in general puts particular emphasis on the social models, training, and environmental, sociological, and personal variables with which an individual comes in contact.

Another very important area in which the principles of social learning apply is in the area of *battered-child syndrome*. There are many questions that can be added that have not been answered yet and that await researching. For example, what kind of models do these battered children have? The physical act of aggression on the part of the parent toward the child creates a very dramatic scene for the child to imitate and model. What can be done to countercondition parents who abuse their children and also to countercondition the negative effects of the aggressive behavior model that is observed and experienced by the child. The studies of Bandura, Ross, and Ross (1961, 1963) have some implications here. If the child observes either a film or an actual model being punished after hitting a doll or a child, the observer (child) is less likely to imitate the behaviors of the model. Punishment of the model has inhibitory effects on the observer.

These are but a few of the implications of the principles of social learning to nursing practice and nursing education. The basic concepts of social-learning theory have vast application to nursing.

Researchable questions

1. What is the effect of observing two types of models—(1) nurturant and (2) aggressive, who is being punished for aggressive behavior—on the aggressive behavior of the battered child?
   a. Independent variable: observation of two types of models
   b. Dependent variable: aggressive behaviors of the battered child
2. In a longitudinal study (15 to 20 years) discover what the effect of battered-child syndrome is on the parental behaviors (provision of nurturance, protection, love, meeting of biological needs of their offspring) of these subjects toward their own offspring? The main rationale of this study is to find out if children who are being abused and battered now by their parents turn out to be parents who in turn abuse their own offspring.
   a. Independent variable: battered-child syndrome, that is, having been physically abused by parents
   b. Dependent variable: parental behaviors of former battered children toward their own offspring

ADDITIONAL LEARNING EXPERIENCES
Highly recommended reading list

Bandura, A., and Huston, A. C. Identification as a process of incidental learning. *Journal of Abnormal and Social Psychology*, 1961, 63:311-318.

Bandura, A., and Walters, R. *Social learning and personality development*. New York: Holt, Rinehart and Winston, Inc., 1963.

Kramer, M. The concept of modeling as a teaching strategy. *Nursing Forum*, 1972, 11:50-51.

Additional recommended reading list
The role of modeling

Bandura, A., Ross, D., and Ross, S. Transmission of aggression through imitation of aggressive models.

Journal of Abnormal and Social Psychology, 1961. 63:575-582.

Bandura, A., Ross, D., and Ross, S. Imitation of film-mediated aggressive models. *Journal of Abnormal and Social Psychology*, 1963, 66:3-11.

Miller, N. E., and Dollard, J. *Social learning and imitation*. New Haven: Yale University Press, 1941.

Child-rearing practices—modeling in dependency behavior

Bandura, A. Relationship of family patterns to child behavior disorders. *Progress Report*, U.S. Public Health Service research grant M-1734, Stanford University, Stanford, Calif., 1960.

Moral development

Aronfreed, J. The origin of self criticism. *Psychological Review*, 1964, 71(3):193-218.

Huckabay, L. M. *A developmental study of the relationship of negative moral-social behaviors to empathy, to positive social behaviors and to cognitive moral judgment*. An unpublished doctoral dissertation, University of California, Los Angeles, Calif., 1971.

Walters, R. H., and Demkow, L. Timing of punishment as a determinant of resistance to temptation. *Child Development*, 1963, 34:207-214.

Nursing role

Pearson, L. E. The clinical specialist as a role model or motivator? *Nursing Forum*. 1972, 11(1):71-77.

INSTRUCTIONS TO THE LEARNER REGARDING POSTTEST

You are now ready to take the posttest to determine the level of achievement of the objectives. Return to the pretest and take it over again as the posttest. Correct your answers using the answer key that is found at the end of this module (p. 164). You need to score 36 correct points (95% level) to proceed to the next module. If your score is less than 36 points, correct the errors, study the text again, and read some of the articles in the recommended reading list. You need to study until you achieve the 95% level of mastery.

ANSWER KEY TO PRETEST AND POSTTEST

1. True (Bandura and Huston, 1961, p. 312)
2. False (Miller and Dollard, 1941, p. 185)
3. True (Bandura and Walters, 1963, pp. 10-11)
4. False (Kramer, 1972, p. 62; Miller and Dollard, 1941, p. 183)
5. False (Bandura and Walters, 1963, p. 224)
6. False (Bandura, Ross, and Ross, 1963, pp. 3-11)
7. True (Bandura, Ross, and Ross, 1963, pp. 3-11)
8. b (Miller and Dollard, 1941, pp. 91-92)
9. c (Miller and Dollard, 1941, pp. 91-92)
10. a (Miller and Dollard, 1941, pp. 91-92)
11. d (Bandura and Walters, 1963, p. 72)
12. e (Bandura and Walters, 1963, p. 72)
13. f (Bandura and Walters, 1963, p. 72)
14. b (Bandura and Huston, 1961, p. 311)
15. a (Bandura and Huston, 1961, p. 311)
16. d (Kramer, 1972, p. 53)
17. a (Bandura and Walters, 1963, p. 110)
18. a (Bandura and Walters, 1963, p. 120)
19. d (Bandura and Walters, 1963, p. 13)
20. d (Bandura and Walters, 1963, p. 44)
21. b (Miller and Dollard, 1941, pp. 18-35)
22. b (Miller and Dollard, 1941, pp. 91-92)
23. d (Kramer, 1972, p. 50)
24. b (Miller and Dollard, 1941, p. 211)
25. a. Superiors in age
    b. Superiors in social status
    c. Superiors in intelligence ranking system
    d. Superior technicians in any field
    (Miller and Dollard, 1941, p. 183)
26. a. Description should include major principles of copying behavior and the variables that influence it. (Text, pp. 158-162)
    1. The process of copying the behavior of the model
    2. Characteristics of the copier and how they affect modeling behavior
    3. Characteristics of the model and how they influence the behavior of the copier
    b. Description should include (1) role of modeling in imitation of aggressive behavior, as in parent (model), battered child (observer); (2) concept of consequences of behavior of the model; for example, mother not being punished for battering child, therefore child will have the tendency to imitate mother when older; (3) concept of counterconditioning to inhibit and/or extinguish this type of behavior; (4) social issues around battered-child syndrome. (Text, p. 162; Bandura, Ross, and Ross, 1961, 1963)

REFERENCES

Allport, F. H. *Social psychology*. Cambridge, Mass.: Riverside Press, 1924.

Anderson, H. H., and Brewer, J. E. Studies of teacher's classroom personalities: I. Dominative and socially integrative behavior of kindergarten teachers. *Applied Psychology Monograph*, No. 6, 1945, pp. 1-157.

Anderson, H. H., and Brewer, J. E. Studies of teacher's classroom personalities: II. Effects of teacher's dominative and integrative contacts on children's classroom behavior. *Applied Psychology Monographs*, No. 8, 1946, pp. 1-128.

Bagehot, W. *Physics and politics*. New York: Appleton and Co. 1873.

Bandura, A. *Relationship of family patterns to child behavior disorders*. Progress Report, U.S. Public Health Service research grant M-1734, Stanford University, Stanford, Calif., 1960.

Bandura, A. Social learning through imitation. In M. R. Jones (Ed.), *Nebraska Symposium on Motivation*. Lincoln, Neb.: University of Nebraska Press, 1962(a), pp. 211-269.

Bandura, A. *The influence of rewarding and punishing consequences to the model on the acquisition and performance of imitative responses*, Unpublished manuscript. Stanford University, Stanford, Calif., 1962(b).

Bandura, A., and Huston, A. C. Identification as a process of incidental learning. *Journal of Abnormal Social Psychology*, 1961, **63**:311-318.

Bandura, A., Ross, D., and Ross, S. Transmission of aggression through imitation of aggressive models. *Journal of Abnormal Social Psychology*, 1961, **63**:575-582.

Bandura, A., Ross, D., and Ross, S. Imitation of film-mediated aggressive models. *Journal of Abnormal Social Psychology*, 1963, **66**:3-11.

Bandura, A., and Walters, R. *Social learning and personality development*. New York: Holt, Rinehart and Winston, Inc., 1963.

Dollard, J., and Miller, N. E. *Personality and psychotherapy*. New York: McGraw-Hill Book Co., 1950.

Gagne, R. *The conditions of learning*. New York: Holt, Rinehart and Winston, Inc., 1970.

Hadley, J. The dynamic interactionist concept of role. *Journal of Nursing Education*, 1967, 6(2):24.

Holt, E. B. *Animal drive and the learning process*, vol. 1. New York: Holt, Rinehart and Winston, Inc., 1931.

Huckabay, L. M. A developmental study of the relationship of negative moral-social behaviors to empathy, to positive social behaviors and to cognitive moral judgment. In B. K. Mitsunaga (Ed.), *Science and direct patient care: II*. Paper presented at the Fifth Annual Nurse Scientist Conference, April 14-15, 1971, School of Nursing, University of Colorado Medical Center, Denver, Colo. pp. 167-183.

Hull, C. L. *Principles of behavior*. New York: Appleton-Century-Crofts, 1943.

Humphrey, B. Imitation and the conditioned reflex. *Pediatric Seminar*, 1921, 28:1-21.

Kahn, M. *A poligraph study of the catharsis of aggression*. Unpublished doctoral dissertation, Howard University, 1960.

Keller, H. *The story of my life*. New York: Doubleday & Co., Inc., 1927.

Kramer, M. Role models, role conceptions and role deprivation. *Nursing Research*, 1968, 17:115-120.

Kramer, M. The concept of modeling as a teaching strategy. *Nursing Forum*, 1972, 11:50-51.

La Piere, R. T., and Farnsworth, P. R. *Social psychology*. New York: McGraw-Hill Book Co., 1936.

Levin, H., and Baldwin, A. L. Pride and shame in children. In M. R. Jones (Ed.), *Nebraska Symposium on Motivation*, Lincoln, Neb.: University of Nebraska Press, 1959, pp. 138-173.

Lovaas, O. I.: Effect of exposure to symbolic aggression on aggressive behavior. *Child Development*, 1961, 32:37-44.

McBrearty, J. F., Marston, A. R., and Kanfer, F. H. Conditioning a verbal operant in a group setting: direct versus vicarious reinforcement. *American Psychologist*, 1961, 16:425.

McDougall, W. *An introduction to social psychology*. London: Methuen, 1908.

Miller, N. E. Acquisition of avoidance dispositions by social learning. *Journal of Abnormal and Social Psychology*, 1961, 63:12-18.

Miller, N. E., and Dollard, J. *Social learning and imitation*. New Haven, Conn.: Yale University Press, 1941.

Morgan, L. C. Habit and instinct. London: Arnold, 1896.

Mowrer, O. H. *Learning theory and the symbolic processes*. New York: Wiley and Sons, Inc., 1960.

Nash, M. Cantel: the industrialization of a Guatemalan Indian community. Unpublished doctoral dissertation, University of Chicago, 1955.

Piaget, J. *The moral judgment of the child*. New York: The Free Press, 1948. (First publication in French, 1932.)

Prince, A. I. Relative prestige and the verbal conditioning of children. *American Psychologist*, 1962, 17:378.

Reichard, G. A. Social Life. In F. Boas (Ed.), *General Anthropology*, Lexington, Mass.: D. C. Health & Co., 1938, pp. 409-486.

Rheingold, H. L., Gerwitz, J. L., and Ross, H. W. Social conditioning of vocalization in the infant. *Journal of Comparative Physiological Psychology*, 1959, 52:68-73.

Sheffield, F. D. Theoretical considerations in the learning of complex sequential tasks from demonstration and practice. In A. A. Lumsdaine (Ed.), *Student response in programmed instruction: a symposium*, Washington, D.C.: National Academy of Sciences—National Research Council, 1961, pp. 13-32.

Skinner, B. F. *The behavior of organisms*. New York: Appleton-Century-Crofts, 1938.

Skinner, B. F. *Science and human behavior*. New York: The Macmillan Co., 1953.

Tarde, G. *The laws of imitation*. New York: Holt, Rinehart and Winston, Inc., 1903.

Thorndike, E. L. *The fundamentals of learning*. New York: Teachers College Press, 1932.

Travers, R. M. *Essentials of learning*. New York: The Macmillan Co., 1967.

Watson, J. B., and Rayner, R. Conditioned emotional reactions. *Journal of Experimental Psychology*, 1920, 3:1-14.

Watson, R. I. *Psychology of the child*. (2nd ed.) John Wiley & Sons, Inc., 1967.

Whiting, J. M., and Child I. L. *Child training and personality*. New Haven, Conn.: Yale University Press, 1953.

PART TWO

Models of instruction

Carroll's model of instruction

DESCRIPTION OF MODULE

This module describes Carroll's model of instruction. The content contains a set of instructional objectives that the learner will be able to demonstrate at the completion of the module. The pretest and posttest is provided for self-evaluation purposes in cognitive areas.

The text of the module presents in an integrated form Carroll's model of instruction as it applies to nursing education and nursing practice. The five areas are: theoretical framework, issues, relevant research studies, application to nursing, and researchable questions.

MODULE OBJECTIVES

At the completion of studying the contents of this module and also having read and studied the required reading list, the student will be able to accomplish the following set of objectives at the 95% level of achievement. The student will be able to:

1. Describe, either in writing or orally, the essential components of Carroll's model of instruction
2. Classify these variables in terms of time needed and time spent
3. Identify those variables that are intrinsic to the individual and those that are extrinsic
4. Describe how Carroll views achievement and underachievement in school learning
5. Describe how Carroll measures degree of learning
6. Describe the advantages (usefulness) of Carroll's model
7. Identify at least one issue in Carroll's model
8. Describe at least two research studies that support aspects of Carroll's model
9. Apply in specific terms each of the components of Carroll's model to nursing education and practice
10. Raise at least one researchable question utilizing Carroll's model, and identify both the independent and dependent variables

PRETEST AND POSTTEST

Circle the correct answers. Each question is worth 1 point. The 95% level of mastery for this test is 19 correct points. Take the test and correct your answers using the answer key found at the end of this module (p. 183).

True or false

1. For Carroll, learning tasks as used in his model concern only educational goals, not goals of attitudes. True or False
2. One hypothesis implicit in the Carroll model is that the degree of learning, other things being equal, is a simple function of the

amount of time during which the pupil engages actively in learning. True or False

3. Carroll views the learner's estimated needed time for learning a given task to be a function of a series of basic aptitudes minus a measure of quality of instruction. True or False

Multiple choice

4. In Carroll's model of instruction, aptitude is described as:
   a. the amount of time a pupil needs to learn a task
   b. one variable unrelated to time
   c. the same for all learning tasks
   d. not related to traits the learner has prior to undertaking the specific learning tasks

5. The correct formula to measure degree of learning according to Carroll's model of instruction is:
   a. degree of learning =
   $$f\frac{\text{(time actually spent)}}{\text{(time needed)}}$$
   b. degree of learning =
   $$f\frac{\text{(time needed)}}{\text{(time actually spent)}}$$
   c. degree of learning =
   $$f\frac{\text{(time not spent)}}{\text{(time actually spent)}}$$
   d. degree of learning =
   $$f\frac{\text{(time actually spent)}}{\text{(time not spent)}}$$

6. The issue of self-pacing versus prescribed amount of time allocated to learning a task affects which variable the most?
   a. aptitude
   b. opportunity
   c. ability to understand instruction
   d. perseverance
   e. quality of instruction

7. Which of the following describe or are factors of aptitude? Circle the correct combination.
   1—amount of time a pupil needs to learn the task under optimal conditions
   2—amount of prior learning that may be relevant to the task under consideration
   3—traits, or characteristics, of the learner
   4—quality of instruction
   a. 1, 2, and 3

   b. 1, 2, 3, and 4
   c. 2, 3, and 4
   d. 3 and 4

8. Carroll's model of instruction is composed of five component elements, some residing in the individual and some stemming from external conditions. Indicate the ones that reside within the individual:
   1—aptitude
   2—ability to understand instruction
   3—opportunity
   4—perseverance
   5—quality of instruction
   a. 1, 2, and 5
   b. 2, 3, and 4
   c. 1, 2, and 4
   d. 3, 4, and 1

9. The five components of Carroll's model of instruction are listed below. Circle the correct combination that stems from external conditions.
   1—aptitude
   2—ability to understand instruction
   3—opportunity
   4—quality of instruction
   5—perseverance
   a. 1, 3, and 4
   b. 2, 4, and 3
   c. 4 and 5
   d. 3 and 4

10. The five components of Carroll's model of instruction are listed below. Which ones are expressed purely in terms of time?
    1—aptitude
    2—ability to understand instruction
    3—opportunity
    4—quality of instruction
    5—perseverance
    a. all of the above
    b. 1, 2, and 3
    c. 1, 4, and 5
    d. 1, 3, and 5

11. Carroll stated that the amount of time that a student needs to learn a given task under optimal learning conditions is a reflection of the learner's:
    a. aptitude
    b. perseverance
    c. motivation
    d. verbal skills

12. Which of the following variables can the nursing instructor manipulate easily in order to produce optimal amount of learning in the nursing student?
    a. aptitude
    b. quality of instruction
    c. perseverance
    d. opportunity
    e. ability to understand instruction
13. Factors that positively affect the student's overachievement, according to Carroll (1963), are:
    1—genetic nature of the student
    2—high quality of instruction
    3—the nature of the task to be learned
    4—high perseverance
    5—ample opportunity for learning
    6—personality traits of the student
    7—cognitive style of the student
    a. all of the above
    b. 1, 2, 3, and 7
    c. 2, 4, and 5
    d. 1, 3, 4, 6, and 7
14. Formative tests include which of the following:
    1—allow for grading and product of learning
    2—denote mastery or nonmastery of a learning task
    3—ensure the thorough mastery of each set of learning tasks before subsequent tasks are started
    4—provide feedback to students as to whether their learning approach and study habits are adequate
    5—provide feedback to the teacher by identifying particular points in the instruction that are in need of modification
    a. 1, 2, 3, and 5
    b. 1, 3, 4, and 5
    c. 2, 3, 4, and 5
    d. 2, 4, and 5

Matching

Part A

_____ 15. Ability to understand instruction
_____ 16. Perseverance
_____ 17. Aptitude
_____ 18. Learning task
_____ 19. Achievement

Part B

a. That which will be attained for a given task when all the time needed is spent, that is, when the ratio of time spent to time needed is unity
b. Amount of time the student is willing to spend to attain instructional objectives
c. Amount of time the student requires to reach a particular instructional objective
d. General intelligence and verbal ability of student
e. Going from ignorance of some specified fact or concept to knowledge or understanding of it, or of proceeding from incapability of performing some specified act to capability of performing it

Discussion question

20. List four methods by which the nursing instructor or the nurse can improve the quality of instruction in teaching a learning task to a student or patient.
    a. _____
    b. _____
    c. _____
    d. _____

TEXT
Theoretical framework
Foreword about models in general

A model is a simplification of reality. It is not reality itself, but is intended to enable the people using the model to organize the way they look at reality. A model provides a vehicle for communication about a certain limited conceptual area, defining elements within its domain, as well as relationships between the elements. It provides a guide for study and research. A model is also intended to distinguish matters of relevance from those outside its province of concern.

A model must be distinguished from a statement of philosophy. Philosophical statements involve description of values about areas of greater scope. However, portions of philosophical statements may be incorporated in the assumptions underlying any specific model.

A familiar example may clarify this point. Medical practice is based on a biological model, which views humans as a system composed of interrelated subsystems (such as the gastrointestinal and cardiopulmonary systems), which in turn are made up of parts having specific functions. However, the practice of medicine also incorporates values about humans and assumptions about the relationships between physicians, patients, and society, with ethical implications for how the biological model is utilized and approached. These values and assumptions are made explicit in such codes or philosophical statements as the Hippocratic oath.

The example of the biological model also illustrates the concept of any open system in which the biological organism (system) interacts with the environment, affecting it and being affected by it. The interdependency of the subsystems is also evident in that a change in the gastrointestinal subsystem's balance may produce changes in the cardiopulmonary subsystem.

There are other types of models, such as mathematical models that describe relationships between aspects of a geometric figure, models that describe interaction between two philosophical concepts, the Parsonian idea of the social system, the conflict paradigm currently gaining strength in sociological circles, political science models describing power distribution, and computer formats.

A model tends to evolve an argot specific to its area of concern. The description of each model should include these terms, as well as the assumptions on which the model is based and the limitations it accepts.

In some circles, the word paradigm is used for the same concept as model. Those interested in further study about models should read the foreword and prefaces to *A Sociology of Sociology* by Robert Friedrichs.

John DeCecco (1968, p. 11) stated that "the best substitute for a theory of teaching is a model of teaching. Teaching models suggest how various teaching and learning conditions are interrelated." Robert Glaser (1962) developed a basic teaching model that was previously explained in the introductory module of this book (p. 15). Carroll's model of instruction is unique in that it is the forerunner of the mastery-learning model of instruction.

Carroll's model of instruction

Carroll's model of instruction is concerned with five basic variables affecting success in school learning and the ways in which they interact. Most of the basic concepts in the model are defined so that they can be measured in terms of time. The model says that the learner will succeed in learning a given task to the extent that the amount of time that is needed to learn the task is spent.

In his model, Carroll implies that if teaching is tailored to the learner's abilities and needs, then the learner can achieve a high level of learning. In one instance in which this model was applied to student learning, with other variables held constant, 90% of the students achieved the same level of accomplishment as "A" students had the previous year, when the model was not applied. In the previous year only 20% of the students received A's. The possibility of attaining this type of high achievement is feasible for students in nursing if the faculty seriously implements Carroll's model of instruction (Wolf. and Quiring, 1971).

The five major variables, or factors, of Carroll's model are: (1) aptitude, (2) ability to understand instruction, (3) quality of instruction, (4) opportunity for learning, and (5) perseverance.

The model is oriented around the definition of a learning task. According to Carroll (1963, p. 723), a *learning task* is defined as ". . . going from ignorance of some specified fact or concept to knowledge or understanding of it, or of proceeding from incapability of performing some specified act to capability of performing it."

The model applies to both cognitive and psychomotor domains. Carroll does not believe that the variables apply as much to the learning of affective domain, such as development of attitudes and disposition, but it does seem to be relevant for affective learning. Carroll stated that affective behavior, such as respect for other races and creeds, respect for parental or legal authorities, and the acquisition of values and drives, is learned by means of emotional conditioning. However, learning tasks may be involved in cognitive support of such attitudes (for example, where the individual learns facts about the different races and creeds). Acquisition of attitudes follows a different paradigm from that involved in learning tasks as Skinner (1953) made the distinction between the two types of learning. Learning tasks involves "operants"; the attitudinal goals of education involve "respondents."

Carroll pointed out that the assumption that the work of the school can be broken down into a series of learning tasks can be questioned in that in actual practice the tasks to be learned may not necessarily be treated as distinct and separate and the process of teaching is organized so that incidental learning can take place in the course of other activities. Nevertheless, he said, "a conceptual model requires certain simplifying assumptions, and the assumption of discrete learning tasks is a useful one to make" (Carroll, 1963, p. 724).

The Carroll model is intended for application to all learning tasks, but it requires that (1) the learning goal be explicitly stated (2) means be available to judge achievement of the learning goal. A pupil's success in learning may be described by summating results of applying the model to component learning tasks in a series of tasks.

The central concepts of this model (Carroll, 1963, p. 725.) are that:

1. The learner will succeed in learning a given task to the extent that the amount of time *needed* for learning that task is spent. (Time in this context means that amount of time *actively spent* in the learning task, not merely elapsed time.)
2. There are certain factors that determine how much time the learner *spends* actively engaged in learning
3. There are certain factors that determine how much time the learner *needs to spend* in order to learn the task

The five variables of the model can be categorized into two headings based on the time factor: (1) determinants of *time needed* for learning and (2) determinants of *time spent* in learning.

DETERMINANTS OF TIME NEEDED FOR LEARNING

Aptitude. Aptitude refers to the amount of time needed to learn the task under optimal conditions. The shorter the time needed, the greater is the learner's aptitude. The longer the time needed to achieve or learn a task, the lower is the learner's aptitude. Variables that affect aptitude are:

1. The *amount of prior learning* that may be relevant to the task that is being learned now
2. *Traits*, or *characteristics* of learners, which may be either genetically determined factors or traits that can be accounted for on the basis of generalized prior learning

Carroll views the learner's estimated needed time (a_t) for learning a given task (t) to be a function of a series of basic aptitudes $(a_1, a_2, a_3 \ldots a_7)$ minus the amount of time saved (S_t) because of prior relevant learning. This concept is presented by the following formula:

$$a_t = f(a_1, a_2, a_3 \ldots a_7) - S_t$$

Ability to understand instructions. The general intelligence and verbal ability of the student influence the ability to understand instructions. Students with high intelligence infer for themselves the concepts and relationships in the material to be learned, should the teacher overlook pointing out this important information; whereas students with low intelligence will be adversely affected by poor quality of instruction. Students with high verbal ability again have the upper hand, because high verbal ability comes into play whenever the instructions utilize language beyond the grasp of the student. It is therefore, essential that students with poor abilities receive instruction in a form that is most usable to them.

Quality of instruction. Quality refers to the degree to which instruction for learning a task is organized and presented in such a way that the learner can learn it as rapidly and efficiently as able. Organization and presentation of such a learning task should include the following steps:

1. The learner must be told in terms that can be comprehended, *what* is to be learned, and *how* it is to be learned
2. The learner must be put into adequate sensory contact with the material to be learned (for example, making sure the student can hear and see the elements of the task to be learned, such as hearing a record player or seeing the slides)
3. Aspects of the learning task should be properly sequenced and presented ·in detail, so that every step of the learning is adequately prepared for by a previous step
4. Instruction must be adapted to the individual learner's characteristics and needs, including stage of learning

These factors or variables determine quality of instruction. The variables apply not only to the quality of the teachers' performance, but also to characteristics of textbooks, workbooks, films, modules, teaching-machine programs, and other resources.

If the quality of instruction is less than optimal, it is possible that students will need more time to learn the task than they would otherwise. Some will be more handicapped by poor instruction than others, depending on their *ability to understand instruction.*

In Carroll's opinion (1963, p. 727) therefore, "The amount of time actually needed by a person to learn a given task satisfactorily is a function not only of aptitude, but also of quality of instruction insofar as it is less than optimal. And the amount of additional time he will need is an inverse function of his ability to understand instruction."

DETERMINANTS OF TIME SPENT IN LEARNING

Opportunity. The amount of time actually allowed by the teacher or the school for learning a given task reflects opportunity for learning. The learning rates of students differ, even when quality of instruction is optimal. Some schools have recognized this fact and have provided the opportunity for students to proceed at their own pace and pursue areas of independent study. Other schools have developed special educational programs for the gifted and for those who need remedial work. Because there are marked individual differences among learners, it may be a good case for the creation of special-ability groupings, however, even this may not be able to meet the individual learner's needs. As pointed out by Wolf and Quiring (1971), the usual baccalaureate program in nursing does not provide for individual pacing of learning.

Perseverance. The amount of time the learner is willing to spend in learning reflects perseverance. Active learning is implied in this definition. The need for perseverance applies to all learners—gifted as well as slow learners. Considering aptitude, quality of instruction, and ability to understand instruction, each learner needs a certain amount of time to learn a given task. There are many reasons for students not being willing or able to put in a certain amount of time to learn the given task to criterion of mastery. Lack of motivation or regarding the task as something very difficult may deter students. They may be distracted or bored or may lose self-confidence. They may go far toward mastery and then overestimate their achievement, thus prematurely terminating efforts to learn. Emotional variability also affects perseverance to learn; for example, one may desire to learn but be unable to endure frustrations, caused by the difficulties of learning the task, or distractions, caused by external circumstances. Some may not have the physical stamina and endurance.

Perseverance in learning also interacts with the quality of instruction. Poor quality of instruction reduces perseverance in learning.

Perseverance is positively affected by motivation, or desire to learn. There are many reasons for wanting to learn something. It may be to please the teacher, to please one's parents and friends, to receive good grades or external rewards, to feed one's own self-esteem, or to avoid disapproval. These are some examples of external incentive factors. In addition to or in place of external incentives, the individual may be intrinsically motivated, such as when the individual perceives the ultimate utility of the thing being learned (Carroll, 1963, pp. 728-729).

The degree of learning is reduced if perseverance is insufficient to attain mastery of the task.

THE COMPLETE CARROLL MODEL—SUMMARY

The following elements are variables that affect success in school learning:

Aptitude	Determine amount
Ability to understand instruction	of time needed for learning a
Instructional quality	specific task

Opportunity (time allowed)	Determine time
Perseverance	actually spent in learning a specific task

Another perspective on the variables is to consider those residing in the individual learner (intrinsic) and those that are part of the environment (extrinsic). The intrinsic variables are aptitude, ability to understand instruction, and perseverance. The extrinsic variables are opportunity (time allowed for learning), and quality of instruction.

These five variables are not static. They interact with each other. Also, they can be manipulated in such a way that each student can achieve optimum levels of learning in relation to individual needs. Carroll stated that if this manipulation of variables is tailored to the individual's needs, then, the student can be expected to achieve mastery. However, this perfect manipulation of variables seldom occurs. As a result there are many cases of underachievement or waste of the student's time by too much repetition (Wolf and Quiring, 1971).

Measurement of variables. Aptitude, perseverance, and opportunity are measurable in terms of time. Ability to understand instruction can be measured in relative terms, by using available tools for measuring general intelligence and verbal ability. Quality of instruction is difficult to measure, although criteria may be established.

Interaction of model components. All elements are interrelated and interdependent. This is expressed in the following equation in which f = function:

Degree of learning =

$$f\frac{\text{(time actually spent in learning)}}{\text{(time needed for learning)}}$$

Time actually spent in learning equals the smallest amount of opportunity, perseverance, or aptitude increased by the amount of time necessary because of poor quality of instruction and poor ability to understand instruction. Time needed to learn after adjustment for quality of instruction and ability to understand instruction is the denominator of the fraction.

Manipulability of elements. Some of the elements of Carroll's model are more readily manipulated than others. Aptitudes based on prior learning may be manipulated; certain other aptitudes may not be easy to manipulate. Ability to understand instruction, or general intelligence, is difficult to manipulate except over very long periods of time in very controlled circumstances; although verbal ability may be stimulated as an aspect of increasing ability to understand instruction. Perseverance—quality of instruction and opportunity to learn are the most available elements for the instructor to manipulate.

• • •

Viewpoints of Carroll's model were found to be primarily positive. The main reasons for the positive viewpoint is in the usefulness of the model. The model has been shown to be very resourceful in clarifying other educational concepts. An example of this is in providing a framework for interpreting the notion of underachievement. *Underachievement* is a situation in which there is discrepancy between actual achievement and that expected on the basis of a certain kind of evidence—evidence concerning the capacity, or aptitude, of the individual to achieve in a particular context (Carroll, 1963, p. 730). This evidence is different from that concerning other factors in achievement, such as motivation and opportunity for learning, and these later factors would not figure in forming expectations. Instead, it is necessary to gather evidence concerning capacity, or aptitude, of the individual, which is the learning rate when all other factors are optimal (Carroll, 1963, p. 730).

ACHIEVEMENT AND EXPECTANCY

Carroll makes reference to his conceptual model and states that the expectation of an individual's achievement in a given task would be that which will be attained when all the time needed is spent, in other words, when the ratio of time spent to time needed is unity. Anything less than this is underachievement (Carroll, 1963, p. 730).

In the framework of the model, underachievement can be seen as a state of affairs that results whenever perseverance is less than some "reasonable value," whenever the quality of instruction is poor, whenever time allowed for learning has not been sufficient, or whenever some combination of these conditions has occurred.

Overachievement occurs when there is a favorable combination of attendant events —high perseverance, ample opportunity for learning, and high quality of instruction (Carroll, 1963).

Another area of usefulness is demonstrated by the fact that Carroll's model inspired Bloom to devise a concept of mastery learning (Module 12).

Relevant research studies

Carroll's model was originally proposed in the context of studies of foreign language learning. Specific research or a test of the model was conducted by Carroll and Spearritt (1967). They applied the model to a simple learning task of the sort that would be found in a school situation. This test of the model will not be explained. A booklet of a programmed-instruction type was developed to test quality of instruction, opportunity for learning, and time to criterion. Simple rules in an artificial foreign language were taught to sixth-grade children by means of the booklet. Several hypotheses were tested, and the results were shown by time to criterion, perseverance, efficiency of learning, and interest in the task.

In general terms, the study (Carroll and Spearritt, 1967, p. 15) indicated that:

. . . . poor quality instruction depressed the performance of children at all intelligence levels, and that it led to reduced perseverance on the part of children of higher intelligence. These findings, if confirmed in other studies, would emphasize the need for good teaching for more able students as well as the less able student. Learning was also shown to be highly inefficient when students had insufficient opportunity for learning. This suggests that learning efficiency measures should be established for children of different intelligence levels for given units of instruction. Such data would allow teachers to assess required amounts of learning time much more accurately than is possible at present.

The variable of Carroll's model are adequately applied by Wolf and Quiring (1971) to new directions in nursing education through curriculum planning and instruction. With application of the model, they show how the first variable—aptitude—influenced nursing education. All nursing students "should be able to achieve a high level of mastery of the material in the nursing program if the time allowed, the instructional method, and the opportunity for learning were in accord with the students' individual needs" (p. 178). Wolf illustrated this with a study conducted by the University of Washington School of Nursing. Students were asked to record the amount of time spent practicing the skills of bedmaking, bathing, and back massage. The time ranged from 0 to 22 hours. Applying this to aptitude, the student who needed 22 hours and had only been allowed to practice 11 hours would not have been able to achieve this skill. Also, the student who needed no practice should not have been required to waste the time.

Several other research groups have studied strategies for achievement that might be generated from Carroll's model of instruction. A *Strategy* is defined by Wolf and Quir-

ing (1971, p. 178) as "the selecting of or focusing on variables in different ways within a research design." Bloom and his students and associates applied Carroll's model in the development and testing of mastery learning. For example, Bloom (1968) took the position that the teacher could and should provide the learner with necessary conditions so that mastery of learning tasks can take place in all students. Airasian (1967), Bloom's student, developed diagnostic progress tests in the form of formative evaluation to be used in conjunction with a course in testing to ensure that all students would start at the same level, in other words, to test the comparability of the entering behaviors of the students. This test, the researchers believed, thus had content sufficiently specific to make this assumption. These formative tests were designed to show the student the extent to which the course objectives were being attained. It provided immediate feedback to the student as well as to the teacher on the level of progression the student was making.

Kim (1968) tested the aptitude component of Carroll's model to determine if students with different aptitudes or capabilities differ in their rate of learning a given task. His subjects were fifth and sixth graders, and he tested the above question in three content areas. Results of his study showed that the time needed to learn a given task was significantly correlated to each student's aptitude. By this study, Kim confirmed Carroll's assumption that any learning task can be achieved by any student, if instruction of the learning task is organized in such a way that it takes into consideration the student's aptitude.

The studies of Behr (1967) and Davis (1967) have shown that spacial perception may be a good predictor of achievement if a course is taught by emphasizing the use of audiovisual media. Also, for students of high verbal ability, a verbal test may be the best predictor of achievement. These studies point out that college students' achievement is maximized when the instructional material is matched to the individual's pattern of abilities.

Application to nursing education and practice

Primary implications of the Carroll model for nursing education lie in manipulation of component elements. Fully applied, the model would stimulate instructional methods that are geared to a variety of aptitudes and abilities to understand instruction. Carroll's model also sheds new light on curriculum planning and instruction. As pointed out by Wolf and Quiring (1971), traditionally, teachers developed a series of pretests that predicted pretty accurately which students would do well in the course. Such an approach to course development and method of instruction views a course as a set of activities to which all students should adjust regardless of their individual capabilities, potentials, and needs. Skillful teachers have just started to adopt Carroll's model to the extent that being "good" in a given learning task may depend greatly on how the content matter is taught and on the material and time available to the student for learning to take place to the mastery level.

When each of the variables is taken into consideration in the planning and implementation of courses, then optimal learning at the mastery level can take place. Examples of other variables are presented in the next section.

Aptitude

How much time does it take for a nursing student to master a given learning task? Since schools of nursing screen their applicants very carefully, it is very likely that all students should achieve the objectives of a given learning task or a program of study at the mastery level, provided that sufficient time

were allowed for all students to study the instructional objectives and the instructional methods and opportunity for learning were tailored according to the individual student's needs. The study of Wolf and Quiring (1971) supports this proposal.

Since aptitude is affected by such factors as previous history of learning and traits, program planning and individual course planning should take these factors into consideration. For example, previous learning, especially that gained in nursing experience and other nursing education, increases aptitude for high levels of nursing education. A program that implements career-ladder concepts can utilize Carroll's model and his concepts of aptitude to design instruction appropriate to various levels of entering behavior both in cognitive and psychomotor domains.

Ability to understand instruction

The determinants of ability to understand instruction are "general intelligence" and "verbal ability." The nursing instructor should take these factors, especially the level of student's verbal ability, into consideration in the planning, implementation, and measurement of a learning task. As pointed out by Wolf and Quiring (1971), some nursing students have very high verbal skills, while others have high spacial and visual skills. The teaching strategy of giving lectures and reading assignments from books and articles is helpful to those students with high verbal ability. These same teaching strategies will put the students with low verbal ability at a disadvantage. With the latter type of students the use of audiovisual and tactual material can help meet the individual needs of the students.

Quality of instruction

This variable is the most manipulatable factor that the nursing instructor can utilize in bringing about a high level of learning in students. This is also an important factor that determines the amount of time a student requires for learning a task. The use of a formative diagnostic test is one way to improve quality of instruction. Formative evaluations that utilize verbal, written, or audio tap feedback enable the student to reduce the time needed to attain a specific level of proficiency in learning a task. Because it provides feedback to student and teacher about the student's areas of strength (areas already mastered) and areas of weaknesses (where additional work is necessary) the student spends the time making up the deficiency instead of overlearning an area that has already been mastered. As a result of such a diagnostic test, time taken to learn a given task or skill is reduced.

Wolf and Quiring (1971) point out a relevant area in which educators have failed in implementing these ideas. Nurse educators emphasize the individualization of patient care but ignore that students need as much individualized instruction. They suggest that instruction should be geared toward a method by which each nursing student learns more efficiently and effectively, and this method should include such strategies as small group discussions, individual tutorial assistance, independent study groups, and the like.

Appropriate *sequencing* of instructional material is another factor that determines quality of instruction. Nurse educators have differing opinions about the order in which to present material in a course or to sequence courses in a curriculum. Some sequence it from the simple to the complex, or expect their students to learn the normal first and then the abnormal. Gagne's (1970) learning hierarchy should provide a framework in organizing and sequencing content in nursing. Wolf and Quiring (1971, p. 178) indicated that further research is needed to determine,

". . . whether there is a correlation between *individual* learners' ability to learn and the different sequences in which materials are presented. Can means be developed to predict which sequences would be most beneficial to individual students?"

They also pointed out that because of the nature of nursing it is not enough for students to attain partial completion in a learning task. For example, a nurse-practitioner who has a low level of nursing knowledge about care plans and medications or a low level of ability to evaluate patients' health-care status and needs is detrimental to patients because proficiency in these areas is vital for the patients' care and safety.

Instruction based on Carroll's model that strives for attainment of mastery level by all students reduces competition for grades; instead the students compete against themselves. This is what is referred to as criterion-referenced evaluation, rather than norm-referenced evaluation. In the latter case, the student is compared with other students in the same class and most probably is graded on the normal curve. In criterion-referenced evaluation, which Carroll's model stresses, many students will be expected to achieve mastery. Furthermore, those students with high aptitude will help classmates with lower aptitude achieve course objectives without themselves being penalized or threatened since they will not be compared to another but will be compared to their own previous performance. Wolf and Quiring (1971) pointed out that such a cooperative attitude should be fostered in nursing students from the very beginning of their program rather than waiting until the senior year when the students have a course in teamwork to provide impetus for this kind of behavior.

Opportunity for learning

Traditionally, nursing curricula are designed either on a quarter (10-week) or semester (16-week) basis. Could it not be possible to develop more flexible time periods to allow students to pace their own learning based on their own needs? It is possible that some students will need less time than others. Why should students be penalized with regard to time to stay longer or shorter than they really need to achieve the objectives of a learning task or course? Independent study kits or modules or different types of programmed instructions have provided for some self-pacing.

Opportunity (time allowed for learning) can also be manipulated when students are regarded individually rather than en masse. Technological advances, study grouping, stimulation of cooperative rather than competitive student relationships, clearly stated behavioral objectives about specific (explicitly stated) learning tasks, provision of resources for individual learning, and more, are implied instructional methods that permit maximum utilization of opportunity for learning without increasing financial costs to the school. Many agencies have gone further in allowing varying periods for students to achieve objectives, recognizing that partial achievement may not provide adequate subordinate hierarchies for future learning; thus, the student who has an adequate, or greater, amount of perseverance but minimal aptitude, or ability to understand instruction, is given greater opportunity and is able to achieve the same objectives as a more gifted student.

Corona (1970) has described some curriculum innovations introduced at Arizona State University College of Nursing that are based on Carroll's model and Bloom's concepts of mastery. She called it the Continuous Progress Curriculum (CPC). The CPC involves a sequential learning process that permits the student to progress according to ability, provides materials and facilities for independent study, and gives freedom to use

initiative in learning. Students are helped to progress at their own rate and assume responsibility for their own learning.

Perseverance

How long is a student willing to spend in learning a task? Perseverance is affected by the student's attitude as well as by physical aspects of the task. Wolf and Quiring (1971) pointed out that the junior-year nursing students at the University of Washington were formerly required to spend a minimum of 6 hours per week on the clinical unit. One instructor found that students were spending between 5 to 15 hours per week on the clinical unit, with the norm being 9 hours. Another teacher reported that students were spending between 8 to 20 hours per week on the unit with 14.1 hours being the mean. These students were not being tested at the end of their work. They were spending this much time optionally. They found out that there were mean differences between the groups. This difference was accounted for because of the physical distance of the facilities from the campus. The first group had to travel 5 miles to reach the clinical area, whereas, the second group utilized the facility on the campus. Wolf and Quiring noted that although the difference might not appear great for one course, factors related to the physical facilities may accumulate and affect perseverance of the students. An implication of these findings is that consideration should be given to the effect of the physical facilities and their availability on the total learning outcomes and times available to the learners to engage in learning.

Summary

To summarize the application of Carroll's model to nursing education we can say that nursing education involves transmission of a complex of theory, interpersonal skills, technical and cognitive skills, and internationalization of values. The very diversity of the nursing content necessitates maximum ability on the part of the nurse educator to manipulate factors that affect student learning. Students cannot be expected to be equally gifted with the intrinsic factors affecting learning in such a variety of tasks. Carroll's model suggests that a student who spends all the time needed should master a given task. The goal of nursing education should therefore be to assist the student by manipulating the instructional components of the educational process. Bloom and Wolf and Quiring have developed a strategy for mastery learning by manipulating the variables. They have found the use of formative evaluation as crucial to the application of mastery learning and have suggested the following methods of applying the variables to nursing education:

1. Given consideration to the student's aptitude, or rate of learning, in planning educational experience
2. Give consideration to each student's aptitude as it relates to instructional methods when planning the method of instruction; those with high verbal ability should be provided verbal instruction, and those high in visual and spacial skills should have instruction utilizing audiovisual methods
3. Sequence course content in such a way that it facilitates student learning
4. Develop formative tests and utilize them in providing feedback to students with regard to their achievement; provide supplementary assistance to those who have not mastered the content
5. Give consideration to student's willingness to engage actively in learning when planning course content and to those factors that affect perseverance, such as physical proximity of learning facilities (Wolf and Quiring, 1971)

Carroll's model also applies to nursing-practice situations because the same principles that apply for student-learning situations also apply to patient-learning situations.

The most obvious situation to which this pertains is the patient-teaching activity of the nurse. Here, measurement of the intrinsic factors is of crucial importance. While some formal assessment measures are available for use in schools, in practice the nurse may need to rely on personal, less-structured assessments. It is helpful to describe some of the aspects of each variable that the nurse will wish to assess. This is a partial list; you should be able to think of others:

APTITUDE

1. What previous knowledge or skills does the patient possess that increases ability to learn the specified task?
2. What misinformation does the patient possess that limits ability to learn this task?
3. What strengths and weaknesses exist in the patient's manual abilities, verbal abilities, and sensory modalities?

ABILITY TO UNDERSTAND INSTRUCTION

1. What is the approximate quality of the patient's general intelligence?
2. What factors may interfere with the patient's ability to understand instruction:
   a. Language most fluently spoken
   b. Pain
   c. Sensory deficits or overloads

PERSEVERANCE

1. What degree of motivation does the patient have toward the specific learning task?
2. What are important rewards and motivators for this patient?
3. Is the patient's willingness to spend time learning the task limited or affected by fatigue or other illness-related variables?
4. Are there specific periods in the day

when the patient is most willing to spend time learning?

EXTRINSIC FACTORS

Based on assessment of such intrinsic factors as described before, the nurse practices patient teaching by assessing the extrinsic factors as well:

1. How much time will be allowed for learning? This will be determined by the patient's and nurse's schedules, including how soon the patient will have to independently utilize the knowledge or skill involved in the learning task.
2. What are the appropriate instructional methods? The nurse will need to know which resources are available, which methods are best related to the patient's aptitude, which resources and methods are most suitable to the content of the learning task, and which methods are most appropriate to the instructor's skills.

Uniformly, the nurse will wish to state explicitly the learning task with related behavioral objectives, and provide concurrent (formative) and final (summative) evaluation of the patient's achievement of the objectives.

Researchable questions

Carroll (1963) pointed out several areas of his model that need researching. He stressed the need for extensive methodological research in developing valid and reliable tools in measuring each of the five variables of the model, especially perseverance and instructional quality. Research is also needed in determining the interaction of the variables with one another; for example, how does instructional quality affect perseverance?

1. More specifically, what is the effect of sequencing a course (simple to complex continuum versus random sequencing of content) on (1) amount of time taken to master the content, (2) degree of cognitive learning, and (3) perseverance (amount of time the student is willing to spend)?
   a. Independent variable: sequencing of course content
   b. Dependent variables: amount of time taken to master the content (aptitude), degree of cognitive learning, perseverance (amount of time the student is willing to spend)
2. What is the effect of opportunity (indefinite versus definite period of time; for example 10 weeks)—time allowed for learning a course on the affective behaviors of students and on perseverance?
   a. Independent variable: opportunity (indefinite versus definite amount of time)
   b. Dependent variables: affective behaviors and perseverance

Conclusion

The description of John Carroll's model of school learning demonstrated the uses of the four components of Robert Glaser's basic teaching model. The instructor of nursing students or patients can utilize this model, realizing that learners do not always need the same degree of exposure to acquire the desired knowledge of a particular subject, or the amount of exposure needed differs with each task and with each individual learner's abilities. The key concept of this model is that any student can learn a specific task, given enough time and high quality of instruction.

ADDITIONAL LEARNING EXPERIENCES—RECOMMENDED READING LIST

Carroll, J. B. A model of school learning. *Teacher's College Record*, 1963, **64**:723-733

Block, J. (Ed.) *Mastery learning*. New York: Holt, Rinehart and Winston, Inc., 1971. (Entire book is excellent, but especially annotated bibliography, pp. 89-147.)

Friedrich, R. *A sociology of sociology.* New York: The Free Press, 1972.

Wolf, V. C., and Quiring, J. Carroll's model applied to nursing education. *Nursing Outlook,* 1971, **19**(3): 176-179.

INSTRUCTIONS TO THE LEARNER REGARDING POSTTEST

Now you are ready to take the posttest to determine the extent to which you have achieved the objectives of this module. Return to the pretest and take it again as the posttest. Correct your errors using the answer key that is found on this page. You need to achieve 19 correct points (95%) to proceed to the next module. Correct your errors, read the text of this module again and some of the articles in the recommended reading list. You need to study until you achieve 95% mastery level.

ANSWER KEY TO PRETEST AND POSTTEST

1. True (Carroll, 1963, p. 724)
2. True (Carroll, 1963, p. 723)
3. False (Carroll, 1963, p. 726)
4. a (Carroll, 1963, p. 725)
5. a (Carroll, 1963, p. 730)
6. b (Carroll, 1963, p. 727)
7. a (Carroll, 1963, pp. 725-726)
8. c (Carroll, 1963, p. 729)
9. d (Carroll, 1963, p. 729)
10. d (Carroll, 1963, pp. 725-729)
11. a (Carroll, 1963, pp. 725-726)
12. b, c and d (Carroll, 1963, p. 731)
13. c (Carroll, 1963, pp. 730-731)
14. c (Wolf and Quiring 1971, pp. 178-179; Block, 1971, p. 58)
15. d (Carroll, 1963, p. 726)
16. b (Carroll, 1963, p. 728)
17. c (Carroll, 1963, p. 725)
18. e (Carroll, 1963, p. 723)
19. a (Carroll, 1963, p. 730)
20. a. State the objectives in terms that the student or patient can understand
    b. Provide for adequate sensory contact

c. Provide for proper sequencing of the task to be learned
d. Adapt instruction to the learner's characteristics, needs and stage of learning (Carroll, 1963, pp. 726-727)

REFERENCES

Airasian, P. *An application of a modified version of John Carroll's model of school learning.* Unpublished master's thesis, University of Chicago, Chicao, 1967.

Behr, M. J. *A study of interaction between structures of intellect factors and two methods of presenting concept modules seven arithmetic.* Unpublished doctoral dissertation, Florida State University, Tallahassee, Fla., 1967.

Block, J., (Ed.) *Mastery learning.* New York: Holt, Rinehart and Winston, Inc., 1971.

Bloom, B. S. Learning for mastery. *UCLA Evaluation Comment,* 1968, **1**:1-12.

Carroll, J. B. A model of school learning. *Teachers College Record,* 1963, **64**:723-733.

Carroll, J. B. and Spearrit, D. *A study of a "Model of school learning."* Center for Research and Development on Education Differences, Cambridge, Mass., 1967.

Corona, D. F. A continuous progress curriculum in nursing. *Nursing Outlook,* 1970, **18**:46-48.

Davis, J. B. *An investigation of the interaction of certain instructional strategies with the structure of basic mental abilities in the learning of some mathematical operations.* Unpublished doctoral dissertation, Florida State University, Tallahassee, Fla., 1967.

DeCecco, J. *The psychology of learning and instruction: educational psychology.* (1st Ed.) Englewood Cliffs, N.J. Prentice-Hall, Inc., 1968, pp. 11-16.

Friedrichs, R. *The Sociology of Sociology.* New York: The Free Press, 1972.

Gagne, R. *The conditions of learning.* (2nd Ed.) New York: Holt, Rinehart and Winston, Inc., 1970.

Glaser, R. Psychology and instructional technology. In R. Glaser (Ed.), *Training research and education.* Pittsburgh, Pa.: University of Pittsburgh Press, 1962, pp. 1-30.

Kim, H. *Learning rates, aptitudes and achievements.* Unpublished doctoral dissertation, University of Chicago, Chicago, 1968.

Skinner, B. F. *Science and human behavior.* New York: The Macmillan Co., 1953.

Wolf, V., and Quiring, J. Carroll's model applied to nursing education. *Nursing Outlook,* 1971, **19**(3): 176-179.

MODULE 12

Bloom's mastery-learning model of instruction

DESCRIPTION OF MODULE

This is a self-contained unit of instruction on Bloom's mastery-learning model of instruction. The content of this module is presented in sequential order. The main text of the module covers five major areas as they relate to mastery learning: theoretical framework, relevant research studies, issues, application to nursing education and practice, and researchable questions. The content is presented in integrated form. In addition to the text, the module contains behavioral objectives for the student to accomplish at the completion of the module and a pretest and posttest to determine the extent to which the student has achieved the objectives.

MODULE OBJECTIVES

At the completion of this module and having studied the recommended reading list, the student will be able to accomplish the following set of objectives at least at the 95% level of mastery:

1. Identify the evolution of the mastery-learning concept from inception to the present
2. Define at least two propositions of mastery learning
3. Differentiate between the work done by Carroll and Bloom

4. Differentiate between mastery learning and other group-based teacher instruction
5. Identify the variables of mastery learning
6. Differentiate between formative and summative evaluations
7. Identify and explain the five components of teaching for mastery
8. Identify two areas of current research in mastery learning
9. Identify at least three issues that can result from the use of mastery-learning concepts
10. Describe at least one area where mastery learning can be applied to nursing education and practice and implement it
11. Select the independent and dependent variables in two researchable questions about mastery learning
12. Identify your own mastery or nonmastery of this unit of instruction

PRETEST AND POSTTEST

Circle the correct answers. Each question is worth 1 point. The 95% level of mastery for this test is 18 correct points. Take the test and correct it yourself using the answer key found at the end of this module (p. 204).

Multiple choice

1. One concept that mastery learning proposes is that:
   a. all students can learn at the same rate
   b. competition is necessary but at a minimal level
   c. mastery and motivation are not linked
   d. almost all students can master what they are taught

2. The earliest work in mastery learning was built on by Carroll who developed:
   a. a conceptual framework to describe mastery
   b. the means to apply mastery learning
   c. formative and summative evaluations
   d. all of the above

3. Both Bloom's work and Carroll's early work fit into which of the following visual models of mastery learning:

a. Degree of learning = f
$$\left(\begin{array}{l} \text{1. Time allowed} \\ \text{2. Ability to understand instruction} \\ \hline \text{3. Perseverance} \\ \text{4. Aptitude} \\ \text{5. Quality of instruction} \end{array}\right)$$

b. Degree of learning = f
$$\left(\begin{array}{l} \text{1. Aptitude} \\ \text{2. Perseverance} \\ \hline \text{3. Time allowed} \\ \text{4. Quality of instruction} \\ \text{5. Ability to understand instruction} \end{array}\right)$$

c. Degree of learning = f
$$\left(\begin{array}{l} \text{1. Time allowed} \\ \text{2. Perseverance} \\ \hline \text{3. Aptitude} \\ \text{4. Quality of instruction} \\ \text{5. Ability to understand instruction} \end{array}\right)$$

d. Degree of learning = f
$$\left(\begin{array}{l} \text{1. Time allowed} \\ \text{2. Aptitude} \\ \hline \text{3. Perseverance} \\ \text{4. Quality of instruction} \\ \text{5. Ability to understand instruction} \end{array}\right)$$

4. According to Bloom's model, aptitude is:
   a. amount of effort required to attain mastery of a learning task
   b. amount of time required to attain mastery of a learning task
   c. amount of motivation required to attain mastery of a learning task
   d. amount of ability required to attain mastery of a learning task

5. Mastery learning is different from regular, group-based instruction because:
   a. mastery is in terms of specified objectives
   b. mastery does not allow for optimal time needed
   c. group-based instruction increases motivation through competition
   d. group-based instruction allows for learning from other students

6. One major distinguishing factor necessary to mastery learning is:
   a. encouraging motivation and competition
   b. motivating the student
   c. keeping the subject whole and varying the time needed for an individual
   d. breaking the subject area into smaller units and accounting for individual differences

7. According to Bloom, the task of instruction is:
   a. to increase motivation and quality of instruction
   b. to define mastery and provide the materials and content that will help students achieve it
   c. to define mastery and make provisions (materials) and allow as much time as needed to achieve it
   d. to increase mastery through some competition

8. Formative evaluation is the process of:
   a. evaluating overall mastery and assigning a letter grade
   b. evaluating mastery of the smaller learning units of a subject
   c. evaluating the amount of time each student needs to achieve mastery
   d. evaluating the amount of motivation a student possesses

9. When a student needs alternative learning experiences, the options include:
   a. small group-study sessions and tutorial assistance

b. specific workbooks and programmed instruction
c. audiovisual material and textbook readings
d. all of the above

10. One of the affective consequences of mastery learning is that:
   a. students believe themselves to be more involved in their learning
   b. students achieve higher grades
   c. students have a feeling of control
   d. students have a decrease in motivation

11. Recent research findings suggest that:
   a. perseverance may be increased by learning success
   b. motivation is increased by the use of competition
   c. the time needed to learn varies little between students
   d. learning success decreases competitiveness

12. Research shows that mastery learning can be most effectively accomplished by:
   a. manipulating competition and motivation
   b. manipulating reinforcement
   c. manipulating quality of instruction
   d. manipulating time allowed and quality of instruction

13. The preconditions for implementing the strategy of mastery learning are:
   1—increasing the aptitude of the student
   2—increasing the positive self-concept of the student
   3—specifying the objectives and the content of instruction, that is, the expectations
   4—translating specifications of instructions into evaluative procedures
   5—setting standards of achievement
   a. 1, 4, and 5
   b. 1, 2, and 3
   c. 3, 4, and 5
   d. 1, 4, and 5

14. The people who believe in mastery learning would agree with which of the following statements:
   1—Mastery learning produces greater student interest in and favorable attitude toward the subject learned than do usual classroom methods.
   2—Students learn more material in more time than with conventional approaches.
   3—Mastery learning enables 60% of all the students to achieve the same high level as the top 25% learning under typical group-based instructional methods.
   4—Mastery learning suggests procedures to manage each student's instruction and learning that will promote the fullest development within the context of ordinary group-based classroom instruction.
   a. all of the above
   b. 1 and 2
   c. 3 and 4
   d. 1 and 4

15. In mastery learning, which of the following strategies are implemented:
   1—The student is appraised individually with respect to performance relative to a fixed standard rather than performance relative to a group of peers.
   2—Grades are never given.
   3—Learning is competitive.
   4—Learning is cooperative.
   5—Summative tests are administered at the completion of each learning unit to help each student pace learning and put forth the necessary effort at the appropriate time.
   a. all of the above
   b. 1, 2, and 3
   c. 1, 4, and 5
   d. 1 and 4

16. Nursing practice would be most influenced by mastery learning in the following area:
   a. feelings toward new learning
   b. awareness of the shortcomings of others
   c. increase in competition
   d. all of the above

17. Those areas in nursing practice that would be suitable to the application of the mastery-learning model would be:
   a. continuing education
   b. learning of new skills
   c. application of principles in practice
   d. all of the above

18. What is the attitude toward competition in nurses being taught by group-based instruction versus mastery learning? In this research-

able question the dependent variable is:

a. student nurses
b. attitude toward competition
c. type of instruction
d. all of the above

19. Based on the type of teaching strategy utilized (mastery learning versus group-based instruction), is there a difference in cognitive ability of nurses at the end of a fundamentals course? In this problem statement the independent variable is:

a. cognitive ability
b. fundamentals course
c. type of instruction utilized
d. all of the above

TEXT
Introduction and historical background

One of the "hottest" issues for discussion today is the delivery of educational services to the consumer. As widespread awareness of the inadequacies of our present educational system develops, other methods and models of instruction will be tried. One of the educational theories being renewed and revitalized is mastery learning. Regarding mastery learning, Bloom (1968, p. 1) writes:

Most students (perhaps over 90%) can master what we have to teach them, and it is the task of instruction to find the means which will enable our students to master the subject under consideration. Our basic task is to determine what we mean by mastery of the subject and to search for the methods and materials which will enable the largest proportion of our students to attain such mastery.

Though mastery learning as described by Bloom (1968) and identification of the five essential variables of the model are new strategies for learning today, the concept of learning to mastery is not new. In the 1920's, the Winnetka plan of Carleton Washburne and Henry Morrison's approach to learning at the University of Chicago laboratory school were two attempts to produce mastery in students. Both of these programs and other early works on mastery learning, which were to become a base for the future had the following features:

1. Mastery was defined in terms of specific educational objectives that each student was to achieve.
2. Instruction was organized into well-defined learning units containing a collection of learning experiences, designed systematically, the purpose of which was to meet the desired objectives.
3. Complete mastery of one unit was required before the student could proceed to the next unit.
4. An ungraded progress test was given at the completion of a unit of learning, the purpose of which was to provide feedback on the adequacy of learning.
5. Original instruction was supplemented with appropriate learning experiences for completion of learning.
6. Time allowed for learning was varied to meet the individual needs of students in their mastery of the unit of instruction.

The idea of mastery learning then seemingly dived into quiescence in the 1930's, primarily because of a lack of technology to sustain a successful strategy, and did not resurface until the late 1950's and early 1960's as a corollary of programmed instruction. A basic idea, utilizing Skinner's studies, was that learning of any behavior, no matter how complex, rested on the learning of a sequence of less complex component behavior. Programmed instruction seemed promising, and two of the most well-known examples were the Individually Prescribed Instruction (IPI) project at Pittsburgh and Stanford's Computer Assisted Instruction (CAI) project. Both broke down subjects into a sequence of major cognitive objectives (Block, 1971).

This initial work, which is a broad base for the present work, disappeared because of its radicalism—that is, it was ahead of its time—and the inadequacy of technology to successfully provide the materials (audio-visual and others) necessary for development of mastery learning experiences for each unit of instruction.

When the concept of mastery learning re-surfaced in the 1950's and 1960's, it was under the cloak of programmed instruction. This format for mastery learning provided a means of breaking down the more complex units of instruction into successive learning experiences, thus providing a building concept into the original concept (Block, 1971).

What programmed instruction did not offer mastery learning was a broad enough scope from which to build in all of the propositions and variables of the original concept of mastery learning.

Prior to the development of Bloom's model, the most encompassing model that clearly incorporated some of the propositions of mastery learning was Carroll's (1963a) model of instruction. The focus of this model is the major factors influencing student success and how these factors interrelate to affect school learning. This model is conceptual in nature (Block, 1971).

The basic model is:

$$\text{Degree of learning} = f\left(\frac{\text{Time actually spent}}{\text{Time needed}}\right)$$

Carroll expanded this basic model to encompass the component parts of time actually spent and time needed.

Time actually spent: time allowed and perseverance

Time needed: aptitude, quality of instruction and ability to understand instruction

These components can be defined in measurable terms. Operationalizing these terms was the major work of Carroll during and after the development of the model. Operationalized, the terms mean:

time allowed actual time span given for learning a specific unit

perseverance combination of time willing to spend on active learning and prior experience of success or failure with similar learning tasks

aptitude amount of time required to learn a task to a given criterion level when ideal instructional conditions are utilized

quality of instruction the degree to which the presentation, explanation and ordering of the elements of a learning task approach the optimum for each learner

ability to understand instruction the basic verbal and conceptual level of the learner, often measured by tests of verbal intelligence

Thus, we have looked at Carroll's basic model, then looked at the components of his basic propositions; now we can see how all of these fit together (Block, 1971).

BASIC MODEL

$$\text{Degree of learning} = f\left(\frac{\text{Time actually spent}}{\text{Time needed}}\right)$$

ACTUAL CONCEPTUAL MODEL

$$\text{Degree of learning} = f\left(\frac{\begin{array}{l}\text{1. Time allowed}\\ \text{2. Perseverance}\end{array}}{\begin{array}{l}\text{3. Aptitude}\\ \text{4. Quality of instruction}\\ \text{5. Ability to understand instruction}\end{array}}\right)$$

Utilization of this model or any application of Carroll's conceptual framework is contingent on the function of the teacher in the instructional process. According to Carroll, the teacher:

1. Specifies what is to be learned
2. Motivates the student to learn it
3. Provides instructional materials
4. Administers learning materials at a rate suitable for each pupil
5. Monitors student progress
6. Diagnoses difficulties in learning and provides proper remediation
7. Gives praise and encouragement for good performance

8. Gives review and practice to maintain learning over long periods of time

Theoretical framework

In developing a strategy for mastery learning Bloom (1968) identified several problems of the current educational system that he contended or implicitly stated that mastery-learning strategy should remedy. These are the rationales on which he based and reasoned out the need for mastery-learning strategy.

First, he pointed out that in general, each teacher begins a course or a new term with the expectation that one-third of the students will learn adequately what is to be taught, another one-third will fail or just "get by," and the other-third will learn a good deal but not enough to be considered "good students." In other words, teachers are accustomed to grading on a "normal curve." Furthermore, this set of expectations supported by school policies and grading systems get transmitted to students through the method of instruction and evaluation policies. Bloom (1968, p. 1) pointed out that such a system creates a self-fulfilling prophecy that "the final sorting of students through the grading process becomes approximately equivalent to the original expectations."

He stated that such a wasteful and destructive educational expectation reduces aspirations and motivations of teachers and students for teaching and learning, and destroys the ego and self-concept of students who are legally required to go to school for 10 to 12 years under these frustrating conditions. Bloom (1968, p. 2) stated that there is nothing sacred about the normal curve. It is the distribution that is most appropriate for random activity and things that happen by chance. He said, "Education is a purposeful activity, and we seek to have the students learn what we have to teach." He also stated that if we teach effectively the distribution of achievement should be very different from the normal curve. In fact, he pointed out that to the extent that the distribution of achievement resembles the normal curve, we have been unsuccessful in our educational efforts of instruction. With mastery learning, most students (over 90%) can master the task. It is the role of instruction to find methods that will enable students to master the subject matter under consideration. Therefore, the main tasks of the mastery-learning method of instruction are (1) to search for the methods and materials that will enable the largest portion of the students to attain mastery and (2) to determine how individual differences in learners can be related to the learning and teaching processes (Bloom, 1968).

Second, some societies and educational systems are concerned more with discovering the talented few who are to be given advanced educational opportunities. Such societies invest more in prediction and selection of talent than in the development of such talent. Bloom pointed out that highly developed nations cannot operate on the assumption that secondary or college education is just for a few, because the complexity of skills and the size of the work force required by these nations is great. Schultz (1963) and Bowman (1966) studied how that investment in the education of humans pays off at a greater rate than capital investment. Bloom pointed out that the problem is not finding people who can succeed, but determining *how* the largest proportion of humans can learn effectively those skills and that subject matter that are essential for their own development in a complex society.

Third, increasingly, the need for continued learning throughout life is becoming a necessity for a large portion of the working population in order to keep abreast of new technology, to renew licenses for work, or to keep their jobs. Bloom (1968, p. 2) pointed out that, "If school learning is regarded as frustrating and even impossible by a sizable proportion of students, then little can be done at later levels to kindle a genuine interest in further learning. School learning must be successful and rewarding as one basis for insuring that learning can continue throughout one's life as needed."

The fourth problem area is concerned with the development of values. Bloom pointed out that in modern society there is malaise about values. As society has become more and more secular, personal values have been restricted to the area of hedonism, interpersonal relations, self-development, and ideas. If the schools frustrate students in the latter two areas, only the first two areas are left open for further exploration. He stressed the fact that it is the role of the school to assure that all students receive successful learning experiences in the areas of ideas and self-development (Bloom, 1968, p. 2). Mastery-learning strategy allows and encourages self-development and ideas.

Bloom does not deny the fact that individual differences exist, but he says that the basic task of education is to find a teaching strategy that takes into consideration the individual-difference variable and promotes the fullest development of the individual. Mastery-learning strategy provides an approach to solving the problem of individual differences.

Therefore, using the above-mentioned rationale for the necessity of an optimum method of teaching strategy, Bloom developed the mastery model of instruction, based on the following set of propositions or premises:

1. That the instructional task is to define mastery of a subject and discover the methods and materials that will help the largest proportion of students reach mastery
2. That learning continues throughout life; therefore, continued learning is most facilitated by successful and rewarding early learning experiences
3. That for successful learning experiences to occur for 90% of the students, major policy, practice, and attitudinal changes must occur in teachers, administrators, and students
4. That to promote the fullest development of the individual, development of teaching strategies that take into account individual differences must be the fundamental task in education

Bloom defined mastery in terms of a specific set of major objectives (content and cognitive behavior) the student is expected to exhibit on completing study of a subject (Block, 1971). Mastery is identified not only in terms of the total instructional content but also in terms of individual units (components) of the larger instructional content. Objectives are established for the larger frame of reference, or content, as well as for the individual component units of instruction. These objectives become the criterion for evaluation since they reflect most clearly the learning that is to take place. Bloom's model proposes:

1. That all or almost all students can master what they are taught
2. That through mastery-learning student learning is more efficient than through conventional approaches
3. That students learn more when sufficient time is allowed
4. That mastery learning produces markedly greater student interest in the subject learned than do conventional methods

The five basic variables of mastery-learning strategy

Bloom has transformed Carroll's conceptual model into a working model of mastery-learning strategy. The components of the model remain the same but their definition and purpose have been expanded or altered. The five factors that Carroll said influenced school learning, Bloom called variables that influence mastery, or the meeting of instructional objectives. Let us now consider these five variables in relation to mastery learning.

APTITUDE FOR PARTICULAR KINDS OF LEARNING

Many research studies have indicated that aptitude tests are good predictors of achievement criteria. The use of such tests and high correlations between such tests and achievement criteria have led many educators to the view that high levels of achievement are possible only for the most capable students. Quite in contrast to this is Carroll's (1963a) view that *"aptitude is the amount of time required by a learner to attain mastery of a learning task"* (Bloom, 1968, p. 3). Bloom pointed out that implicit in this definition of aptitude is the assumption that given enough time, all students can master a learning task. If this concept is correct, then mastery learning is available to all.

Evidence for this viewpoint is provided by Glaser (1968) and Atkinson (1967). They both showed that most students reached mastery on each learning task, but some reached it faster or sooner than others. Another type of support is provided by the standardized achievement tests. These norms demonstrate that criterion scores achieved by bright students at an earlier grade level are achieved by the majority of students at later levels (Bloom, 1968, p. 3).

Bloom asked whether all students can learn a subject equally well, that is, whether all students can master a highly complex learning task. He stated that as they study attribute distributions (1% to 5%) there are individuals with special disabilities for particular learning. For example, tone-deaf individuals will have difficulty learning music, or the color-blind person learning art; or the in-

dividual who thinks in concrete forms will have difficulty thinking in abstract concepts. However, Bloom said these constitute less than 5% of the distribution and will vary with the subject and the aptitudes. In between these two extremes are the other 90%. Where given enough time and optimum method in instruction, 95% (the top 5% and the next 90%) can learn the task to mastery level. Bloom believes, as does Carroll, that aptitudes are predictive of rate of learning rather than the level or complexity of the learning that is possible (Bloom, 1968, pp. 3-4).

The greatest *issue*, whether mastery learning is worth this great effort for the students who may take a long time to achieve mastery, is highly questionable. Groff (1974) argued this point and stated that it is not worth the effort and is not possible. Bloom (1968) and his associates at the University of Chicago have provided sufficient proof to substantiate the validity of mastery learning (Block, 1971). Bloom does point out, however, that one of the biggest problems of mastery-learning strategy is to find a way of reducing the time it takes a student to reach mastery, especially for the slow students, so that it is not a prohibitively long and difficult task for them.

Aptitude for a learning task is not absolutely stable. The studies of Bloom (1964) and Hunt (1961) show that aptitude can be changed and modified by environmental conditions or home and school learning experiences. Therefore, the major task of education is to produce positive changes in the students.

QUALITY OF INSTRUCTION

We have used the group-based teacher instruction as a frame of reference for years. Quality may not have been achieved in the group-based instruction since, as Carroll conceptualizes, individual students may need different qualities and types of instruction to learn the same subject content to meet the instructional objectives for mastery.

Bloom defined quality of instruction as the degree to which the presentation, explanation, and ordering of the elements of a learning task approach optimum for a given learner.

Bloom based the statement of definition on Congreve's (1965) research and suggested that some students need more active involvement in learning than others and that some students will need more concrete instructional cues, additional practice, and increased reinforcement.

In addition to the basic definition, Bloom stated that it is essential that quality be developed with respect to the needs and characteristics of individual learner rather than groups of learners.

Bloom (1968) noted that if it were possible to provide a very good tutor for each student, most of them would accomplish the learning task to a high degree of achievement. A good tutor, he stated "attempts to find the qualities of instruction (and motivation) best suited to a given learner" (p. 4). The study by Dave (1963) demonstrated that middle-class parents tutor their children when they believe that quality of instruction at school is poor. Bloom also had similar findings to those in Dave's (1963) study. Students in an algebra course received high grades. For these students, the relationship between mathematical aptitude tests at the beginning of the course and their achievement in algebra at the end of the course was almost zero. In contrast to those who did not receive home tutoring, the relationship of aptitude test and achievement scores was (+.90). This research points out that home tutoring was providing the type of quality instruction needed by these students to learn algebra.

ABILITY TO UNDERSTAND INSTRUCTION

Bloom (1968, p. 5) defined ability to understand instruction as "the ability of the learner to understand the nature of the task he is to learn and the procedures he is to follow in the learning of the task." Ability to understand instruction is determined by verbal ability and reading comprehension of the learner. These two measures of language ability are highly related (+.50 to +.60) to grade-point average and achievement in a majority of subjects. Therefore, verbal ability determines to a certain extent some general ability to learn from teachers and instructional materials. Bloom (1964) pointed out that changes in verbal ability are produced more at preschool and elementary-school age levels and decrease as the learner gets older.

The greatest help will come when dealing with the ability to understand instruction and from modifications in instruction in order to meet individual student's needs. Bloom stated that the ability to understand instruction can be enhanced through the use of a variety of instructional materials; for example, an alternative textbook, small group-study sessions, tutorial help, programmed instruction, and audiovisual methods. A particular material or method need not be used by a particular student throughout the course, but it should help the individual student at selected points in the learning process or as the student encounters different types of difficulties.

Whether one uses alternative methods of instruction or instructional material, it should be kept in mind that these are ways by which to improve the *quality of instruction* in relation to the student's ability to understand instruction. As students learn the task and also learn which method of instruction is most suited for them, they should be encouraged to be independent learners. That is, when confronted with a difficulty, they should be able to identify those methods and alternative materials they might resort to in order to accomplish the learning.

Group study methods. Group study is

most helpful and effective when two or three students meet regularly to go over difficult points in the learning task. The composition of this small study group is very important because of the opportunities it gives each person to expose difficulties and have them corrected without demeaning one person or elevating another. It has to be a cooperative rather than a competitive group.

Tutorial help. Tutorial help is very expensive and should be used as a last resort when other methods have failed. The tutor should be someone other than the regular teacher so that there will be a fresh viewpoint. The tutor must be skillful in detecting areas of difficulty in the student's learning and helping the student to be free of continued dependence on the tutor.

Alternative textbooks. Textbooks vary in the clarity with which materials are presented. The important factor to remember here is for the teacher to determine where, specificially, the learner is having difficulty in understanding instructions and then provide alternative textbook explanations that are more effective in explaining that specific point.

Workbooks and programmed instruction. Programmed instruction is helpful with students who cannot grasp the ideas and procedures of the textbook. Some of them may need the drill and practice sessions of specific tasks that workbooks provide; others may need the small steps and frequent reinforcements that programmed instruction provides. Such resources may be needed at the beginning of a course or as students encounter specific difficulties.

Audiovisual methods and academic games. Some students learn better by means of concrete illustrations, by actual demonstration, or by tactual contact. It is very likely that filmstrips and slides can be used by individual learners, as needed, and may be very effective. Academic games and puzzles can be used to enact a situation or a role.

PERSEVERANCE

Carroll (1963a) defined perseverance as the time the learner is willing to spend in learning. It is directly related to attitudes toward and interest in learning as well as to the rewards associated with past efforts. The International Study of Educational Achievement conducted by Husén (1967) showed that the relationship between the number of hours spent on homework per week (measure of perseverance), as reported by students, and the number of years of further education desired by the students was $+.25$.

The premises underlying the application of perseverance—whether they will enhance or inhibit perseverance—are that (1) sooner or later the learner will give up if a task is too painful, (2) perseverance can be increased if there is an increase in reward and evidence of learning success, and (3) the need for perseverance is decreased when the quality of instruction is at an optimum level.

Bloom's (1968) research supports the premise that demands for perserverance are reduced when students are provided with instructional resources most appropriate for them. Also, the use of frequent feedback accompanied by specific help in instruction and material reduced the time and perseverance required.

TIME ALLOWED FOR LEARNING

For Carroll, the time actively spent in learning is the key to mastery. Therefore, the student must be *allowed* enough time and must be given the opportunity for learning to take place.

The amount of time students need for a particular kind of learning has not been tested directly. However, the International Study of Educational Achievement done in 12 countries with 13-year-old students (Husén, 1967), showed that the ratio of time required to learn the same task between the fastest and the slowest learner was roughly

6:1. That is, some students spent six times as much time on mathematical homework as did others.

Bloom (1968) pointed out that if instruction and students' use of time became more effective, it is possible to lower the ratio between the slow learner and fast learner from 6:1 to 3:1, having the slow learner learn the task to mastery at a much reduced rate. Bloom further stated that it is not the sheer amount of time that accounts for the level of learning, but that each student should be allowed the time needed to learn a subject. The time needed to learn a subject is determined by the student's aptitude, verbal ability, quality of instruction received in class, and type of help received outside.

The task of mastery-learning strategy is, therefore, to find ways of altering the time that individual students need for learning, as well as ways of providing whatever time is needed by each student.

Strategy for implementation of mastery learning

Whatever strategy is chosen to incorporate the concept of mastery learning into a teaching-learning situation, the strategy must take into account the aforementioned five variables. Approaches run the gamut from incorporating mastery-learning principles into group-based instruction to altering instructional techniques to meet all of the components of the mastery-learning model. No matter what the strategy chosen, it must incorporate not only the five variables but also certain preconditions, operating procedures, and outcomes to indicate when a student has attained mastery. These factors are considered here (Block, 1971).

PRECONDITIONS

Specification of the behavioral objectives, the content of instruction, and the evaluation process. It is extremely important to clarify what is expected so that both the student and teacher understand it.

Distinction between the teaching-learning process and the evaluation process. Teaching-learning process prepares the student in the subject area. Evaluation process appraises the extent to which this teaching-learning process has succeeded. The teacher and student must have a mutual understanding of what the achievement criteria are, and both must be able to secure evidence of progress toward these criteria.

If the criteria are set up on a competitive basis, then the student will seek evidence of standing in comparison to classmates. However, it is preferable in terms of intrinsic motivation for learning to set up absolute standards of mastery and excellence apart from interstudent competition, followed by efforts to bring as many students as possible to the set standard of mastery.

Evaluation against a student's own previous performance and in terms of set standards. Rather than evaluations being based on a normal curve or some arbitrary standard, what Bloom (1968) has recommended is the development of realistic performance standards developed for each school, group, or unit of instruction, followed by instructional procedures that will enable the majority of students to accomplish the set criteria.

Bloom (1968) tested and implemented this strategy and found out that when achievement standards were set, the students were able to work together cooperatively, helping each other without being concerned about giving special advantages or disadvantages to other students.

OPERATING PROCEDURES

The operating procedures have to do with the actual implementation of the teaching-learning process. This is the time when teachers instruct and students learn. The operating procedures that Bloom (1968) has used are intended (1) to provide detailed feedback to teachers and students with regard to the extent and success of learning (formative evaluations) and (2) to provide specific supplementary instructional resources (alternative learning resources).

Formative evaluation. One useful operating procedure is the utilization of formative tests that are diagnostic in nature. It is accomplished by:

1. Breaking the subject into small learning elements or units—such as a chapter in a textbook, a well-defined content portion of a course, or a particular time unit—that may take about 1 or 2 weeks of learning.

2. Analyzing each unit of learning on the basis of simple to complex learning tasks; for example, terminology and facts at the simple level and concepts, principles, problem solving, and implementation of principles at the higher level.

3. Constructing a brief diagnostic-progress test that can be used to determine the extent to which the student has mastered that specific unit of learning and whether there is an area of difficulty that the student has not mastered. *Formative evaluation* refers to these diagnostic-progress tests, which should be administered at the end of each unit of learning.

4. Marking tests as mastery or nonmastery rather than giving a specific grade. The rationale for this is, according to Bloom (1968), that the use of grades on repetitive progress tests prepares the student for accepting less than mastery. For example, a student who constantly receives a grade of C will come to accept the C as "fate" for that course, and this will reduce motivation to progress. It should be stressed that formative evaluation tests should be regarded as part of the learning process and should not be confused with the judgment of student's capabilities or be used as a part of the grading process. There is limited evidence on this point.

The purpose of formative evaluation is:

1. To help the student pace learning
2. To pinpoint particular learning difficulties and prescribe alternative instructional materials and processes that can be used to overcome the learning difficulties
3. To assist the teacher in identifying particular points of instruction that need modifying
4. To serve as a means of quality control in future replications of the course—relevant and irrelevant as well as clear and unclear areas are identified (This particular purpose is achieved by the scoring process, which looks at the questions that are incorrect for the individual and for a group of students. Consistently wrong answers can identify shortcomings or misunderstandings in the instructional content.)

Alternative learning resources. Bloom suggested that one of the best ways to motivate students to complete learning is to provide specific suggestions about what they need to do.

When the initial teaching process is completed, and evaluation uncovers deficits in learning, or when a student needs additional resources to master the unit, the following corrective learning procedures can be used:

1. Providing small group-study sessions, meeting regularly, reviewing formative test results, cooperatively overcoming identified difficulties
2. Providing tutorial assistance
3. Rereading particular pages of the original instructional material
4. Studying specific explanations in alternative textbooks and other sources
5. Using specific pages of workbooks or programmed instruction
6. Using selected audiovisual materials

The function of these procedures is to provide each student with instructional cues, active participation and practice, and the amount and type of reinforcement needed to complete the learning.

OUTCOMES

Cognitive outcome of mastery-learning strategy. Cognitive outcomes can be measured both by means of formative and summative evaluations. Summative evaluation is the achievement test that is usually given at the end of a course or a sequence of instruction. It is for grading and judgmental purposes. Formative evaluations are predictors of summative evaluation in that a student who consistently performs at mastery level in the formative evaluations is likely to perform at the mastery level—"A level" of performance on the summative evaluation. Results of research studies conducted by Bloom (1968) and his associates are very optimistic and supportive of the outcomes of mastery-learning strategy.

Affective consequences of mastery learning strategy. Mastery learning must be both subjective recognition by the learner of his capabilities and competence in a given field and public recognition by the school or society. The latter must provide this recognition in the form of certification. No matter how much the student has learned, if the school and the society denies the student this public recognition, the student will come to think of himself as inadequate. However, when the student receives both objective and subjective evidence of mastery, there will be profound changes in self-perception and perception of the outer world.

It is important for a student to feel control over ideas and skills and realize the ability to do what the subject requires. Through the mastery-learning process, as mastery over a subject occurs, the student will have a feeling of control that often creates or generates more interest in learning. Thus, as a result of mastery, students have an increased motivation for further learning, which is a major goal of modern education. In addition, mastery learning affects the self/concept of the student:

1. It offers positive recognition of worth; the student views himself as adequate in areas where mastery has occurred

2. Mastery plus public recognition yield in a student reassurance and reinforcement of self-worth, which Bloom believes, is one of the more positive aids to mental health and is an objective evaluation of self-development

Relevant research studies

Findings of important research studies will be presented under the heading of the major variables of the mastery-learning model of instruction.

Aptitude and rate of learning

The research studies of Ausubel (1964), Behr (1967), Carroll (1963b), Davis (1967), Green (1969), and Kim (1968) have all demonstrated a positive relationship between aptitude and rate of learning. Their work has focused on the difference in rate of learning among students as well as some empirical evidence of aptitude being predictive of learning rate. The relationship between aptitude and learning rate is more clearly predictive for initial or lower-level skills.

Ability to understand instruction

The research studies of Coleman (1966) and Cronbach and Snow (1969) have indicated that ability to understand is mainly determined by verbal ability, student comprehension of instruction, and to some extent intelligence. Block (1971, p. 93) discussed a major work, Aptitude-Instructional Treatment Interaction research (Cronbach and Snow, 1969), which has shown that by modifying the instructional mode of the first presentation of information to fit the learner's aptitude, the teacher optimizes the level of achievement and learning rate. There is evidence that use of only a single mode of instruction hampers learning by students who are weak in the aptitudes required to learn by that mode.

Quality of instruction

The definition of quality of instruction has been enlarged to include:

1. Clarity and appropriateness of individual cues
2. Amount of participation in and practice of learning
3. Amount and types of reinforcement

These factors affect both student learning rate and achievement level. Research studies (Airasian, 1967; Coleman, 1966, Cronbach and Snow, 1969; Feather, 1966) also have indicated that two major methods can be utilized to improve quality of instruction: (1) construction of methods and materials to meet different students' aptitude patterns and (2) building feedback and corrective techniques into group-based instruction.

Perseverance

Research studies (Sears, 1940; Seashore, 1942; Thornton, 1939; Weiner, 1965) have identified an important and pertinent individual trait that affects perseverance: persistence.

Perseverance may be increased by some form of external positive reinforcement or learning success. Research suggests that perseverance also may be increased or decreased by the quality of instruction.

Time allowed for learning–opportunity

Block (1971) summarized the findings of several research studies (Block, 1970; Glaser, 1968; Green, 1969; Sjogren, 1967; Wright, 1967), indicating that most students can achieve mastery if they are *allowed* and do spend the necessary amount of time on a learning task. As was also indicated by Husén's (1967) International Study of Educational Achievement, the difference between the fastest and slowest group of learners is the ratio of 6:1, that is, the slow learners take six times as much time as the fast learners.

Affective consequences

Research (Block, 1970; Brookover, Shailer, and Paterson, 1964; Modu, 1969; Sears, 1940; Thorshen, 1969) has shown a clear relationship between a student's academic progress and self-concept and mental health. A history of successful and rewarding experiences in a given task can yield: increased confidence to perform related tasks, increased aspiration to learn, and increased actual performance.

Use of mastery-learning concepts and strategies

Research (Airasian, 1967; Anthony, 1967; Block, 1970; Collins, 1969; Feather, 1966) suggests that mastery learning has a marked effect on the student's cognitive and affective development and learning rate. It enables 95% of the students to learn to criterion level of performance. Research indicates, "Mastery of the earliest units in a school subject appears to facilitate the learning of the subsequent units, especially where the learning units are sequentially arranged" (Block, 1971, p. 97).

Issues in mastery learning (Bloom's model)

One of the most vocal critics of mastery-learning strategy is Groff (1974). He criticized mastery learning as describing learning in very simplistic and naive terms. Groff views teaching as very complex. He also criticized the feasibility of implementation of mastery learning. He said the teacher does not have the spare time to develop the many formative diagnostic tests; whereas Bloom had advocated that a couple of teachers can develop a series of diagnostic tests for a course of 2 to 3 weeks by spending a day on it (Groff, 1974).

Groff also stated that advocates of mastery learning do not accept that individuals differ in aptitude. However, Groff has misunderstood what the advocates of mastery learning are saying about aptitude. According to Bloom (1968) and Carroll (1963a) it does not matter what the aptitude of the individual is; as long as enough time and appropriate quality of instruction are provided to the students, most students should accomplish the learning task at the mastery level.

Groff said that it is overly optimistic to assume that developing learning units, alternative learning materials, or diagnostic tests is an easy task. Groff further asserted that mastery learning does not explain how the teacher would know in advance which students would require alternative learning materials; also, if there are such successful materials, why shouldn't students use these resources in the first place. Mastery learning never implied that such alternative resource materials should not be available to the students in the first place. What was said was that if the student does not understand the learning task with what the teacher has available, then the teacher should find other methods and resources. Not all students need all the resources. These are too expensive to make readily available. However, there should be enough for those students who are experiencing learning difficulty.

Groff further criticized the mastery-learning proposition that the task to be learned must be explained to the learner in terms of behavioral objectives. He said that Simon (1973) and Duchastel and Merrill (1973) have found that behavioral objectives are not valid determiners of student learning; therefore, the extra effort it takes to write behavioral objectives is futile.

He also criticized and disagreed with the proposition that mastery learning enhances the self-concept of the student. He wrote, "Note the bait mastery learning offers students who fail: Try one more time and you

will master it. For students truly unable to cope with a certain subject (there are such students, mastery learning notwithstanding), this 'encouragement' is just one more signal of their inferiority" (Groff, 1974, p. 90). Bloom (1968) proposed that mastery learning has positive affective consequences and contributes to an increase in positive self-concept. The studies of Block (1970); Brookover, Shailer, and Paterson (1964); Modu (1969); Sears (1940); and Thorshen (1969) all support Bloom's proposition. Groff criticized mastery learning, but seldom did he give any research evidence to support his criticism; whereas Bloom attempted to support most of his propositions with empirical evidence.

In general, therefore, in spite of the criticism and some of the shortcomings of mastery learning, it is by far one of the best models of instruction. Any new theory or concept is subject to criticism, which helps to sharpen and clarify the unclear aspects. A good theory and model of instruction will endure criticism; time will tell if mastery learning will endure. The probability is, it will.

Application to nursing education and practice

Nursing education and practice are presently at a pivotal point. Not only are new dimensions being added to nursing practice, but also valid questions are being asked by administrators about the product that nursing education is delivering. It is possible that mastery learning may be one fulcrum to consider for the rocky plank on which nursing education is wavering.

Schools of nursing are changing their philosophies to meet the needs of the changing community and the subsequent changing focus of nursing. As curriculum committees are formed and faculties discuss philosophies and objectives, they must also decide on a method of instruction. Acceptance of the view that almost all students can learn to high levels is basic to the development of an effective strategy of mastery learning for three reasons: first, this acceptance stimulates teachers, administrators, and, ultimately students to strive for high levels of learning; second, this acceptance provides a touchstone for the solution of most procedural problems encountered during a strategy's development and implementation, that is, what course of action will provide learning for all students; third, its acceptance helps justify modification of school grading policies and practices so that all students who attain mastery can be appropriately rewarded for their efforts (Block, 1971).

One example of mastery learning in nursing education is at Arizona State University, where the baccalaureate and R.N. programs are planned around a continuous-progress concept. It involves a learning process that permits each student to progress according to individual ability, provides materials and facilities for independent study, and gives freedom to use self-initiative in learning. On a smaller scale, mastery has been used in modified form in a course at the University of Texas entitled Leadership and Management in Nursing. The students were given a list of objectives to be met by the end of the course; four small informal conferences were conducted throughout the course to provide feedback; students were graded individually on their ability to meet objectives; and a variety of learning activities such as films, programmed units, study guides, references, and others were made available. One conclusion of the study was that it is possible to make allowances for individual differences in learning modes and rates and still have students achieve as well as those taught by more traditional methods (Langford, 1972).

Nursing educators adopting the mastery-learning model would be required to refocus their thinking. No longer would power and control of learning rest solely with the instructor. The power and control would be a mutual responsibility. The teacher would be required to provide objectives and enough time and learning experiences for almost all students to achieve mastery of a learning task. Each student would have power and control over individual mastery. Each would be responsible for utilizing the content and experiences available and making the necessary time adjustments to achieve mastery.

The career-ladder concept in nursing education and practice offers a useful area for considering the strategies of mastery learning. Using the concepts of mastery learning, each nursing program would set major objectives. Once the major objectives are established, then the program can set up units, each with objectives appropriate for that unit. The individual would attain mastery of each of the units, and once the major objectives of the program were realized by the student, the student then could become eligible for a more advanced nursing program. Theoretically, it would be possible to enter nursing at the aide position and have the opportunity for education completed at the master's level. Pragmatically, however, there would be students stopping at various points along the continuum of nursing education.

Mastery learning has application to nursing practice both in general terms and in specific patient-teaching situations. Generally speaking, as new concepts and skills are introduced, the nurse operating or learning under the mastery-learning model will feel comfortable enough to master the skill. The time and competition elements will be absent.

Practice would be affected by the kinds of students entering as graduates. If the new graduates are from a program incorporating mastery-learning concepts, the new labor force would include workers who consider learning a positive, rewarding experience. These workers also would be more likely to seek further learning. Their attitude and example hopefully would influence the other nurses with whom they practice.

If nursing education utilized the mastery-learning model, then institutions employing new graduates would have concrete, baseline data regarding the skills of the new employee.

Mastery learning would enhance and clearly define objectives for continuing education, nursing practice, and the specific skills required to complete a task. Mastery learning then would provide an opportunity for nursing practice and education to unify standards and expectations. It would provide some of the concreteness that has been in demand.

More specifically, principles of mastery learning are extremely applicable to the teaching-learning process at the teacher-student and nurse-patient teaching levels. The following specific example illustrates how mastery learning could be applied. Let us assume that the learner is a junior nursing student or a female adult patient. The task to be learned is self-examination of the breasts for detection of lumps.

The sequence of mastery learning entails the following basic four steps: (1) identifying the *preconditions* necessary to learn this specific learning task and planning and preparing them, (2) determining what the *operative procedures* should be and preparing them, (3) determining what measures will be used to evaluate the *outcome*, and (4) looking over and evaluating the *instructional strategy* to determine if it has taken into consideration the five basic variables of the mastery-learning model. Now let us take each point and go through it step by step.

Preconditions

The nurse-teacher identifies the preconditions necessary to learn the task of breast self-examination for detection of abnormal lumps by doing the following:
1. Explaining the objective of the learning task in terms that the student or patient can understand and in behavioral or measurable terms; for example:

   Objective: At the completion of this instructional period, given enough time (as long as it will take the learner to reach mastery) and optimal quality of instruction, the learner will be able to demonstrate the correct procedure for self-examination of the breasts for detection of abnormal lumps

2. Developing the criteria of acceptable performance, so that the teacher and the student have a mutual understanding of these criteria, such as through the use of an observation checklist that includes the appropriate steps in proper sequence; for example:
   a. Position of the arm that is not doing the examination
   b. Position of the body
   c. Rotating movement of the examining hand
   d. Position of the hand on the breast
   e. Reasons for all these different positions and other information
3. Assessing the entering behavior of the student or patient to discover if the learner possesses all the necessary entering behaviors to conduct a breast self-examination; if not then determining the areas that are lacking and teaching those concepts prior to starting the self-examination procedure
4. Assuring the student or patient that there will be no evaluation during learning and that performance will be compared to and evaluated against previous performance and the set standards will not be compared to the achievement level of other students or patients

Operative procedure

During the operative procedures, implementation of the mastery-learning strategy takes place. It is the time when the learner attempts to learn.

First the nurse-teacher may give the content matter or explain the learning task utilizing many different approaches. In this situation the nurse-teacher may first explain verbally the gross anatomy and physiology of the breast (the student nurse may learn this in greater depth than the patient). Then the teacher may show photographs and diagrams of the breast and how the procedure is carried out—the direction of the motion and position of body. Then the nurse-teacher may actually demonstrate the procedure either on herself or on the student or patient. Then the teacher asks the learner to demonstrate the correct procedure for learning purposes first (not for evaluation purposes).

Next, if the learning task were a long and complicated task, the teacher would have analyzed the content to be learned and divided it into units of learning on the basis of simple to complex learning tasks. In this situation of breast self-examination, the whole task can be considered as one unit of learning.

Third, the teacher constructs a formative diagnostic test in order to give immediate feedback to the learner. In this situation, it can be given at the end of one position, such as self-examination in the lying position. The teacher may utilize the observation checklist or the student or patient may utilize an illustration that shows step-by-step progression, so the learner compares her performance to the set criteria and can determine what she has done correctly and where she is having difficulty.

Finally, if the student or patient is having difficulty with a specific area, then the nurse-teacher may provide the learner with alternative learning materials and resources. The student or patient may study the procedure in a small-group situation with two or three students or patients learning cooperatively.

Hopefully, the selection and composition of the other members of the group will be such that they will be able to help the learner with specific problem areas. The teacher may provide a motion picture, a film strip, slides, or other audiovisual aids to help the learner with the difficulty. The teacher may want the student to reread or restudy the particular pages of the original instructional material or may provide alternative textbooks or workbooks. Other tutorial assistance may also be provided. The important point to keep in mind is that the student should be provided with or *allowed* enough time to learn the task (self-examination of breast) to mastery level.

Outcome

Cognitive outcome, or in this case both cognitive and psychomotor skills (procedure), of the task (breast self-examination) can be done when the student or patient is ready for evaluation. Summative evaluation in this case is the evaluation of achievement (of performing the correct procedure for self-examination of the breasts for detection of abnormal lumps) at the end of learning. The nurse-teacher may also want to know or evaluate the affective behaviors of the student or patient, for example, how does the patient or student feel about the procedure? Is she confident that she can do it at home? Does she express any feelings about the worthwhileness of learning such a procedure? How does she see or perceive herself.

Evaluation of instructional strategy

Evaluation is done to determine whether the five major variables have been taken into consideration. This the nurse-teacher can do by asking pertinent questions about each of the variables.

1. *Aptitude.* Since aptitude is determined by the amount of time required by the learner to attain mastery of a learning task, the teacher can ask the following questions:

a. Have I allowed enough time for the learner to learn this task?
b. Does the learner have special disabilities that will adversely affect the task to be learned? In this situation, can the patient or student feel with her hands?
c. Have I taken the learner's history of previous learning (entering behavior) into consideration?

In the example used, the role of aptitude has been taken into consideration.

2. *Quality of instruction.* Since quality of instruction is determined by the "degree to which the presentation, explanation and ordering of elements of the task to be learned approach the optimum for a given learner" (Bloom, 1968, p. 4), the teacher can ask the following questions:

a. Have I presented and explained the learning task the best way I can?
b. Have I ordered the units of learning in proper sequence?
c. Have I taken into consideration the needs of individual learners?
d. Are my methods of instruction suitable for each learner?
e. Have I constructed formative evaluations so that learners can receive immediate feedback?
f. Are my formative-evaluation tests valid and reliable so the learners and I can detect areas of difficulty?
g. Have I provided for alternative instructional materials and resources for those students who have difficulty?

3. *Ability to understand instruction.* Ability refers to the learner being able "to understand the nature of the task he is to learn and the procedures he is to follow in the learning of the task" (Bloom, 1968, p. 5).

Since the learner's ability interacts with the instructional material and the instructor's ability to teach, it is important to evaluate the student's or patient's verbal ability and reading comprehension. (This may be done when the teacher evaluates the learner's entering behavior.) The teacher may ask the following questions to find out if the learner's ability to understand instruction has been taken into consideration:

a. Can the learner (especially the patient) read?
b. To what extent has the learner comprehended the instructions, or understood what is required?
c. Have the objectives been clear?
d. If the learner (patient or student) speaks English as a second language, have I made my instructions simple and clear?
e. Have I taken into consideration the individual learner's background (entering behavior, special abilities, disabilities, and so on)?
f. Have I modified the instructions to meet the needs of students?
g. Have I utilized alternative instructional materials or methods of instruction that are appropriate to the needs of the specific student or patient?

4. *Perseverance.* Since perseverance deals with the amount of time the learner is willing to spend actively in learning, and since it is related to attitudes toward and interest in learning, it is therefore important that the teacher find out whether motivational variables have been taken into consideration. This can be done by asking the following questions:

a. Is the task that the student or patient is learning rewarding?
b. Are reinforcements frequently given for desirable behavior (learning of task), especially at the beginning and during the shaping phase of the behavior?
c. Is the learning situation too frustrating or painful to the student? If so, how can I reduce the frustration?
d. Is the student experiencing success as the task is mastered?
e. Are the feedbacks for correct behaviors

and mastery of learning units frequent enough?

f. Does the learner value what is being learned?

g. Is the student happy with the method of instruction?

5. *Opportunity.* These questions can be used to check whether adequate time has been allowed for learning:

a. Have the students or patients been allowed enough time to learn the task to mastery?

b. Have I allowed for approximately a 6:1 ratio of time between the fastest and slowest learners?

c. How can I reduce the time needed for the slowest learner? What teaching strategy or alternate instructional resources should I use to lower the amount of time needed by the slow learner?

These are but sample questions that the nurse-teacher can ask to find out if the five basic variables in the implementation of the mastery-learning strategy has been taken into consideration. In the example of teaching breast self-examination to detect any abnormal lumps, most of these strategies have been used and have taken into consideration the five basic variables.

The same principles and step-by-step application of principles of mastery learning can be done for the teaching of a course, a lecture situation, a specific patient-teaching situation, and an entire program in curriculum. There is no denying that it takes a lot of work—time, effort, and knowledge—but it is all worth it if 95% of the students or patients master the tasks to be learned.

Researchable questions

What, then, can be done to add to the body of knowledge about the concepts and application of mastery learning. In nursing there are several ways to contribute to the foundations of mastery-learning research. Here are some problem statements with the independent and dependent variables defined. There are many questions; these are but a few:

1. What are the attitudes of student nurses toward nursing practice as a result of mastery learning versus group-based teacher instruction?

a. Independent variable: teaching technique

b. Dependent variable: attitudes toward nursing practice

2. What is the attitude toward competition in nurses taught by mastery learning versus group-based instruction?

a. Independent variable: teaching technique

b. Dependent variable: attitudes toward competition

3. Is there a difference in cognitive ability and affect of nurses at the end of a continuing-education course based on the teaching strategy utilized—mastery learning versus group-based instruction?

a. Independent variable: teaching technique

b. Dependent variable: differences in cognitive ability and affect

Again, not only can these three questions be changed by changing the variables, but a host of other questions can be raised.

ADDITIONAL LEARNING EXPERIENCES—RECOMMENDED READING LIST

Block, J. H. *Mastery learning: theory and practice.* New York: Holt, Rinehart and Winston, Inc., 1971.

Corona, D. F. A continuous progress curriculum in nursing. *Nursing Outlook,* Jan. 1970, **18:**46-48.

Groff, P. Some criticisms of mastery learning. *Today's Education,* Nov.-Dec. 1974, **63:**88-91.

Langford, T. Self-directed learning. *Nursing Outlook,* Oct. 1972, **20:**648-651.

Wolf, U. C., and Quiring, J. Carroll's model applied to nursing education. *Nursing Outlook,* Mar. 1971, **19:** 176-179.

INSTRUCTIONS TO THE LEARNER REGARDING POSTTEST

Now you are ready to take the posttest to determine the extent to which you have achieved the objectives. Return to the pretest and take it again as a posttest. Correct your answers using the answer key that is found on this page. You need to score 18 correct points in order to qualify for 95% mastery level. If your score is less than 18 correct points, correct your errors, study the content of this module again, and read some of the articles in the recommended reading list. You need to study until you achieve the 95% mastery level or better before proceeding to the next module.

ANSWER KEY TO PRETEST AND POSTTEST

1. d (Bloom, 1968, p. 1)
2. a (Bloom, 1968, pp. 1-7)
3. c (Block, 1971, p. 6)
4. b (Bloom, 1968, p. 3)
5. a (Bloom, 1968, p. 8)
6. d (Bloom, 1968, pp. 8-9)
7. c (Bloom, 1968, p. 7)
8. b (Bloom, 1968, pp. 9-10)
9. d (Bloom, 1968, p. 10)
10. c (Bloom, 1968, p. 11)
11. a (Bloom, 1968, pp. 6-7)
12. d (Bloom, 1968, pp. 3-11)
13. c (Bloom, 1968, pp. 8-9)
14. d (Bloom, 1968, pp. 10-11)
15. d (Bloom, 1968, pp. 9-10)
16. a (Bloom, 1968, p. 11)
17. d (Bloom, 1968, p. 1)
18. b (Text, p. 203)
19. c (Text, p. 203)

REFERENCES

Airasian, P. W. An application of a modified version of John Carroll's model of school learning. Unpublished master's thesis, University of Chicago, Chicago, 1967.

Antony, B. C. M. The identification and measurement of classroom environmental process variables related to academic achievement. Unpublished doctoral dissertation, University of Chicago, Chicago, 1967.

Atkinson, R. C. Computerized instruction and the learn-ing process. Technical Report No. 122, Institute for Mathematical Studies in the Social Sciences, Standford, Calif., 1967.

Ausubel, D. P. How reversible are the cognitive and motivational effects of cultural deprivation? Implications for teaching the culturally deprived child. *Urban Education*, 1964, **1**:16-38.

Behr, M. J. A study of interactions between "Structure-of-intellect" factors and two methods of presenting concepts of modulus seven arithmetic. Unpublished doctoral dissertation, Florida State University, Tallahassee, Fla., 1967.

Block, J. H. The effects of various levels of performance on selective cognitive, affective and time variables. Unpublished doctoral dissertation, University of Chicago, Chicago, 1970.

Block, J. H. (Ed.) *Mastery learning: theory and practice.* New York: Holt, Rinehart and Winston, Inc., 1971.

Bloom, B. S. *Stability and change in human characteristics.* New York: John Wiley & Sons, Inc., 1964.

Bloom, B. S. Learning for mastery. *UCLA Evaluation Comment*, 1968, **1**(2):1-12.

Bowman, M. J. The new economics of education. *International Journal of Educational Sciences*, 1966, **1**:29-46.

Brookover, W. B., Shailer, T., and Paterson, A. Self-concept of ability and school achievement. *Sociology of Education*, 1964, **37**:271-278.

Carroll, J. A model for school learning. *Teachers College Record*, 1963a, **64**:723-733.

Carroll, J. Programmed instruction and student ability. *Journal of Programmed Instruction*, 1963b, **2**:7-11.

Coleman, J., and others. *Equality of educational opportunity*, Final report, U.S. Office of Education, Report No. 38001, United States National Center for Educational Statistics, Washington D.C., 1966.

Collins, K. M. A strategy for mastery learning in freshman mathematics. Unpublished study, Purdue University, Division of Mathematical Sciences, Lafayette, Ind., 1969.

Congreve, W. J. Independent learning. *North Central Association Quarterly*, 1965, **40**:222-228.

Cronbach, L. J., and Snow, R. E. *Individual differences in learning ability as a function of instructional variables*, Final report, U.S. Office of Education, Contract No. OEC4-6-061269-1217, Standford University School of Education, Standford, Calif., 1969.

Dave, R. H. The identification and measurement of environmental process variables that are related to educational achievement. Unpublished doctoral dissertation, University of Chicago, Chicago, 1963.

Davis, J. B., Jr. An investigation of the interaction of certain instructional strategies with the structure of basic mental abilities in the learning of some mathematical operations. Unpublished doctoral dissertation, University of Chicago, Chicago, 1967.

Duchastel, P. C., and Merrill, P. F. The effect of behavioral objectives on learning: a review of empirical studies. *Review of Educational Research*, 1973, **43**: 53-69.

Feather, N. T. Effects of prior success and failure on expectations of success and subsequent performance. *Journal of Personality and Social Psychology*, 1966, 3:287-298.

Glaser, R. Adapting the elementary school curriculum to individual performance. In Proceedings of the 1967 invitational conference on testing problems. Education Testing Service, Princeton, N.J., 1968, pp. 3-36.

Green, B. N., Jr. *A self-paced course in freshman physics*. Cambridge, Mass: Massachusetts Institute of Technology, Education Research Center, 1969.

Groff, P. Some criticisms of mastery learning. *Today's Education*, Nov.-Dec. 1974, **63**:88-91.

Hunt, J. McV. *Intelligence and experience*. New York: Ronald Press Co., 1961.

Husén, T. (Ed.) *International study of educational achievement in mathematics: a comparison of twelve countries*. New York: John Wiley & Sons, Inc., 1967.

Kim, H. Learning rates, aptitudes and achievements. Unpublished doctoral dissertation, University of Chicago, Chicago, 1968.

Langford, T. Self-directed learning. *Nursing Outlook*, 1972, **20**:648-651.

Modu, C. C. Affective consequences of cognitive changes. Unpublished doctoral dissertation, University of Chicago, Chicago, 1969.

Schultz, T. W. *The economic value of education*. New York: Columbia University Press, 1963.

Sears, P. S. Level of aspiration in academically successful and unsuccessful children. *Journal of Abnormal Social Psychology*, 1940, **35**:498-536.

Seashore, H. B., and Bavelas, A. A study of frustration in children. *Journal of genetic psychology*, 1942, **61**:279-314.

Simons, H. D. Behavioral objectives: a false hope for education. *Elementary School Journal*, 1973, **73**:173-181.

Sjogren, D. D. Achievement as a function of study time. *American Educational Research Journal*, 1967, 4:337-344.

Thornton, G. R. A factor analysis of tests designed to measure persistence. *Psychological Monograph*, 1939, **51**:1-42 (whole no. 229).

Thorshen, K. The relation of classroom evaluation to students' self-concepts. Unpublished manuscript, University of Chicago, Chicago, 1969.

Weiner, B. The effects of unsatisfied achievement motivation on persistence and subsequent performance. *Journal of Personality*, 1965, 33:428-442.

Wright, W. Achievement as a function of time: an analysis of selected Standford Achievement Test battery results. Unpublished manuscript, University of Chicago, Chicago, 1967.

Wolf, U. C., and Quiring, J. Carroll's model applied to nursing education. *Nursing Outlook*, 1971, **19**: 176-179.

MODULE 13

Skinner's (S–R) model of instruction

DESCRIPTION OF MODULE

This module is an independent unit of instruction that explains Skinner's stimulus—response (S–R) model of instruction. The content of this module is presented in sequential order. It contains the student's objectives and the pre- and posttest with the answer key of correct answers. The text of this module is presented in an integrated form. It covers five major areas: (1) theoretical framework, (2) research studies, (3) issues, (4) application to nursing education and practice, and (5) researchable questions.

Prerequisites to studying this module are knowledge of all the conditions of learning.

MODULE OBJECTIVES

At the completion of this module, having studied the content of this module and the recommended reading list, the student will be able to accomplish the following set of objectives at the 95% level of accomplishment. The student will be able to:

1. Describe Skinner's (S–R) model of instruction
2. State the steps of the model of instruction in proper sequential order
3. Describe the theoretical framework of the S–R model of instruction
4. Define teaching machines and programmed instruction

5. Identify the four types of programmed instruction
6. Discuss both the disadvantages and advantages of teaching machines
7. State the variables that compose the contingencies of reinforcement
8. Cite relevant research studies to support the model
9. Apply Skinner's model of instruction to a specific patient or student teaching situation
10. Raise at least one researchable question and identify both the dependent and the independent variables
11. Identify issues in or criticisms of Skinner's model

PRETEST AND POSTTEST

Circle the correct answers. Each question is worth 1 point except the last question, which is worth 10 points. The 95% level of mastery for this test is 25 correct points out of 26 points. Take the test and correct your answers using the answer key found at the end of this module (p. 218).

Multiple choice

1. In order to reinforce a behavior, the teacher must first make sure that the behavior occurs. The two ways that Skinner believed are best

in arranging for the initiation of the first instance of a behavior are:

   1—physically forcing the behavior to occur (making *not* doing it aversive)

   2—waiting for the behavior to occur spontaneously

   3—shaping approximations of the behavior until the desired behavior has been attained

   4—using stimuli that will elicit the desired response

  a. 1 and 2
  b. 2 and 3
  c. 1 and 4
  d. 2 and 4

2. When Skinner speaks of the problem of the first instance he is referring to:
  a. the problem of handling an incorrect response
  b. the problem of getting the student's interest in the subject
  c. the problem of initially establishing the desired response

3. In Skinner's model of learning, he identifies variables that compose the contingencies of reinforcement under which learning takes place. The correct variables are:

   1—an occasion on which the behavior occurs

   2—the behavior itself

   3—the time spent learning the behavior

   4—the consequence of the behavior

  a. all of the above
  b. 1, 2, and 3
  c. 2, 3, and 4
  d. 1, 2, and 4

4. According to Skinner, a repertoire of behavior is acquired because behavior is naturally reinforced when it resembles behavior that has just been observed in others. This is an example of:
  a. product duplication
  b. movement duplication
  c. forced behavior
  d. nonduplicative repertoire

5. Demonstrating for the patient with a mastectomy how to exercise and asking the patient to return the demonstration is an example of:

  a. product duplication
  b. movement duplication
  c. shaping of a behavior
  d. nonduplicative repertoire

6. Skinner's model of instruction consists of five consecutive steps. These steps are listed in mixed order. Arrange them in proper sequence.

   1—noting the problem of the first instance

   2—prompting the behavior

   3—sequencing

   4—programming complex behavior

   5—defining the terminal behavior

  a. 5, 1, 2, 4, 3
  b. 1, 2, 3, 4, 5
  c. 4, 1, 2, 5, 3
  d. 2, 1, 3, 5, 4

7. Skinner cited two factors that need to be taken into consideration in devising the contingencies of reinforcement. These are:
  a. using the appropriate reinforcement
  b. gradually elaborating extremely complex patterns of behavior
  c. using a variable-ratio schedule of reinforcement
  d. maintaining the behavior in strength at each stage

Matching

Part A

    ___ 8. Teaching machines
    ___ 9. Terminal behavior
    ___10. Movement duplication
    ___11. Vanishing
    ___12. Nonduplicative repertoire
    ___13. Prompting
    ___14. Product duplication

Part B

a. An expectant mother performing a return demonstration on how to bathe a newborn baby

b. A nurse instructing a patient to take three deep breaths before coughing, and then reinforcing the patient when the task is accomplished

c. Any device that arranges the contingencies of reinforcement

d. Stating objectives within a course or a lesson plan

e. Fragment of a prime

f. Using a tape recorder that has the model's voice recorded on it, and having the patient listen to the tape recorded and try to pronounce similarly

g. Reducing the extent of a prompt in a teaching situation

Discussion questions

15. Give two advantages of using teaching machines in teaching a course or a lesson plan:

    a. _____

    b. _____

16. List two objections to the use of teaching machines in classroom teaching situations:

    a. _____

    b. _____

17. Select a specific patient- or student-learning situation and implement Skinner's model of instruction.

TEXT
Theoretical framework
Introduction

Skinner (1968, p. 2) termed education as "the culture of the *intellect* or *mind.* A student grows in *wisdom.* He behaves more successfully when *concepts* emerge in his thinking."

The stimulus-response (S–R) model views the learning process in terms of curves of acquisition. The teacher assumes the active role of the transmitter. This, the teacher does by sharing experiences. If the student assumes the passive role of the recipient of information, the teacher gives and the student takes. The teacher *impresses* facts on the student, *drills* ideas into the student, or *inculcates* good taste or love of learning. However, if the student assumes a more active role, then the student grasps the *structure* of facts or ideas. In a teaching-learning situation, "the teacher does not actually pass along some of his own behavior. He is said to impart *knowledge,* after subdividing it into *meanings, concepts, facts,* and *propositions.*" (Skinner, 1968, p. 3.)

Skinner considers instruction as a cognate construction. The teacher *informs* the student; through this process, the student's behavior is given *form* or *shape.* Skinner (1968, p. 5) defined teaching as "simply the arrangement of contingencies of reinforcement"—circumstances under which a particular bit of desired behavior is rewarded or reinforced to make sure it will be repeated—so the student will learn more quickly. This is the main theme on which he developed his model of instruction. There are three variables that compose or determine the contingencies or reinforcement under which learning takes place:

1. An occasion on which behavior occurs —the stimulus
2. The behavior itself—the response
3. The consequences of behavior—the reinforcers

Gagne described Skinner's notion of contingencies of reinforcement as the central part of Skinner's theoretical view of learning. He noted that while reinforcement is a name for particular arrangements of stimulus and response conditions and that while a response is deliberately contingent on the occurrence of some other response, they all involve a common characteristic: learning is preceeded systematically by the occurrence of a chosen event. To be effective, learning conditions must be organized so that a satisfying activity closely follows the occurrence of a desired behavior (Gagne, 1970, pp. 81, 119).

While it is not within the context of this text to discuss operant conditioning in depth, some considerations seem appropriate to include in this discussion. Skinner attributes much of operant conditioning to Thorndike's Law of Effect and those ideas that have emerged because of it have permitted the shaping of the behavior of an organism by the arrangement of particular types of consequences (reinforcements) in particular sequences so that effects do occur (Skinner,

1968, pp. 10, 81). Of considerable importance is the construction of various schedules of intermittent reinforcement, which Skinner describes as crucial in the transfer of learning and the shaping and maintenance of behavior (Skinner, 1968, p. 11).

The application of operant conditioning to education is simple and direct. Since teaching is the arrangement of contingencies of reinforcement under which students learn, the teacher's role is to arrange the special contingencies that facilitate and expedite learning; hasten the appearance of the desired behavior, which would otherwise take a long time to be learned; and assure the appearance of the desired behavior, which might otherwise never occur (Skinner, 1968, pp. 64-65).

Skinner pointed out that teaching can be improved if appropriate reinforcements are used, and if they are made contingent on desired behavior. He stated that the sheer control of nature is itself reinforcing. The net amount of reinforcement is not that important. A very small reinforcement may be tremendously effective in controlling behavior if it is wisely used. There are two considerations in devising the contingencies of reinforcement for desired behavior: (1) the gradual elaboration of extremely complex patterns of behaviors and (2) the maintenance of the behavior in strength at each stage (Skinner, 1968, p. 21).

There are many ways in which the necessary contingencies of reinforcement may be arranged. They may be mechanical or electrical in nature. Teaching machines are means by which such contingencies of reinforcements can be given. Skinner defined a teaching machine as any device that arranges contingencies of reinforcement (Skinner, 1968, p. 65). He invented the machine in 1954 after a visit to his daughter's fourth-grade arithmetic class. The purpose of the teaching machine is to present pupils with a succession of easy steps. At each step, a correct answer to a question brings instant reinforcement to a printed statement, telling the pupil that the answer is correct.

The important features of the teaching machine are that reinforcement for the correct answer is immediate; manipulation of the device is probably reinforcing enough to keep most students at work for a suitable period each day; children can work at their own speed, even though the teacher can supervise an entire class at the same time; children who have been absent can, on returning, pick up where they left off; and aversive control is minimized or absent.

There are a couple of other important features of teaching machines. One is that they require students to *compose* their responses rather than select them from a set of alternative answers, as is done in multiple-choice question. According to Skinner, the reasons for this are that: (1) recalling the correct answer is preferable to recognizing it because students make responses and also see that they are right and (2) multiple-choice questions that are effective contain plausible wrong responses, which Skinner believes to be out of place in the delicate process of "shaping" a behavior because they strengthen unwanted forms. Green (1963, p. 117) defended Skinner's type of programming by noting that if learners can construct responses, then they can certainly recognize them, but that the reverse is not necessarily true.

Another positive aspect of teaching machines is that students pass through a carefully designed sequence of steps in order to acquire complex behavior. The machine itself does not teach, but it puts the student in contact with the person who composed and programmed the material. According to Skinner (1968, pp. 33-39) it acts like a private tutor in many respects in that the machine:

1. Provides constant interchange between

the program and student, unlike lectures or textbooks, and sustains activity, so the student is always alert, busy, and taking an active part

2. Enables the student to master and understand one given point before moving on to the next

3. Presents just the materal the student is ready to handle at that moment

4. Enables the student to come up with the correct answer

5. Positively reinforces every correct response, and by doing so gives immediate feedback to the student and maintains interest

Programming good material for the teaching machine is very important. Skinner (1968, p. 48) suggested that in composing material for the machine the programmer should go directly to the source—to define the field and to collect technical terms, facts, laws, principles, and cases. These then need to be arranged in proper sequential or developmental order—linear if possible, branching if necessary.

According to Skinner, there are at least four different kinds of programming. The first is concerned with generating new and complex patterns, or "topographies," of behavior. He goes on to say that "it is the nature of operant conditioning that a response cannot be reinforced until it has occurred" (Skinner, p. 65). A method of shaping a topography of response was used by Wolf, Mees, and Risley (1964) to help shape the responses of a young boy who had refused to wear glasses after surgery for cataracts. He had severe temper tantrums that included self-destructive behavior. Two principles of operant conditions were applied: (1) the tantrums were extinguished by making sure they were never reinforced and (2) contingencies of reinforcement were used to shape the desired behavior of wearing glasses, although it was necessary to let the boy go hungry in order to

use food as an effective reinforcer. This method can also be used in treating autistic children.

Another case history involved the use of teaching machines with a 40-year-old microencephalic with a mental age of 18 months. With candy as the reinforcer, form discrimination was taught, and it was reported that the intellectual accomplishment following the programmed instruction was more than in all his 40 years (Sidman and Stoddard, 1966, pp. 151-208).

A second kind of programming is used to alter temporal or intensive properties of behavior. An example of this would be an athletic coach programming a high jumper by moving the bar higher by small increments and permitting some successful jumps to occur at each setting (Skinner, 1968, pp. 68-71). Another example would be a nurse programming a cerebrovascular-accident (C.V.A.) patient to walk longer distances by increasing the distance between the starting point to the goal and also increasing the pace.

The third kind is concerned with bringing behavior under the control of the stimuli. This technique can be used in discrimination learning; for example, in teaching a diabetic patient how to read the results of urine tests correctly. When the patient says "plus four" (+4) to the test result that indicates orange color solution with precipitation (S^D), the nurse positively reinforces the patient by giving the feedback that the answer is correct. The patient is not reinforced for saying "plus three" (+3) which is an S^Δ. In this way the patient's behavior of correct recognition and identification of test results will be brought under the control of the discriminative stimuli (S^D). Such a teaching procedure can be programmed to be taught by a teaching machine.

The fourth method of programming has to do with maintaining behavior under partial reinforcement. The effective scheduling of reinforcement is an important element of educational design. An example of this would be in teaching an autistic child how to maintain the use of words in asking for an object. At first, when the behavior is newly being acquired every correct response is reinforced positively. However, once the behavior is within the child's repertoire, then partial-reinforcement techniques in the form of fixed- or variable-ratio schedules can be used to maintain the behavior at the desired level. Such a teaching procedure can easily be programmed for and taught by a teaching machine.

Skinner acknowledges some of the criticisms of the work done on behavioral responses using lower animals. He himself admitted that "pigeons aren't people" but pointed out that his ideas have already been put to practical use in schools, mental hospitals, and penal institutions.

Another objection is that the contingencies of reinforcement used are not realistic. If the reinforcement can expedite learning and is the most effective, then Skinner believes it justifies its use and one can substitute a more realistic reinforcement at a later date. Still another objection to programmed instruction is that it does not teach a student to explore, to do problem solving, and to study. However, if used wisely, programmed instruction could make the student skillful, competent, and informed. Programmed instruction is effective in transmitting knowledge and in teaching skills; in this way it relieves the teacher of these tasks, so attention can be directed to other areas, such as problem solving, thinking, and exploring, as well as supervising and counseling students.

Skinner's view of teaching thinking

According to Skinner (1968, p. 117), the traditional view of thinking is an "obscure, intellectual, cognitive activity, something which goes on in the mind and requires the use of rational powers and faculties." He stated that the cognitive psychologist explains thinking by means of structure of expressed thoughts. They confine themselves to the outcome of thinking rather than thinking itself. Skinner, on the other hand, views "thinking" as behaving. In this sense, one is said to think verbally or nonverbally, mathematically, musically, socially, politically, and so on. He also identified thinking with certain behavior processes, such as learning, discriminating, generalizing, and abstracting. These, he has called changes in behavior and are not actually behaviors.

Related to thinking is attending, or paying attention. Skinner (1968, pp. 121-122) stated that some selective mechanisms are genetic. Individuals respond to energies and stimuli that affect their receptors. To attend to something is to respond to it in such a way that the subsequent behavior is likely to be reinforced. Students can be induced to act selectively to special features of the environment by arranging contingencies of reinforcements. They can be taught that some aspects and features of the environment are "worth responding to." The central process is discrimination, and instruction consists of arranging appropriate contingencies of reinforcement.

Thinking is also often referred to as problem solving. According to Skinner, almost everything we do is relevant to problem solving. We cannot learn problem solving as we learn to pay attention or study, just by learning or acquiring a few techniques. He stated that there are many ways of altering a situation so that it can be responded to more effectively. We can clarify stimuli, change them, rearrange them for comparison purposes, group and regroup them, and organize them until an expression appears that can be solved in some way already learned. Skinner believes that this entire repertoire of the process of problem solving is essentially a verbal one and is easily represented and taught with the help of available systems of notation, as in solving a mathematical problem. He also stated that both verbal and nonverbal problem-solving repertoires may recede to the covert level, where analysis of them becomes difficult, but they are taught at the overt level (Skinner, 1968, p. 133).

Skinner's view of creativity and originality is also very interesting. Since Skinner (1968, p. 170) views teaching as the arrangement of contingencies of reinforcement that control the learner's behavior, it appears that by its very nature teaching is inimical to inquiry and originality. A technology of teaching that is based on an experimental analysis of the external variables must confine itself to a more mechanical transmission of standard material. He stated that we cannot teach original behavior to students because of course, it would not be original if taught. But it is possible to maximize the probability that an original response will occur, if we go about teaching the student to arrange the environment appropriately. The student can then learn not only to take advantage of the accidents, but also to produce them. "He can generate new ideas by arbitrarily rearranging words, altering established propositions in mechanical ways. Subtle activities of this sort are probably part of all exploratory thinking" (Skinner, 1968, p. 188).

Skinner's model of instruction

Skinner based his model of instruction on the basic principles of operant conditioning. He took the implications of the Law of Effect very seriously in designing his model of instruction. His main theme is: teaching is simply the arrangement of contingencies of reinforcement. Skinner's model of instruction follows this sequencing: identifying the terminal behavior, initiating the first instance of its occurrence, prompting the behavior, programming complex behavior and sequencing instruction.

IDENTIFYING THE TERMINAL BEHAVIOR

The first step in designing instruction is to identify the terminal behavior; in other words, to state the objective for the student or the patient to accomplish at the end of instruction. Skinner pointed out that to use such words as adapting, adjusting, or surviving do not describe specific forms of behavior. They refer to consequences of teaching that may result from educational policy rather than method. Also, terms referring to mental or cognitive processes fail to specify the terminal behavior that is useful to the teacher and to the student; for example, words such as understand, recognize, or have a knowledge of are not useful. He further stated that to point to the ultimate utility of an education is not enough. To impart knowledge, according to Skinner (1968, p. 203) "is to bring behavior of given topography under the control of a given variable."

Therefore, the first step in designing instruction is to identify the terminal performance, or the behavior. One example would be that at the completion of instruction the female student or patient will demonstrate correctly the procedure of self-examination of the breasts for detection of lumps or tumors. Another example would be, at the completion of instruction, the C.V.A. patient will demonstrate correctly the performance of hand exercises.

INITIATING THE FIRST INSTANCE OF BEHAVIOR

When the learner objective has been stated, or the terminal behavior has been specified, arrangement must be made to strengthen the behavior through reinforcement. Skinner pointed out that just waiting for the behavior to occur so that it can be reinforced is an inefficient technique because it may take a long time before the learner gives the first correct response, if ever. Also, shaping the behavior by progressive approximation can be a very tedious procedure. He stated that there are several more efficient ways of producing the first behavior and solving the problem of the first instance:

Behavior is sometimes physically forced, as in the situation of teaching a child how to write. The child's hand is squeezed around a pencil and is moved to write a letter. In the examples used before, the instructor may place the student's or the patient's hand in the correct position on the breast and move it in the correct direction and rotation to examine the breast. Or, the C.V.A. patient's hand may be squeezed around a toy or an exerciser and moved back and forth or pressed up and down. Another example of physically forcing the first behavior to occur is when a judge orders the parent who has battered a child to attend a therapy group. Once the first behavior occurs, then it can be reinforced.

The second method by which the problem of the first instance can be solved is by using stimuli that elicit or evoke the response to be reinforced. Konorski and Miller (1937, p. 207) applied this concept to a dog. The dog's foot was shocked, and the resulting flexion of the leg was reinforced with food. After several practice sessions with operant conditioning, the operant response simulating the reflex eventually appeared in the absence of the shock. Skinner pointed out that when a teacher induces a student to pay attention to an object by moving the object conspicuously, the attention evoked (operant) in the student is not the attention that the student eventually learns to pay. In our example of the breast-examination situation, a photograph or diagram that shows the procedure of the breast examination step by step can evoke the first correct response, which can then be positively reinforced. In the C.V.A. patient, the seeing the exerciser or the toy or viewing a motion picture of another person doing the exercise may evoke the first behavior to occur.

Skinner (1968) pointed out that these solutions to the problem of the first instance are relevant only to a small part of standard terminal behaviors. There are other ways the teacher can evoke behavior to be reinforced, such as by using a stimulus that, because of its effect, is called a *prime*. A familiar example of primed behavior is imitation. There are three types of imitative learning that enable the initiation of the first instance so that it can then be reinforced.

1. *Movement duplication.* A small part of movement-duplication behavior may be innate. It is also possible that such an imitative repertoire is acquired because when a behavior resembles the behavior that is being observed in others, it is reinforcing. Most imitation is learned. "The teacher can use the imitative repertoire resulting from such contingencies, but he usually extends it, reinforcing a student when his behavior resembles that of a model, often the teacher himself" (Skinner, 1968, p. 208). When the model is conspicuous, the movement-duplicating contingencies are very effectively acquired. The model, who may be the teacher, responds slowly and repeats and exaggerates the distinctive features of the behavior to be observed and performed. The contingencies are improved if the learner is first taught to discriminate between the subtle features of the behavior.

An example of movement duplication would be when the nurse-teacher actually models and demonstrates the correct procedure of the self-examination of the breast while the student or the patient observes. Or, the student or the patient may see a motion picture of a model doing the procedure of self-examination of the breast. Similarly, when the C.V.A. patient actually observes the nurse or the physiotherapist demonstrating the correct procedure of hand exercise is an example of movement duplication. Other examples of movement duplication are when the public health nurse demonstrates to a new mother how to wash the baby, and the mother, having observed the nurse, imitates the procedure. Almost all basic nursing procedures or skills can be learned first by means of movement duplication.

2. *Product duplication.* Movement cannot be easily duplicated if the learner cannot see the behavior of the model, but its effects may be duplicated. Imitation of vocal behavior is an example of product duplication. Speech as such, and the movements that produce the speech cannot be seen, but the speaker (learner) is often reinforced when a speech pattern resembles that of the model. Most product duplications can be traced to environmental contingencies (Skinner, 1968, p. 209).

The application of product-duplication principles to produce the first instance of the desired behavior can be done, as in teaching the above-mentioned C.V.A. patient how to pronounce words correctly in speech therapy. The model's voice also can be taped, and the C.V.A. patient can listen to it and practice. The patient's own voice can be recorded, so the patient can listen to it and hear if the words resemble those of the speech therapist. This gives immediate feedback to the patient. As the patient's speech and pronunciation come to resemble the model's, it is very reinforcing for the patient.

Imitation by means of product-duplication methods can be used in teaching autistic children how to pronounce and learn words and enhance speaking behavior.

3. *Nonduplicative repertoire.* Nonduplicative repertoire is the third type of imitative behavior that will produce the first instance. In this situation, the behavior is primed with the help of preestablished repertoires in which neither the response (behavior) nor their products resemble the controlling stimuli (Skinner, 1968, p. 210); for example, verbal instruction that is given to the learner in performing an act or behavior, as in drilling a squad of soldiers, or calling a square dance.

The nonduplicative-repertoire type of imitation can apply to the previous nursing examples. When the teacher or the nurse gives instruction or asks the patient or the student to demonstrate self-examination of the breasts, instruction from the teacher can be given to the student or the patient either orally or in written form, as in test questions. The stimulus in this situation is either the spoken word or the written question. The response or the behavior is actual demonstration of the procedure of self-examination of the breasts. In this situation, the response does not resemble the stimulus; consequently, this type of imitative behavior is called nonduplicative repertoire.

The same thing applies to the C.V.A. patient. Instructions (written or oral) may tell the patient to demonstrate arm exercises. Here again, the response of exercise is not the same as the spoken or written words of "using the exerciser, demonstrate the correct procedure of the arm exercise," which is the stimulus.

Skinner (1968) pointed out that nonduplicative repertoires are not taught by natural contingencies. They must be taught by verbal communication.

PROMPTING BEHAVIOR

Prompting refers to the situation in which the teacher provides some hints, or cues, often referred to as "primes," to help the student recall the expected behavior. Skinner (1968) pointed out that in traditional fact-to-fact teaching situations, the teacher uses as many primes as needed to evoke a response from the student. An example of prompting behavior is when parents want to teach a child the name of an object. First they say it loud, then the child echoes back, Then the parents only whisper the word or the first syllable of the word (part of the prime), and the child echoes again, until the child learns how to pronounce the word correctly. Fragments of a prime have a special effect on the recall of the word. They are referred to as "prompts." The stimulus encourages the prompt appearance of behavior that already exists to some degree. To reduce the extent of a prompt is referred to as "vanishing," that is one causes the prompt, or cue, to "vanish" or "disappear." Israel's (1960) experiment utilized the principles of prompting in teaching students English-German vocabulary. Initially, priming procedures were used, then prompting; then they vanished the prompt, too. By so doing the students learned the German words.

Skinner (1968) thought that in order to help a student, the teacher must, as far as possible, refrain from helping with the response. Priming and prompting procedures should be used as a last resort, when the student cannot recall the behavior. He stated that teachers tend to make the mistake of prompting because they are reinforced immediately when the student responds correctly, but only after a delay when the student demonstrates the ability to make the similar correct response independently. Immediate priming of correct responses on the part of the teacher deprives the student of the chance to respond with minimal help and to learn to respond without any help (Skinner, 1968, pp. 215-216).

Examples of prompting behavior follow. In teaching a student or a patient the correct procedure of breast self-examination, the teacher may cue (prime) the student or patient by saying: "Where is the starting point?" "What should you do with the left arm if the left breast is to be examined in a lying position?" Or the teacher may provide the prime by the use of a photograph or dia-gram that shows the procedure step by step. Another example of a prime can be a written word that is a key concept that reminds the student or the patient of the events that follow. Similarly, the C.V.A. patient can be prompted for performing (exercising) correctly.

Other examples of prompting may be used in written examinations; for example, fill-in-the-blank questions may prompt the student by utilizing the first letter of the correct word. An example of this is, "The fragment of a prime has the special effect to which the term p _____ has been given." The answer to this fill-in question is "prompt." The letter "p" is a prompt. The prime in this situation would have been if the teacher whispered the word "prompt" or if it had been written in the margin of the examination question. It is important to keep in mind that the learner must first be given the opportunity to recall the correct behavior without either prompting or priming. These should be used only when the student cannot recall or when the student performs inaccurately.

PROGRAMMING COMPLEX BEHAVIOR

Complex behaviors cannot be reinforced all at once, neither can they simply be divided and reinforced part by part. Skinner says they must be programmed. Different techniques of priming and prompting can be used to evoke operants of specific topography so that they can be reinforced in the presence of specific stimuli. Other techniques are required to condition complex and extensive terminal behaviors; for example, by means of a course in school.

Skinner (1968, pp. 219-220) pointed out that programming is "not simply a matter of teaching one thing at a time. A subject is not a mere collection of responses and the steps in a program are more than the pieces of a final pattern . . . nor is programming simply a matter of proceeding in small steps." He stated that "whether a student can take a step in a program is as much a matter of earlier preparation and current help as of the physical size of the step. Small steps are necessary in order to keep the student within reach of reinforcement. He further stated that in programming, it is necessary to make sure that the student understands one step before taking another. In a good program, a student stays at one stage until ready to move to the second stage, but the student learns only those things that are needed in order to move on. The student does not necessarily learn the stage thoroughly.

Green (1963) developed a scheme and a specific sequencing of steps by which a programmed instruction can be developed.

The application of programming principle can be done both to the example of breast self-examination and that of the C.V.A. patient. As described in the beginning of this module, the characteristics, types, and methods of programming material must be taken into consideration in order for the content (behavior) to be taught by teaching machines. The same principles apply to these two situations. Let us first take the breast-examination situation:

The programmer needs (1) to define the field—in other words, what will be taught—and identify the terminal performance (student or patient's ability to self-examine her breasts,) and (2) to collect the information (such as terms, facts, laws, principles, and others) and list the steps of the procedure in proper sequential or developmental order—linear if possible, branching if necessary.

Then the programmer selects the type of programming that is appropriate for the task to be taught. In this situation, the first type is very appropriate, that is, the programming that generates new and complex patterns of behavior. This is done by means of operant conditioning. The teacher arranges the procedure in small steps so that the student or patient receives positive reinforcement as each stage is correctly learned.

The other three types of programming could also be used, both in the breast-examination situation and with the C.V.A. patient. With the C.V.A. patient it can be used in getting him first to learn how to exercise correctly and then—proceeding to the second type of programming that is concerned with altering temporal and intensive properties of behavior—for increasing the amount of time used to exercise the hand or the distance for walking.

The third type of programming can also be used in both situations. For example, if the student or the patient is not able to discriminate between the correct method of self-examination and the wrong method, then programming has to be designed to bring the behavior under the control of specific stimuli. The same is true with the C.V.A. patient. The patient has to discriminate between the correct position of the exerciser or between correct posture and incorrect posture.

The fourth type of programming can be used to maintain the learned behavior by stretching the ratio (schedule) of reinforcement.

SEQUENCING

The last step of Skinner's model of instruction is sequencing of instruction. Skinner (1968, p. 221) stressed the point that the steps in a program must not only be of the proper size but they must also be sequenced properly and effectively. He also stated that the student works in the single dimension of time, but what is learned is multidimensional. All programs branch, and the student must cover many different segments of a subject matter.

Skinner (1968, p. 221) proposed two types

of sequencing in order for effective and efficient learning to take place:

1. Steps in a segment must be arranged in order

2. Segments must be arranged in such a way that the student is properly prepared for each segment or step when it is reached

The teacher who works directly with the student has the advantage not only of using primes and prompts but also of arranging sequences. The teacher knows what the entering behavior of the student is and knows in what direction the student is able to move. Skinner considers the arrangement of effective sequences of content matter or behavior to be learned to be part of the art of teaching (Skinner, 1968, p. 223).

Sequencing techniques can be followed by utilizing Gagne's (1970) hierarchy of conditions of learning that progresses from the simple to the complex, in which a subordinate hierarchy of knowledge and content are essential for the learning of higher-order knowledge and should be programmed and sequenced accordingly. Let us apply this principle of sequencing to the examples.

In teaching the student or patient the correct procedure of self-examination of the breasts, the teacher first determines the entering behavior of the learner. Then, the teacher analyzes the procedure to be learned and places the steps of the procedure in correct order, or sequence, taking into consideration that a lower-order hierarchy of knowledge may be necessary in order for the learners to understand and perform the procedure correctly. In the implementation phase of the procedure, the teacher also pays attention to the fact that the steps are practiced in order and also ensures that the student or the patient is properly prepared for each step when it is reached. In a similar fashion, the principles of sequencing can be applied in teaching the C.V.A. patient how to exercise the arm correctly or to walk or speak correctly.

Skinner handles individual differences as follows: if these are genetic differences, different methods of instruction may be needed, as in the case of blind or mentally retarded persons. If the differences can be traced to early or current environmental contingencies, remedial action may be taken. A careful arrangement of contingencies of reinforcement would greatly reduce the effects of differences of this kind.

Researchable questions

1. What is the effect of different types of teaching strategies (for example, teaching child-feeding patterns to parents, utilizing programmed instruction versus presentation in a verbal form) on the cognitive behavior (amount learned) of the parents?

   a. Independent variable: teaching strategy—programmed instruction versus verbal presentation

   b. Dependent variable: cognitive behavior—amount learned

2. What is the effect of prompting versus no prompting of a concept on the retention of that concept after 6 weeks, 1 year, and 2 years.

   a. Independent variable: prompting versus no prompting

   b. Dependent variable: amount of retention after 6 weeks, 1 year, and 2 years

OTHER LEARNING EXPERIENCES—RECOMMENDED READING LIST

Skinner, B. F. *The technology of teaching*. New York: Appleton-Century-Crofts, 1968. (Read especially Chapter 10, "A review of teaching").

INSTRUCTIONS TO THE LEARNER REGARDING POSTTEST

At this stage of your learning process you are ready to take the posttest to determine the extent to which you have achieved this module's objectives. Return to the pretest of this module and take it over again as the posttest. Correct your own answers by using the answer key found on this page. You need to achieve 25 correct points to have reached the 95% mastery level. If your score is less than 25 points, correct your errors, study the content of this module again, and read the article in the recommended reading list. Take the posttest again. You need to study until you achieve the 95% mastery level or better.

ANSWER KEY TO PRETEST AND POSTTEST

1. c (Skinner, 1968, p. 208)
2. c (Skinner, 1968, pp. 206-214)
3. d (Skinner, 1968, p. 65)
4. b (Skinner, 1968, p. 208)
5. b (Skinner, 1968, p. 208)
6. a (Skinner, 1968, pp. 199-224)
7. b and d (Skinner, 1968, p. 21)
8. c (Skinner, 1968, p. 65)
9. d (Skinner, 1968, pp. 199-206)
10. a (Skinner, 1968, pp. 208-210)
11. g (Skinner, 1968, p. 214)
12. b (Skinner, 1968, pp. 209-210)
13. e (Skinner, 1968, p. 214)
14. f (Skinner, 1968, 209-210)
15. Any two of these is correct. The teaching machine:
    a. Allows constant interchange between the program and the student
    b. Induces sustained activity
    c. Insists that a given point be completely understood before proceeding
    d. Presents just the material for which the student is ready
    e. Helps the student come up with the right answer
    f. Reinforces the student for every correct response and through this feedback shapes behavior and sustains interest (Skinner, 1968, pp. 37-39, 65)
16. a. The contingencies of reinforcement used are not realistic.
    b. The use of the lower animals in their experiments has been criticized, and it is argued that the results are not applicable to humans.
    (Skinner, 1968, pp. 83-91)
17. Compare your answer with the answers that are explained under the heading of "Skinner's Model of Instruction" (p. 00), which is explained in this module. You should include specific implementation under each of his steps, such as:
    a. Identifying the terminal behavior
    b. Initiating the first instance
    c. Prompting behavior
    d. Programming complex behavior
    e. Sequencing

REFERENCES

Gange, R. *The conditions of learning.* (2nd Ed.) NY: Holt, Rinehart and Winston, Inc., 1970.

Green, E. *The learning process and programmed instruction.* New York: Holt, Rinehart and Winston, Inc., 1963.

Israel, M. Variably blurred prompting: I. Methodology and application to the analysis of paired-associate learning. *Journal of Psychology*, 1960, **50**:43-52.

Konorski, J. A., and Miller, S. M. On two types of conditioned reflex. *Journal of genetic psychology*, 1937, **16**:264-272.

Sidman, M., and Stoddard, L. T. Programming perception and learning for retarded children. *International Review of Research in Mental Retardation*, 1966, **2**:151-208.

Skinner, B. F. *The technology of teaching.* New York: Appleton-Century-Crofts, 1968.

Wolf, M., Mees, H., and Risley, T. Application of operant conditioning procedures to the behavior problems of an autistic child. *Behavioral Research Therapy*, 1964, **1**:305-312.

MODULE 14

Gagne's model of instruction

DESCRIPTION OF MODULE

This is an independent unit of instruction. This module describes in great detail Gagne's model of instruction. The text of the module covers five major areas: (1) theoretical framework, (2) relevant research studies, (3) issues, (4) application to nursing education and practice, and (5) researchable questions.

The content of the module is presented in sequential order. In addition to the text, the module contains student objectives, a pretest and posttest, an answer key, and instructions to follow.

MODULE OBJECTIVES

On completing this module, having studied and read the content of the module and the required reading list, the student should be able to accomplish the following:

1. Identify or define in written form all of the following terms: productive learning, knowledge, instructions, learning, learning programming, learning sets, entering behavior, and learning sets in a hierarchy
2. Identify in writing the relationship of instructions and subordinate capabilities (independent variable) to changes in human performance (dependent variable) in Gagne's theory of productive learning
3. Identify or list in writing the four func-

tions or steps of instruction necessary for knowledge to be acquired
4. List and define in writing all eight of Gagne's behavior categories or types of learning, beginning with the simplest category and ending with the most complex
5. State in writing how Gagne identified the subordinate learning sets required to perform successfully on an entire class of specific tasks, rather than on one member of the class
6. Identify in writing the four criteria necessary for the positive transfer of learning sets
7. Identify or list in writing the two stipulations Gagne cited as necessary to attain each new learning set in the process of positive transfer
8. Identify in writing the independent and dependent variables in Gagne's two hypotheses regarding learning sets in a hierarchy
9. Identify or list in writing the three elements that constitute the learning event
10. Discuss orally or in written form the theoretical framework of Gagne's model of instruction
11. Discuss two research findings relating to Gagne's model
12. Give two specific examples in nursing

education to which you can apply Gagne's model of instruction
13. Give two specific examples in nursing practice to which you can apply Gagne's model of instruction
14. Identify in writing or discuss orally two issues in the areas of nursing education and practice
15. Raise two researchable questions utilizing Gagne's model and indicate both the independent and dependent variables

PRETEST AND POSTTEST

Circle the correct answers. Each question is worth 1 point. The 95% level of mastery for this test is 26 correct points. Take the test and then correct it yourself using the answer key found at the end of this module (pp. 233-234).

Multiple choice

1. According to Gagne, in productive learning, there are two categories of variables. These are:
   1—learning to learn
   2—knowledge
   3—ability to understand
   4—instruction
   a. 1 and 2
   b. 2 and 3
   c. 3 and 4
   d. 2 and 4
2. According to Gagne's model of instruction, transfer from one learning set to another above it in the hierarchy is:
   1—0% if the lower one cannot be recalled
   2—100% if most of the lower-level learning sets can be recalled
   3—100% if all the related lower learning sets can be recalled
   4—0% if the lower learning set can be recalled
   a. 1 and 3
   b. 2 and 4
   c. 1 and 2
   d. 3 and 4
3. If the higher-level learning set has been failed

and if all the related lower-level learning sets have been passed, then the absence of positive transfer would be the result of:
   a. individual differences
   b. each student's ability to understand instruction
   c. deficiency in instruction
   d. student's lack of mediators for positive transfer
4. Which of the following functions, or steps of instruction necessary for knowledge to be acquired, are included in Gagne's model? Instructions make it possible for the learner to:
   1—identify the required entering behavior
   2—identify the required terminal performance
   3—identify the elements of the response situation
   4—identify the elements of the stimulus situation
   5—establish social-learning teachniques
   6—establish high recallability of learning sets
   7—establish guidance of thinking
   a. all of the above
   b. 1, 3, 4, and 7
   c. 2, 4, 5, and 6
   d. 2, 4, 6, and 7
5. Attaining each new learning set depends on a process of positive transfer. Gagne cited two stipulations necessary for this positive transfer process to take place. They include which of the following:
   1—the effects of instruction
   2—identification of the terminal performance
   3—recall of relevant subordinate learning sets
   4—the ability to pass higher-level learning sets when one lower-level task has not been passed
   5—lateral transfer
   a. 1 and 4
   b. 2 and 4
   c. 1 and 3
   d. 2 and 5
6. The three distinct elements Gagne cited as constituting the learning event include which of the following:
   1—mediation

2—learner
3—guidance
4—stimulus situation
5—response
6—instructor
   a. 1, 3, and 6
   b. 2, 4, and 5
   c. 3, 5, and 6
   d. 3, 4, and 5

7. The theoretical framework of Gagne's model includes which of the following concepts:
   1—hierarchy of knowledge
   2—productive learning
   3—categorizing social learning
   4—identifying terminal performance
   5—guidance of thinking
   6—identification of the elements of the stimulus situation
   7—establishing high recallability of learning sets
   8—creative thinking
   a. all of the above
   b. all but 3 and 5
   c. 1, 2, 5, 7, and 8
   d. 1, 4, 5, 6, and 8
   e. all but 3 and 8

8. Constructing a learning program that would begin each individual at the point of lowest successful learning set and bring the student to successful achievement of the final class of tasks would be another application of Gagne's model of nursing education. The method, according to Gagne, would have frames that would include which of the following functions:
   1—ensure high recallability of relevant learning sets on which achievement has been demonstrated
   2—make possible identification of expected performance
   3—make possible identification of new stimuli for each newly presented task
   4—guide thinking so as to suggest proper directions for hypotheses, associating subordinate learning sets with each new one
   a. all of the above
   b. 1
   c. 1, 2, and 4
   d. 2 and 4

Matching

Gagne lists four criteria necessary for the transfer of learning sets. Choose from part B the one best answer to successfully describe each criterion in part A. Fill in each blank with the appropriate answer.

Part A

9. If a higher-level learning set is passed, _____ related lower-level tasks must have been passed.
10. If _____ lower-level tasks have been failed, the related higher-level tasks must be failed.
11. If a higher-level task is passed, _____ related lower-level tasks must have been failed.
12. If a higher-level task has been failed, even though all related lower-level tasks have been passed, the absence of positive transfer would be attributable to a deficiency in _____ and does not contradict the notion that lower-level sets are essential to the achievement of higher-level ones.

Part B
   a. Related
   b. All
   c. One or more
   d. No
   e. Instructions

In the blank place the letter of the response in part B that best defines the concept in part A. There is only one correct answer for each item.

Part A
_____13. Productive learning
_____14. Knowledge
_____15. Instructions
_____16. Learning
_____17. Programmed learning
_____18. Learning set
_____19. Entering behavior
_____20. Learning sets in a hierarchy

Part B
a. Inferred capability that makes possible the successful performance of a class of tasks that could not be performed before learning was undertaken
b. One particular form of the ordering of stimulus and response events designed to bring about productive learning

c. Class of tasks

d. Generally takes the form of sentences that communicate something to the learner

e. Mediators of positive transfer from lower-level learning sets to higher-level tasks

f. The kind of change in human behavior that permits the individual to perform successfully on an entire class of specific tasks rather than simply on one member of the class

g. A relatively permanent change in a behavioral tendency and is the result of reinforced practice

h. The present status of the student's knowledge and skill before instruction begins in reference to a future status the teacher wants attained

i. The process of measuring the student's auxiliary and terminal performances during and at the end of instruction

Two research findings that have been investigated relating to Gagne's model are given in part A. Relating to Gagne's model, from part B choose the most appropriate concept of Gagne's model that relates to these two research findings and fill in the blank space to the left of the margin in part A. Choose one best answer only.

Part A

_____21. Harlow's concept of learning to learn

_____22. Maltzman's habit-family hierarchies

Part B

a. Social learning

b. Learning set

c. Chaining

d. Knowledge hierarchy

e. Programmed learning

f. Guidance of thinking

Sequencing

23. From the list identify *in correct sequence* Gagne's eight learning types (behavior categories) by writing the numbers 1 to 8 in the blanks provided. Remember to begin with the simplest and end with the most complex. Place an X before the ones that are *not* part of Gagne's behavior categories.

_____a. Discovery

_____b. Problem solving

_____c. Discrimination

_____d. Mastery

_____e. Principle

_____f. Chaining

_____g. Stimulus-response

_____h. Concept

_____i. Guidance

_____j. Verbal association

_____k. Rule and example

_____l. Signal

_____m. Creative

_____n. Social

Discussion questions

24. State in writing the *key* question Gagne asks in order to obtain the necessary learning sets or subordinate capabilities.

25. Specific transfer from one learning set to another above it will be zero if the lower one cannot be recalled and will range up to 100% if it can be.

a. Independent variable(s): _____

b. Dependent variable(s): _____

26. Stating and writing instructional objectives for each nursing course taught would be one example of the application of Gagne's model of nursing education. List Gagne's three reasons for instructional objectives:

a. _____

b. _____

c. _____

27. What would a test of entry behavior given to students on any nursing procedure determine? Your answer should be brief and explicit.

28. Write one example of your own to which you can apply Gagne's model of instruction to nursing practice.

Text
Theoretical framework

Gagne's model of instruction is aimed at producing "productive learning" in students. By this Gagne means "the kind of change in human behavior which permits the individual to perform successfully on an entire *class* of specific tasks, rather than simply on one member of the *class*" (Gagne, 1966, p. 116). The degree of productive learning is dependent on two important variables: (1) knowledge and (2) instruction.

Gagne (1966, p. 117) defined knowledge as "that inferred capability which makes possible the successful performance of a *class of tasks* that could not be performed before learning was undertaken." Therefore, knowledge indicates the level of capability a person possess at a given stage of learning.

Instruction is defined as "the content of the communications presented within the frames of a learning program" (Gagne, 1966, p. 117).

It is important to distinguish between Gagne's conditions or types of learning and his model of instruction. He views learning as a change in human disposition or capability, which can be retained and which is not simply ascribable to the process of growth. This learning exhibits itself as a change in behavior (Gagne 1965, p. 3).

Gagne distinguishes eight types of learning arranged in hierarchical order: (1) signal learning, (2) stimulus-response learning, (3) chaining, (4) verbal association, (5) discrimination learning, (6) concept learning, (7) rule learning, and (8) problem solving. This hierarchy begins with the simple forms of learning and ends with the complex. His model stresses primary interest in the observable behavior and performance that are products of each type of learning. These he calls the conditions of learning.

Gagne has identified three elements of a learning event: the learner, the stimulus or stimulus situation, and the response. The learner, a human being, consists of sense organs, a central nervous system, and muscles. It is the learner's past learnings and experiences and present set of capabilities at any given point in time that are considered the learner's external conditions of learning

(Gagne 1970, p. 4). Gagne has stated that it is these prior capabilities that are of crucial importance in drawing distinctions among the varieties of conditions needed for learning. The second element is the stimulus, an event in the environment, or the stimulus situation, which is several events in the environment, that stimulates the learner's senses. The third element, the response, is the action that results from stimulation and subsequent nervous activity; it is often called the performance.

To quote Gagne, "A learning event, then takes place when the *stimulus situation* affects the learner in such a way that his *performance* changes from a time *before* being in that situation to a time *after* being in it. The change in performance is what leads to the conclusion that learning has occurred" (Gagne, 1970, p. 5).

In searching for and identifying these learning conditions, Gagne has said that one must look first at the capabilities internal to the learner and then at the stimulus outside the learner. These have been stated in other words as the knowledge or capabilities the individual possesses at any given stage in the learning. This capability is internal to the learner. Instruction, on the other hand, is the stimulus outside the learner. As defined previously, it is that content of communication that is presented to the learner within the frames of the learning program.

Gagne's model of instruction is based on a theory of productive learning. To develop his theory of productive learning, Gagne thought that the independent variables in the categories of (1) knowledge and (2) instruction must be identified.

Knowledge: subordinate capabilities —learning sets

In beginning with the knowledge category, Gagne found it possible to identify the variables in this class by beginning with the final task (the desired knowledge) and asking his *key* question: "What would one have to know in order to be capable of doing this task without undertaking any learning, but given only instruction?" The answer to this question, he found, identified a new set of tasks, which identified a new set and so on, until a hierarchy of subordinate knowledges and capabilities essential to the performance of the more specific final task was developed. Also, "this task" determines the entering behavior and the subordinate capabilities in the form of learning sets known as a class of tasks (Gagne, 1966, p. 118-119).

The most important characteristic of a subordinate task is that it is directly measurable as a performance, yet it is not the same performance as a final task from which it was derived. Also, it is simpler and more general. Gagne repeats his key question with this newly defined task, establishing a hierarchy of subordinate knowledges growing increasingly simple. These subordinate hierarchies are mediators for positive transfer to the next level up.

From this systematic analysis of hierarchies of knowledge (subordinate categories), Gagne (1966, p. 118) proposed two major hypotheses:

1. "No one can perform the final task without being able to perform the subordinate tasks or capabilities."

2. "Any superordinate task in the hierarchy could be performed by one provided suitable instruction were given, and provided the relevant subordinate knowledges could be recalled by him."

Gagne speculated that his concept of hierarchy of knowledge may have some resemblance to Maltzman's (1955) habit-family hierarchies, which are conceived to mediate problem solving and are affected by instruction. He also speculated that his hierarchy might be similar to Kataona's (1940) "organizations," which are viewed to be put together by the learner into new knowledge by the help of instruction, without repetitive prac-

tice. Gagne also noted some resemblance between his hierarchy of knowledge and Harlow's (1949) concept of learning sets. Harlow demonstrated that his monkeys acquired the capability of solving oddity problems (class of tasks). Harlow also suggested that there may be hierarchy of more complex tasks than oddity problems, which his monkeys were able to perform. Gagne said that "there is a continuity between the relatively complex performances described here and the simpler ones performed by monkeys, we are inclined to refer to these subordinate capabilities as 'learning sets.'"

As mentioned previously, through the systematic analysis of subordinate categories of knowledge and by asking his key question, Gagne formulated his theory or concept of transfer. He viewed the subordinate categories of knowledge as the mediators for positive transfer to the next level up. He then tested the following predictions (Gagne, 1966, pp. 124-125) that were derived from his two major hypothesis:

1. If a higher-level learning set is passed, *all* related lower-level tasks must have been passed.

2. If *one or more* lower-level tasks have been failed, the related higher-level tasks must be failed.

3. If a higher-level task is passed, *no* related lower-level tasks must have been failed.

4. If a higher-level tasks has been failed, related lower-level tasks may have been passed. The absence of positive transfer in this instance would be the result of a deficiency in instructions, and does not contradict the notion that lower-level sets are essential to the achievement of higher-level ones.

Instruction

Instruction is the second major variable of Gagne's theory of productive learning, which is the basis for his model of instruction. Instruction, as Gagne perceived it, implies communicating something of value to learners and allowing them to progress from a point in the learning sequence at which they can perform one set of tasks to a point at which they achieve, for the first time, a higher-level class of tasks (learning sets).

In formulating his model of instruction, Gagne (1966, p. 120) asked the following question: "What functions must a theory of knowledge acquisition account for if it is to encompass the effects of instruction?" He identified four functions of the effect of instruction that he thought his theory of knowledge acquisition (model of instruction) must account for:

1. *Making it possible for the learner to identify the required terminal performance,* that is, defining the goal of what it is the student has to do. The statement of the terminal performance is in the form of an instructional objective, for example, at the end of 2 hours of instruction, the nurse will be able to demonstrate how to make a bed.

2. *Fostering proper identification of the stimulus situation.* For example, suppose that problems are to be presented using the symbols g, mg, and mcg; the student must be able to identify each symbol as a unit of weight and distinguish the difference in weight between each unit. Instruction has to establish this identification through trials and provision for contrasting feedback for right and wrong responses.

3. *Establishing high recallability of learning sets.* This is done by using repetition in the form of presenting additional examples of a class of tasks. For example, on the ward the student could be given the opportunity to give a medication in grams(g) and one in milligrams(mg) and would be required to identify the meaning of each unit and explain the difference between them.

4. *Providing guidance of thinking.* This provision obviously is initiated following completion of the other three, with the pur-

pose of suggesting how to approach the solution of a new task without, however, actually telling the learner the answer. An example would be: There is 1 g of a specified medication, but the physician has ordered only 100 mg to be given to the patient. What portion of the 1 g would you administer to the patient? How much of 1 g is equal to 100 mg?

Several factors determine the proper selection or design of instructional objectives. One is that student behaviors the teacher can observe and measure identify the end product of instruction (terminal behavior or performance), which is the outcome of behavior (DeCecco, 1968, p. 33). The second factor is entering behavior, defined as the present behaviors (performances or accomplishments) the student must have acquired *before* acquiring specific new terminal behaviors. Entering behavior, therefore, is where the instruction must always begin; terminal behavior is where the instruction concludes. Additional factors guiding the proper selection of instructional procedures are called the conditions of learning (DeCecco, 1968, p. 239; Gagne, 1970), and they distinguish between two categories of learning conditions: internal and external conditions. The internal conditions are the level of the student's entering behavior—present capabilities; in other words, the initial capabilities possessed by the learner exist outside the student. The teacher's task is to indicate the specific procedures and materials to be used from the learning types involved and their associated conditions. In this organization of material it is the learning type that determines the internal and external conditions of learning. Gagne formed a hierarchy of eight categories of learning types as previously mentioned (p. 223), with the simplest learning near the base and the most complex near the apex. It is important to keep in mind the distinction between learning and performance (DeCecco, 1968, p.

244). We can observe a performance but we cannot observe learning. This is why Gagne's theory is concerned with observable performances; they can be measured, whereas learning can only be inferred. The presence of the performance does not make it possible to conclude that learning has occurred. It is necessary to demonstrate that there has been a *change* in performance (Gagne, 1970, p. 22). The incapability of exhibiting the performance before learning must be taken into account as well as the capability that exists after learning (Gagne, 1970, p. 23).

The important thing to note is that the conditions of learning, both internal and external, are not the same in each learning type. Each type of learning starts from a different point of internal capability and is also likely to demand a different external situation in order to take place effectively.

Gagne (1965a) provides three persuasive reasons for the careful, explicit definition of instructional objectives:

1. To provide guidance in the planning of instruction
2. To assess performance
3. To let the student know beforehand what must be achieved in any given unit of instruction; thereby better enabling the student to direct efforts and attention

Relevant research studies

Brown and Gagne (1961) performed an experiment with ninth-grade boys, using a series of test items, with the final task being "to derive formulas for the sum of n terms in number series" (p. 122). Based on the previous discussion that attaining each new learning set depends on a process of positive transfer, which is dependent on the recall of revelant subordinate learning sets and the effects of instruction, they hypothesized that (1) no individual could perform the final task without having the identified subordinate capabilities and (2) any subordinate task in

the hierarchy could be performed by an individual provided suitable instructions were given and the revelant subordinate knowledge could be recalled. The data supported the hypothesis. It showed that there were quite different capabilities of the boys entering the task, that no boy who was able to perform the higher-level learning was unable to perform the lower-level learning sets associated with it, and that there was a greater number of instances in achieving the task after appropriate, adaptive instruction was given than before.

Another study by Airasian (1969) using algebra and chemistry textbooks broken into a hierarchy of elements following Gagne's model found that 75% of the students who missed lower-level elements in the hierarchy also missed the related higher-level items.

As mentioned previously, Gagne's knowledge hierarchy resembles the hypothetical constructs of Maltzman's habit-family hierarchy, Katona's (1940) organization, and Harlow's (1949) learning set. A brief description of these experiments will be given in this section.

Maltzman and his associates (1956) conducted an experiment to determine whether task instructions would still have the effect of inducing a given set when prior instruction and training had induced a different set. Ninety-six volunteer subjects from introductory psychology classes received instructions to look for a particular kind of solution to anagrams that would induce a disposition for these solutions when previous training and instructions were incongruent with such a set. The results indicated that a set may be established by task instructions despite the incongruence of previous training and instructions. A theoretical analysis of a set induced by training and by instructions was outlined by Maltzman and his associates (1956).

Maltzman (1955) elaborated on an interpretation of problem solving that may incorporate the phenomena traditionally described as mental set and determining tendency. Briefly, the theory assumes that mental sets established through training produce a change in the compound habit-family hierarchy by increasing the habit strength of a particular class of responses. Sets, or determining tendencies, established by task instructions produce a change in the compound habit-family hierarchy by increasing the reaction potential of a class of responses through arousal of their anticipatory goal response. Sets developed through training are based on the growth of habit strength, and therefore develop relatively slowly and have a degree of permanence. In contrast, sets induced by instructions are labile, are aroused rapidly, and need not persist. The results of this experiment seem to be in accord with the theoretical interpretation (Maltzman, 1955).

A series of experiments by Henry Harlow and his associates (1949), using both monkeys and children as subjects, provided some of the most convincing evidence for the usefulness of the concept of learning to learn, which is often at the base of Gagne's learning structures. Harlow demonstrated that the learning of primary importance to primates, at least, is the formation of learning sets. It is learning how to learn efficiently in the situations the animal frequently encounters. This learning to learn transforms the organism from a creature that adapts to a changing environment by trial and error to one that adapts by "seeming hypothesis and insight" (Harlow, 1949, p. 51).

We frequently observe that our capacity to learn new tasks increases when we have practiced similar tasks. For example, after an individual practices solving linear equations for several days, speed and accuracy increase in solving new linear equations. This progressive improvement in performance is called "learning to learn" (Harlow, 1949, p. 52). Harlow's monkeys acquired a general capability of successfully performing a class of

tasks, such as oddity problems, and accordingly are said to have acquired a learning set. There is also the suggestion in one of Harlow's research studies that there may be a hierarchical arrangement of tasks more complex than oddity problems that monkeys can successfully perform (DeCecco, 1968, p. 119).

Since Gagne thinks it is important to imply a continuity between complex performances and simpler ones, the performances demonstrated by Harlow's monkeys are referred to as learning sets (subordinate capabilities) (DeCecco, 1968, pp. 68-72).

A comparison of Harlow's concept of learning to learn and Gagne's learning sets suggests the following conclusions:

1. The capabilities in learning to learn are frequently at the base of Gagne's learning structures and are the most basic and general capabilities the learner requires.

2. Learning sets differ from learning to learn in two ways:

   a. They are more specific and are defined in relation to a specific instructional objective.

   b. They are hierarchically related. The concept that some learning sets are more basic than, or are subordinate to, other sets, is an important expansion of the concept of learning to learn.

Both concepts allow entering behaviors to be described as classes of performances.

In Katona's card-trick experiment he distinguished between senseless and meaningful learning, largely by contrasting the results of rote memorization with those of learning by understanding. Sixty high school students were assigned to two groups (a memorization group and an understanding group). The experimentation was done individually. The following results were obtained:

1. More time was required to teach the problems initially to the understanding group than to the memorization group.

2. Overnight retention was equal for both groups, although many retention errors were made even over this short interval. After the first retention task was relearned, the retention test for the second task favored the understanding group.

3. Transfer to a task requiring simple transposition was achieved more successfully in the understanding group than in the memorization group.

4. Transfer to three tasks requiring problem solving all favored the understanding group by significant amounts.

5. Large numbers of errors were made by members of the memorization group. According to Hilgard (1953, pp. 288-292), these are attributed to (a) reliance on rote memory when logical solution was possible, (b) careless errors within an understood approach, and (c) confusion because of partial understanding that was insufficient to mediate more difficult transfer.

Katona's original investigations demonstrated the relative ineffectiveness of memorizing and of "verbal principle learning" in the solution of matchstick pattern problems as well as card-trick problems, as compared to what Katona refers to as understanding (Melton, 1964, p. 293).

The organizations proposed by Katona (1940) resemble Gagne's knowledge hierarchy in that both Katona and Gagne stress that a major distinction between problem solving and other learning is that problem solving has high generalizability, or transferability. They are both interested in the student's solving a type of problem rather than solving single problems. The measurement of how much learning has occurred in problem solving is the student's ability to solve new problems of the same class. Successful solutions to similar problems is the evidence of positive transfer of learning as well as of successful problem solving that should result in immediate transferability (DeCecco, 1968, pp. 431, 442, 450-451).

We can relate guided discovery to Gagne's fourth function of instruction, that is, "guidance of thinking" in which thinking is guided by suggestions that progressively limit the range of hypotheses considered by the student. In this way the number of incorrect solutions is decreased until the final solution is obtained.

Experiments on the outcome of direction in the pendulum problem by Maier (1930) are a special case of productive thinking in that instructions and demonstrations are employed to increase the reaction potential of the anticipatory goal response and individual response members of the habit families leading to a correct solution. The problem was to make two pendulums that would make chalk marks on two different places on the floor. In Maier's experiment one group of subjects was given only the statement of the problem plus various additional instructions. Table 1 describes the in-

Table 14-1. Description of experimental groups in the Maier (1930) study (From DeCecco, John P. The psychology of learning and instruction: educational psychology © 1968, p. 450.) Reprinted by permission of Prentice-Hall, Inc., Englewood, Cliffs, N.J.

Group	Instructions
1 (control)	Statement of problem
2	Statement of problem and demonstration of three principles
3	Statement of problem, demonstration of principles, and verbal direction A (to use parts)
4	Statement of problem and verbal direction B
5	Statement of problem, demonstration of principles, and verbal directions A and B (A and B are verbal direction to guide the student's thinking, short of telling them the solution to the problem.)

structions given to the groups in the study.

The results demonstrated that with the exception of one student, only those students in group 5 were able to solve the problem.

Maier's instructions fulfilled many of the principles in Gagne's model of instruction (Maier, 1930; DeCecco, 1968, pp. 443-452). For example, Maier's instructions as a whole to Group 5, the only group that was able to solve the problem, involved the following principles:

1. Described for the student the terminal performance (behavioral objective)
2. Analyzed the problem (task analysis hierarchically arranged) to determine the lower-order principles the students must know to solve the problem and to find out whether the students knew them
3. Provided for recall of the principles involved in the solution of the problem by actually demonstrating each one
4. Provided guidance of thinking through verbal direction, short of telling the students the solution to the problem

Melton (1950) indicated that initial discovery may be the main problem in some kinds of learning (such as problem solving), while it plays little part in others (such as serial rote memorization). The controversy between trial and error and insight in the interpretation of learning hinges in part on the nature of this initial discovery of the correct solution. Melton noted that two other forms of initial discovery have played less systematic roles in learning theories, yet they should not be neglected. One of these is *guidance*. The discovery of the correct response can be facilitated by the teacher or trainer through appropriate manipulation of the environment or the learner. Therefore guided learning is intermediate between rote learning (with no discovery) and problem solving (with unguided discovery). An extensive research program on guided learning to demonstrate

its effectiveness was carried out by Carr and his students (1930) and was later summarized by him.

The guidance of thinking is Gagne's fourth function of instruction and perhaps is the most interesting from the standpoint of the questions it raises for research. Duncan (1959) conducted experimental and theoretical studies that dealt with the problem-solving performances of normal human adults. Once the subordinate learning sets had been recalled, instructions were used to promote their application to the performance of an entirely new task as far as the learner was concerned. Thinking was guided by suggestion, hints, or aids given subjects just before or during work on a problem to facilitate and guide the learner toward a solution. For example, Duncan cited several research studies, all done on human problem solving, in which various hints or aids to instruction were given to the subjects just before or during work on a problem to facilitate solution. His study based on "explication of the goal" (Duncan, 1959, p. 411) is one good example. Several experiments were done having human adults work on two problems: (1) making triangles out of matches and (2) fitting together pieces of wood to form a tetrahedron. Experimental groups received hints at regular intervals while working, each successive hint making the goal increasingly more explicit. The hints for control groups were not intended to explicate the goal. In general, each successive hint to experimental subjects increased the number of subjects solving the problem. Significantly more experimental subjects eventually solved the problems in all the experiments and on both problems.

Issues

Some of the issues relating to Gagne's model of instruction revolve around the following concepts:

There are many pros and cons regarding

Gagne's insistence on the use of behavioral objectives. The positive aspects, as mentioned before, include their helpfulness in the following:

1. Providing guidance in the planning of instruction
2. Assessing performance
3. Providing the student beforehand with the knowledge of what must be learned in any given unit of instruction

The arguments against the use of behavioral objectives include the following:

1. That instructional objectives should be concerned with the development of processes as well as products (Ebel, 1963). Gagne (1965b, p. 6) in repudiating this complaint, uses two objectives to illustrate it: (1) The student should acquire a developing awareness of the magnitude of the solar system and the universe, or (2) the child should become increasingly confident in extemporaneous oral expression. In evaluating these objectives, Gagne (1965b, p. 6) related:

It is difficult to know what to say about such statements except that they are weasel-worded. Why is it not possible to say exactly what one wants the student to do in showing his awareness of solar system magnitudes? Why is it not possible to state what kind of extemporaneous oral expression one expects the child to perform? The answer may be, of course, that the latter kind of objectives can indeed be stated, but not all students will attain them. Unfortunately, this is probably true under present circumstances. It would be good, though, if we could amend the statement to read: "Not all students will attain them *with the same speed.*" Then they would still remain objectives which any intelligent person could identify, rather than descriptions which if not deliberately hedging are at least ambiguous.

2. That instructional objectives, being explicit, well-defined statements involve the danger of overemphasis on conformity. Robert Ebel (1963, p. 34) said:

For, if the goals of education are defined in terms of narrowly specific behavior desired by curriculum makers and teachers, what need is there for critical judgment by the student; what freedom is there for creative innovation; what provision is there for adaptive behavior as the cultural world changes?

Those persons repudiating this position say that it is ridiculous to claim that the acquisition of knowledge and performances results in conformity to the past, because a uniformity of achievement has never been obtained or recorded by any teacher or school, given the initial differences in the entering behavior of the students. In addition, this claim ignores the well-documented observation that those persons who provide creative contributions in the sciences and the arts are those who are the most knowledgeable about their fields.

3. That we cannot determine what the student may be able to do at the end of a course of instruction. By this is meant that long-range educational goals are of interest; that is, what the student will be able to do years after a course of instruction is completed. The student may be able to do something no one ever anticipated. Gagne's reply was to encourage longitudinal studies researching this area of complaint. As for unanticipated learning, such as changes in performance other than those specified in the behavioral objective, Gagne stated that we can even specify these if we are to supply evidence that these changes have occurred (DeCecco, 1968, pp. 40-41). In rebuttal to this criticism Gagne (1965) suggested that teachers strive for instructional objectives such as these:

"Reads a French newspaper," rather than "reads French"; "solves problems requiring the use of sine, cosine, and tangent," rather than "understands trigonometry"; "makes a quantitative description of dispersion errors in observations," rather than "knows statistics" (DeCecco, 1968, p. 41).

Another argument revolves around entering behavior. After the differences in entering behavior had been determined, how would one go about getting every student in the class started at the same time? This would be difficult and would involve time and individual attention that perhaps might not be practical (DeCecco, 1968, pp. 38, 54-82).

Application to nursing education and practice

Stating and writing instructional objectives for each course taught would be one example of the application of Gagne's model to nursing education. Gagne (1965a) gives three important reasons for making explicit statements of instructional objectives. They are the following:

1. To provide guidance in the planning of instruction of any kind, since a careful statement of terminal performance enables the teacher to plan the steps the learner must take to achieve it
2. To assess performance because educators have discovered that by using explicit, well-defined instructional objectives they can more easily construct tests and text items that would accurately determine to what extent the objectives had been accomplished.
3. To inform the student beforehand what must be learned in any specified unit of instruction; therefore, better enabling the student to channel attention and efforts (Considering how often students are unable to make even an approximate statement of what the teacher is attempting to explain, the vital significance of this practice becomes clear.)

Constructing a learning program that would begin each individual at the point of lowest successful learning-set achievement and bring that learner to successful achievement of the final class of tasks would be

another application of Gagne's model to nursing education. The method, according to Gagne, should include frames with the following functions:

1. Ensuring high recallability of relevant learning sets on which achievement has been demonstrated
2. Making possible identifications of expected performance and of new stimuli for each newly presented task
3. Guiding thinking so as to suggest proper directions for hypotheses associating subordinate learning sets with each new one

An example would be for the nursing instructor to evaluate each student's entering behavior regarding a certain task or skill by giving a pretest. In this way the teacher would be able to diagnose individual learning needs and construct a learning program beginning at the level at which the student first attained success on learning-set tasks. The learning program would be a type of mediated instructional system to be used in independent study, similar to this module. Students would manage their own participation and practice at their own pace to accomplish the cognitive and manual aspects of learning the specified skill or task. The instructional objectives would be explicit, indicating the content to be learned. The program could be in the form of a teaching machine consisting of the content material typed on cards. After writing the answer to each successive frame on a numbered answer sheet, the student could be provided with immediate feedback by turning over the card to see the correct answer on the back. If the answer were wrong, instructions would be given to read the content (frame) again until the student could identify and see in writing what the answer was. Additional items of the same type would be given after each learning set was mastered, and then the student's thinking would be guided by instruction and cues to another learning set in either a co-ordinate or higher-level position in the hierarchy. The process would continue until learning of the final task was achieved, at which time the posttest would be taken to inform the learner of mastery of the task. The learning frames in the instructional program would be constructed to ensure high recallability of relevant learning sets in the following ways: by repetition, by presenting additional examples of a class of tasks, and by asking the learner to practice the subordinate activities in one or more trials (De Tornyay, 1971, pp. 132-133; Gagne, 1966, pp. 125-126; DeCecco, 1968, pp. 124-130).

Once behavioral objectives are stated, consider how much time and frustration could be saved if a test of entering behavior were given to nursing students on any nursing procedure. The results of such a test would measure previous rather than present learning and would indicate to the student nurse and the instructor the student's level of capability before instruction (DeCecco, 1968, p. 81). If a student had more than adequate entry behavior, perhaps instruction could begin at a more advanced point. If a student lacked the required entry behavior, either measures could be taken to increase behavior by review exercises, which would help the student to recall material learned previously but forgotten, or more instruction could be given at an earlier point than was originally intended. In any case Gagne related that the results of the assessment of entering behavior must become a component of instruction, since how else would one discover whether or not a student had acquired a behavior for a specific behavioral objective.

For inservice education much time and frustration would be saved by assessing the level of present knowledge required for the specific behavioral objectives (type of work expected of the nurse or any other employee). In most hospitals today, an entire group as a whole is oriented to the institution and its nursing practices, without consideration of the individual differences that exist regarding knowledge of individuals.

The challenging examinations given in the various schools of nursing enabling a nurse to *demonstrate* present capabilities without having to take a specific course is another example of Gagne's principle of the value of assessing levels of performance. Many nurses have successfully moved quickly up the career ladder in this way.

Gagne's model of hierarchy of learning skills could be used to teach all nursing procedures and courses. By identifying the learning sets necessary for a particular task, the concept of learning sets can be applied to the nursing curriculum. For example, consider the skill of catheterization. By working backward from the task to the prerequisite capabilities, one could identify the sets necessary for learning this task in the following way. By beginning with the final task (instructional objective), one would ask what capability the student would need to perform this task successfully. The answer would identify a new task that would be simpler and more general than the final task from which it was derived. The process would continue, disclosing increasingly more simple and general capabilities that when combined with the higher capabilities would form a hierarchy of learning. Analyzing a task in this manner reminds us of the necessity of analyzing all subject matter, task or otherwise, before presenting it to students (DeCecco, 1968, pp. 45-52). Within public health settings, the formulation of a hierarchical model of the knowledge required for the instruction and learning of the basic health practices, based on the life-style of the individual in such care situations as nutritional food balance, infant bathing, and immunizations, could assist the nurse in finding the present knowledge of the individual, making the material applicable and learnable, and eliminating cross-cultural biases and lack of knowledge.

Researchable questions

Determination of subordinate categories of knowledge within the body of knowledge called "nursing," ranging from simple nursing skills (motor) and facts (cognitive) to more complex and higher-order skills, or hierarchies of knowledge, requires extensive research.

1. What is the effect of teaching strategy based on Gagne's model of instruction as opposed to traditional (no model) methods of instruction on the cognitive learning of the four basic food groups when taught to a Mexican-American mother?
   a. Independent variable: teaching strategy (Gagne's model versus no model)
   b. Dependent variable: cognitive learning (amount)
2. What is the effect of a curriculum in a B.S. program in nursing that is based on Gagne's model of instruction versus no model of instruction ("Smorgasbord approach") on the affective (attitudes, feeling of unpreparedness) and cognitive behavior of students?
   a. Independent variable: model of instruction (Gagne's model versus no model of instruction)
   b. Dependent variable: affective and cognitive behavior

ADDITIONAL LEARNING EXPERIENCES—RECOMMENDED READING LIST

Gagne, R. The acquisition of knowledge. In R. Anderson and D. Ausubel (Eds.), *Readings in the psychology of cognition.* New York: Holt, Rinehart and Winston, Inc., 1966, pp. 116-132.

INSTRUCTIONS TO THE LEARNER REGARDING POSTTEST

At this stage of your learning process you are now ready to take the posttest. Return to the pretest of this module and take it as a posttest. Correct your answers using the answer key found on pp. 233-234. You need to score 26 correct points to qualify for the 95% level of mastery. If your score is less than this, correct your errors, study the content of this module again, and read the article in the recommended reading list. Take the posttest again. You need to study in this fashion until you score 95% or better.

ANSWER KEY TO PRETEST AND POSTTEST

1. d (Gagne, 1966, p. 117)
2. a (Gagne, 1966, p. 112)
3. c (Gagne, 1966, pp. 124-125)
4. d (Gagne, 1966, pp. 120-121)
5. c (Gagne, 1966, p. 122)
6. b (DeCecco, 1968, pp. 246-247; Gagne, 1970, pp. 4-5)
7. e (Gagne, 1966, pp. 116-132)
8. a (Gagne, 1966, pp. 125-126; DeCecco, 1968, p. 72)
9. b (Gagne, 1966, p. 122)
10. c (Gagne, 1966, p. 122)
11. d (Gagne, 1966, p. 122)
12. e (Gagne, 1966, p. 122)
13. f (Gagne, 1966, pp. 116, 129)
14. a (Gagne, 1966, p. 117)
15. d (Gagne, 1966, p. 117)
16. g (DeCecco, 1968, pp. 243-246)
17. b (Gagne, 1966, p. 116)
18. c (Gagne, 1966, pp. 120-122; DeCecco, 1968, pp. 54-67)
19. h (DeCecco, 1968, pp. 54-67)
20. e (Gagne, 1966, p. 122)
21. b (DeCecco, 1968, pp. 68-73; Harlow, 1949, pp. 51-65)
22. d (DeCecco, 1968, pp. 433-436; Maltzman, I., and others, 1956, pp. 418-420)
23. a. X
    b. 8
    c. 5
    d. X
    e. 7
    f. 3
    g. 2

h. 6

i. X

j. 4

k. X

l. 1

m. X

n. X

(Gagne, 1970, pp. 35-62; DeCecco, 1968, pp. 47-50)

24. What would the individual have to be able to do in order to attain successful performance on this task, provided his is given only instruction?

(Gagne, 1966, pp. 117, 122)

25. a. Recall of learning sets
    b. Transfer

26. a. To provide guidance in the planning of instruction
    b. To aid in performance assessment
    c. To indicate to the student beforehand what must be learned in any specified unit of instruction; therefore, better enabling the student in channeling attention and efforts (DeCecco, 1968, pp. 36-39)

27. A test on entering behavior would measure previous rather than present learning. (A pretest will measure terminal performance before instruction begins; a test of entering behavior tells the level of the student before instruction begins.)

(DeCecco, 1968, p. 81)

28. Answer should include and implement these four steps:
    a. Identify the terminal behavior
    b. Foster proper identification of the stimulus situation
    c. Establish high reliability of learning sets
    d. Provide guidance of thinking (Gagne, 1966, pp. 116-132)

REFERENCES

Arasian, P. W. "Formative evaluation instruments: a construction and validation of tests to evaluate learning over short time periods. Unpublished doctoral dissertation, University of Chicago, Chicago, 1969.

Brown, L., and Gagne, R. Some factors in the programming of conceptual learning. *Journal of Experimental Psychology*, 1961, **62**(4):313-321.

Carr, H. A. Teaching and learning. *Journal of Genetic Psychology*, 1930, **30**:189-219.

DeCecco, J. *The psychology of learning and instruction: educational psychology.* (1st Ed.) Englewood Cliffs, N.J.: Prentice-Hall, Inc., 1968.

De Tornyay, R. *Strategies for teaching nursing.* New York: John Wiley & Sons, Inc., 1971.

Duncan, C. P. Recent research on human problem solving. *Psychological Bulletin*, 1959, **56**(6):397-429.

Ebel, R. L. The relation of testing programs to educational goals. In *The Impact and Improvement of School Testing Programs*, Part 2 of the 62nd Yearbook of the N.S.S.E., Chicago: University of Chicago Press, 1963, pp. 28-44.

Gagne, R. The analysis of instructional objectives for the design of instructions. In R. Glaser (Ed.), *Teaching machines and programmed learning. II: Data and directions.* Department of Audiovisual Instruction, National Education Association, Washington, D.C., 1965a, pp. 21-65.

Gagne, R. Educational objectives and human performance. In J. D. Krumboltz (Ed.), *Learning and the educational process.* Chicago: Rand McNally & Co., 1965b, pp. 1-24.

Gagne, R. The acquisition of knowledge. In R. Anderson and D Ausubel (Eds.), *Readings in the Psychology of Cognition.* New York: Holt, Rinehart and Winston, Inc., 1966, pp. 116-132.

Gagne, R. *The conditions of learning.* (2nd Ed.) New York: Holt, Rinehart and Winston, Inc., 1970.

Harlow, H. The formation of learning sets. *Psychological Review*, 1949, **56**:51-65.

Hilgard, E. *Theories of learning.* (2nd Ed.) New York: Appleton-Century-Crofts, 1956.

Hilgard, E., Irvine, R., and Whipple, J. E. Rote memorization, understanding and transfer: an extension of Katona's card trick experiments. *Journal of Experimental Psychology*, 1953, **46**:288-292.

Katona, G. *Organizing and memorizing: studies in the psychology of learning and teaching.* New York: Hafner Publishing Co., Inc., 1967.

Maier, N. Reasoning in humans. I. On Direction. *Journal of Comparative Psychology*, 1930, **10**:115-143.

Maltzman, I. Thinking from a behavioristic point of view. *Psychological Review*, 1955, **66**:275-286.

Maltzman, I., Eisman, E., Brooks, L., and Smith, W. Task instructions for anagrams following different task instructions and training. *Journal of Experimental Psychology*, 1956, **51**:418-420.

Melton, A. W. Initial discovery of the adequate response. In W. S. Monroe (Ed.), *Encyclopedia of educational research.* New York, The Macmillan Co., 1950, pp. 668-690.

Melton, A. W. *Categories of human learning.* New York: Academic Press, Inc., 1964.

MODULE 15

Discovery-learning model of instruction

DESCRIPTION OF MODULE

This module is an independent unit of instruction on discovery learning. The content is presented in sequential order. The content matter covers five major areas in integrated form. They are: (1) theoretical framework, (2) research studies, (3) issues, (4) application to nursing education and practice, and (5) researchable questions. In addition to the content matter, the module contains a pretest and posttest, additional learning experiences, and a key to guide the learner in correcting the pre- and posttest.

MODULE OBJECTIVES

On completion of this module, given that the content of this module and of the required reading list is carefully studied, the learner will be able to accomplish the following set of objectives at the 95% level of accomplishment. The student will be able to:

1. Define discovery learning, guided discovery learning, induction, deduction, and expository teaching
2. Explain the theoretical framework of discovery learning
3. Identify both the disadvantages and advantages of discovery learning
4. Identify the issue
5. Explain research studies that are supportive of discovery learning and guided discovery learning
6. Apply the principles of discovery learning to patient and student teaching-learning situations
7. Raise at least two researchable questions and identify both the independent and dependent variables

PRETEST AND POSTEST

Circle the correct answers. Each question is worth 1 point except the last question, which is worth 10 points. The 95% level of achievement for this test is 25 points. Take the test and correct your answers using the answer key found at the end of this module (p. 250).

Multiple choice

1. In different research studies, discovery learning is viewed as:
   a. the dependent variable
   b. the independent variable
   c. the intervening variable
   d. all of the above
2. According to Bruner, discovery learning has all the following advantages *except:*
   a. increasing intellectual potency
   b. increasing intrinsic motivation
   c. speeding up the learning process

d. teaching the student the techniques of discovery

3. When the instructor provides examples, and the student is expected to derive the principle, the student is utilizing:
   a. an inductive approach
   b. a deductive approach
   c. unguided teaching

4. The teaching strategy of discovery learning should not be used in teaching contraceptive technique in planned-parenthood classes because:
   a. it takes a long time to learn
   b. the retention of the technique is not good
   c. it employs errorful learning
   d. women cannot transfer what they have learned in actual practice

5. In teaching-learning situations, when the teacher provides the principle and applies it to a specific situation, the teaching strategy is referred to as:
   a. guided discovery
   b. seminar
   c. expository teaching
   d. transfer in problem solving

6. The ability to search out and find regularities and relationships within the environment, to ask questions that attempt to locate the constraint within the problem, to perceive connectivity in data collected, and to protect overloading of cognitive thinking are characteristics of:
   a. intrinsic motivation
   b. heuristics of discovery
   c. intellectual potency
   d. conservation of memory

7. Discovery-learning strategy of teaching favors:
   a. impulsive students
   b. reflective students
   c. children between the ages of 5 to 7 years
   d. children from age 9 years and up
   e. students who have already learned how to discover

8. The strategy of learning by discovery is utilized in:
   a. all types of situations (conditions of learning)
   b. problem-solving situations only

c. simple associative learning and verbal associates
d. concept learning and problem solving
e. principle learning, but it is not absolutely essential

Matching

Part A

_____ 9. Discovery learning
_____10. Guided discovery
_____11. Induction
_____12. Deduction
_____13. Intrinsic motivation

Part B

a. A problem-solving situation where the teacher provides the principle and asks the student to supply the example

b. A teaching-learning situation where the teacher provides either the rule or the example

c. A teaching-learning situation in which the student achieves the instructional objectives with limited or no guidance from the teacher

d. A problem-solving situation where the teacher provides specific examples, and the student produces the general proposition or the principle

e. The student's tendency and desire to carry out learning activities and rewards independently

Discussion questions

14. List *three* characteristics of discovery learning.
    a. _____
    b. _____
    c. _____

15. Identify at least *three* disadvantages of discovery learning.
    a. _____
    b. _____
    c. _____

16. Identify at least *four* conceptual issues in discovery learning.
    a. _____
    b. _____
    c. _____
    d. _____

17. Take a specific patient or student teaching-

learning situation and apply the principles of discovery learning.

TEXT

"When I use a word," Humpty Dumpty said, in a rather scornful tone, "it means just what I choose it to mean—neither more nor less."

"The question is," said Alice, "whether you *can* make words mean so many different things."*

Theoretical framework
Introduction

The conversation between Humpty Dumpty and Alice appears to be analogous with the dialogue that exists currently among educational psychologists, teachers, and other interested parties regarding the definition, merits, applications, and implications of the discovery-learning method of instruction. Many different claims have been made with regard to its uses, purpose, advantages, and disadvantages; but the majority of these claims have not been empirically tested. Wittrock (1966) furthermore pointed out that there is confusion with regard to the meaning of discovery learning. For example, is it a method of learning, a method of teaching, or something one learns? In other words, discovery is given a wide variety of meanings ranging from an intervening process in the learning (searching for and deriving relationships to all forms of obtaining knowledge for oneself) to an independent variable (for example, something the teacher does, such as withhold answers from the pupils) to an dependent variable (for example, what the learner learns to do, such as formulation of relationships discovered in one's own language, assimilation or reconstruction of an accepted framework, induction and errorful learning).

---

*From Carrol, Lewis. *The Annotated Alice, Alice's Adventures in Wonderland & Through the Looking Glass.* New York: Branhall House, 1960, p. 209.

Both Cronbach (1966) and DeCecco and Crawford (1974) pointed out that even when there is agreement that it is something learned, there are questions raised with regard to the nature of this "something" that is supposed to be learned. Whether it is a specific principle or a problem solution, or ability to solve problems by using a single principle, or a structure of knowledge within a given discipline, or a technique of discovery or an interest in the satisfaction of the creative urge, is not very clear. Different authors and researchers have used the meaning of discovery learning the way they see it fit into their own framework and research interests.

Both Wittrock (1966) and Bruner (1966) consider learning by discovery still as a hypothesis. Bruner, who is one of the leading proponents of discovery learning, still considers it as a hypothesis, in spite of the fact that he cited the four major advantages of discovery learning as being greater intellectual potency, intrinsic motivation, memory processing, and learning of the heuristics of discovery. He implied that in spite of moderate advances that have been made in the area of discovery learning, learning by discovery is still in the hypothetical stage of development. He stated it as:

It is, if you will, a necessary condition for learning the variety of techniques of problem solving, of transforming information for better use, indeed for learning how to go about the very task of learning. Practice in discovering for oneself teaches one to acquire information in a way that makes the information more readily viable in problem solving. So goes the hypothesis. It is still in need of testing. But it is an hypothesis of such important human applications that we can not afford not to test it— and testing will have to be in schools (Bruner, 1961, p. 26).

Bruner pointed out that in the abovementioned hypothesis, the dependent variable is the solving of problems to index the results of discovery learning. The independent variable is practice at problem solving.

Definition of discovery learning

Glaser (1966, p. 15) defined learning by discovery as "teaching an association, a concept, or rule which involves 'discovery' of the association, concept, or rule."

Gagne (1966, p. 149) referred to discovery learning as an act of learning, that is said to occur when "the performance change that is observed requires the inference of an internal process of search and selection. What is sought for and selected varies with the kind of learning that is taking place."

Wittrock (1963) and DeCecco and Crawford (1974) defined discovery learning as those teaching situations where the learner achieves the instructional objectives with limited or no guidance from the teacher. The main characteristic is the *amount of guidance* the learner receives from the teacher (Kersh and Wittrock, 1962).

Wittrock (1963) has developed a useful framework for classifying the amount of instructional guidance the teacher provides in problem solving.

1. The teacher may give the principle or the rule and the problem solution. This situation is often referred to as expository teaching where both the rule and example are given; it is abbreviated as "ruleg."
2. The teacher may give the rule or the principle that applies but not the problem solution or the example. This is often referred to as the deductive approach, where the student solves the problem or gives an example by utilizing the principle; it is the application of the principle.
3. The teacher may not give the principle but may give the problem solution or examples. This is often referred to as the inductive approach, where the student derives the principle from the examples, in other words, makes generalizations.

4. The teacher may give neither the principle nor the problem solution. This is often referred to as either "complete discovery," or "unguided discovery," whereas the second and third conditions (where either the rule or the example is given) are referred to as "guided discovery."

Characteristics of discovery learning

The first characteristic of discovery learning, as mentioned in the previous section, is the *amount of guidance* given to the learner (Kersh and Wittrock, 1962).

The second major characteristic that Glaser (1966) pointed out is that discovery learning employs *errorful learning*. In the course of self-teaching, the student undoubtedly makes mistakes. This is often referred to as trial-and-error learning. Glaser pointed out that in discovery-learning method of instruction, the teacher does not impose a structured sequence of instruction. The student is provided with a relatively unguided sequence onto which the learner imposes structure. This methodology, or sequence of instruction, allows the student to explore blind alleys and find negative instances and, therefore, to make mistakes. Discovering implies a low probability of correct responses and a high probability of errors (Glaser, 1966, p. 15).

The third characteristic of discovery learning according to Glaser (1966) is *induction*. This is the procedure of giving specific examples, and the student then induces the general proposition or the principle involved. Evaluation of accomplishment is tested by having the student verbalize the principle derived and apply it to new situations and examples.

Wittrock (1966) on the other hand indicated that it does not matter whether an *inductive* or *deductive* approach is used; both are methods of guided discovery technique. Wittrock (1966, p. 73) stated:

Induction-deduction is a variable commonly confused with the discovery hypothesis. The learner can discover from either very general or very specific cues, one presented before the other. When applied to independent variables, induction-deduction pertains to the order in which general and specific cues are presented. When applied to hypothetical, logical processes, the learner can still discover a principle or generalization by either procedure. It depends on where he starts and what he is asked to discover.

Wittrock also pointed out that whether the individual succeeds or fails in the process is not only a function of the treatment given, but also of the individual's previous history; in other words, individual differences affect success and failure.

The nature of discovery learning: what is it ?

Bruner (1961) described discovery learning as a way of finding out things that were previously unknown. He also thought of discovery learning as including all forms of obtaining knowledge for oneself by using one's own mind.

Discovery learning favors the well-prepared mind. The act of discovery, according to Bruner (1961, p. 22), is in its essence "a matter of rearranging or transforming evidence in such a way that one is enabled to go beyond the evidence so reassembled to additional new insights. It may well be that an additional fact or shred of evidence makes this larger transformation of evidence possible. But it is often not even dependent on new information."

Bruner also pointed out that a child, when left alone, will go about discovering things, within limits. Also, he noted that the home atmosphere positively or negatively affects whether a child becomes a discoverer or not.

Bruner made a distinction between the *expository* mode of teaching and the discovery method, which he calls the *hypothetical* mode. In expository teaching, the decisions concerning the mode, pace, and style of exposition are determined mainly by the teacher, who is the expositor. The student is the listener. In the discovery, or hypothetical, method of instruction, the teacher and the learner are in more cooperative positions with regard to the pacing, style, and decisions. The student is not a passive "bench-bound listener," but takes an active main role in the teaching-learning process. The student will be aware of alternatives and will have an "as if" attitude toward them; as further information is obtained the learner may evaluate it as it comes.

Wittrock (1966) summarized some of the concepts of what discovery is as viewed from the early proponents of discovery learning, such as Montessori (1912, 1917) and Dewey (1910). They viewed discovery learning both as an end and a means. Through discovery a student is supposed to learn regularities, concepts, and how to solve problems and go beyond the data and almost act like a junior scientist. The learner is supposed to be motivated and enthusiastic about the discipline because of the discovery method of learning. The learner is also supposed to derive personal satisfaction from determining the sequence of problems. Through taking an active role and responding, the learner has succeeded at solving these problems. Wittrock pointed out that these propositions have not been carefully tested, even though they sound attractive.

Wittrock (1966) also made a distinction between discovery as a way to learn and as an objective of learning. He stated that as a way to learn or to teach, discovery may not be an effective treatment in producing learning, retention, transfer, affectivity, and time, when measured by these criteria. It depends on the meaning of treatment. Treatments may be viewed as "the way a teacher uses verbal stimuli—their sequence, nature, and variety. It may also refer to the learner's use of verbal stimuli. The results also depend upon the dependent variable sample, e.g., learning or transfer" (Wittrock, 1966, p. 73).

For example, as a way to learn, discovery may be inferior to more highly directed procedures. Wittrock (1966, p. 73) indicated that "when the criterion is the learning of concepts and hierarchically ordered subject matter, discovery may fare better. If the criteria are transfer to new concepts, originality, and learning by discovery, learning by discovery as a treatment may fare well. There are no carefully gathered experimental data on this last issue."

Discovery as an objective of learning (ability to discover) is important in its own right. Wittrock (1966, p. 74) raised the following question as an agreed on objective for teaching: "whether learning by discovery as a treatment is as effective at producing learning by discovery as are other treatments. In other words, is practice an important variable?" Many researchers believe that it is. Wittrock and others think that alternatives to practicing the terminal behavior needs researching. He suggested that a sequence of verbal materials and some practice at discovering would be better than an equal amount of time devoted only to practice at discovering. It also depends on many subject-matter factors. This issue needs definite researching (Wittrock, 1966, p. 74).

Relevant research studies

Research studies range from support for unguided discovery methods to support for guided discovery.

One of the major advocates of discovery learning is Bruner (1961). He listed the role of mediation in discovery learning. He used three groups of 12-year-old children who were to learn a list of paired associates. One group was told to remember the words; a second group was asked to select their own mediators; and a third group was given the mediators selected by the second group. Group 2 learned the greatest percent (95%) of paired associates in a one-trial test. Bruner concluded that discovery is the superior method. From this experiment he also concluded that discovery learning has four benefits: (1) developing greater intellectual potency; (2) receiving intrinsic reward, thereby reducing the need for extrinsic reward; (3) learning the art of inquiry through practicing discovery; and (4) making information more readily accessible in memory.

Haslerud and Meyers (1958) conducted a study on the effect of discovery-learning strategy on transfer of learning. College students were divided into two groups, an experimental and a control group. The experimental group was given two coding tests (power) a week apart; the control group received only the second test. The first test consisted of 20 problems, half of which had no directions given and half of which had the code printed above the problems. The second test was multiple choice and used the same 20 codes that appeared in the first test. The experimental group performed significantly better than the control group. On the first test there were more correct answers when the rule was given rather than derived, but on the second test, there were more correct answers with the reverse. The conclusion that was drawn was that those principles independently derived are more transferable.

Kersh (1958) tested the adequacy of "meaning" as an explanation for superiority of learning by independent discovery. College students were divided into three types of groups: no-help, direct-reference (given perceptual aids indicating relationships), and rule-given (without reference to relationships). The task was to learn the arithmetical and geometrical relationships involved in an odd-numbers rule and a constant-difference rule. Not all students learned the two rules to criterion. A test was given immediately following the learning period and 4 weeks later. On the retest Kersh was not interested in whether the problems were solved correctly, but how they were solved. The no-help and not the hypothesized direct-reference group gave the superior performance. Kersh explains the superiority of the no-help group not in terms of their understanding but in terms of their motivation to continue learning. (He had no objective evidence for motivation— only the written and verbal reports to the experimeter.) Cronbach (1966) attributed the effect to novelty and thought it would vanish in a long-term treatment.

Qualified support for discovery learning was provided by the studies of Hilgard, Irvine, and Whipple (1953); Craig (1956); Gagne and Brown (1961); and Corman (1957).

The study by Hilgard, Irvine, and Whipple (1953) consisted of 60 high-school students who were divided into two groups: memorization (the card order for two tricks was given and memorized) and understanding (subjects were taught a rational method for deriving card orders). All subjects learned the initial tasks to perfect performance. The following day retention and transfer tests were given to both groups. There was no difference between groups on overnight retention nor on the simple transposition task. However, the understanding group had the advantage on the more complex transfer tasks because the memorization group did not have the wherewithal to solve the problems; yet the understanding group still performed relatively poorly. The conclusions were that there is greater transfer with understanding, but there is no advantage to it in terms of ease of acquisition (the understanding group took much longer on all tasks).

Craig's (1956) study used college graduates whose task was to choose the word that did not belong to a series of items on the basis of some dimension. Three groups were given different amounts of guidance (clues), and one group was given none. Craig defined discovery and transfer in terms of the number of principles recognized and stated. The results were that the three groups given guidance made fewer errors than the group given none; progressively fewer errors were made as the number of clues increased; the maximum guidance group transferred more. The conclusions were that guidance is necessary for efficient discovery. Adult learners of high ability benefit more from more guidance and transfer more.

Support for guided discovery was also provided by Gagne and Brown (1961). Their subjects were boys in ninth and tenth grades. Their task was to state and use formulas for the sum of any number of terms in a number series. Three treatments were used: rule and example (correct formulas for all cases were printed on the answer sheet); discovery (students were asked for the rule; student worked alone but could ask for hints); and guided discovery (relevant relationships were pointed out). The measures used in the learning and transfer tests were time to solve and number of hints used. The results showed that all groups learned according to the criteria. On the transfer test the guided-discovery group did best, followed by the discovery group, and then the rule and example group. Conclusions made were that *what* has been learned is of greater effect than *how* it is learned. The discovery method gains its effectiveness from the fact that it requires the learner to reinstate (practice) concepts that will be used later.

Corman (1957) tested the effect of varying amounts and kinds of information as guidance in problem solving. He tested nine groups of high school students. The groups represented all possible combinations of two kinds of information (rule and method information) and three amounts of information (none, some, and much). The materials used were Katona's matchstick tasks. Both the success in solving problems and the success in verbalizing the rule were measured. Results showed that on the instruction problems, the more method information given, the greater the number of problems solved, particularly for high-ability students. On the transfer problems, high-ability students were helped most by more direct information, and low-ability students by less implicit information. Only information about the rule led to significant differences in the success of stating the rule; statement of rule and success in solving problems were not correlated. However, success on initial tasks was correlated with success on succeeding tasks. The conclusion was that success in solving problems is dependent on the amoung of guidance given as well as on student ability. Some appropriate guidance is better than none.

Advantages and disadvantages of discovery learning—a critique
ADVANTAGES

Bruner (1966) cited four major advantages of discovery learning.

Increase in intellectual potency. By means of discovery learning, the student acquired information in such a way that the information gathered is readily available in problem solving. Bruner (1961, 1966) made the following observations and inferences with regard to the effect of discovery learning on the intellectual potency of the learner:

1. In order for people to search out and find regularities and relationships in the environment or problem situation they must have the expectancy and the belief that there will be something to find and, once aroused by expectancy, must devise methods of searching and finding.

2. The type of question asked in discovering the problem solution is important. One may distinguish between two types of questions asked: (a) the question that is designed to locate a constraint in the problem—constraints that will eventually give shape to a hypothesis and (b) the question that is the hypothesis. For example, if a child is given a hypothetical story that a car has gone off the road and hit a tree and is told to ask questions that can be answered by "yes" or "no" to discover the cause of the accident. One child may ask, "Was there anything wrong with the driver?" Another child may ask, "Was the driver rushing to the doctor's office for an appointment, and the car got out of control?" Bruner pointed out that there are children (as in his experiment) who precede hypotheses with efforts to locate constraints, and there are those who are "pot-strollers," who string out hypotheses noncumulatively one after another (pp. 24-25).

3. Another element of strategy in discovery learning is its connectivity of information gathering, referring to the extent to which questions asked utilize, ignore, or violate previously obtained information. Bruner has observed that children who employ constraint location as a technique prior to formulating their hypotheses tend to be far more connected in their seeking of information.

4. Persistence is another element of the strategy. It has two components: (a) doggedness, that is, need for achievement, and (b) organized persistence, which is a method of protecting overloading of cognitive thinking. For example, a child who acquires tremendous amounts of disconnected information gets frustrated and confused. The important point is the recognition that the value of information is not simply in getting it, but in being able to carry it. The persistence of the organized child stems from knowledge of how to organize questions in cycles, how to summarize things (Bruner, 1961, p. 25). In the form of a hypothesis, Bruner postulated that discovery-learning method of instruction enables the learner to be a "constructionist, to organize what he is encountering in a manner

not only designed to discover regularity and relatedness, but also to avoid the kind of information drift that fails to keep account of the uses to which information might have to be put" (p. 26). He also viewed it as a necessary condition for learning a variety of problem-solving techniques, for transforming information for better use, and for learning to learn. Practice in discovering makes information viable for problem solving.

Discovery learning increases intrinsic motivation. Discovery learning increases and strengthens the students' tendency and desire to carry out learning activities and rewards on their own. The act of discovering may in itself be a reward.

Bruner (1961, p. 29) proposed that "the degree to which competence or mastery motives come to control behavior, to that degree the role of reinforcement or 'extrinsic pleasure' wanes in shaping behavior. The child comes to manipulate his environment more actively and achieves his gratification from coping with problems. Symbolic modes of representing and transforming the environment arise and the importance of stimulus-response-reward sequence decline."

Discovery learning teaches the techniques of discovery, the heuristics of discovery. Problem solving through discovery develops a style of solving problems by the very act of engaging in problem solving or inquiry.

Bruner (1961, p. 31) stated, "It is only through the exercises of problem solving and the effort of discovery that one learns the working heuristics of discovery." He further stated that, "Practice in inquiry, in trying to figure out things for oneself is indeed what is needed, but in what form? Of only one thing I am convinced. I have never seen anybody improve in the art and technique of inquiry by any means other than engaging in inquiry" (p. 31).

Conservation of memory. Discovery learning results in a better retention system. It develops in the student a better memory-processing method, which results in better retention, since the student has organized the information and stored it in a cognitive storage system and knows where to find and retrieve it when needed.

Bruner (1961) proposed that any organization of information that reduces the complexity of material by embedding it into the cognitive structure of the person will make the material more accessible for retrieval. He asked how information could be "placed" in a person's memory so that it would be available on demand. His view is that material should be organized in terms of the person's own interests and cognitive structure. If so done, it has the best chance of being accessible to memory. "It is more likely to be placed along routes that are connected to one's own ways of intellectual travel" (p. 32). Bruner further asserted that "the very attitudes and activities that characterize 'figuring out' or 'discovering' things for oneself also seems to have the effect of making material more accessible in memory" (p. 32).

DISADVANTAGES AND CRITICISMS OF DISCOVERY LEARNING

Ausubel (1963) criticized the proponents of discovery learning as making comments without backing it with research. For example, such unsupportable claims as: discovery learning produces the best method of problem solving in students; it is the best method of transmitting knowledge, it produces self-confidence and high motivation in students; problem solving is the primary aim of education; every child can become a creative and critical thinker; and expository teaching is authoritarian. Ausubel believes that the primary aim of teaching is to present a body of knowledge in a systematic way. The organization of content matter should be specific and should be given to the students in an explicit way. He does not believe that creative and critical thinking can be taught outside the context of a specific discipline. Such thinking, can be accomplished by "adopting a precise, logical, analytical and critical approach to the teaching of a particular discipline, an approach which fosters appreciation of scientific method in that discipline" (Ausubel, 1963, p. 158). Ausubel further stated that learning by discovery has its rationale—it uses and advantages at the appropriate time and place (such as in the early stages of learning any abstract subject matter)—and its mystique—its unwarranted assumptions (such as, all real knowledge is self-discovered), overstated claims, and inadequately tested propositions. The basic issue for him is not whether discovery learning enhances learning, retention, and transferability but whether it does so sufficiently to warrant the time spent in it and whether it is a feasible technique for mature learners.

Gagne (1970) also criticized the claim that discovery-learning method of instruction if constantly used will enable the individual to make great discoveries. He viewed such thinking as wishful thinking.

Kagan (1966) stated the following points against the discovery method: (1) many students do not have the initial motivation to exert the effort required to make inferences; (2) young children, 5 to 7 years of age, do not have sufficient appreciation of what a problem to benefit from discovery learning; (3) impulsive students are apt to settle on the wrong conclusions and become vulnerable to developing feelings of intellectual impotence; and (4) impulsive students make more errors of inductive reasoning than reflective students do.

Wittrock (1966) pointed out that "only those students who have already learned how to discover may learn by discovery" (p. 36). Wittrock (1966), Bruner (1966), and de Tornyay (1971) all agree that discovery learning favors the well-prepared mind. Wittrock also criticized discovery learning in that the hypothesis of learning by discovery confuses means with ends. For example, to enable the student to discover (an end) may involve more than simple practice at discovering (a means). He stated that discovery learning is time consuming. It tends to repudiate the nature of culture, since "the essence of culture is that everyone need not discover for himself everything anew but that he can profit from the experiences of others as summarized in language" (Wittrock, 1966, p. 36). Furthermore, he stated that problem-solving ability is important as an end, but it is not the only end. An individual must learn to acquire and understand much of the culture as well as learn to discover new knowledge and to solve problems.

Theoretical issues in discovery learning

Wittrock (1966) has identified six conceptual issues in discovery learning.

A way to learn subject matter versus an end in its own right. Wittrock pointed out that discovery is viewed to be not only a way to learn the structure of a subject matter, but also a way to teach problem solving. Therefore, no matter what subject matter students learn, it is thought to be important that they discover it. Wittrock suggested that these two ends should be kept separate. They can and should be operationally measured as dependent variables.

Related to this issue is the confusion between the view of discovery learning as a dependent or independent variable. Wittrock (1966, p. 35) called this a dilemma, saying:

Herin lies the crux of the dilemma among educational psychologists about discovery learning. When learning and discovery are measured by one event, discovery cannot be given as a cause for learning. It does no good to say tautologically that those who discover learn. For example, the desired result is an event named *learning by discovery*. The treatment designed to produce the result is also an event named *learning by discovery*. A tautological conclusion easily followed. The discovery learners learned by discovery, therefore their treatment was the better one, regardless of the data.

He suggested that treatment and its results must be kept separate. The treatment is an independent variable. It may or may not necessarily produce transfer, retention, savings, or ability to discover that is as good as or better than other treatment measures.

What is to be discovered? There is confusion as to whether the thing to be discovered is a rule, a generalization, or more specific information. Wittrock suggested that an attempt should be made to define the difference between verbal statements of generalizations and more specific information. The uses of discovery learning may be different to learn these ends.

Induction versus deduction. As mentioned in the beginning of this module, induction approach is commonly equated with discovery learning, where the learner makes generalizations from specific situations. The thinking proceeds from the specific to the general. Wittrock (1966, pp. 42-43) pointed out that:

It is just as plausible to assume that the learner begins with a higher order generalization, from which he derives more specific conclusions and thus discovers answers and even generalizations. That is, there are probably several different processes involved in discovery. Induction has no exclusive identity with discovery learning. Discovery should be viewed as a set of very complex processes.

Depreciation of verbal learning. Wittrock (1966) pointed out that, in general, research on discovery learning has been very critical of a teacher's use of words. They argue that students should derive their own verbalizations rather than receiving them from the teacher.

Control of rate and sequence of stimuli. In general, learning by discovery refers to a previously determined sequence that begins with problems and examples rather than with rules and generalizations. Wittrock (1966) noted that for some unknown reason the effect of letting the student control the rate and sequence of stimuli are not studied in the literature.

Variety of dependent variables. There are a variety of dependent variables, such as transfer, savings, retention, and ability to solve problems, that have been studied that are supposed to measure learning by discovery. The ability to verbalize rules and conclusions is viewed as an index of discovery. The affective behaviors of positive emotions and the increased interest in subject matter and problem solving are also viewed as dependent variables. Wittrock pointed out that it is alright and healthy to have so many different types of dependent variables, provided that the results of the study are carefully related to the specific dependent variables sampled in the study. He cautioned against comparing and contrasting the different findings with one another unless they pertain to the same types of dependent variables.

Methodological problems

There are several methodological problems raised by the research in discovery learning:

1. Ambiguity, impreciseness, and bias in defining terms and treatments, such as treatments given different labels in different experiments are often indistinguishable

2. Lack of replicability of treatments

3. Unwarranted extrapolation of results (tenuous conclusions about learning by discovery because of the great variety of complex treatments, subject matter, students, and indices of discovery that make it difficult to compare results across studies)

4. Confusion of means and ends, of learning by discovery and learning to discover, as well as confusion of treatments and results, that is, labeling treatments in terms of the re-

sponses they are said to produce (Wittrock, 1966)

5. Confusion of teacher and learner roles, which results in opposing views such as the following:

a. Hawkins (1966)—the teacher can only prepare the child to discover by bringing the student to the point of readiness; the teacher can neither guide nor teach discovery because of the multiplicity of paths it may take

b. Glaser (1966)—the teacher is totally responsible for the occurrence of discovery as a means and as an end; it is simply a matter of identifying the component behaviors, setting the appropriate behavioral objectives, carrying out objectives through inductive processes, and structuring the instruction as little as possible

There is also the issue that if discovery is to be meaningful, it must somehow be structured. Who is to order the material and determine the rate of presentation, the teacher or the students? If the teacher, how are the students to create their own structure and derive their own verbalizations?

Use of discovery-learning method

With which conditions of learning can discovery learning method of instruction be used? Gagne (1966) indicated that in the act of learning, discovery occurs when the observed performance change requires the inference of an internal process of search and selection. What is sought for and selected varies with the type of learning that is taking place.

Discovery processes occur as part of most types of learning, ranging from the simple to the complex. In this sense, Gagne said that discovery may be considered a "dimension" of learning. Discovery processes take longer time than the processes of acquiring and storing information. Therefore, he noted that

discovery-learning methodology is not more efficient than other methods.

Gagne (1966) pointed out that the role of discovery is different with different conditions of learning.

Discovery in simple associative learning. The learning of simple connections (such as pronouncing foreign words) involves the process of discovery in searching for and selection of the kinesthetic part of the stimulus complex, which necessitates the need for practice (Gagne, 1966, p. 149).

Discovery in verbal associate learning. In verbal associate learning, the thing to be discovered is the mediating link between two verbal members. Bruner's (1966) study demonstrated that self-generated links are more favorable to learning and retention than links that are externally supplied. For example, Bruner showed that 95% of the associations were recalled when learners had supplied their own mediating links, whereas less than 50% were recalled when the mediator was supplied by someone other than the learner.

Discovery in concept learning. According to Gagne (1966, p. 149) concept learning requires to a certain extent a process of discovery in the sense that an internally generated process of representation is involved. He stated:

In adults, who have available suitable verbal mediators, concept formation in a novel situation appears to be a most rapid kind of learning. Laboratory studies of effective conditions for concept learning in children seem to be singularly lacking. But the employment of a high degree of guidance, verbal or otherwise, seems to be a necessity for efficient learning.

Discovery in principle learning. Principle learning can take place with or without discovery. When principles are learned by utilizing discovery method of instruction, evidence (McConnell, 1934; Anderson, 1949; Craig, 1956) indicates that learned principles are retained better and transferred more. Gagne (1966) suggested that guided discovery method of instruction serves to reduce the time of search while maintaining the advantages of internal selection.

Discovery in problem solving. Gagne (1966) pointed out that problem solving, as a form of learning, requires discovery because the learner is expected to generate a new way of combining previously learned rules or principles. Guidance in problem solving also reduces the time for search.

• • •

Learning to discover, or the heuristics of discovery, is possible. People can learn strategies of solving particular classes of problems. For example, Katona (1940) demonstrated that subjects learned how to solve matchstick problems. Gagne and Brown (1961) showed that high school students were able to learn how to discover the solution to number-series problems. The study of Bruner, Goodnow, and Austin (1956) demonstrated that strategies of discovery are learned and are transferred to a variety of card-coding problems. Gagne (1966) furthermore noted that there is no convincing evidence that one can learn to be a discoverer, in a general sense, but this proposition is open for investigation.

Gagne (1966, p. 150) is convinced that discovery learning has important implications for educational practice. He stated:

First is the idea that discovery learning is an integral process for several varieties of learning. It is not a panacea for learning effectiveness, nor is it an essential condition for all kinds of learning. But it can be identified widely in school learning situations. Second, when discovery does occur, it is obviously dependent upon internal events generated within the learner. This means that if one is interested in promoting the occurrence of discovery to achieve some educational objective, he must somehow see to it that prerequisite capabilities have been established. In other words, there must certainly be a lot of attention to the preparation phase of instruction, if discovery is going to take place.

DeCecco and Crawford (1974) pointed out a very important point that the teacher needs to take into consideration prior to subscribing to any specific method of instruction. They stated that instrinsic to the concept of teaching is the assumption that the selection of teaching procedures should be based on prior statement of instructional objectives and a description and assessment of the prerequisite entering behavior. The complex relationship among objectives, learners, and procedures should make all a priori claims about the universal applicability and suitability of a specific instructional procedure for all objectives and all students very questionable.

DeCecco and Crawford suggested that the teacher's selection of teaching procedures should be guided by the instructional objectives and the entering behavior of the learner. Objectives tell what is to be learned and what type of learning is to be used. Entering behaviors indicate what the students need to know and how much they do know. Knowledge of the type of learning and the entering behavior enables the teacher to select the appropriate instructional procedure to accommodate the necessary internal and external conditions of learning. Also, with the use of performance evaluations, the teacher can receive feedback on the efficiency and success of the instructional procedure and the effect it has on student learning. DeCecco and Crawford also suggested that the teacher should ask the following question prior to subscribing to any specific model of instruction. "For what purposes and for which students and under what learning conditions should I employ and any one method or combination of methods of instruction." (DeCecco and Crawford, 1974, p. 362).

After asking this important question, should the teacher decide that discovery method of instruction utilizing either the complete discovery or the guided discovery method of instruction is most appropriate, then the teacher can utilize Bruner's (1966) suggestions of methods by which the teacher can aid the student to discovery learning. These are:

1. Arrange learning in such a way as to encourage students to stop and think about what they are doing and saying so that they recognize that when they have information they can go beyond it and that there is connectedness between the facts they have learned and other data and situations

2. Get the students to approach new material in such a fashion that they fit it into their own organizational system by helping the students to find connections or mediators between the new material and already-known material

3. Activate the students so that they can experience their own capacity to solve problems and have enough success to feel rewarded for the exercise of thinking (Bruner believes that the reward for thinking is intrinsic to the activity and students can be corrupted if they are only working for grades.)

4. Give the students practice in the skills related to the use of information and problem solving

5. Get the students to reflect on their behavior and to put the reasons for the behavior into words

6. Engineer discovery so that it takes place in a context of problem solving—so that the students can retrieve and combine information in an appropriate setting rather than under the spell of inspiration such as by getting the students to explore contrasts

Application to nursing education and practice

Can discovery learning be used in nursing? de Tornyay (1971) offered a very good answer. She stated that the learning of specific facts or a way of handling a specific patient situation would make this method less useful. But if the objective is to help students acquire and incorporate new concepts into their cognitive structure—to "learn to learn"—then teaching by means of discovery will enhance the learning process.

An example of a specific patient-teaching situation is teaching a group of people effective family planning, or the use of different methods of contraception. Since the use of learning by discovery entails a high degree of errorful learning, that is, the probability of making errors is very high, the use of discovery-learning method of instruction is inappropriate.

However, if the instructional objective is to learn a specific nursing concept or to apply a specific health-care principle to the planning and implementation of a specific patient-care situation (where problem solving is involved), then the discovery method of instruction is appropriate. The teacher needs to incorporate Gagne's (1966), DeCecco and Crawford's (1974), Bruner's (1966) suggestions in:

1. Stating instructional objectives, identifying and classifying the type or condition of learning that the task to be learned entails
2. Assessing the prerequisite entering behaviors necessary to solve the problem
3. Assessing the entering behavior of the student
4. Selecting the appropriate method of instruction; for example, using the guided discovery method for some objectives and complete discovery for others
5. Implementing Bruner's six-step method of aiding the student to discover

The same teaching strategy can be applied to patient-teaching situations.

Researchable questions
What should be the proper direction of research?

Either discovery in learning will simply cease to be a topic of interest in research, or it will need to go through a process of redefinition and reformulation.

We need a terminology change—some terms, such as discovery and rote are too emotionally loaded. They need new names or need to be broken down into more fundamental components. All terms need to be operationally defined. Treatments and measures need to be standardized. Cronbach (1966) proposed that each treatment be optimized in its own terms, so that each has a fair chance to show what it can do within a fixed time.

Researchers have differing opinions about where the appropriate place is to begin. Hawkins (1966) and Bruner (1966) advocated finding and producing the best practice found in the classroom. They denied the relevence of formal learning experiments to classroom learning. On the other hand, many more researchers advocate asking limited questions and then extending the scope of inquiry where possible. An intermediate strategy suggested by Cronbach (1966) is to make the experimental task part of school work and elongate the experimental time to get cumulative effects.

The all-or-none issue of rote versus discovery learning is essentially dead and needs to be replaced with questions such as what kind and how much guidance is best under what circumstances? A continuum of guidance specified by the subject matter, the objectives, and learner characteristics could be developed, starting out with the limited generalizations proposed by Cronbach (1966, p. 77):

With subject matter of this nature, inductive experience of this type, in this amount, produces this pattern of responses in pupils at this level of development.

A great deal of research still needs to be done on the learner variable—history, personality, and individual differences. These will interact differently with various teaching methods. A future goal would be to develop individual profiles to indicate the kind of experience each child needs.

Another important research need is to determine the effects of group problem solving using a discovery method on individuals in the group. For example, are there differences in transfer between the passive and active participants in the discussion?

Specific researchable questions

1. What is the effect of past experience of the learner—past exposure to discovery learning versus traditional expository teaching—on the learning and motivation of the student?
   a. Independent variable: past experience of the student—exposure to discovery learning versus expository teaching
   b. Dependent variables: learning and motivation
2. What are the long-term (1 year after learning, 5 years after learning) effects of transfer and retention of concepts when student learning is facilitated by a teaching strategy designed to foster discovery of generalization, as opposed to when generalization is given by means of expository teaching?
   a. Independent variable: teaching strategy—discovery versus expository
   b. Dependent variables: transfer and retention of concepts after 1 year and 5 years

ADDITIONAL LEARNING EXPERIENCES—RECOMMENDED READING LIST

Bruner, J. S. The act of discovery. *Harvard Educational Review*, 1961, 31:21-32.

DeCecco, J., and Crawford, W. *The psychology of learning and instruction: educational psychology.* (2nd Ed.) Englewood Cliffs, N.J.: Prentice-Hall, Inc., 1974, pp. 353-366.

Shulman, L. S., and Keislar, E. R. (Eds.) *Learning by discovery: a critical appraisal.* Chicago: Rand McNally & Co., 1966.

Wittrock, M. C. The learning by discovery hypothesis. In. L. S. Shulman and E. R. Keislar (Eds.), *Learning by discovery: a critical appraisal.* Chicago: Rand McNally & Co., 1966, pp. 33-76.

INSTRUCTIONS TO THE LEARNER REGARDING POSTTEST

You are now ready to take the posttest to determine the extent to which you have achieved the module objectives. Return to the pretest of this module and take it over again as the posttest. Correct your answers using the answer key found on this page. You need to score 25 correct points to qualify for 95% mastery level. If your score is less than this, correct your errors, study the content of this module over again, and read some of the articles found in the recommended reading list. Take the posttest again. You need to study in this fashion until you achieve the 95% mastery level before moving on to the next module.

ANSWER KEY TO PRETEST AND POSTTEST

1. d (Wittrock, 1966, pp. 45-71)
2. c (Wittrock, 1966, p. 33; Bruner, 1961, p. 23)
3. a (Glaser, 1966, p. 15)
4. c (Glaser, 1966, p. 15)
5. c (DeCecco and Crawford, 1974, pp. 356-360)
6. c (Bruner, 1961, pp. 23-24)
7. b, d, and e (Kagan, 1966, pp. 151-161; Wittrock, 1966, p. 36)
8. c, d, and e (Gagne, 1966, pp. 136-150)
9. c (DeCecco and Crawford, 1974, p. 355)
10. b (DeCecco and Crawford, 1974, p. 355)
11. d (Glaser, 1966, p. 15)
12. a (Wittrock, 1963, pp. 42-43)
13. e (Bruner, 1961, p. 29)
14. a. Amount of guidance varies
    b. Errorful learning
    c. Inductive and deductive approach is utilized
    (Kersh and Wittrock, 1962, pp. 282-292; Glaser, 1966, pp. 14-22; Wittrock, 1966, p. 73)
15. a. It is time consuming
    b. It employs errorful learning
    c. Many students do not have the initial motivation to exert the necessary effort required to make inferences
    d. Impulsive students make more errors of inductive reasoning

(Kagan, 1966, pp. 151-161; Wittrock, 1966, pp. 36-37; DeCecco and Crawford, 1974, pp. 360-362)
16. a. Discovery as a way to learn subject matter versus as an end in its own right
    b. The issue of what is to be discovered—a rule, a generalization, or more specific information
    c. The issue of induction versus deduction
    d. The issue of depreciation of verbal learning
    e. The issue of control of rate and sequence of stimuli
    f. The issue of variety of dependent variables
    (Wittrock, 1966, pp. 42-43)
17. The answer should include the following points:
    a. The instructional objectives
    b. The entering behaviors of the student
    c. How to assess entering behavior and objectives
    d. Reasons for selecting discovery strategy
    e. Application of Bruner's six-point strategy in aiding the student to discover
    (DeCecco and Crawford, 1974, p. 362; Bruner, 1966, pp. 101-113; Text, pp. 257)

REFERENCES

Anderson, J. L. Quantitative thinking as developed under connectionist and field theories of learning. In E. J. Swenson, and others. *Learning theory in school situations.* Minneapolis: University of Minnesota Press, 1949, 40-73.
Ausubel, D. P. Learning by discovery: rationale and mystique. *Bulletin of the National Association of Secondary School Principals,* 1961, **45**:18-58.
Ausubel, D. P. *The psychology of meaningful verbal learning.* New York: Grune and Stratton, Inc., 1963.
Bruner, J. S. The act of discovery. *Harvard Educational Review,* 1961, **31**:21-32.
Bruner, J. S. Some elements of discovery. In L. S. Shulman and E. R. Keislar (Eds.), *Learning by discovery: a critical appraisal.* Chicago: Rand McNally & Co., 1966, pp. 101-114.
Bruner, J. S., Goodnow, J. J., and Austin, G. A. *A study of thinking.* New York: John Wiley & Sons, Inc., 1956.
Corman, B. R. The effect of varying amounts and kinds of information as guidance in problem solving. *Psychological Monographs,* 1957, **71**(2):(whole no. 431, pp. 59-61, 85, 88).
Craig, R. C. Directed versus independent discovery of

established relations. *Journal of Educational Psychology*, 1956, **57**:223-234.

Cronbach, L. L. The logic of experiments on discovery. In L. S. Shulman and E. R. Keislar (Eds.), *Learning by discovery: a critical appraisal*. Chicago: Rand McNally & Co., 1966, pp. 76-92.

DeCecco, J., and Crawford, W. *The psychology of learning and instruction: educational psychology*. (2nd Ed.) Englewood Cliffs, N.J.: Prentice-Hall, Inc., 1974.

de Tornyay, R. *Strategies for teaching nursing*. New York: John Wiley & Sons, Inc., 1971.

Dewey, J. *How we think*. Lexington, Mass. D. C. Heath & Co., 1910.

Gagne, R. Varieties of learning and the concept of discovery. In L. S. Shulman and E. R. Keislar (Eds.), *Learning by discovery: a critical appraisal*. Chicago: Rand McNally & Co., 1966, pp. 135-150.

Gagne, R. *The conditions of learning*. (2nd Ed.) New York: Holt, Rinehart and Winston, Inc., 1970.

Gagne, R., and Brown, L. T. Some factors in the programming of conceptual learning. *Journal of Experimental Psychology*, 1961, **62**:313-321.

Glaser, R. Variables in discovery learning. In L. S. Shulman and E. R. Keislar (Eds.), *Learning by discovery: a critical appraisal*. Chicago: Rand McNally & Co., 1966, pp. 13-26.

Haslerud, G. M., and Meyers, S. The transfer value of given and individually deprived principles. *Journal of Educational Psychology*. 1958, **49**:293-298.

Hawkins, D. Learning the unteachable. In L. S. Shulman & E. R. Keislar (Eds.), *Learning by discovery: a critical appraisal*. Chicago: Rand McNally & Co., 1966, pp. 3-12.

Hilgard, E. R., Irvine, R. P., and Whipple, J. E. Rote memorization, understanding and transfer: an extension of Katona's card trick experiments. *Journal of Experimental Psychology*, 1953, **46**:288-292.

Kagan, J. Learning, attention and the issue of discovery. In L. S. Shulman and E. R. Keislar (Eds.), *Learning by discovery: a critical appraisal*. Chicago: Rand McNally & Co., 1966, pp. 151-161.

Katona, G. *Organizing and memorizing*. New York: Columbia University Press, 1940.

Kersh, B. Y. The adequacy of "meaning" as an explanation for superiority of learning by independent discovery. *Journal of Educational Psychology*, 1958, **49**:282-292.

Kersh, B. Y., and Wittrock, M. C. Learning by discovery: an interpretation of recent research. *Journal of Teacher Education*, 1962, **13**:461-468.

McConnell, T. R. Discovery vs. authoritative identification in the learning of children. *Studies in Education*, 1934, **9**(5):13-60, 81-82, 86, 89, 145.

Montessori, M. *The Montessori method*. New York: Frederick A. Stokes Co., 1912.

Montessori, M. *The advanced Montessori method: spontaneous activity in education*. New York: Frederick A. Stokes Co., 1917.

Wittrock, M. C. Effect of certain sets upon complex verbal learning. *Journal of Educational Psychology*, 1963, **54**:85-88.

Wittrock, M. C. The learning by discovery hypothesis. In L. S. Shulman and E. R. Keislar (Eds.), *Learning by discovery: a critical appraisal*. Chicago: Rand McNally & Co., 1966, pp. 33-76.

MODULE 16

Bruner's model of instruction

DESCRIPTION OF MODULE

This independent unit of instruction describes Bruner's model of instruction and how it applies to actual patient- and student-teaching situations. Prerequisite entering behavior necessary to study this module is knowledge of all the conditions of learning. The text of this module presents five major areas in an integrated form. These five areas are: (1) theoretical framework, (2) relevant research studies, (3) application to nursing education and practice, (4) issues, and (5) researchable questions. The module also contains student objectives with instructions to the learner, a pretest and posttest, an answer key, and other learning experiences.

MODULE OBJECTIVES

At the completion of this module, having studied the content presented in this module and in the recommended reading list, the student will be able to accomplish the following set of objectives at the 95% level of mastery. At the completion of the module the learner will be able to:

1. Explain Bruner's model of instruction
2. Identify the basic components of the model and give examples of each
3. Cite research studies that support the different aspects of the model
4. Identify and discuss the issues inherent in Bruner's model
5. Apply each aspect of Bruner's model of instruction in teaching a specific task or concept to either a patient or a nursing student

PRETEST AND POSTTEST

Circle the correct answers. Each question is worth 1 point except the last question, which is worth 10 points. The 95% level of mastery for this test equals 32 correct points. Take the test and correct it yourself using the answer key found at the end of this module (p. 261).

Multiple choice

1. According to Bruner, a theory of instruction:
   a. must be specific
   b. must describe learning
   c. is perscriptive and normative
   d. is the same as theories of learning and development
2. The characteristic listed below that is *not* a characteristic of a theory of instruction is:
   a. a set of rules for the most effective way of achieving knowledge or skill
   b. a standard for criticizing or evaluating teaching or learning
   c. a set of criteria and conditions for meeting them
   d. a set of rules for the most efficient way of learning in a defined content area
3. For Bruner, the concept of "readiness" for learning:
   a. does not apply since he believes anyone can be taught anything

b. is a developmental stage

c. is taught for and opportunities are provided for its acquisition and growth

d. is a basic activity that must be present before something can be taught

4. For Bruner, mastery of a skill or learning task is:

a. the highest goal for teachers

b. self-rewarding

c. the basis for his model of instruction

d. a secondary means of reinforcement

5. The aspects of exploration of alternatives, according to Bruner are:

a. activation, motivation, and direction

b. activation, motivation, and freedom to explore

c. freedom to explore, maintenance, and direction

d. activation, maintenance, and direction

6. Mode of representation, economy, and effective power are three characteristics of which basic component of Bruner's model?

a. predisposition

b. structure

c. sequence

d. reinforcement

7. Activation of the exploratory behavior necessary for learning is dependent on:

a. high anxiety levels

b. a state of confusion regarding the subject

c. routinization of the knowledge or skill

d. an optimal level of uncertainty

8. Direction of exploration is dependent on:

a. random alternative testing

b. a sense of the goal of a task

c. rewards and punishment

d. insightful, spontaneous learning

9. In order to maintain the exploration for alternatives:

a. the benefits of the exploration must exceed the risks of learning

b. consequences of error should be kept great

c. anxiety must remain high

d. curiosity should be maintained

10. Research on instruction and learning according to Bruner:

a. should be concerned with the application of developmental theory to learning

b. has led to most of the major changes in teaching methods

c. should focus on how to arrange environments for optimal learning according to various criteria

d. is best carried out by educational psychologists in arranged environments

11. The major features of Bruner's model of instruction are:

1—specification of the experiences that most effectively implant in the student a predisposition toward learning

2—specification of the structure and form of knowledge so that it can readily be grasped by the student

3—specifications of economy

4—specification of the most effective sequencing of material to be learned

5—specification of the effective power

6—specification of the nature and pacing of rewards and punishment

a. all of the above

b. 1, 2, and 3

c. 1, 3, and 5

d. 1, 2, 4, and 6

12. A nursing instructor teaching pharmacology made a study of the nursing class and discovered that most of the students could not work out simple fractions. She was faced with a problem of:

a. readiness

b. maturation

c. lack of attentional set

d. unmotivated students

13. Mary, a senior nursing student, needed to give 40 units of regular insulin to a patient. She called her instructor in a fit of despair stating that she could not possibly give the insulin because the only syringes on the unit were 3-ml syringes and TB syringes. This is an example of:

a. lack of problem-solving ability

b. lack of ability for transposition

c. functional fixedness

d. lack of subordinate learning set

Matching

In the following questions you are asked to differentiate between the three types of presentations that the teacher uses in teaching strategy. Match the example in part A with the type of presentation from part B by placing an a, b, or c in the blanks.

Part A

_____14. Demonstrating how a patient can give a self-injection of insulin

_____15. Using diagrams to teach how to properly locate various injection sites

_____16. Using a patient dummy to practice making an occupied bed

_____17. Using words to describe the procedure of rotating tourniquets

_____18. Using photographs and diagrams to show how blood returning to the heart (volume of blood) is decreased by the rotating-tourniquets technique

_____19. Demonstrating how to apply the tourniquets to the extremities

_____20. Giving a lecture in which the principles for taking vital signs are given

_____21. Teaching the nurse-practitioner's role through role models

_____22. Having students write on proper body mechanics to be used for transferring patients from bed to chair

_____23. Showing a film on how to do physical assessment of a patient

_____24. Conducting a class discussion on the proper techniques for interviewing patients

Part B

a. Enactive
b. Ikonic
c. Symbolic

Discussion question

25. As a nurse on a surgical unit, you are assigned the task of planning for preoperative teaching of patients of your choice. Using Bruner's model of instruction, how would you plan this teaching. Include dependent and independent variables to be considered.

TEXT
Theoretical framework
Introduction

In describing a theory of instruction and in comparing it to a theory of learning and a theory of development, Bruner (1964) identified two differentiating characteristics of the nature of a theory of instruction. First, a theory of instruction is *prescriptive* because it provides guidelines and rules to enable an individual to acquire knowledge and skills in the most effective way. It also provides a measuring device, or yardstick, to evaluate and criticize any method of teaching or learning. In contrast to this, theories of learning and development are descriptive. That is, they tell what is occurring at a stage or time, but not how to create the change that is wanted. The prescriptive nature of a theory of instruction prescribes "how best to learn what one wishes to teach, with improving, rather than describing, learning" (p. 307).

The second characteristic of a theory of instruction is its *normative* nature. In other words, it sets up a criteria and indicates the conditions for meeting them. By this, Bruner means that general criteria are set up for efficient learning. These criteria, Bruner states, must have a high degree of generality. There is emphasis on the word general. This is because the theory should cover all types of instruction at all levels rather than specific areas, such as the teaching of specific nursing assessment for junior baccalaureate students. The specifics can be derived from the general once the general concepts are understood and stated. A more general concept would be how to bring about learning of the nursing process that would include nursing assessment to all levels of nursing students.

Components of Bruner's model of instruction

The four major features of a theory of instruction are:

1. *Predisposition toward learning.* A theory of instruction must specifically state the conditions and the learning experiences that in the most effective way implant in the learner the desire, willingness, or predisposition toward learning.

2. *Structure of knowledge.* A theory of instruction must indicate specifically how best to structure the body of knowledge so that it can be easily grasped and understood by the learner. It is here that the student's entering behavior (ability and knowledge base) is taken into consideration. Bruner (1964, pp. 307-308) stated, "the goodness of a structure depends on its power for simplifying information, for generating new propositions, and for increasing the manipulability of a body of knowledge, structure must always be related to the status and gifts of the learner."

3. *Sequencing of knowledge.* A theory of instruction must specifically indicate the best and the most effective way of ordering, or sequencing, and presenting a body of knowledge so that it can be learned by the student.

4. *Nature and pacing of rewards and punishments.* A theory of instruction must indicate specifically the nature and pacing of positive and negative reinforcements and punishments in the process of learning and teaching. Bruner (1964) pointed out that extrinsic reinforcement, such as praise from the teacher, should be replaced eventually with intrinsic reinforcement, which is inherent in actual learning. It is also important for immediate reward for performance to be replaced by differed reward.

Each of these four major features of Bruner's model are discussed separately in greater detail and are applied to the teaching of nursing.

PREDISPOSITION TOWARD LEARNING

Traditionally, predisposition to learning has been looked at from cultural, motivational, personal, and environmental points of view as they affect an individual's willingness to learn and desire for problem solving. Bruner (1964) noted that even though these variables are important, his model of instruction pays more attention to predisposition for

searching behavior, that is, exploration of alternatives. It deals more on the cognitive level.

Exploration of alternatives is essential if learning and problem-solving behavior are to occur. It is affected by cultural and motivational factors. The task of instruction is to facilitate and guide this exploratory behavior of the learner. The mechanisms that initiate, maintain, and guide the exploratory behavior are *activation*, *maintenance*, and *direction*. In other words, the teacher must enable the learner to begin the exploration, then use methods to keep the learner seeking alternatives, and guide the learner against going haphazardly and on the wrong paths in this seeking.

Activation. Activation refers to the initiation phase of the exploratory behavior. The role of instruction is to get the learner started in exploring alternatives. Bruner pointed out that an optimum level of uncertainty creates curiosity in the learner and is an essential condition for initiating, or activating, exploration of alternatives in problem solving. Berlyne (1960) supported Bruner's notion that curiosity is a response to uncertainty and ambiguity. Let us take the example of a student nurse trying to find out (problem solve) why patients with breast cancer do not find the breast lump at an early stage and consult their physicians. Implicit in Bruner's model of instruction is the statement of the terminal behavior that the student is to perform. In this situation, the terminal behavior is for the student nurse to state by means of problem-solving techniques the reasons why a breast cancer patient delays finding out if there is a lump in her breast, and why such patients do not consult their physicians at an earlier stage.

The role of instruction (teacher) is to get the student nurse (learner) started, or activated, in an exploratory behavior. Since an optimal level of uncertainty and ambiguity creates curiosity in the learner, which in turn prompts the learner to explore alternatives, the teacher, therefore, has to create this optimal level of curiosity (a desire to know) in the student. The teacher can instill this type of behavior in the student by asking such questions as: What would have happened if the lump in Mrs. X's breast had been discovered 2 years ago while it was only 1 cm in diameter? How much difference would it have made in her life span? In what ways can the public health nurse change the statistics on "the size of lump" first discovered in patients and the cure rate in patients where the lump is discovered early? Why do patients fear to consult their physicians? What type of taboos are associated with the role of the breast in women? These types of questions and many others help to create curiosity in the student nurse. There are other methods of motivating the student to get started in exploring behavior. Some of these methods may be more anxiety producing and some frustrating. For example, lack of structure or lack of information given to the student to start investigating this problem may cause a certain amount of anxiety and frustration. The optimal amount of anxiety and frustration is good, and it is conducive to initiation of exploratory behavior in the student; however, strong anxiety or drive inhibits the problem solver in using the information correctly. The studies of Postman and Bruner (1948); Easterbrook (1950); Bahrick, Fitts, and Rankin (1952); and Longnecker (1962) supported this finding.

Maintenance. The second aspect of the behavior of searching for alternatives is maintenance of exploration. Once the teacher has helped the student begin, then the responsibility shifts to keeping the learner going. This is accomplished by having the benefits from exploring alternatives exceed the risks. Bruner (1964) pointed out that if instruction is effective, learning a task or solving a problem with the aid of the teacher should be less risky, and the consequences of an error should be less grave. Consequently, the yield from exploration of correct alternatives should be greater than if the student had learned it independently.

In the previous example, the teacher can maintain the student's exploratory behavior by utilizing intermittent schedules of positive reinforcement in the form of praise, or knowledge of results that what the student is doing is correct, and any other secondary positive reinforcements. Also, as the student investigates the problem area (whether at the stage of doing literature research as to why breast cancer patients avoid fear-producing subjects or at the stage of testing the hypothesis), cues from the teacher or the subjects that the selected alternatives are correct, or are in the right direction, act as reinforcement and maintain exploratory behavior.

Direction. Direction of exploration constitutes the third aspect of exploratory behavior. Bruner (1964, p. 309) cited two important factors that affect the direction of exploration: one is the "sense of the goal of the task," and the second is the "knowledge of the relevance of the tested alternatives to the achievement of that goal." When this principle is applied to the example, the teacher's task becomes one of directing the student's exploratory behavior while maintaining learning activity. The goal that is sought must be clearly stated. The student must recognize when the alternatives that are being tested are going to lead to the goal and when they are not.

STRUCTURE OF KNOWLEDGE

One of Bruner's (1961, p. 33) most widely quoted statements holds the key to his philosophy on structuring of information. He stated:

We begin with the hypothesis that any subject can be taught effectively in some intellectually honest form to any child at any stage of development. It is a bold hypothesis and an essential one in thinking about the nature of the curriculum. No evidence exists to contradict it; considerable evidence is being amassed to support it.

This would seem to be contrary to Piaget's (1952) age-bounded notion of "state of readiness." Bruner, however, believes that readiness consists of mastery of simpler skills that will enable one to reach higher skills. Therefore, while it may be difficult for a student to grasp a concept, the teacher has to prepare the student for it by teaching ideas that prepare the student to grasp it. Also, the teacher must provide opportunities for the student to develop the skill.

According to Bruner (1964), the structure of any area of knowledge is characterized in three ways: (1) the mode of representation, (2) its economy, (3) its effective power. Each of these ways influences the learner's ability to master the area. These three characteristics vary in appropriateness to different ages, to different learner styles, and to different content areas.

Mode of representation. Any concept, problem area, or domain of knowledge can be presented in three ways:

1. By *enactive representation*, which is a set of actions that will achieve the result. An example of this would be demonstration and practice of a skill. In the previous problem-solving example, enactive representation would be when the learner actually demonstrates by actions the method of collecting data, testing the hypothesis, and so on to demonstrate the carrying out of certain aspects of the research project.

2. By *ikonic representation*, which is the use of summary images or graphics that stand for a concept but do not fully define it. Pictures, diagrams, illustrations, and graphs that represent a concept or a topic are examples of ikonic representation. In the example, if the student nurse places the results of the study on a chart or a graph that indicates a trend, this would be an example of ikonic representation.

3. By *symbolic representation*, which is a "set of symbolic or logical propositions drawn from a symbolic system that is governed by rules or laws for forming and transforming propositions" (Bruner, 1964, p. 310). Formulation of hypotheses, presentation of concepts in the form of a formula, and the use of words are all examples of symbolic representation.

As mentioned previously, these can be used at any age but are most effective at certain ages or stages of comprehension. For example, the young child learns difficult things best by doing or by active manipulation of an object. As the child gets older, pictures can be used effectively. When the ability to grasp written or spoken symbols is present, this method alone may be used. Some tasks are very difficult for most people to learn just by symbolic representation. Knowledge of these three modes of representation should help the teacher in planning a strategy for teaching specific concepts.

Economy. Economy of representation is the second characteristic of the structure of knowledge. It refers to the amount of information a student must keep in mind and process in order to achieve the task and understand it. The larger the amount of information the person has to keep in mind in order to solve a problem or understand a concept, the less economical it is because the individual has to subject that much information to successive steps of processing in order to understand it. Bruner pointed out that economy varies with representation and is also a function of the sequence in which material is presented or the manner in which it is learned.

One of the functions of the teacher in presenting the structure of content more economically is to eliminate the tangential material that is distally related to the core concepts that are currently being taught, in order not to confuse the student and overload the processing of information. Another method of structuring a content area in more economical terms is to present the concepts in diagrammatical forms. For example, the nursing student who is trying to design a study to investigate and identify the reasons why breast cancer patients do not discover lumps at an early stage and why they do not consult their physicians immediately would find it very difficult to keep these many concepts in mind and to process them simultaneously. One way of making this structure more economical is by having the design of the study presented diagrammatically; for example, how many groups of subjects is the student planning on investigating, what are the dependent and independent variables, and what are the predictions.

Yet another method of structuring the content area of this study to be more economical is to list the key concepts of the study—anxiety, cancer, fear of death, coping mechanisms, and others—and to use arrows to indicate relationships between these concepts in diagrammatical form as illustrated below.

Stimulus →	Reaction →	Coping mechanism
Cancer (?) (lump in breast)	↑ Fear of death ↑ Anxiety	Avoidance behavior Will not consult physician Will ignore lump Confronting (approach) behavior Will consult physician Will check lump frequently

There are of course many other ways that such a complex set of concepts can be structured in economical terms.

Effective power. The third characteristic of structure is its effective power. This refers to "the generative value of a set of learned propositions" (Bruner, 1964, p. 321). Power

of a representation is also described as its "capacity, in the hands of a learner, to connect matters that, on the surface, seem quite separate" (Bruner, 1964, p. 313). The teacher has to structure the information so the student can see relationships between material. This may be hard to do in things that have seemingly obscure relationships. But to be effective, the teacher must do this for the student if the student cannot do it alone. The structure should account for how it will be done. One method of doing this in the above example is by the use of a diagram that shows the relationships between the concepts. It may also generate other types of relationships and new hypotheses.

SEQUENCING OF KNOWLEDGE

Sequencing, the third major component of Bruner's model deals with the order in which material is presented. "Instruction consists of leading the learner through a sequence of statements and restatements of a problem or body of knowledge that increase the learner's ability to grasp, transform, and transfer what he is learning" (Bruner, 1964, p. 313). Sequencing of content matter determines the extent to which the learner will have difficulty mastering the subject matter. There is no unique sequence for all learners. Optimal sequencing depends on the learner's past learning experiences, the learner's stage of development, the complexity and nature of the material, and individual differences.

Bruner indicated that intellectual development progresses from enactive to ikonic to symbolic representation. He suggested that it is probable that optimal sequencing should progress in the same order. An important concept to keep in mind is the need to program, or sequence, the structure of material from the simplest to the most complex. Sequencing must also take into consideration the limited capability of the learner to process the material or the information.

In the example, proper sequencing of the knowledge base is necessary to conduct a study of such a nature. It consists of (1) finding out if the student nurse has basic knowledge about the important concepts, such as cancer, fear, anxiety, coping mechanisms, and others; (2) finding out if the student has basic knowledge about the process of problem solving (scientific method); and (3) learning concepts, then learning the relationships between the concepts. The teacher should sequence the content matter in a hierarchical form, so lower-order skills in the hierarchy (subordinate knowledge base or tasks) are mastered before moving to higher-order tasks. This concept of the hierarchy of learning has been explicitly explained by Gagne (1970).

Bruner also commented that optimal sequencing cannot be specified independently of the criterion by which final learning is evaluated. The classification of criteria, according to Bruner (1964, p. 314), is as follows:

1. Speed of learning
2. Resistance to forgetting
3. Transferability of what has been learned to new situations
4. Form in which presentation of what has been learned is to be expressed
5. Economy of what has been learned in terms of cognitive strain
6. Effective power of what has been learned in terms of its generativeness for new hypotheses

THE NATURE AND PACING OF REINFORCEMENTS

Bruner stated that learning depends on knowledge of results, which is a form of reinforcement, when it is given at a time when and at place where the learner can use this knowledge for corrective purposes. The role of instruction is to increase the appropriateness of timing and placing of corrective information.

According to Bruner, the effectiveness of knowledge of results is dependent on:

1. When and where the learner will be able to put the corrective information to work
2. The conditions under which corrective information can be used by the learner
3. The form in which corrective information is received by the learner

Appropriate timing of knowledge of results in a problem-solving situation should come when the learner is comparing own results with the criterion of what is to be achieved. Bruner thinks that knowledge of results given before this point cannot be understood by the learner. However, if knowledge of results is given after this point, it may be too late to guide the learner in making a new hypothesis. He therefore asserted that knowledge of results, in order to be useful, must provide information not only about whether a particular act produced success, but also whether the act is in fact leading one through the hierarchy of goals one is seeking to achieve (Bruner, 1964, p. 316).

Instruction, therefore, should provide learners with information about the higher-order relevance of their efforts. In time, Bruner stated, learners must develop their own techniques of obtaining corrective information because instruction will eventually come to an end.

Bruner also believes that as individuals learn, they will get more rewards from within and need fewer from outside. The shift from external to internal rewards occurs as students find learning itself rewarding. Bruner (1966) discounted Thorndike's "law of effect" as not being of any long-term importance in learning (pp. 157-158). This is because while it may help learning to begin or actions to be repeated as rewards are given, it is not in the long run necessary to satisfy individuals from without to get them to learn. To really be effective, students must learn because there is inner satisfaction, desire, and curiosity. This is what Bruner (1966, p. 133) said differentiates humans from other beings. Humans, said have an "almost involuntary . . . will to learn." The teacher must, after activating the learner, lead the student to getting satisfaction from within rather than without. Also the teacher must help the student delay reward. Knowledge of the results of learning must be given to the student. Its effectiveness, however, depends on its timing. It must not come before it will be of benefit or be understood or after it is useful.

One state in which corrective information is least useful is when the person is very anxious and is impelled by strong drive. The studies of Postman and Bruner (1948), Easterbrook (1950), and Longnecker (1962) support this statement.

Another such state is "functional fixedness." It refers to the situation when the student can only see one way of solving a problem, only one way of using available information or material. The studies of Maier (1930), Luchins (1942) and Dunker (1945) all point to the fact that during such a period there is significant intractability or incorrigibility to problem solving. It has also empirically been shown that high drive and anxiety lead the organism to be more prone to functional fixedness (Bruner, Matter, Papanek, 1955; Bruner, and others, 1958).

The form and pacing of reward in the nursing example can be given to the student nurse in the form of knowledge of results when the results obtained are compared to the hypothesis made. This type of knowledge of results at this stage of investigation can be self-initiated. Knowledge of results provided by the teacher would be of specific importance in terms of timing when the student has designed the study and before implementing it, so that in case there are errors, corrective actions can be taken prior to its implementation. The student may seek from the teacher cues acknowledging the correct proceeding of the study while it is being planned (such as while the proposal is being written, the problem area is being established by means of literature review, and the scientific argument for the existence of the problem is being developed). The teacher's corrective feedback to the student at this stage is of great importance.

Once the process of conducting a scientific research study (problem solving) has been learned, the student will be able to provide her own corrective feedback. The shift from an external reward system to an internal reward system will occur.

• • •

In summary, therefore, Bruner's model has four basic components. These are: (1) specification of the experiences that most predispose a person to learn, including the concepts of activation, maintenance, and direction; (2) specification of how the knowledge that is to be presented can be structured so that it is more readily grasped, including the modes of representation (enactive, ikonic, or symbolic), economy, and effective power of the body of knowledge; (3) specification of the sequence in which the material that is to be taught should be presented; and (4) specification of the type of rewards and punishment that are to be used and how they will be paced.

Issues in Bruner's model

Issues regarding Bruner's model are basically centered around the concept of readiness, or rather the lack of it as being necessary for learning. Bruner's concept of readiness is different from the generally accepted ideas of Piaget (1952) and Gagne (1970). There is much disagreement as to how far Bruner can support the concept of teaching almost anything to just about everyone.

There is little evidence to support Bruner's concepts as being applicable to the philosophy of education currently held in the United States. That idea is that education should be available to the masses. His ideas and concepts may lend themselves more to limited educational settings. This is at issue.

Bruner's concept of rewards is also open to question. Can rewards for learning really be shifted to intrinsic sources, especially in initiating a new behavior, or is this rather an unrealistic idea.

Researchable questions

1. What is the effect of the use of different models of instruction (Bruner's model versus mastery model) on the type of reinforcements (intrinsic versus extrinsic) used by the learner?

  a. Independent variable: the use of different models of instruction (Bruner's versus mastery)

  b. Dependent variable: the type of reinforcements sought by the learners (extrinsic versus instrinsic)

2. What is the effect of different modes of representation on the speed of learning and retention of material learned?

  a. Independent variable: different modes of representation (enactive, ikonic, and symbolic)

  b. Dependent variables: speed of learning and retention of material learned

ADDITIONAL LEARNING EXPERIENCES—RECOMMENDED READING LIST

Bruner, J. S. Some theorems on instruction illustrated with reference to mathematics. In E. R. Hilgard, (Ed.), *Theories of Learning and Instruction*, The 63rd Yearbook of NSSE, Part 1. Chicago: The University of Chicago Press, 1964, pp. 306-335.

Bruner, J. S. *Toward a theory of instruction.* Cambridge, Mass.: Harvard University Press, 1966.

INSTRUCTIONS TO THE LEARNER REGARDING POSTTEST

Now you are ready to take the posttest to determine the extent to which you have achieved this module's objectives. Return to the pretest of this module and take it over again as the posttest. Correct your answers using the answer key found on this page. You need to achieve 32 correct points to qualify for 95% mastery level. If your score is less than this, correct your errors, study the content of this module again, and read the articles in the recommended reading list. Take the posttest again and try to achieve a score of 32 correct points or better. You need to study in this fashion until you obtain the 95% mastery level or better.

ANSWER KEY TO PRETEST AND POSTTEST

  1. c (Bruner, 1966, p. 40)
  2. d (Bruner, 1966, p. 40)
  3. c (Bruner, 1966, p. 29)
  4. b (Bruner, 1966, p. 114)
  5. d (Bruner, 1966, p. 43)
  6. b (Bruner, 1966, p. 44)
  7. d (Bruner, 1966, p. 43)
  8. b (Bruner, 1966, p. 44)
  9. a (Bruner, 1966, pp. 43-44)
10. c (Bruner, 1964, pp. 306-335)
11. d (Bruner, 1964, pp. 307-308)
12. a (DeCecco, 1968, p. 61; Bruner, 1961, p. 33; Bruner, 1964, pp. 307, 309-313)
13. c (Bruner, 1966, p. 52; Bruner, 1964, p. 317)
14. a (Bruner, 1964, p. 310)
15. b (Bruner, 1964, p. 310)
16. a (Bruner, 1964, p. 310)
17. c (Bruner, 1964, p. 310)
18. b (Bruner, 1964, p. 310)
19. a (Bruner, 1964, p. 310)
20. c (Bruner, 1964, p. 310)
21. a (Bruner, 1964, p. 310)
22. c (Bruner, 1964, p. 310)
23. b (Bruner, 1964, p. 310)
24. c (Bruner, 1964, p. 310)
25. An answer for question 25 at the level of mastery will include discussion of all four of the major components of the model and how they relate to this problem. Inclusion of elements within the major components will be determined as greater than an 95% level of learning. The answers will vary but should have the following framework:

  a. Specify the experiences that most effectively predispose the patient to learning of this type and how these predispositions can be arranged for effective teaching; mention how it will be activated and when, plans for maintenance, the direction of the teaching, and the variables to learning

b. Tell how the information will be structured, including the mode of presentation to be used, why it was chosen, how it relates to economy, and its effective power

c. Include the sequence in which the material will be arranged

d. Include discussion of the type of reinforcement to be used and the frequency with which it will be given

(Bruner, 1964, pp. 306-335)

REFERENCES

Bahrick, H. P., Fitts, P. M., and Rankin, R. E., Effect of incentives upon reactions to peripheral stimuli. *Journal of Experimental Psychology*, 1952, 44:400-403.

Berlyne, D. E. *Conflict, arousal and curiosity.* New York: McGraw-Hill Book Co., 1960.

Bruner, J. S. *The process of education.* Cambridge, Mass.: Harvard University Press, 1961.

Bruner, J. S. Some theorems on instruction illustrated with reference to mathematics. In E. R. Hilgard (Ed.), *Theories of Learning and Instruction*, The 63rd Yearbook of NSSE, Part 1. Chicago: The University of Chicago Press, 1964, pp. 306-335.

Bruner, J. S. *Toward a theory of instruction.* Cambridge, Mass.: Harvard University Press, 1966.

Bruner, J. S., Mandler, J. M., O'Dowd, D., and Wallack, M. A. The role of overlearning and drive level in reversal learning. *Journal of Comparative and Physiological Psychology*, 1958, 51:607-613.

Bruner, J. S., Matter, J., and Papanek, M. L. Breadth of learning as a function of drive level and mechanization. *Psychological Review*, 1955, 62:1-10.

DeCecco, J. *The psychology of learning and instruction: educational psychology.* (1st Ed.) Englewood Cliffs, N.J.: Prentice-Hall, Inc., 1968.

Duncker, K. On problem-solving. *Psychological Monographs*, 1945, 58(5):1-111 (whole no. 270).

Easterbrook, J. A. The effect of emotion on cue utilization and the organization of behavior. *Psychological Review*, 1950, 56:183-201.

Gagne, *The conditions of learning.* (2nd Ed.) New York: Holt, Rinehart and Winston, Inc. 1970.

Longnecker, E. D. Perceptual recognition and anxiety. *Journal of Abnormal and Social Psychology*, 1962, 64:215-221.

Luchins, A. S. Mechanization in problem-solving—the effect of Einstellung. *Psychological Monographs*, 1942, 54(6):(whole no. 248).

Maier, N. R. F. Reasoning in humans. I. On direction. *Journal of Comparative Psychology*, 1930, 10:115-143.

Piaget, J. *The child's conception of number.* New York: Humanities Press, 1952.

Postman, L., and Bruner, J. S. Perception under stress. *Psychological Review*, 1948, 55:314-323.

PART THREE

Transfer of learning and behavior modification techniques

MODULE 17

Transfer of learning

DESCRIPTION OF MODULE

This is a self-contained unit of instruction on transfer of learning. The content is presented in sequential order. The module contains instructions to the learner, specific objectives that need to be accomplished, a pretest to measure the student's entering behavior, and a posttest to determine the extent to which the objectives were accomplished. The main text of the module is designed so that the learner attains the objectives. It covers five areas pertinent to transfer of learning that are presented in an integrated form. These are: (1) theoretical framework, (2) relevant research studies, (3) issues, (4) application to nursing education and practice, and (5) researchable questions.

MODULE OBJECTIVES

On completing this module on transfer of learning and having studied the content of this module and the recommended reading list, the student will be able to accomplish the objectives at the 95% level of accomplishment. The student will be able to:

1. Define operationally the term "transfer of learning" and be able to give examples of situations where positive, negative, and zero transfer occur
2. Describe the four main theories of transfer of learning and cite relevant research studies that support each theoretical framework

3. Identify four issues or problem areas pertinent to transfer of learning
4. Apply the principles of transfer of learning to nursing education and practice
5. Identify at least one researchable question and indicate the independent and dependent variables

PRETEST AND POSTTEST

Circle the correct answers. Each question is worth 1 point except the last question, which is worth 8 points. The 95% level of mastery for this test is 38 correct points. Correct your own test by using the answer key found at the end of this module (pp. 284-285).

Multiple choice

1. Susan, a nursing student in the operating room (O.R.), learned how to hand instruments to the physician with her right hand. Later in her O.R. experience, Susan also found herself able to hand the instruments to the physician with her opposite hand. This example best illustrates the principle of:
   a. early task learning
   b. bilateral transfer
   c. response similarity
2. Barbara Cook, a student nurse, has learned to open a variety of packages of sterile dressings in the nursing laboratory. While working on the nursing unit one day, Barbara's team leader asked her to bring a sterile Foley catheter and open it. Although Barbara has never opened this type of package before, she does

265

so without contaminating the catheter. This example best illustrates the transfer principle of:

  a. discrimination learning
  b. insightful learning
  c. positive transfer
  d. warm-up effect

3. Mrs. Katz likes to play word-association games with her nursing students to help them learn new medical terminology. She hopes that during these games intervening processes will serve to bridge the gap between the questions she poses and the final answers her students produce. In selecting this type of learning experience for her students, Mrs. Katz is basing her rationale on which of the following transfer principles?
  a. stimulus predifferentiation
  b. warm-up
  c. learning-to-learn
  d. mediated transfer

4. A student responding to a new discrimination based on relationships of stimuli is exhibiting:
  a. positive transfer
  b. stimulus predifferentiation
  c. learning set
  d. transposition

5. The factor that does *not* particularly influence transfer from one task to another is:
  a. the time elapsing between the original task and the transfer task
  b. the kind of mediating responses available to the learner
  c. the degree of similarity between the stimuli of each task

6. The primary internal condition for vertical transfer is:
  a. motivation
  b. verbal mediation
  c. mastery of subordinate capabilities
  d. practice with a variety of situations

7. A generalization that spreads over a broad set of situations at approximately the same level of complexity is called:
  a. vertical transfer
  b. lateral transfer
  c. learning
  d. stimulus generalization

8. Mary, a senior nursing student, needed to give 40 units of regular insulin to her patient. She called her instructor in a fit of despair stating that she could not possibly give the insulin because the only syringes on the unit were 3-ml syringes and tuberculin syringes. This is an examples of:
  a. lack of problem-solving ability
  b. lack of ability for transposition
  c. functional fixedness
  d. lack of subordinate learning set

9. Positive transfer can occur in paired-associate learning. It consists of which two distinct stages:
  a. transposition and stimulus discrimination
  b. response integration and associative hook-up
  c. associative cues and identifying responses

10. Which of the following factors influencing transfer, if used in instruction, can aid in the student's learning:
  1—providing adequate experience with the original task
  2—providing variety when teaching concepts and principles
  3—maximizing similarity between teaching and testing situations
  4—identifying or labeling important features of a task
  5—ensuring understanding of general principles before expecting much transfer
  a. all of the above
  b. 1, 2, and 4
  c. 3, 4, and 5
  d. 1, 3, 4, and 5

11. The greater the similarity of the stimuli:
  a. the greater the amount of negative transfer
  b. the closer it will come to zero amount of transfer
  c. the greater the amount of positive transfer
  d. similarity and transfer are not related

12. If a new response is expected from a stimulus similar to another stimulus that evoked an opposite response:
  a. a higher degree of positive transfer is expected
  b. a low degree of positive transfer is expected
  c. transfer does not operate in this case

13. An ophthalmic nurse shows the patient a videotype of how to self-administer eye drops. Providing a preliminary experience with the stimulus aspects of the task and identifying the important elements of the stimulus situation before having the patient actually try to self-administer the eye drops is called:
    a. warm-up
    b. learning to learn
    c. stimulus predifferentiation
    d. mediated transfer

Fill in the blanks

The following is a transfer design used by a nursing instructor to determine the type of transfer between tasks that might occur if the students learned task A (setting up enema equipment) before learning task B (setting up intravenous equipment).

The design:
Experimental group: Learns task A then learns task B
Control group: Learns task B only

Fill in the blanks with the terms (a) positive, (b) negative, or (c) zero as they apply to the examples.

14. If the nursing instructor found that the experimental group performed inferiorly to the control group on task B, then _____ transfer probably occurred.
15. If the experimental and control groups performed equally well, then _____ transfer probably occurred.
16. If the control group performed inferiorly to the experimental group, then _____ transfer probably occurred.
17. If the control group performed better than the experimental group, then _____ transfer probably occurred.

Mildred Horen, R.N., M.S.N., is a fundamentals instructor who uses the following scheme of selecting learning experiences for her students. In each of the examples, is Mildred correctly utilizing the available empirical knowledge about the transfer of learning? Answer *yes*, if she is correctly utilizing this knowledge, or *no*, if she is not utilizing this knowledge correctly.

_____18. Mildred tries to make the training tasks that students learn in the nursing laboratory as similar as possible to the tasks that they will be doing on the nursing unit.
_____19. When giving her students new tasks to learn, Mildred usually calls their attention to or helps them discover the principle involved.
_____20. Mildred gives her students mostly complex tasks to learn because she knows that transfer of learning will be greater than if she gave them only easy tasks to learn.
_____21. Mildred utilizes group learning experiences as much as possible for her students because transfer of problem-solving skills is promoted from the group experiences to individual situations.
_____22. During the original learning sessions, Mildred gives her students a variety of tasks to learn, knowing it should increase the amount of positive transfer.
_____23. Mildred always has her students learn a transfer task within 1 or 2 days of learning the original task, even when the transfer task does not require the student to remember specific aspects of the original task.
_____24. To maximize the amount of transfer of learning, Mildred makes her nursing students spend greater effort mastering the early series of related tasks.
_____25. Mildred is not worried when her students have only limited practice on an original task because she knows that any amount of practice (except zero practice) helps to prevent negative transfer.

Matching

Match the theories of transfer (part A) with the major concepts (part B) that describe them by placing the letters of the concepts in the blank before the appropriate theory.

Part A
_____26. Mediation
_____27. Stimulus predifferentiation

____28. Paired-associate learning

____29. Mathematical model

____30. Learning-set theory

____31. Transposition

____32. Gagne's theory of transfer

Part B

a. Has the advantage of increased ability to predict behavior accurately and more simply

b. May lead to greater flexibility in problem solving through practice with various tasks in which cue reversal occurs

c. Proposes that individuals improve their ability to learn new tasks when they have practiced a series of related or similar tasks

d. Intervening processes serve to bridge the gap between the question presented and the final answer produced

e. Responding to a new discrimination task on the basis of relationships among stimuli

f. Focuses the learner's attention on relevant cues

g. Has two distinct stages: the first being response integration

h. Using labels to make similar stimuli more distinctive

i. If a learner has passed or attained the higher-order learning set, then *all* related lower level learning sets must have been passed

Discussion question

33. List the four major issues or problems in the area of transfer today and pose one researchable question for each issue or problem as it might relate to nursing education or practice

Issues or problems   *Researchable questions*

a.

b.

c.

d.

TEXT
Theoretical framework
Introduction

Transfer of learning generally refers to the influence that past or present learning has on future learning. Wittrock (1968) takes the position that transfer of training is one of the most important products of education, and the identification of the conditions of transfer is as an essential area for basic research in school learning.

Transfer is considered to be one of the most important and common dependent variables of problem solving. Traditionally, the topic of problem solving has been treated separately from that of transfer (Duncan, 1959). A recent analysis, however, has shown that many studies of problem solving can, in fact, be treated as transfer (Schulz, 1960).

To reiterate further the importance of transfer, Deese (1958) stated that there may be no topic in the psychology of learning that is more important than the transfer of learning. Ellis (1965) contends that there is very little adult learning that is not affected by previous learning.

Certainly, many formal education and training programs are based on the assumption that what one learns in the training period will transfer to daily living situations. The purpose of this module, therefore, is to present the major concepts and principles related to the transfer of learning and to enable students to apply the principles and concepts of transfer of learning to nursing education and practice.

Definition, designs, and measurement of transfer
DEFINITION

Barbara Myers, R.N., recently graduated from nursing school and is now working on a medical-surgical unit in a small community hospital. Lately, Barbara has been performing dressing changes for one of her patients who has a severe leg ulcer. Although Barbara has never changed dressings on patients with leg ulcers before, she is able without difficulty to apply the principles of sterile technique that she learned in school to this new learning situation.

This example generally describes what is meant by the *transfer of learning*. What Barbara learned in school appears to have carried over into her new nursing-practice situation, even though her original learning tasks were different from her present ones.

Ellis (1965, p. 3) described the meaning of the transfer of learning in much this same way: "that experience or performance on one task influences performance on some subsequent task."

Operationally defined, transfer is said to have occurred when there is a reliable difference between the experimental and the control group's performance on task B in Fig. 17-1. The difference will be attributed to the effect of task A on the experimental group's performance on task B, assuming that the two groups have not been differentially treated in any relevant respect other than exposure versus nonexposure to task A. Positive transfer is demonstrated when the experimental group's performance is superior to that of the control group. Negative transfer is said to have occurred when the control group's performance is better than that of the experimental group. Zero transfer is said to have occurred when there is no difference in performance between the control and the experimental groups (Schulz, 1960).

For example, if one were to design a transfer experiment to measure the effect that learning task A (such as how to catheterize a female patient) has on learning task B (such as how to start an I.V.), using nursing students as subjects, the experiment might be diagrammed as shown in Fig. 17-1. The experimental group of nursing students would learn task A, while the control group rested or did some nonrelated task. After the experimental group learned task A, both groups would learn task B.

If the experimental group performed superiorly to the control group on task B, then *positive transfer* probably occurred. If the control group performed superiorly to the experimental group on task B, then *negative transfer* probably occurred. If both groups performed equally well on task B, then *zero transfer* probably occurred.

In the transfer design just mentioned, it must be noted, however, that at least two assumptions were made. First, it was assumed that the experimental and control groups of student nurses were equally intelligent. Second, as was mentioned earlier, the control group had to be resting or learning some unrelated task while the experimental group learned task A.

DESIGNS

There are several designs for transfer of learning, but only three commonly used designs are presented here. For detailed presentation of designs and formulas, the reader is referred to Ellis (1965, pp. 9-14).

The most common design of transfer is the one presented in Fig. 17-2. In this design, the experimental group learns the original task, task A, while the control group rests. Later, both groups learn task B, which is the transfer task. The differences between the two groups is commonly attributed to the effect of task A. However, Ellis (1965, p. 9) pointed out that this design suffers from a major weakness that one is not sure if the superior performance of the experimental group is entirely the result of the specific features of task A, the result of the more general effects of learning to learn and warm-up, or the summation of all three of these effects.

Group	Task A	Task B
Experimental	X	X
Control		X

Fig. 17-1. Operations for defining transfer (design 1).

Nursing students	Female catheterization	Starting I.V.
Experimental group	Learn task A	Then learn task B
Control group		Learn task B only

Fig. 17-2. Example of design 1.

Group	Learning	Transfer test
Experimental	Learn task A	Then learn task B₁
Control	Learn task A	Then learn task B

Fig. 17-3. Transfer design 2.

Group	Learning	Transfer test
Experimental	Learn task A	Then learn task B
Control	Learn task B	Then learn task A

Fig. 17-4. Transfer design 3.

To control for these differences, one can use another design in which both the experimental and the control groups learn task A first. The experimental group then learns task B_1, while the control group learns task B. One of the assumptions of this design is that B_1 and B are equivalent to each other. The difference between the experimental group and the control group on B tasks should be attributed to the differences in transfer caused by features of task A, and not to warm-up or learning-to-learn effects. This design can be illustrated diagramatically (Fig. 17-3).

The third design is useful when one wants to determine how transfer from task A to task B might differ from the transfer from task B to task A. In this design, the experimental group learns task A followed by task B. The control group learns task B first, followed by task A. Design 3 can be illustrated as:

One of the assumptions of this model is that practice effects from task A to task B are the same as from task B to task A. This type of design is useful in studies of intersensory transfer.

MEASUREMENT OF TRANSFER—TRANSFER FORMULAS

Formulas for computing percentages of transfer have been developed to enable educators, researchers, and practitioners to determine the effect (transfer effect) of one task on another and also, more specifically, to enable researchers to compare results across transfer studies, using different problems, task, and measures.

Three basic transfer formulas are presented. These formulas are similar in that they compare experimental and control groups on performance on the transfer test.

Ellis (1965, p. 12) pointed out that in order to use these formulas, some measure of transfer performance must be taken. These can be such measures as: "(1) the number of trials required to reach a given level of mastery; (2) the amount of time required to reach a given level of mastery; (3) the level of mastery reached after a given amount of time or number of trials, such as the number of correct responses; and (4) the number of errors made in reaching a given criterion of mastery."

Formula 1 compares the performance on the transfer task between the experimental and the control groups.

$$\text{Percentage of transfer} = \frac{E - C}{C} \times 100 \quad \textbf{(1a)}$$

where

E = Mean performance of the experimental group on the transfer task (task B)
C = Mean performance of the control group on the transfer task (task B)

This formula (1a) is appropriate when the measure of performance is such that *the larger* the value of the measure, *the better* the performance (Ellis 1965, p. 12). For example, if the measure of performance is the number of correct responses, then the use of this formula is correct, because the number of correct responses becomes larger with better performance.

If the measure of performance is such that *the smaller* the value of the measure, *the better* the performance, as for example, in the case of number of errors (as measure of performance), then the previous formula is modified by reversing the numerator to C − E, such as in 1b:

$$\text{Percentage of transfer} = \frac{C - E}{C} \times 100 \quad \textbf{(1b)}$$

Formula 2 was proposed by Gagne, Foster, and Crowly (1948). This procedure compares the difference between the experimental and control groups with the maximum amount of improvement possible on the transfer task. The maximum improvement possible is designated by the difference between the total possible score on task B and the control group's performance on task B. If the measure of performance is number of correct responses, as in the first formula (1a), then the formula is:

$$\text{Percentage of transfer} = \frac{E - C}{T - C} \times 100 \quad \textbf{(2a)}$$

where

T = Total possible score
E = Mean performance of experimental group on transfer test
C = Mean performance of control group on transfer test

The denominator and numerator of this formula (2a) are reversed (2b) if the measure of performance is time, trials, or errors, as in formula 1b.

$$\text{Percentage of transfer} = \frac{C - E}{C - T} \times 100 \quad \textbf{(2b)}$$

Ellis (1965, p. 13) pointed out that the main difficulty with formulas 2a and 2b is that it is not always possible to know the total possible score (T), and its determination may be difficult or impossible.

Formula 3 was proposed by Murdock (1957) and has advantages over the first two types. It produces symmetrical positive and negative transfer values that range from plus 100% transfer to minus 100% transfer. This is accomplished by making the denominator of

the formula include the performance of the experimental and the control groups. The formula (3a) is:

$$\text{Percentage of transfer} = \frac{E - C}{E + C} \times 100 \quad \textbf{(3a)}$$

As in formula 1a, this formula is appropriate if the measure of performance is such that the larger the value of the measure, the better the performance. However, if the reverse is true, that is, if the measure of performance is such that the smaller the value the better the performance, the numerator is reversed as C − E. The formula (3b) becomes:

$$\text{Percentage of transfer} = \frac{C - E}{E + C} \times 100 \quad \textbf{(3b)}$$

Wittrock (1966) pointed out that if a researcher in education wants to compare the percentage of transfer in one study with that obtained in another study, it is important that the researcher find out which formula of transfer has been used in the other study. This is because in most cases each formula gives a different answer and will give values different from the other formulas.

Conceptual approaches to transfer of learning—theories of transfer

Different authors classify transfer theories into different categories. For example, Wittrock (1968) classified them into three major categories: (1) stimulus-response approach to transfer, which includes the transfer theories of stimulus predifferentiation, transposition, paired-associate verbal learning, learning-set theory, and warm-up effect; (2) mediational approach to transfer; and (3) Gagne's theory of transfer. Ellis (1965) classified theories of transfer into six categories: (1) mediational theory; (2) stimulus predifferentiation, which contains four hypotheses; (3) transposition; (4) paired-associate verbal learning; (5)

learning-set theory; and (6) mathematical theory of transfer.

This module integrates Wittrock's (1968) and Ellis' (1965) classifications and categorizes them into four major conceptual approaches to transfer of learning: (1) stimulus-response approach, which includes stimulus predifferentiation, transposition, paired-associate verbal learning, and learning-set theory; (2) mediational theory; (3) mathematical model; and (4) Gagne's (1962) model of hierarchical learning-set theory.

Currently, an impressive amount of investigation is being done in the area of transfer of learning that is showing considerable progress in the development of theories or conceptual models.

A problem in transfer, until recently, has been the lack of systematic theory that would serve to organize the diverse empirical findings and to predict new relationships. Certainly, a number of functional relationships have been established; however, they have not always been easily integrated within the framework of systematic theory.

STIMULUS-RESPONSE APPROACH TO TRANSFER OF LEARNING

Stimulus predifferentiation. Stimulus predifferentiation is one of the areas in which the stimulus-response approach has been the most productive in adding to the body of knowledge about the conditions that increase transfer, more specifically, position transfer.

A variety of theories to account for the positive transfer effects resulting from stimulus predifferentiation have been proposed. These have been described in several sources (Arnoult, 1957; Wittrock, 1965; Ellis and Muller, 1964; Gibson, 1940; Gibson and Gibson, 1955; Jeffrey, 1969).

1. The first of these hypotheses is *acquired distinctiveness of cues* (Goss, 1955; Miller and Dollard, 1941; Ellis, 1965), which states that attaching different verbal labels to similar stimuli tends to increase their "distinctiveness." Labeling is treated as an intervening variable and is inferred from the ease with which one attaches new instrumental responses to stimuli following labeling practice or in the improvement in recognition or discrimination following labeling practices. Studies that have used relevant stimulus-response pretraining have uniformly shown positive transfer as compared with other kinds of pretraining (Gagne and Baker, 1950; Goss and Greenfeld, 1958; Norcross and Spiker, 1958). In an elaborate study, Goss and Greenfeld attempted to examine in great detail the various conditions influencing transfer of predifferentiation. Their basic findings revealed that subjects given the various labeling tasks were superior on the transfer task to those given instructions that involved various combinations of looking at, discriminating, and naming overtly or covertly. In addition, all conditions led to superior transfer when compared with groups who only saw the stimuli. The pronounced superiority of the various labeling groups over the "seeing" group was quite striking. The authors viewed their results as being consistent with the hypothesis of response-produced cues, namely, that attaching verbal responses to the stimuli generated additional cues that served to make them more distinctive.

2. The second type of stimulus predifferentiation was proposed by Ellis and Muller (1964). They suggested that learning how to make *identifying responses* (naming) in training tasks may aid in the making of new identifying responses in the transfer task, even though the responses are qualitatively different. In other words, relevant-stimulus training, may in fact produce two effects: one being to increase the distinctiveness of the stimuli, and the other, to facilitate a learning-how-to-learn process in which sub-

jects acquire skill in making identifying responses. They further pointed out that if indeed labeling practice does increase the distinctiveness of the stimuli, that such increase ought to be reflected in a perceptual task such as recognition as well as in a learning task that requires differential motor responses (Ellis, 1965).

In their study, subjects were given pretraining tasks of either labeling or observing a series of random shapes. The subjects were then tested on either a *learning task* (subjects had to learn to make new responses to stimuli) or a *perceptual task* (subjects had to "discriminate or recognize stimuli rather than learn to make new responses in their presence") (Ellis, 1965, p. 51). Ellis and Muller found that labeling the random shapes (the stimulus aspects) in the pretraining sessions helped their subjects make new responses to the stimuli (transfer task 1), but did not seem to help them much when they were required to recognize or discriminate between the stimuli (transfer task 2).

3. Gibson (1940) proposed a third hypothesis to account for the findings of stimulus predifferentiation in terms of *reduction of intralist* generalization. Accordingly, the effect of pretraining is to reduce the amount of stimulus generalization among the stimulus items in a list. As the amount of generalization among stimuli is reduced, the amount of positive transfer in learning a new task is increased.

4. The *attention-to-cues* hypothesis has been suggested by several researchers (Robinson [1955], Jeffrey [1969], and Wittrock [1965]).

• • •

In summary, no single theory appears adequate in accounting for the empirical phenomenon of stimulus predifferentiation. Part of this difficulty may lie in inadequate or incomplete conceptualization of the events involved. It is conceivable that all of the proposed theories may be adequate for limited sets of data and that a more comprehensive theory will emerge as a result of better integration of the theories.

Some of the assumptions of these four hypotheses seem to overlap each other, and it is very hard to draw a distinct line between the two, such as the distinctiveness of cues hypothesis and attention to cues hypothesis. The former one seems to be a prerequisite for the latter, that is, if you make the stimulus distinctive or the relevant stimulus more obvious, the subject will pay more attention to that cue than to an irrelevant cue. The important question is what kind of cues will draw more attention, and how can they be made more distinctive, so that the learner will be able to transfer more?

Suppose a nurse was planning to teach a new mother how to bathe her baby. Before having the mother practice the activity herself, the nurse encourages the mother to go over to the table where the bath equipment has been placed and just look at it and identify and label the items. This opportunity for the new mother to become familiar with, or look at, the stimulus components of the task is an instance of stimulus predifferentiation. If the nurse had shown the new mother a movie demonstration of another person bathing a baby and identifying the parts, this too would provide the new mother with preliminary experiences with the stimulus aspects of the task. Attention-focusing activity, says Ellis (1965, p. 49), helps a person "to 'predifferentiate' the task so whatever is learned subsequently will be learned with greater ease."

The use of verbal cues seems to be one of the most prominent ways of producing transfer; for example, Maier (1930) found that providing a verbal cue ("Observe how easy the solution would be if you could only hang the pendulum from two nails from the ceiling." [Wittrock, 1965]) helped people to solve his double-pendulum problem. Ewert and Lambert (1932) found that instructions increased the subject's ability to solve problems that involved moving circular cardboard disks from a given arrangement to a second specified arrangement. Irwin and associates (1934) found that learning was best when a rule or principle was rehearsed and its application was practiced. Kittell (1957) found that presenting rules to learners enhanced retention and transfer and provided the background that promoted discovery of new principles. Wittrock (1963) taught college students to decipher transpositional cryptograms by one of four treatment conditions: (1) rule and answer given; (2) rule given, answer not given; (3) rule not given, answer given; and (4) rule and answer not given. The treatment that presented rules and answers produced the greatest learning, but the treatment that presented rules and required the subjects to apply the rules to unanswered examples produced the greatest retention and transfer to new examples. These results were in close agreement with Craig (1956) and Kittell (1957) and were later supported by Wittrock and Twelker (1964). Further experiments by Wittrock (1964); Wittrock, Keislar, and Stern (1964); and Wittrock and Keislar (1965) have concluded that verbal instructions enhance retention and transfer by eliminating incorrect responses that produce negative transfer. Both retention and transfer were facilitated by explicit verbalizations by the experimenter of the name for the correct concept, followed by practice in and reinforcement for applying the label.

Transposition. Transposition is transfer that is presumed to result from responding to relationships among stimuli, rather than to an absolute quality of a stimulus. A strict stimulus-response approach (Spence, 1946) to learning assumed that all stimuli acting on the receptors when a reinforced response is initiated become associated with that response, and that this association is strengthened with each subsequent reinforcement of that response in the presence of those stimuli. Such a conception suggests that an organism would not ordinarily learn to respond to a relationship between the stimuli, but only to their absolute stimulus attributes (Jeffrey, 1969).

Kohler (1925) tested the concept of transposition with chickens. He trained the chickens to respond to the darker of the two gray disks (stimulus) and rewarded them when they responded to the darker stimulus and did not reinforce them when they responded to the lighter disk. This is a form of discrimination training. After this discrimination was reliably established, the chickens were given a new discrimination task in which they had to choose between the original gray that was reinforced and a new darker gray disk. In the new task (transfer task) the animals responded to the darker of the two grays even though they had always been rewarded for choosing the other gray.

In another experiment on transposition, Kuenne (1946) found that seven children with mental ages of 3 years failed to respond consistently on test trials presenting a transposed size discrimination, whereas 27% of the 4-year mental-age group, 52% of the 5-year mental-age group, and 100% of the 6-year mental-age group responded consistently to the smaller stimulus of the test pair. No children transposed who did not either spontaneously verbalize or respond to questioning with the correct basis for solution, whereas 43% of those who verbalized the correct basis for solution also showed transfer to the transposed stimuli. This correlation of verbalization and transposition was taken as support for the proposition that the verbal response mediated the transfer by permitting a relational response (Jeffrey, 1969).

Paired-associate verbal learning. A recent development in verbal learning has been the construction of a two-stage theory of paired-associate learning (Hovland and Kurtz, 1952; Underwood and Schulz, 1960). Ellis (1965) stated that although this theory was initially developed to interpret certain features of paired-associate learning, it appears to be applicable to the analysis of transfer phenomenon. This theory regards paired-associate learning as consisting of two fairly distinctive stages: *response integration* and *associative "hook-ups."* Accordingly, the first stage in learning a list of paired-associates is response integration. In this stage, the subject learns to differentiate each response in the list from the others. In other words, the response becomes highly available to the subject. After the response becomes integrated, the subject learns to associate it with its appropriate stimulus (Ellis, 1965).

The following is a nursing example of paired-associate learning. If a nurse first learned that erythromycin (A) is an antibiotic (B), and then learned that garamycin (C) is also an antibiotic (B); the response integration that occurs when learning erythromycin is an antibiotic (A–B) should also make it easier to associate, or "hook up," with garamycin is an antibiotic (C–B).

Ellis and Burnstein (1960) have extended this theory to the learning of two successive paired-associate lists and have analyzed the transfer of learning. They have analyzed the A–B, C–B paradigm in which the same responses are made to new stimuli in the transfer task. This study has enabled them to interpret their findings, which involved transfer as a function of the time elapsing between the original and transfer tasks. First, with paired-associate tasks containing highly meaningful responses, such as adjectives, transfer was found to remain roughly constant with the passage of time. This finding has suggested that the constancy of the transfer-time function is largely dependent on the operations of the associative, or the

hook-up, stage, since the responses were already well integrated. Next, they found that if the responses are low in meaningfulness, such as nonsense syllables, transfer declines with the passage of time (Ellis and Burnstein, 1960).

Learning-set theory. It is commonly observed that individuals improve in their ability to learn new tasks when they have practiced a series of related tasks; for example, a person who practices solving linear equations each day for several days becomes progressively more efficient in solving linear equations. Not only does the work become more accurate, but also the problems are solved much faster. This progressive improvement in performance indicates that the student has "learned how to learn," that is, has acquired a learning set (Ellis, 1965; Harlow, 1949).

The findings from Harlow's study (1949) on the formation of learning sets have significant implications for education. Learning-set theory implies that important aspects of learning how to learn to solve problems are built up over many practice trials on related problems. It is only after extensive practice that the student becomes proficient in executing complex skills and in solving problems. In the development of learning sets, Harlow has sometimes arranged the experimental situation so that the cues are reversed, that is, if the positive cue was originally the cube instead of the triangle, the triangle is now made the positive cue. According to Osgood's (1949) theory of transfer, this is a condition for producing negative transfer. At first, this is precisely what happens; the animal has some difficulty in dealing with the reversed cues and continues to select the original cue. Later after considerable practice in dealing with reversals, it acquires a facility for handling them and learns to shift with relative ease. In short, the animal learns to become flexible in dealing with discrimination reversals. One educational implication stemming from this finding is that if we wish to teach children to be flexible in problem solving, then they must be given practice with various tasks in which cue reversals occur (Ellis, 1965).

Later, in another study, Harlow (1959) noted that the early trials are extremely significant in establishing a reliable learning set. He contended that if practice with a particular type of problem is discontinued before it is reliably learned, then little transfer will occur to the next series of problems. Therefore, he concluded, considerable time and effort should be spent on the early problems before moving on to more securely developed stages, where relatively few trials are necessary on new problems. Harlow's findings have also been supported by Duncan (1958), whose study showed that: (1) transfer is a direct function of a degree of variation in training, and (2) the amount of transfer increases as a result of increased amount of practice.

Where do we see these principles being demonstrated in nursing education and practice? A number of examples can be cited that may help to make the point. In nursing school, most students have a number of patients with whom they must learn to communicate effectively. Process recordings are often used as practice activities to help students learn about interpersonal relations. After doing a number of these process recording, most students develop a reliable learning set for approaching patient-nurse communications. This reliable learning set involves looking at (1) what was said or was not said, (2) how the problem was interpreted at the time, (3) what nursing intervention was made, and (4) how the effectiveness of that intervention was evaluated. In other words, the reliable learning set is to use the nursing process in approaching nurse-patient communication problems. Students learn how to learn, and ease in dealing with future nurse-

patient communication problems is probably influenced by how much effort is spent in mastering early nurse-patient communication problems (early task learning).

MEDIATION THEORY

Mediation theory was described by Wittrock (1965, p. 4) as the theory that

hypothesizes mediating stimuli and responses (r–s) which intervene between initiating Si (S) and terminating responses (R). The operational model for this series (S–r–s—R) is often represented by the series (A–B–C), with the B term as the operational equivalent of the mediating response (r) and the mediating stimulus (s). Each B may also be associated with a specific R, or with several Rs (C). In this case, the B term is the common mediating term for the several A terms, and is probably most important in concept learning studies, where there is a hierarchical arrangement of many Si to a common R.

Mediating responses are regarded as mechanisms for producing transfer. In other words, the ease or difficulty with which a person learns a new task depends in part on the kind of mediating responses that are available, these in turn being a function of earlier learning experiences. Much of the ability of humans to learn new tasks with ease stems from the use of language, a major source of mediating responses.

A series of studies by Birge (1941), Cantor (1955), Dietze (1955), Kendler and Kendler (1961, 1962), Norcross and Spiker (1957), and Murdock (1960) have all shown that the distinctive labels for stimulus objects have a greater transfer effect than a condition that specified no distinctive names for the stimuli. The researchers listed interpreted their findings in terms of the hypothesis of "acquired distinctiveness of cues" and at the same time mediational theory. Verbal labels produce mediating responses that can help the children to discriminate and transfer. Furthermore, the study by Spiker, Gerjuoy, and

Shepard (1956) found that children who verbalized the concept "middle-sizedness" learned a relational task more readily than did those who did not know this concept (Wittrock and Hill, 1968).

MATHEMATICAL MODEL

During the past few years there has been a rapid growth of mathematical models in psychology. In evaluating different models, Ellis (1965) concluded that mathematical models have some advantages in that they have increased conceptual rigor, increased likelihood of detecting unstated assumptions, and increased ability to predict events in an unequivocal fashion. Only a very brief account of one mathematical model is given. Bower's model (1962) is used mainly for predicting performance in paired-associate learning tasks. This model has been extended to apply to the study of paired-associate transfer by Rickert (Ellis, 1965).

Bower's model* for predicting performance in paired-associate task learning (as quoted in Ellis, 1965, pp. 81-82) is:

$$q_n = (1 - \frac{1}{N}) \, (1 - C)^{n-1}$$

where q_n = The probability that a subject will make an error on a given trial

$(1 - \frac{1}{N})$ = The probability of an incorrect guess

$(1 - C)^{n-1}$ = The probability that a stimulus item will fail to be conditioned

GAGNE'S HIERARCHICAL LEARNING-SET THEORY OF TRANSFER

Gagne's (1962) theory of hierarchical learning set explains a phenomena that occurs in productive learning. "Productive learning" refers to transfer across a class of behaviors,

---

*For more extensive information, the reader is advised to refer to the original source.

such as solving linear algebraic equations. Gagne called these classes of behavior learning sets, and they are the components of knowledge.

For Gagne, knowledge consists of subordinate capabilities called learning sets, which are arranged in a hierarchy. Each learning set may have its own group of subordinate learning sets. Together, the subordinate learning sets mediate positive transfer to the superordinate learning set that is immediately above it. Gagne (1962) predicts that: (1) if the learner cannot recall one or more of the subordinate learning sets, transfer to the next higher order of learning set is zero; (2) if a learner has passed or attained the higher-level learning set, then *all* related lower-level learning sets must have been passed; (3) if a learner has passed the higher-level learning set, then *no* related lower-level tasks must have been failed; and (4) if a learner cannot pass or attain a higher-level task, even though all the related lower-level learning sets have been passed and attained, then the absence of positive transfer would be attributed to a deficiency in instruction and does not contradict the notion that lower-level learning sets are essential to the achievement of higher-order ones.

Learning sets, along with instructions, comprise the two essential variables of Gagne's theory, and they predict transfer in instructions. The detailed explanation of Gagne's model of instruction is provided in a previous module (pp. 219-234).

Wittrock (1968) pointed out that Gagne's theory of transfer is better than the previously mentioned theories of transfer in that it involves ability and achievement measures in predicting transfer from lower-order sets to higher-order sets. Gagne's model also predicts correlations between individual differences, general intelligence, irrelevant basic abilities, number and pattern of relevant learning sets, and measure of rate and achievement of transfer to the higher level of a learning-set hierarchy.

Gagne has researched his own theory. The study by Gagne and Paradise (1961) supported all of his predictions about transfer. The subjects were seventh-grade students, and the learning set involved the task of solving linear algebraic equations.

Learning sets, then, are one of the two major variables that affect transfer; the other is instruction. Gagne (1962, pp. 357-358) stated that instructions, which are the content of communication, mediate positive transfer in one or more of the following four ways:

1. Identifying the required terminal performance
2. Identifying elements of the stimulus situation
3. Establishing high recallability of learning sets
4. Guiding the thinking of the learner

Wittrock (1968) pointed out that research is lacking in testing the effects of these instructional variables in producing transfer.

Gagne (1965) also presented conditions for producing transfer of learning. First, he distinguished between *lateral transfer* and *vertical transfer*. Lateral transfer refers to the broad application of previous learning sets. Vertical transfer refers to the situation where subordinate learning sets mediate positive transfer to superordinate learning sets.

The important conditions for inducing lateral transfer are the individual differences among the learners, including relevant learning sets and basic intellectual abilities. Practice in a variety of situations and reinforcement for application of principles and knowledge to a broad variety of situations are two external conditions that contribute to lateral transfer.

Vertical transfer, which can be measured by rate of learning, is mediated by mastery of subordinate learning sets. Basic abilities and variety of previous knowledge are important internal conditions that mediate a certain amount of vertical transfer. The external conditions are similar to those required for lateral transfer; namely, practice, variety, verbal cues, and application of previously learned rules in novel combinations (Wittrock, 1968).

Variables that affect transfer of learning

Some of these variables are treated as principles of transfer that have been empirically derived. Again, the major emphasis here is to summarize these findings and the effect of these variables on transfer of learning, so that they can be applied or used as guidelines for nursing education and practice.

OVERALL TASK SIMILARITY

Transfer research has shown that a high degree of similarity between the original and the transfer tasks will produce greater amounts of positive transfer. According to Ellis (1965), however, this principle is not as uncomplicated as it sounds because it is dependent on how one defines similarity, or in other words, how one measures transfer.

One approach to defining similarity is to analyze a learning task into its stimulus and response components. In other words, says Hall (1966), researchers can study the kind and amount of transfer obtained when (1) an old response is attached to a new stimulus (A–B, C–B) and (2) when a new response is attached to an old stimulus (A–B, A–C).

Ellis (1965) cited one of his own research studies in which he looked at the effect of stimulus similarity on the transfer of learning. The stimulus aspects of the original and transfer tasks were varied, but the responses for each task were kept the same. In this study, Ellis used a definition of similarity that was developed by Haagen (1949). Haagen had rated pairs of adjectives as being very high to very low in similarity. An example of a word pair might be agile-modest, where agile would be the stimulus aspect of the task, and modest would be the response aspect (Ellis, 1965, pp. 16-20).

In his experiment, Ellis had groups of subjects learn an original list of eight pairs of adjectives. Two days later, Ellis had his subjects learn a second list of word pairs. This time, however, the groups of subjects received second lists of word pairs whose stimulus aspects varied in their degree of similarity between the stimulus aspects of the word pairs on the original lists. Ellis found that the subjects who learned the transfer lists that contained stimulus words highly similar to the stimulus words of the original list learned faster than the other subjects. The other subjects had learned transfer lists of words where the stimulus aspects were only of moderate or low similarity to the stimulus aspects of the original list of word pairs. In other words, Ellis found that the greater the degree of stimulus similarity, the greater the amount of positive transfer.

We have just mentioned stimulus similarity as being a factor involved in the transfer of learning, but what happens when a subject is required to make new responses to the same stimuli?

A study by Porter and Duncan (1953) found that both positive and negative transfer effects can occur when subjects are required to make new responses to old stimuli. According to Ellis (1965), however, negative transfer is seen more in motor skill learning than in verbal learning where people are required to make new responses to the same stimuli.

The following is a nursing example to illustrate the correct usage of the empirical findings about task similarity. In general, a nurse who tries to teach a hospitalized patient self-care activities under circumstances that are highly similar to those that will be encountered at home is at least trying to use this principle of overall task similarity correctly. A nurse, on the other hand, who has a hospitalized patient learn self-care activities that cannot possibly be performed in the same manner at home (in other words, the response aspects of the task have been changed) is *not* utilizing the empirical findings about task similarity and the transfer of learning. This example may help to emphasize the importance of assessing the patient's home situation before trying to set up a discharge teaching plan.

WARM-UP EFFECT

According to Ellis (1965, p. 35), warm-up is related to learning-to-learn, but its transfer effects are "more transitory or short-lived."

In Hamilton's (1950) study, subjects were given a list of meaningful paired words to learn. At varying time intervals after learning the original list of paired words, the subjects were then given another list of paired words to learn. Hamilton found that it was easier for subjects to learn the second list if they had received this test list within 60 minutes of learning the first list. After this 60-minute time interval, the facilitating effects of warm-up were found to be minimal.

What would a nursing example of warm-up be? If, at the beginning of a class period, a nursing instructor had the students learn task A (such as how to recognize a set of surgical instruments) and then about 30 to 60 minutes later had them learn task B (such as how to recognize a different set of surgical instruments), the instructor might expect to obtain some warm-up effects from task A to task B. If the time interval between task A and task B was greater than 60 minutes, however, the nursing instructor should not expect to see many, if any, facilitating transfer effects as the result of warm-up.

TIME INTERVAL BETWEEN TASKS

The time interval between tasks has been studied by a number of investigators (Bunch, 1936; Bunch and McCraven, 1938; Bunch and Lang, 1939) who wanted to know if varying the time interval between learning two related tasks affected the transfer of learning from one to the other. In these studies, subjects were given original tasks to learn, and afterward, at varying time intervals, were given a transfer task to learn. The results of each of these studies showed that the transfer of learning from the original task to the transfer task remained roughly the same regardless of the time elapsing between the tasks as long as the performance on the transfer task did not depend on memory for the specific items of the original task.

TASK CHARACTERISTICS

Task characteristics have been the object of study of other investigators (Mandler, 1962; Underwood, 1949; Postman, 1962; and many others). They have studied the effect that the *degree of original learning of a task* had on transfer. Findings of these studies show that in general, positive transfer increases with increasing practice on the original task, and also that the greatest amount of negative transfer occurs after relatively little practice on the original task. In other words, if one practices extensively on an original task, negative transfer is less likely to occur (Ellis, 1965, pp. 42-43).

Does *task variety* influence transfer? Duncan (1958) found that it did. In a study investigating this factor of task variety, Duncan had his subjects practice perceptual motor tasks in which the stimulus aspects of the transfer tasks were different from those of the original task. The results of Duncan's study showed that

. . . (1) the amount of transfer increased as a result of increased amount of practice, and (2) transfer increased as a direct function of increased variety of original training. . . . In other words, the increased positive transfer due to task variety occurred with only a small increase in the number of training tasks. (Ellis, 1965, pp. 44-45.)

What about *task difficulty;* does it influence transfer? Studies (Day, 1956; Lordahl and Archer, 1958; Nobel, 1959; Lawrence, 1952) summarized by Ellis (1965, pp. 45-47) show contradictory results. Each has used different types of tasks, and they have defined task difficulty in a variety of ways. The investigators also came up with a variety of inconsistent results. For these reasons, says Ellis, it has been very difficult to generalize about the effect of task difficulty on transfer.

If one were to illustrate the correct usage of these four principles that have just been reviewed, one would have to say that a nursing instructor should not be worried that transfer effects will decline if long intervals occur between original learning and new related learning. They will not decline as long as memory of specific aspects of the original learning task is not involved. A nursing instructor should provide students with adequate experience with the original task to prevent negative transfer. The instructor should give students opportunities to learn a variety of related tasks in order to ensure positive transfer to new tasks. And finally, the instructor should know that, as of now, no clear-cut generalizations about task difficulty can be made. There is not enough empirical evidence to support giving students all simple or all complex tasks to learn in order to promote transfer.

EFFECTS OF GROUP LEARNING ON TRANSFER

Although group problem-solving activity has been shown to be superior to individual problem-solving activity (Ellis, 1965, p. 68), the study by Taylor and Faust (1952) has shown that skills learned in a group will not necessarily transfer to the individual situation. Another study by Hudgins (1960) gave support to this viewpoint. In this study, fifth-grade students were selected by Hudgins to practice solving arithmetic problems for three days either in groups or individually. Hudgins found that there was no significant difference in the performance on a transfer task between students who had practiced solving arithmetic problems in groups and those who had practiced solving problems on their own.

The implications of this finding to nursing situations are clear. If a nurse likes to have diabetic patients learn self-care skills in groups rather than in individual learning sessions, would it be correct to assume that self-care skills acquired in the group situation will automatically transfer to the individual situation? The answer is no. This nurse may possibly economize time, and the patients may benefit socially; but it is not certain that transfer of learning in individual patients will occur just because self-care skills were learned in a group.

EFFECTS OF UNDERSTANDING ON TRANSFER

According to Ellis (1965, p. 74), the general principle relating to understanding and transfer is that "transfer is greater if the learner understands the general rules or principles which are appropriate in solving new problems." To apply this idea to nursing education and practice, nurse instructors must be sure that patients, students, or staff members understand the principles involved in the content material being presented before they can expect much transfer. A nursing student who is learning how to set up intravenous equipment, a patient who is learning to irrigate a colostomy, or a nurse who is trying to discover why a patient's tube feeding is not functioning properly all must understand the principle of fluid flow by gravity before this knowledge can transfer to new situations.

INDIVIDUAL DIFFERENCES

Several learner characteristics, such as intelligence, and motivational factors, such as anxiety and preferences, are also known to influence transfer. Studies by Craig (1953) and Werner (1930) have shown that more intelligent students show greater transfer. A typical finding by Werner was that those students who were above average in intelligence were able to profit from foreign language studies when tested on their ability in English, whereas students of average intelligence were not. A reasonable interpretation of this and similar findings were made by the authors in that brighter students tend to seek out relationships and are more likely than less bright students to have a set for transfer.

CHILDREN'S PREFERENCES

The study by Wittrock and Hill (1968) demonstrated the role of dimensional preferences in transfer. Children whose preferred dimension is relevant to the problem solve the transfer problem more quickly than children whose preferred dimension is irrelevant to the problem. The facilitation of learning was shown to exist in both initial learning and transfer. Furthermore, they also showed that when a problem has two relevant dimensions and the child prefers one (such as form) over the other (such as brightness), training that reinforces the child for choosing the less preferred but still relevant dimension (brightness) increases transfer, compared with a procedure that reinforces choosing only the preferred dimension. From this study the authors pointed out important implications for instruction: (1) instruction and teaching involve interaction between children's preferences—the previously acquired and proactive factors the subject brings to the learning situation—and the training appropriate to teach problem solving; and (2) measures of the learner's preferences should be obtained, and then these measures should be used to locate the less frequently chosen but relevant dimensions, which are the ones that should be trained to enhance transfer (p. 56).

FUNCTIONAL FIXEDNESS

The term functional fixedness refers to a situation in which the subject has become so "fixed" in the perception of an object as to be unable to perceive new or unusual uses for it. Schulz (1960) cited two experiments conducted by Adamson (1952) and Birch and Rabinowitz (1951), who have demonstrated that a functionally fixed group (the experimental group) could not solve Maier's two-string pendulum problem, whereas the control group was able to solve the problem.

Issues in transfer of learning

In looking at the research trends in the area of transfer of learning, one cannot help but notice some of the problem areas or issues of transfer that remain unsolved today. As Ellis (1965) indicated, there are four major problem areas: (1) transfer research methodology and developing precise ways to measure transfer, (2) problems in identifying variables that influence transfer and discovering *how* they do it, (3) problems in developing adequate theories or conceptual models to organize empirical knowledge and to help predict transfer effects, and (4) lack of adequate educational technology to help deal with the training problems that exist.

Summary and conclusion

Transfer of learning was explained in terms of four different theoretical approaches, namely: stimulus-response approach, which included the concepts of stimulus predifferentiation, transposition, paired verbal association, and learning set; mediation theory; mathematical models; and Gagne's model. No single theory appeared adequate in accounting for the total empirical phenomenon of transfer. Part of the difficulty may lie in the incomplete conceptualization of the events involved. In addition, failure to specify precisely the meaning of various constructs employed in the theories may also account for some of the difficulty. It is conceivable that all of the proposed theories may be adequate for limited sets of data and that a more comprehensive theory will emerge as a result of better integration of the theories.

However, based on the results of the previously mentioned research, one can conclude that transfer of learning will be aided by any pretraining procedures that:

1. Establish learning sets
2. Help define the problem or the task for the learner
3. Increase the likelihood of attending responses to appropriate cues
4. Maximize the similarity between teaching and the ultimate testing situation.
5. Provide adequate experience with the original task
6. Provide for a variety of examples when teaching concepts and principles
7. Make sure that general principles are understood before expecting much transfer
8. Label and identify important features of a task

Application to nursing education and practice

Let us take a specific patient- or student-teaching situation and apply the above-mentioned recommendations to produce transfer of learning.

The example that is used is how to give an injection. This can be a situation where a student nurse is learning how to give an injection, a patient is learning how to self-administer an injection, or a family member is learning to give an injection to a patient.

1. *Establish learning sets.* According to Gagne (1962), learning sets are subordinate categories of knowledge that the learner needs to know in order to perform a task and transfer it to other situations. An example of establishing learning sets for "giving an injection" could be as follows:

   a. Learning sets for stimulus items, such as vial, calibration on vial, syringe, needle, cotton, alcohol, medication, and concepts and principles associated with these items that are relevant for giving an injection

b. Principles and concepts dealing with medication, such as type of drug, appropriate dosage, actions of drug

c. Sterilization techniques, such as boiling or using the autoclave and concepts and principles associated with these techniques that are relevant for giving an injection

d. Method or procedure of giving an injection; for example, how to put the syringe together without contaminating it, how to draw medication from the vial, how to select the appropriate body site for the injection, how to clean the skin, how to give the injection, and how to take care of the equipment after it has been used

Once these subordinate hierarchies of knowledge are identified, then the learner is given a chance to practice each of the steps, until adept at the procedure; in other words, until the stage is reached where the learner has learned how to learn. This can be observed in the student's dexterity in handling the items and how long the procedure takes. As the student becomes more adept, the task will be performed easier and faster.

2. *Define the task or the problem* to the learner. This is another principle that induces transfer of learning. This can be done by identifying the stimulus elements involved in the problem situation. In step 1a, this has been done. Another way of defining the problem can be to tell the student or the patient the *type* of solution that is necessary to solve the problem. (Remember, it is *not* the solution that is given, but the solution model.) For example, the teacher can tell the nurse, "You have to think of a way to get the solution into the syringe without contaminating it."

3. *Increase the likelihood of attending responses* to appropriate cues. This can be done by focusing the student's or patient's attention on important elements of the procedure by drawing it, demonstrating it, or saying, "Look, this is very important," or at times exaggerating a point in order to impress the learner and get his attention.

4. *Label and identify important features of a task.* As the learner identifies the features of a stimulus situation, ask the learner to label them, or name them, since according to mediation theory of transfer, labeling, or naming, the important features of a task produces positive transfer.

5. *Maximize the similarity between the teaching situations and the ultimate testing situation.* Let us assume that the teacher provides oranges or apples on which student nurses or patients can practice giving injections. However, in order to maximize the similarity between the teaching and testing situations, the teacher needs to provide the students or patients with learning experiences (practice) with a dummy, then a patient, then another patient, and then maybe themselves. If the testing situation is to give an injection to a patient, then the practice situation has to induce giving injections to patients.

6. *Provide adequate experiences with the original task.* If the task is to give different types of injections (hypodermic, intramuscular, and others), then practice with the original task can be the type of injection students first learned to give. For example, if they started giving hypodermic injections, then enough practice must be done with this original task before asking them to give other types of injections. Practice should be set up for approximately 50% overlearning (Kreuger, 1929).

7. *Provide for a variety of examples when teaching concepts and principles.* Once the learner has mastered well the original task, then a variety of situations should be given.

For example, the students or patients can give injections at different body sites, or the students can give injections to people of different age groups, use different types of syringes, or handle other situations.

8. *Ensure that general principles are understood before expecting much transfer.* The teacher can find out if the learner has understood the underlying principles and concepts of the task by having the learner answer, in own words, such questions as: What is the principle? Why is it important to sterilize the needle? Can you give other examples utilizing the principle? What would you do if you did not have sterile cotton in the house? How could you sterilize a piece of gauze or cloth using the kitchen oven?

In conclusion, therefore, these principles can be used with any task or problem-solving situations to produce transfer of learning.

Researchable questions

1. What is the effect of teaching patients how to change their colostomy dressing in the home compared to in the hospital on transfer of learning (that is, carrying out the correct procedure) after they are discharged from the hospital?

   a. Independent variable: teaching patients in their home setting as opposed to the hospital setting

   b. Dependent variable: transfer of learning (that is, carrying out the correct procedure)

2. What is the effect of teaching strategy (that takes the patients' as opposed to the nurse's preferences for foods into consideration in teaching patients about food exchanges) on transfer of learning (calculating the correct exchanges) after the patient is discharged from the hospital?

   a. Independent variable: teaching strategy utilizing the patient's preferences for food versus the nurse's preferences

   b. Dependent variable: transfer of learning (the ability to calculate the correct exchanges of food)

ADDITIONAL LEARNING EXPERIENCES—RECOMMENDED READING LIST

Ellis, H. C. *The transfer of learning.* New York: The Macmillan Co., 1965.

Wittrock, M. C. Three conceptual approaches to research on transfer of training. In R. Gagne and W. J. Gephart (Eds.) *Learning research and school subjects.* Itasca, Ill.: F. E. Peacock Publishers, Inc., 1968.

INSTRUCTIONS TO THE LEARNER REGARDING POSTTEST

You are now ready to take the posttest to determine the extent to which you have achieved the objectives of this module. Return to the pretest and take it over again as the posttest. After completing the test correct your answers using the answer key found at the end of this module (pp. 284-285). You need to achieve 38 correct points to obtain mastery at the 95% level. If your score is less than this, correct your mistakes, study the content of this module over again, and read some of the references found in the recommended reading list. Take the posttest again. You need to study in this fashion until you achieve the 95% mastery level prior to moving to the next module.

ANSWER KEY TO PRETEST AND POSTTEST

1. b (Ellis, 1965, pp. 6, 38, 73)
2. c (Ellis, 1965, pp. 3-4)
3. d (Ellis, 1965, pp. 36-38, 73)
4. d (Ellis, 1965, p. 76)
5. a (Ellis, 1965, pp. 20, 36, 40)
6. c (Gagne, 1965, p. 337)
7. b (Gagne, 1965, p. 335)
8. c (Bruner, 1967, p. 52)
9. b (Ellis, 1965, p. 79)
10. a (Ellis, 1965, p. 72)
11. c (Ellis, 1965, pp. 15-16)
12. b (Ellis, 1965, p. 23)

13. c (Ellis, 1965, pp. 48-60, 73)
14. b (Ellis, 1965, pp. 3-4)
15. c (Ellis, 1965, pp. 3-4)
16. a (Ellis, 1965, pp. 3-4)
17. b (Ellis, 1965, pp. 3-4)
18. yes (Ellis, 1965, pp. 72-73, 15-31)
19. yes (Ellis, 1965, p. 74)
20. no (Ellis, 1965, pp. 45-47, 74)
21. no (Ellis, 1965, pp. 68-69, 74)
22. yes (Ellis, 1965, pp. 44-45, 73)
23. no (Ellis, 1965, pp. 39-41, 73)
24. yes (Ellis, 1965, pp. 42-44, 73)
25. no (Ellis, 1965, pp. 73-74)
26. d (Ellis, 1965, pp. 36-38)
27. f and h (Ellis, 1965, pp. 48-60)
28. g (Ellis, 1965, pp. 78-80)
29. a (Ellis, 1965, pp. 81-82)
30. b and c (Ellis, 1965, pp. 32-35, 80-81, 119-139)
31. e (Ellis, 1965, pp. 76, 78)
32. i (Gagne, 1962, pp. 355-365)
33. The order of the issues may vary but should include:
    a. Research methodology and transfer measurement—must relate to research methodology and measurement of transfer in nursing education or practice, that is, how can one measure the amount of transfer that occurs between nursing tasks learned in a laboratory setting and related tasks performed on the nursing unit
    b. Variables influencing transfer and how they do it—must relate to transfer variables in nursing education or practice, that is, determine whether nursing students should only be given complex, rather than simple, tasks to learn in order to maximize transfer
    c. Development of conceptual models or theories of transfer—must relate to conceptual models or theoretical frameworks of transfer as they relate to nursing education and practice, that is, determine which theories of transfer are more applicable to the learning involved in schools of nursing
    d. Development of educational technology to deal with educational and training problems—must relate to educational technology that will help to deal with transfer problems occurring in nursing education and practice, that is, how to sequence nursing courses in order to ensure positive transfer in students (Ellis, 1965, pp. 7-8)

REFERENCES

Adamson, R. E. Functional fixedness as related to problem-solving: a repetition of three experiments. *Journal of Experimental Psychology*, 1952, **44**:288-291.

Arnoult, M. D. Stimulus predifferentiation: some generalizations and hypotheses. *Psychological Bulletin*, 1957, **54**:339-350.

Birch, H. G., and Rabinowitz, H. S. The negative effect of previous experience on productive thinking. *Journal of Experimental Psychology*, 1951, **41**: 121-125.

Birge, J. S. The role of verbal responses in transfer. Unpublished doctoral Dissertation, Yale University, 1941.

Bower, G. An association model for response and training variables in paired-associate learning. *Psychological Review*, 1962, **69**:34-55.

Bruner, J. *Toward a theory of instruction.* Cambridge, Mass.: Harvard University Press, 1967.

Bunch, M. E. The amount of transfer in rational learning as a function of time. *Journal of Comparative Psychology*, 1936, **22**:325-337

Bunch, M. E., and Lang, E. S. The amount of transfer of training from partial learning after varying intervals of time. *Journal of Comparative Psychology*, 1939, **27**: 449-459.

Bunch, M. E., and McCraven, V. Temporal course of transfer in the learning of memory material. *Journal of Comparative Psychology*, 1938, **25**:481-496.

Cantor, G. N. Effects of three types of pretraining on discrimination learning in preschool children. *Journal of Experimental Psychology*, 1955, **49**:332-342.

Craig, R. C. *The transfer value of guided learning.* New York: Teachers College Press, 1953.

Craig, R. C. Directed versus independent discovery of established relations. *Journal of Educational Psychology*, 1956, **47**:223-234.

Day, R. H. Relative task difficulty and transfer of training in skilled performance. *Psychological Bulletin*, 1956, **53**:160-168.

Deese, J. *The psychology of learning.* New York: McGraw-Hill Book Co., 1958.

Dietze, D. Facilitating effects of words on discrimination and generalization. *Journal of Experimental Psychology*, 1955, 50, 255-250.

Duncan, C. P. Transfer in motor learning as a function of degree of first-task learning and inter-task similarity.

Journal of Experimental Psychology, 1953, **46**:445-452.

Duncan, C. P. Transfer after training single versus multiple tasks. *Journal of Experimental Psychology*, 1958, **55**(1):63-72.

Duncan, C. P. Recent research on human problem solving. *Psychological Bulletin*, 1959, **56**:397-429.

Ellis, H. C. *The transfer of learning*. New York: The Macmillan Co., 1965.

Ellis, H. C., and Burnstein, D. D. The effect of stimulus similarity and temporal factors in perceptual transfer of training. *Technical Report* No. 1, Sandia Corp., Albuquerque, New Mex, 1960.

Ellis, H. C., and Muller, D. G. Transfer in perceptual learning following stimulus predifferentiation. *Journal of Experimental Psychology*, 1964, **68**:388-395.

Ewert, P. H., and Lambert, J. F. The effect of verbal instructions upon the formation of a concept, Part 2. *Journal of Genetic Psychology*, 1932, **6**:400-412.

Gagne, R. M. The acquisition of knowledge. *Psychological Review*, 1962, **69**:355-365.

Gagne, R. M., and Baker, K. E. Stimulus predifferentiation as a factor in transfer of training. *Journal of Experimental Psychology*, 1950, **40**:439-451.

Gagne, R. M., Foster, H., and Crowly, M. E. The measurement of transfer of training. *Psychological Bulletin*, 1948, **45**:97-130.

Gagne, R. M., and Paradise, N. E. Abilities and learning sets in knowledge acquisition. *Psychological Monographs*, 1961, **75**(14): (whole no. 518).

Gibson, E. J. A systematic application of the concepts of generalization and differentiation to verbal learning. *Psychological Review*, 1940, **47**:196-229.

Gibson, E. J., and Gibson, J. J. Perceptual learning: differentiation or enrichment. *Psychological Review*, 1955, **62**:32-41.

Goss, A. E. A stimulus-response analysis of the interaction of cue producing and mediating responses. *Psychological Review*, 1955, **62**:20-31.

Goss, A. E., and Greenfeld, N. Transfer to a motor task as influenced by conditions and degree of prior discrimination training. *Journal of Experimental Psychology*, 1958, **55**:258-269.

Haagen, C. H. Synonymity, vividness, familiarity and association value rating of 400 pairs of common adjectives. *Journal of Psychology*, 1949, **27**:453-463.

Hall, John F. *The psychology of learning*. Philadelphia: J. B. Lippincott Co., 1966, pp. 472-546.

Hamilton, C. E. The relationship between length of internal separating two learning tasks and performance on the second task. *Journal of Experimental Psychology*, **40**:613-621.

Harlow, H. F. The formation of learning sets. *Psychological Review*, 1949, **56**:51-65.

Harlow, H. F. Learning set and error factor theory. In S.

Koch (Ed.), *Psychology: a study of science 2*. New York: McGraw-Hill Book Co., 1959, pp. 492-537.

Hovland, C. I., and Kurtz, K. H. Experimental studies in rote-learning theory: X pre-learning syllable familiarization and the length difficulty relationship. *Journal of Experimental Psychology*, 1952, **44**:31-39.

Hudgins, Bryce B. Effects of group experience on individual problem solving. *Journal of Educational Psychology*, 1960, **51**(1):37-42.

Irwin, F. S., and Kaufman, K., Prior, G., and Weaver, H. B. On learning without awareness of what is being learned. *Journal of Experimental Psychology*, 1934, **17**:823-827.

Jeffrey, W. E. Transfer. 1969 (mimeograph copy). Chapter to be published in Reese, H. W. and Lipsitt, L. P. (Eds.), *The scientific study of child behavior and development*.

Kendler, H. H., and Kendler T. S. Effects of verbalization on reversal shifts in children. *Science*, 1961, **134**:1619-1620.

Kendler, H. H., and Kendler, T. S. Vertical and horizontal processes in problem solving. *Psychological Review*, 1962, **69**:1-16.

Kittell, J. E. An experimental study of the effect of external direction during learning on transfer and retention of principles. *Journal of Educational Psychology*, 1957, **48**:391-405.

Kohler, W. *The mentality of apes*. New York: Hartcourt, Brace and World, 1925.

Kreuger, W. C. F. The effect of overlearning on retention. *Journal of Experimental Psychology*, 1929, **12**:71-78.

Kuenne, M. R. Experimental investigation of the relation of language to transposition behavior in young children. *Journal of Experimental Pschology*. 1946, **36**:471-490.

Lawrence, D. H. The transfer of a discrimination along a continuum. *Journal of Comparative and Physiological Psychology*, 1952, **45**:511-516.

Lordahl, D. S., and Archer, E. J. Transfer effects on a rotary pursuit task as a function of first-task difficulty. *Journal of Experimental Psychology*, 1958, **56**:421-426.

Maier, N. R. F. Reasoning in humans: I. On direction. *Journal of Comparative Psychology*, 1930, **10**:115-143.

Mandler, G. From association to structure. *Psychological Review*, 1962, **69**:415-427.

Miller, N. E., and Dollard, J. *Social learning and initiation*. New Haven,. Conn.: Yale University Press, 1941.

Murdock, B. B., Jr. Transfer designs and formulas. *Psychological Bulletin*, 1957, **54**:313-326.

Murdock, B. B., Jr. Response factors in learning and transfer. *American Journal of Psychology*, 1960, **73**:355-369.

Noble, C. E. Meaningfulness *(m)* and transfer phenomena in serial verbal learning. Paper presented at the 31st meeting of the Midwestern Psychological Association, Chicago, 1959.

Norcross, K. J., and Spiker, C. C. The effects of type of stimulus pretraining on discrimination performance in preschool children. *Child Development*, 1957, **28**:79-84.

Norcross, K. J., and Spiker, C. C. Effects of mediated association on transfer in paired-associate learning. *Journal of Experimental Psychology*, 1958, **55**:129-134.

Osgood, C. E. The similarity paradox in human learning: a resolution. *Psychological Review*, 1949, **56**:132-143.

Postman, L. Transfer of training as a function of experimental paradigm and degree of first list learning. *Journal of Verbal Learning and Verbal Behavior*, 1962, **1**:109-118.

Robinson, J. S. The effect of learning labels for stimuli on their later discrimination. *Journal of Experimental Psychology*, 1955, **49**:112-115.

Schulz, R. W. Problem solving behavior and transfer. *Harvard Educational Review*, 1960, **30**:61-429.

Spence, K. W. The nature of discrimination learning in animals. *Psychological Review*, 1946, **43**:427-449.

Spiker, C. C., Gerjuoy, C. R., and Shepard, W. O. Children's concept of middle sizedness and performance on the intermediate size problem. *Journal of Comparative and Physiological Psychology*, 1956, **49**:416-419.

Taylor, D. W., and Faust, W. L. Twenty questions: Efficiency in problem solving as a function of size of group. *Journal of Experimental Psychology*, 1952, **44**:360-368.

Underwood, B. J. Proactive inhibition as a function of time and degree of prior learning. *Journal of Experimental Psychology*, 1949, **39**:24-34.

Underwood B. J., and Schulz, R. W. *Meaningfulness and verbal learning*. Philadelphia: J. B. Lippincott Co., 1960.

Werner, O. H. The influence of the study of modern foreign language on the development of desirable abilities in English. *Studies in Modern Language Teaching*, 1930, **17**:97-145.

Wittrock, M. C. Verbal stimuli in concept formation, learning by discovery. *Journal of Educational Psychology*, 1963, **54**:183-190.

Wittrock, M. C. *Transfer through verbal cuing in concept identification.* U.S. Office of Education, Cooperative Research Project No. 1684, University of California, Los Angeles, 1964.

Wittrock, M. C. *The effects of verbal cues on transfer of training.* U.S. Department of Health Education and Welfare, Title VII, Project No. 1107, University of California, Los Angeles, 1965.

Wittrock, M. C. Three conceptual approaches to research on transfer of training. In R. M. Gagne and W. J. Gephart (Eds.), *Learning, research and school subjects.* Itasca, Ill.: F. E. Peacock Publishers, Inc., 1968.

Wittrock, M. C., and Hill, C. E. *Children's preferences in the transfer of learning,* U.S. Department of Health, Education and Welfare, Project No. 3264, University of California, Los Angeles, 1968.

Wittrock, M. C., Keislar, E. R., and Stern, C. S. Verbal cues in concept identification. *Journal of Educational Psychology*, 1964, **55**:195-200.

Wittrock, M. C., and Keislar, E. R. Verbal cues in transfer of concepts. *Journal of Educational Psychology*, 1965, **56**:16-21.

Wittrock, M. C., and Twelker, P. A. Prompting and feedback in the learning retention and transfer of concepts. *British Journal of Educational Psychology*, 1964, **34**:10-18.

Behavior modification: initiating or acquiring behavior

DESCRIPTION OF MODULE

This is an independent unit of instruction on initiating or acquiring behavior. Understanding the content of this module is dependent on the student's level of knowledge in conditions of learning and models of instruction and content on transfer of learning. The content of this module covers five major areas that are presented in an integrated form: (1) theoretical framework, (2) relevant research studies, (3) application to nursing education and practice, (4) issues, and (5) researchable questions. In addition to the main content of the module, it also contains the module objectives, a pretest and posttest, an answer key, and additional learning experiences.

MODULE OBJECTIVES

On completion of this module and the content listed in the recommended reading list, the student will be able to accomplish the following objectives at the 95% level of accomplishment:

1. Describe in own words the theoretical framework of initiating or acquiring a behavior
2. Identify the steps involved in initiating a behavior
3. Select a specific patient- or student-learning situation and apply the principle of initiating behavior
4. Identify one issue
5. Raise one researchable question
6. Cite research studies that support the theoretical framework

PRETEST AND POSTTEST

Circle the correct answers. Each question is worth 1 point except questions 10, 11, and 12, which are worth 5, 6 and 10 points, respectively. The 95% level of mastery for this test is 29 correct points. Take the test and correct your answers using the answer key that is found at the end of this module (pp. 296-297).

Multiple choice

1. There are preconditions that must be established and must precede the learning event itself and that operate to determine the probability of learning; these preconditions are:
   1—attentional set
   2—I.Q.
   3—motivation
   4—developmental readiness
   a. all of the above
   b. 1, 3, and 4
   c. 1 and 3
   d. 2, 3, and 4

2. A nursing instructor teaching pharmacology made a study of the nursing class and discovered that most of the students could not work out simple fractions. The instructor was faced with a problem of:
   a. readiness
   b. maturation
   c. lack of attentional set
   d. unmotivated students
3. According to Bruner (1964), uncertainty is the major condition for:
   a. activation
   b. maintenance
   c. direction
4. According to Skinner, two techniques for initiating behavior more effectively are:
   a. making the model more apparent to the learner
   b. making certain that the student responds to the stimulus situation
   c. helping the student to discriminate between the subtle features of the stimulus situation
   d. having the student always initiate the behavior
5. In initiating behavior, Skinner believes that:
   a. priming is the most important force in learning
   b. reinforcement is the key to learning
   c. reinforcement and priming are equally important in learning
6. Which one of the following statements indicates that acquisition of a behavior has occurred?
   a. The individual cannot do a particular performance but would like to.
   b. The individual can verbalize items in the stimulus configuration that is being attended.
   c. The individual can execute some performance that could not be done previously.
7. Before learners can respond to a stimulus, they must first:
   a. perceive and code the stimulus correctly
   b. know that a reward is in store that is concrete in nature
   c. none of the above
8. Giving the learners information about the type of behavior expected at the completion of instructional event serves the function of:
   a. reducing the learners' anxiety
   b. providing direction to their learning
   c. enabling the students to match their own responses with a response class previously learned
   d. delineating the students' responsibility
9. According to Bruner (1964), curiosity and drive to achieve are:
   a. genetically determined
   b. extrinsic motives
   c. intrinsic motives
   d. the determinant of exploratory behavior

Discussion questions

10. Briefly describe the methods the teacher can use in gaining and controlling the students' attention.
11. Explain the uses and function of the pretest in instruction.
12. Select a specific patient- or student-teaching situation and initiate the behavior in the learner. Specify the steps you will follow.

TEXT
Theoretical background

Initiating behavior may be operationally defined as enabling an individual to perform an act or response so the behavior or the response learned and performed becomes a part of the individual learner's own repertoire. The behavior gets integrated into the internal organization system of the individual and can be viewed as a relatively permanent change in an observable behavior.

According to Gagne (1970) learning entails three components: (1) the learner, or the subject; (2) the stimulus or the stimulus situation; and (3) the response, or behavior. In order to obtain the response, the instructor manipulates the stimulus situation by altering the conditions and the timing of the presentation of the stimulus. "Control of the external events in the learning situation is what is typically meant by the word 'instruction.' These are events that are manipulated by the teacher, the textbook writer, the designer of films or television lessons, the developer of self-instructional programs" (Gagne, 1970, p. 303).

The external events of instruction are a part of the total set of instructional events, but they are not all that comprise the instructional sequence. Instruction may be seen as being comprised of a set of separate events, each of which has a distinctive effect on the learner.

Identification of the expected response, or the terminal behavior, expected of the learner is the first step in initiating any behavior. This can be done by identifying verbally or in written form the type of behavior, or performance, expected of the learner on completion of the instructional events. This is often referred to as a statement of objectives that are observable or measurable. By giving the learner information about the class of responses expected at the completion of the instructional events, the learner gets (1) direction to the learning, that is, an internal set that allows the learner to reject extraneous and irrelevant stimuli and (2) knowledge of expected performance, which enables the student to match personal responses with a response class the learner remembers, so reinforcement functions can occur. The research studies of Maier (1930) and Ausubel (1960) support these propositions.

The learner comes to the stimulus situation with a specific level of knowledge. This is often referred to as the student's level of entering behavior, in other words, in the events of instruction the first aspect of the learner's behavior that must be assessed is that of entering behavior. Assessment of the entering behavior of the student constitutes the second step in the process of initiating a behavior. A list of entering behaviors has two characteristics: the statements are explicit and refer to specific, observable performances; and the list, as a whole, is generally more comprehensive than the corresponding

list of terminal performances (DeCecco, 1968, p. 61).

Gagne (1970) stated that there are three preconditions that are internal to the learner and are controllable through environmental changes that can be made prior to the arrival of the learner in the stimulus situation. These three preconditions affect the acquisition of behavior by the learner. They include: (1) developmental readiness, (2) motivation, and (3) attentional set.

1. Gagne stressed the learner's state of *readiness* in terms of the learner's entering behavior. The relevant prerequisite skills necessary to perform a task are the subordinate level of knowledge that the learner must possess before any learning or transfer of learning is expected to occur at the higher level. If the learner possesses these relevant subordinate levels of knowledge—Gagne also calls them prerequisite "learning sets" —then the learner is viewed as being in a "state of readiness."

2. *Motivation* is the second precondition for initiating behavior. Motivation refers to those factors that increase and decrease the vigor of an individual's activity. It determines the degree or level of activity that will be initiated, and by strengthening an individual's motivation, there is an increased likelihood of the learner making the response that has been learned best (DeCecco, 1968, p. 132). Motivation is an important aspect of learning. It is possible, however, to instruct unmotivated individuals and enable them to learn, with the hope that acquisition of knowledge will generate an intrinsic desire for more knowledge, Bruner (1964) and Berlyne (1960) agree that in order to activate an individual to perform a task or explore alternatives in a task, a certain optimal amount of uncertainty in the situation is necessary. Berlyne has demonstrated that curiosity is a response to uncertainty and ambiguity. Bruner pointed out that a routine task arouses little explora-

tory behavior, a task that is too uncertain may arouse confusion and anxiety, with the effect of reducing exploration. Bruner also suggested that curiosity and drive to achieve are intrinsic motives that attract and sustain the learner's attention to something that is somewhat unclear, unfinished, or uncertain. Thus Bruner implies that curiosity creates what Gagne refers to as the attentional set.

3. The *attentional set* allows the learner to select and apprehend appropriate stimuli. Gagne (1970) indicated that every learning act requires an apprehending phase, which is dependent on attention. Attending to relevant stimuli is facilitated by having the stimulus situation contain elements of change, novelty, intensity of stimulation, and so on. Gagne believes that to provide continuously for such external "attention getters" would be an impossible task for instruction in school settings. He, therefore, suggested that there must be a mechanism whereby attending is internally controlled and enables the learner to select stimuli to be apprehended at the appropriate time. Such an internal state is referred to as *set* by Hebb (1966) and *attentional set* by Gagne (1970).

Gagne (1970) further pointed out that young children initially learn certain stimulus-response chains that govern their own behaviors in observing stimuli that form the external conditions of learning. Children must also learn to direct their sense organs toward the source of stimulation in order to discriminate the distinctive features of the stimulus, to maintain the internal cues that determine sequence of action, and to continue doing their specific act in face of internal or external distractions. These capabilities Gagne classified as aspects of attentional sets. Learning appropriate kinds of attentional sets can be achieved and explained by means of basic kinds of learning, connections, and chains.

A third step that needs to be mentioned in the realm of acquiring new behavior is the *presentation of the stimulus situation*. The general forms of stimuli are determined by the type of learning that must be undertaken. For simple forms of learning stimuli are those features of stimulus objects that are to serve as cues to the stimulus-response connections. In discrimination learning, contrasting stimuli presented during "contrast practice" are necessary for the establishment of connections that differentiate among these stimuli. For concrete concepts, a variety of stimulus objects are needed to represent the class being learned. Finally, for defined concepts and rules, verbal stimuli presented in the proper sequence are usually employed to arouse the concepts that are being combined to form them.

In gaining attention, the function of verbal direction is to direct attention to the object or characteristic that is to become the stimulus in a learned connection. In the simpler forms of learning, the instructor may say, "Now watch this," while holding up a stimulus object or pointing to a stimulus event. In the acquisition of concepts and principles, since the content itself is represented verbally, methods are sought to distinguish this content from the directions. It is common to find the concepts italicized, underlined, or printed in bold type.

The fourth step in the process of initiating behavior is *to get the learner to emit or elicit the response*, in other words, to perform the task. Once the terminal behavior has been specified, arrangements must be made to strengthen it through reinforcement. If the learners have the appropriate response capability in their repertoire, association of the response with a previously unrelated stimulus can be accomplished through the use of principles of operant or classical conditioning or the use of reinforcement theory in general. As mentioned previously, the technique utilized to initiate the behavior will depend on the nature of the behavior or the task to be performed by the learner. For example, if the behavior to be initiated is a good habit, classical conditioning principles can be used. If it is an instrumental response that has to be initiated (for example, getting an autistic child to label objects or getting catatonic patients to leave their rooms) then principles of operant conditioning can be utilized. Each of the seven basic conditions of learning require specific approaches to getting them started. In general however, according to Skinner (1968), the acquisition of the change in behavior is most efficiently achieved through the use of simple techniques of reinforcements, that is, making reinforcements contingent on desired behavior. The skill required of the teacher is the ability to arrange the contingencies of reinforcement. Once behavior is initiated, it can be sustained by means of a specified schedule of reinforcement.

As mentioned previously, once the terminal behavior is specified, appropriate arrangements must be made to initate the first behavior and strengthen it through reinforcement. Appropriateness of this arrangement depends on the *learner's characteristics,* such as whether the learner is a child or an adult, of normal intelligence or retarded, whether the learner is able to follow verbal instructions or not, and whether the learner possesses the motivation and capabilities required for the task to be performed. Another factor that determines the appropriateness of the arrangements and interventions to be used to initiate the first instance is the *nature of the task.* For example, does the task require a motor performance or a more cognitive (abstract concept) performance. Does the stimulus situation require that the learner be able to see, touch, and hear in order to perform the task, or does it only require one of the sensory channels? Another factor that determines the appropriateness of

the arrangements to initiate the first instance of behavior is the *type of schedule of reinforcement* to be used. Does the reinforcement have an incentive value for the subject? Skinner does not use the word motivation or drive to get the learner to perform the first instance of behavior. He stated that the incentive value of the reinforcement used, the contingencies, and the schedule of reinforcement determine whether a behavior will occur or not.

Therefore, having these determinants of contingencies of reinforcements and appropriate arrangement of conditions of interventions in mind, the teacher, the therapist, or the nurse can initiate the first instance of behavior by the following methods. First, the teacher can wait until the behavior occurs, then reinforce it. However, Skinner (1968) pointed out that simply waiting for the desired behavior to occur so that it can be reinforced is inefficient because it may take a very long time for the learner to emit the correct response—if ever. If time is of essence, then this method is inappropriate.

Shaping behavior by means of progressive approximation is another method of initiating the first instance. It utilizes operant-conditioning principles. For example, if the subject or the learner is a mentally retarded or autistic child and the behavior desired is correct labeling of objects or reading from a book, then the technique of "shaping" behavior can be utilized. The initiation of the desired behavior in this case is the initiation of a response that is related to the final response. As each successive stimulus-response connection is learned, the reinforcement is changed and is associated with the next stage in the acquisition of the first behavior. The previous stimulus-response link is no longer reinforced. This approximation procedure continues until the final desired behavior is emitted by the learner. For example, in teaching an autistic or mentally retarded child to read, the procedure of shaping behavior entails the following steps: reinforcement is given when the child makes the first move toward the book; then only when the child touches the book; then only for opening the book; then, when the child attempts to verbalize what is seen on the open page, no matter how wrong the pronounciation (although the correction is made); then reinforcement is withheld until the responses are more accurate, until at last the child correctly identifies what is on the page.

The reinforcement used must have incentive value for the learner. It may be candies —primary reinforcement—at first. Then the learner may graduate to secondary social reinforcements, such as praise, hug, gold star, or others. Secondary social reinforcement must be paired with primary reinforcement until the former acquires the incentive values (properties) of the primary reinforcers. Then they can be used without the primary reinforcement. During the acquisition phase of the behavior, the reinforcement has to be on a 100% level, that is, reinforcement has to be given after every response.

The technique of shaping behavior is appropriate with certain types of behavior, such as whenever instrumental type of learning is involved. Skinner (1968, p. 207) noted that shaping behavior through progressive approximation can be tedious. There are better ways of solving the "problem of the first instance."

Skinner (1968) suggested that at times the behavior is physically forced; for example, when a child's hand is squeezed about a pencil and moved to make a form. Other situations in which such a technique can be used is in teaching a patient how to walk correctly with crutches. The nurse can place the crutches under the arm pits of the patient and place the patient's hands in the center portion of the crutches; then the nurse can move the right leg forward, then the left, and

so on. In addition to physically placing ("forcing") the crutches at the appropriate places of the body and physically moving the legs in forward movements, the nurse utilizes verbal directions. As the behavior is performed by the patient (that is, appropriate use of crutches in walking motions), reinforcement is given by the nurse to strengthen the desired behavior. Other examples where such a technique of physically forcing the behavior to occur can be utilized are when the surgical nurse teaches a preoperative chest patient how to cough. For example, the nurse may place pillows underneath the diaphragm of the patient (or may place the patient's hands over the diaphragm), then ask the patient to cough, and so on. Here again, the nurse may also use verbal directions and demonstration in addition to getting the patient to do it. Positive reinforcement is given when the correct behavior is performed by the patient. Another example of physically forcing the behavior to occur may be in a situation where a judge forces a parent who batters a child to attend rehabilitation (corrective) classes.

Another technique that can be used in initiating the first instance of behavior is to use stimuli that will elicit, or evoke, the response to be reinforced. For example, use of stimuli that attract the learner's attention. A teacher may induce a student to pay attention to whatever is being written on the blackboard or to the chart on the board by moving the object about conspicuously or by saying, "Look at this bone." The behavior expected of the learner in this case may be the correct identification of the name of the bone in the chart. The stimuli used by the teacher— "Look at this bone" or "what is the name of *this* bone?"—will evoke the correct response of labeling "tibia". That is then reinforced. The studies of Konorski and Miller (1937) support this proposition. In their experiment, a dog's foot was shocked, and the resulting flexion by the dog was reinforced with food. The operant response of flexion eventually appeared in the absence of the shock. Skinner cited another example of smearing food on the lever a rat is to press, or fastening a grain of corn to the key a pigeon is to peck. Skinner also pointed out that these techniques of inducing the first instance of behavior are relevant only to a small part of standard terminal behavior.

There are still other techniques that the teacher can utilize to evoke behavior in the student. One such technique is that of *priming*. Imitation is a form of primed behavior. The three types of imitative learning that could be utilized to evoke the first instance of the behavior are movement duplication, product duplication and nonduplicative repertoire.

1. *Movement duplication*. As the name implies, in movement duplication the learner reproduces the type of behavior that is observed in the model. The type of behaviors that can be produced by movement-duplication technique are those that involve motor performance as the learner imitates the movements of the model. Skinner (1968) pointed out that a small part of imitative behavior may be innate, but learning of such behaviors is mostly acquired because behavior is naturally reinforced when it resembles the behavior of the model. Imitation through movement-duplicating contingencies are most effectively learned or acquired when the model is conspicuous. Such is the case when the model exaggerates the specific important aspects of the behavior or repeats it slowly. Movement-duplicating contingencies are improved if the learner is first taught to discriminate between subtle features of behavior.

An example of this would be when the nurse (model) demonstrates to the new mother how to bathe her infant. When the nurse demonstrates and emphasizes the proper positioning of the head by repeating slowly and exaggerating a little, then the new mother can discriminate between proper versus improper positioning of the baby's head during bathing. As a result of such movement-duplicating contingencies, the mother can acquire the new behavior (bathing the newborn baby) more quickly and more accurately.

The studies of Bandura, Ross, and Ross (1961, 1963) have demonstrated the acquisition of aggressive behaviors in children as a result of observing a model demonstrate aggressive behaviors.

Movement-duplicating techniques can be utilized to initiate behaviors that can be performed by observing a model do it. Most nursing skills, especially procedures, are a series of behaviors that could be initiated and acquired by this technique.

2. *Product duplication*. The type of imitation involved in product duplication is the imitation of vocal behavior. Skinner (1968, p. 209) pointed out that "movement cannot be easily duplicated if the behavior of the model cannot be seen, but its effects may be. For example, movements involved in speech cannot be seen; but their effect can be duplicated, and it is reinforcing when the speaker's own speech resembles the speech that has just been heard. Imitation by means of product duplication can be utilized in speech therapy. The same may apply to stroke patients who are in the process of rehabilitation because their speech center has been affected by the stroke. They can hear a speech therapist or a nurse pronounce a word, then they can repeat it. They can record their own voices and then listen to determine if their speech resembles that uttered by the model.

Product duplication can also be used in microteaching. This is form of simulated experience where students present their lectures and a videotape recording of their lecture is taken. Afterward, they can hear their voices on the replay and analyze whether what they have said is clear and makes sense.

3. *Nonduplicative repertoire.* The third imitative situation that could be used to create the first instance of the behavior is nonduplicative repertoire. This is the situation where verbal instruction or direction is given to produce a behavior. Skinner (1968) referred to this situation as a form of primed behavior that is acquired with the help of pre-established repertoires in which neither the responses nor their products resemble controlling stimuli. Behaviors initiated by means of nonduplicative repertoire are like instructions telling the learner what to do at any given point in time. In this sense, they are like the directions printed on packages to tell purchasers how to open them; for example, the directions may state, "first, pull tab, then press with thumb." In a similar way, in verbal directions to the learner one may say, "First remove the cap from the needle, then insert the needle into the skin at a 90-degree angle, aspirate, inject fluid, withdraw, and apply pressure." These are verbal instructions given to the student nurse learning to give an intramuscular injection. Of course the events of instruction can be controlled without verbal directions, and they may have to be with a young child or with emotionally disturbed or retarded adults who do not understand the words. But typically, verbal communication is the preferred mode of instructional direction.

In summary, therefore, a behavior can be initiated by having the teacher or the nurse follow these steps:

1. Identify the terminal behavior that the learner is to exhibit or perform at the completion of instruction or intervention

2. Assess the entering behavior of the learner to determine if the learner possesses the subordinate capabilities required to perform the task, taking into consideration the developmental readiness of the learner, the motivation, and the attentional set

3. Present the stimulus situation, that is, under what circumstances the learner will be able to perform the task (Is the stimulus situation a problem to be solved, or a procedure to be performed?)

4. Get the learner to emit the response, that is, to perform, again taking into consideration the learner's characteristics, the nature of the task, and the type of schedule of reinforcement used and utilizing one or more of the following procedures to elicit the first instance of behavior depending on the nature of the task:

   a. Waiting until the subject acts or behaves and then reinforcing the learner

   b. Shaping behavior

   c. Physically forcing the behavior to occur

   d. Using priming behavior: (1) movement-duplication technique, if the task to be performed is a physical or motor performance; (2) product-duplication technique if the behavior required is of verbal or speech in nature; or (3) nonduplicative repertoire if the task to be performed can be done by means of verbal directions or communication

Measurement of acquired behavior

Kimble (1961) pointed out that acquisition of behavior is the basic process assumed to operate in learning studies. Whether a behavior is acquired or not is reflected in changes in several different response measures. The most common of which are the following:

1. *Probability of occurrence*—expressed as the percentage of trials with which a given subject produces a conditioned response, or the percentage of subjects giving a conditioned response on a given trial

2. *Latency*—the time between the presentation of a signal and the occurrence of a conditioned response

3. *Rate of responding*—the number of conditioned responses produced in some standard period of time

4. *Response magnitude*—some measure that reflects the vigor of response on trials when it occurs
5. *Response speed*—the reciprocal of some time measure such as latency
6. *Response to extinction*—the number of unreinforced responses that occur before the attainment of some criterion of extinction, measures the strength of conditioning

Almost any of these measures will reflect the process of acquisition, at least under certain circumstances (Kimble, 1961, p. 82). Depending on the type of behavior initiated and acquired by the learner, some of these measures could be used by the teacher or the nurse to evaluate the success of instruction and intervention in initiating a behavior.

Issues in initiating behavior

Issues in the area of initating behavior through behavior modification deal with the explanation of the underlying process of initiating behavior. For example, Skinner (1968) would say that motivation, or drive, is not an important concept in initiating behavior. His strategy is to arrange the contingencies and schedules of reinforcement. Other behavioral scientists, such as Kimble (1961) and Harlow (1950) would explain the causes, or underlying mechanism, of initiating behavior terms of drive reduction.

Researchable questions

1. What is the effect of different types of teaching strategies (independent-study techniques versus traditional lecture and discussion) on initiating the desire for continued education after graduation?
   a. Independent variable: teaching strategies (independent-study versus lecture-discussion technique)
   b. Dependent variable: initiation of the desire for continued education after graduation

2. What is the effect of different types of reinforcements used (positive or negative) on initiating and maintaining a "dieting" behavior in diabetic patients (newly discovered versus long-time diabetics)?
   a. Independent variables: (1) negative and positive reinforcements and (2) newly discovered versus long-time diabetics
   b. Dependent variable: initiating and maintaining the diabetic dieting behavior

ADDITIONAL LEARNING EXPERIENCES—RECOMMENDED READING LIST

DeCecco, J., and Crawford W. *The psychology of learning and instruction: educational psychology.* (2nd Ed.) Englewood Cliffs, N.J. Prentice-Hall, Inc., 1974, pp. 47-69.

Gagne, R. *The conditions of learning.* (2nd Ed.) New York: Holt, Rinehart and Winston, Inc., 1970, pp. 302-380.

Skinner, B. F. *The technology of teaching.* New York: Appleton-Century-Crofts, 1968, pp. 199-226.

INSTRUCTIONS TO THE LEARNER REGARDING POSTTEST

At this point in the learning process you are ready to take the posttest to determine the extent to which you have achieved the objectives of this module. Return to the pretest and take it again as the posttest. Correct your answers by using the answer key that is found on this page and the next. If your score is less than 29 correct points, correct your errors and study the content of this module and some of the references found in the recommended reading list. Take the posttest again. You need to study in this fashion until you achieve the 95% mastery level.

ANSWER KEY TO PRETEST AND POSTTEST

1. b (Gagne, 1970, pp. 277-279)
2. a (DeCecco 1968, p. 61)
3. a (Bruner, 1964, p. 309)
4. a and c (Skinner, 1968, p. 206)

5. b (Skinner, 1968, p. 212)
6. c (Gagne, 1970, p. 74)
7. a (Gagne, 1970, p. 72)
8. b and c (DeCecco 1968, pp. 47-69)
9. c and d (Bruner, 1964, pp. 308-309)
10. Guideline to answer:
    a. Verbal directions
    b. Gestures made by the teacher
    c. Sudden movement of an object
    d. Variety of illustrations used as a part of instruction
    e. Distinguishing concepts by italicizing, underlining, printing in bold type, and other means.
    f. Setting content apart by color by use of a surrounding box
    (Gagne, 1970, pp. 305-306)
11. Pretests are a way of helping the teacher assess the level of knowledge that the student has on entering the class, or the patient before learning. It helps the teacher know where the gaps in information are and then helps to determine in which areas the student may need more help. Hopefully, this method will help the teacher see the individual differences in students and plan information-giving and teaching accordingly.
    (DeCecco and Crawford, 1974, pp. 48-51)
12. Answer should include the following steps in given sequence:
    a. Identify the terminal behavior
    b. Assess the entering behavior
    c. Present the stimulus situation
    d. Initiate the first instance by means of:
       (1) Shaping
       (2) Physically forcing the behaviors to occur
       (3) Priming behaviors—3 types of initiation:
           (a) Movement duplication
           (b) Product duplication
           (c) Nonduplicative repertoire
    e. Evaluate

REFERENCES

Ausubel, D. P., *Educational psychology: a cognitive view*. New York: Holt, Rinehart and Winston, Inc., 1968.

Bandura, A., Ross, D., and Ross, S. Transmission of aggression through imitation of aggressive models. *Journal of Abnormal Social Psychology*, 1961, **63:** 575-582.

Bandura, A., Ross, D., and Ross, S. Imitation of film-mediated aggressive models. *Journal of Abnormal Social Psychology*, 1963, **66:**3-11.

Berlyne, D. E. *Conflict, arousal and curiosity*. New York: McGraw-Hill Book Co., 1960.

Bruner, J. Some theorems on instruction illustrated with reference to mathematics. In E. R. Hilgard (Ed.), *Theories of learning and instruction*. The 63rd Yearbook of NSSE. Chicago: The University of Chicago Press, 1964, pp. 306-335.

DeCecco, J. P. *The psychology of learning and instruction: educational psychology*. (1st Ed.) Englewood Cliffs, N.J.: Prentice-Hall, Inc., 1968.

DeCecco, J., and Crawford, W. *The psychology of learning and instruction: educational psychology*. (2nd Ed.) Englewood Cliffs, N.J.: Prentice-Hall, Inc., 1974.

Gagne, R. *The conditions of learning*. (2nd Ed.) New York: Holt, Rhinehart, and Winston, Inc., 1970.

Harlow, H. F. Learning and satiation of response in intrinsically motivated complex puzzle performance by monkeys. *Journal of Comparative Physiological Psychology*, 1950, **43:**289-294.

Hebb, D. O. *A textbook of psychology*. (2nd Ed.) Philadelphia: W. B. Saunders Co., 1966.

Kimble, G. A. *Hilgard and Marquis' conditioning and learning*. New York: Appleton-Century-Crofts, 1961.

Konorski, J. A., and Miller, S. M. On two types of conditioned reflex. *Journal of Genetic Psychology*, 1937, **16:**264-272.

Maier, N. R. F. Reasoning in humans: I. On direction. *Journal of Comparative Psychology*, 1930, **10:**115-143.

Skinner, B. F. *The technology of teaching*. New York: Appleton-Century-Crofts, 1968.

MODULE 19

Behavior modification: eliminating, or extinguishing, behavior

DESCRIPTION OF MODULE

This module on eliminating behavior is a self-contained unit of study. It is an aspect of behavior-modification technique to eliminate undesirable behavior. The contents of this module are presented in sequential order. The text of the module covers five major areas presented in an integrated form. They include: (1) theoretical framework, (2) relevant research studies, (3) issues, (4) application to nursing education and practice, and (5) raising researchable questions. In addition to the text, the module contains learner objectives, pre- and posttest, and an answer key for correcting your answers and for feedback purposes. Additional learning experiences are also provided.

MODULE OBJECTIVES

At the completion of this module, having studied the content very carefully and read the additional recommended reading list, the student will be able to accomplish the following set of objectives at the 95% level of accomplishment. The student will be able to:
1. Explain in written form or orally the different methods of eliminative behavior
2. Describe the different theoretical frameworks that attempt to explain the basic

mechanism underlying the extinction procedure
3. Identify the pros and cons of at least one issue in the area of eliminating behavior
4. Explain the difference between extinction and forgetting
5. Select a specific case study that demonstrates a maladaptive behavior and apply to it the principles of behavior-modification technique pertinent to eliminating behavior
6. Raise at least one researchable question and identify both the independent and dependent variables

PRETEST AND POSTTEST

Circle the correct answers. Each question is worth 1 point, except questions 39 through 41, which are each worth 5 points. The 95% mastery level for this test is 50 correct points. Take the test and correct your answers, utilizing the answer key found at the end of this module (pp. 311-312).

Multiple choice

1. A woman comes to an out-patient clinic with the following situation. She is 30 years old and married. Her relationship with her spouse is good. She had always enjoyed driving a car.

However, since seeing a terrible accident 3 years ago, she developed increased apprehension about driving. Now, the fear is even present when her husband drives the car. Presently, she panics and tries to avoid being in a car at all costs, and this is interfering with her life. Which theoretical framework accounts for the acquisition of the maladaptive behavior?
a. operant conditioning
b. classical conditioning
c. discrimination learning
d. negative reinforcement

2. In the above example which method of eliminating behavior is most appropriate?
a. use of punishment
b. broncobusting
c. method of toleration (desensitization)
d. regular extinction procedure

3. Which of the following methods of eliminating undesirable behaviors have the most potential for producing undesirable side effects?
a. aversive stimulation
b. extinction
c. withdrawal of positive reinforcement
d. satiation

4. Which of the following methods of eliminating behavior produces the most rapid result in decreasing self-destructive behavior?
a. aversive stimulation
b. withdrawal of positive reinforcement
c. counterconditioning
d. extinction
e. satiation

5. Satiation technique in eliminating unwanted behaviors should *not* be used:
a. when a child is lighting matches
b. to reduce incessant talking
c. to reduce hoarding of items such as towels
d. to reduce excessive eating behaviors by an overweight person

6. In order to eliminate a behavior by means of extinction, an important criterion must be met to make this procedure effective. The criterion is:
a. a willing subject
b. omission of all reinforcements for the undesirable behavior
c. having an incompatible desirable behavior to replace the desirable one

d. the behavior that is to be eliminated must have been learned on a continuous schedule of reinforcement

7. Evidence from studies in animal learning indicates that responses resist extinction more when they have been reinforced on a:
a. delayed schedule
b. partial schedule
c. continuous schedule
d. immediate schedule

8. In signal learning, behavior is eliminated by:
a. presentation of the conditioned stimulus without the unconditioned stimulus
b. presentation of the unconditioned stimulus without the conditioned stimulus
c. lack of reinforcement of the response

9. The difference between forgetting and extinction is:
a. extinction occurs when a response is not rewarded, whereas, forgetting occurs when a response is not practiced
b. there is no difference between forgetting and extinction
c. extinction refers to permanent elimination of behavior, whereas, forgetting is temporary

10. Extinction in discrimination learning is a result of:
a. learning subsequent chains in the same situation
b. insufficient practice
c. not varying the reinforcement schedule

11. In multiple discrimination tasks, extinction occurs:
a. from failing to reinforce any particular chain
b. in the correct response as well as the incorrect
c. if there is hesitation in repetition

12. In verbal learning, extinction of previously learned material is considered to be:
a. the basic phenomenon of interference
b. often produced by the act of making an initial mistake
c. different from other forms of learning

13. A person has been a fingernail biter for some time now, but wants to stop. In order to eliminate this behavior, which of the following should occur:

a. must receive punishment for biting the nails
b. must not receive internal or external satisfaction (reward) for nail biting
c. must not be allowed to complete the satisfying last link in the chain of biting the nails

14. Correct statements about extinction would include which of the following:
   a. The probability that a response will occur is decreased each time it is not reinforced.
   b. A way to weaken or to eliminate a response is to make two responses incompatible.
   c. If a teacher does not reinforce the correct responses that a student makes, the forces of extinction may work to weaken both correct and incorrect student responses.
   d. all of the above

Fill in the blank

15. One of the theories of extinction is that it is an active process of _____, generated by the act of responding that depresses the strength of the learned response.
   a. inhibition
   b. fading
   c. diminishing reactions
   d. delineation

16. Another theoretical explanation for eliminating learning is that it is mainly a matter of learning other connections that _____ with the initially learned one.
   a. conflict
   b. interfere
   c. disagree

Matching

Match the following types of learning with their corresponding ways to extinguish the behavior.

Part A
____17. Signal learning
____18. Operant conditioning
____19. Skill learning
____20. Discrimination learning

Part B
a. Not reinforcing final link of chain or preventing final link from occurring

b. Learning chains that interfere with originally learned chains
c. Presenting conditioned stimulus along without its unconditioned stimulus over a period of time
d. Removal of reward after a response

Match the following activities to indicate if they are part of assessment (A), intervention (I), or evaluation (E).

____21. Defining the target behavior in operational terms
____22. Making observations of frequency of behavior
____23. Using the differential reinforcement method
____24. Recording baseline data
____25. Applying intervention
____26. Monitoring the patient's progress during intervention
____27. Determining if the undesirable behavior is decreasing
____28. Identifying the antecedents
____29. Designating the contingency between target behavior and reinforcers
____30. Using instruction (if used)
____31. Using shaping
____32. Ascertaining if the observation made about the patient's behavior is accurate

Match the following terms and definitions:

Part A
____33. Discrimination
____34. Generalization
____35. Reinforcing other behavior
____36. Spontaneous recovery
____37. Deprivation
____38. Satiation

Part B
a. Identification of cues that differentiate the circumstances for response in one way under one set of circumstances but not another
b. Lack of a particular reinforcement for a long period of time
c. Process by which one response can come under the influence of other situations and provide opportunity for a specific behavior to occur
d. Receipt of large amounts of reinforcement

e. Administration of positive reinforcers only when an adaptive behavior occurs that is incompatible with the maladaptive behavior

f. Recurrence of the undesirable behavior after a period of extinction

Discussion questions

39. What is spontaneous recovery, and what is its implication to eliminating behavior?

40. According to Gagne, what function does practice play in extinguishing certain responses during chain learning?

41. Describe how parents could use the theory of extinction to get a child to eliminate tyrant-like tantrum behavior.

TEXT
Theoretical background
Methods of eliminating behavior

Extinction is operationally defined as the process whereby a response that has been previously learned through reinforcement is permitted to occur and recur without reinforcement, by so doing, the response undergoes progressive decrement and eventually dies out. This process is called *extinction.*

Behavior can be eliminated by means of several different methods; for example, (1) extinction procedures, (2) counter-conditioning, (3) bronchobusting, or flooding techniques, and (4) the use of punishment. These are the most popular and most tested methods. There are other techniques, such as by means of modeling or discrimination teaching and psychotherapeutic techniques that have been partially successful in redoing the maladaptive behaviors rather than completely extinguishing them. In this module only the first four major techniques will be presented.

EXTINCTION

The conditions of extinction for different types of learnings vary. For example, any behavior that has been learned by means of classical conditioning can be extinguished by not pairing the conditioned stimulus (CS) (such as the bell in Pavlov's experiment) with the unconditioned stimulus (US) (such as the meat powder). The conditioned response (CR) of salivation will be extinguished after several trials of the unpaired conditioned stimulus.

A behavior that has been learned by means of operant conditioning can be eliminated simply by cutting out the reinforcement that follows the behavior. In other words, when a reinforcing stimulus no longer occurs following a response, the response becomes less and less frequent until it dies out. It is generally known that when one engages in behavior that no longer pays off, one is less inclined to behave in that way again. For example; if one continuously gets no answer when making a telephone call, one eventually stops telephoning that person. The behavior has not been positively reinforced; therefore, there is a good probability that it will be eliminated. Therefore, in the case of behaviors that are maintained by positive reinforcement, elimination can sometimes be accomplished simply by withdrawing the reinforcer.

Furthermore, in operant conditioning, the occurrence or the nonoccurrence of a behavior is determined by the consequences that follow that behavior; therefore, the *elimination of a given behavior is based on altering the consequences.* A vivid example of eliminating the maladaptive behavior of a young retarded girl who frequently vomited in the classroom was eliminated by changing the consequences that followed the behavior (Franks, 1969). Ordinarily, the child was returned to the hall when she vomited. In order to eliminate that behavior, the girl was not returned to the hall when she vomited, and the class continued to operate normally. In addition, praise and candy were used as reinforcers in an attempt to shape desirable behaviors. After a short spurt upward, the vomiting later dropped to zero and remained there. In this example, discontinuing the positive reinforcement, and reinforcing positively for the desirable behavior were used in eliminating the undesirable behavior.

In everyday situations it is sometimes difficult to achieve generalized elimination of behavior because different social agents are inconsistent in their reinforcement practices. For example, if parents no longer reward temper tantrums, but other significant adults continue to do so, a child will, in all likelihood, exhibit a discriminative pattern of negative behavior toward others in accord with their customary reinforcement practices. For example, Williams (1959) cited a case of a child who had been ill for some time and required special care and attention. After he had recovered from his illness, the parents attempted to withdraw some of their attention; but the child responded with tantrums, crying spells, and demands, especially at bedtime. They were instructed to put the child to bed in a nonpunitive manner and to ignore the child's screaming and crying. An immediate marked drop in the duration of tantrums occurred, followed by almost complete extinction of tantrums within a few days. However, the child's aunt began putting the child to bed, and the tantrums started again. The aunt stayed with the child and held him while he cried; therefore, the behavior was reinstated because the child had learned to discriminate his responses. Behavior of this kind is liable, if intermittently reinforced, to generalize and to become very troublesome.

An important point to keep in mind is the variable schedule of reinforcement and its effect on ease of extinction. It has been amply demonstrated that behaviors that are learned and maintained by means of intermittent schedule of reinforcement are extremely resistant to extinction; whereas, behaviors that are learned and maintained on a continuous schedule of reinforcement are easier to extinguish (Skinner, 1968).

Eliminating behavior through extinction may not always be the most effective and economical method of eliminating deviant behavior. It requires complete environmental control since the agents may unwittingly reinforce the behaviors that are being eliminated. However, when relevant reinforcers in the person's natural setting are willing to cooperate, eliminating of behavior by extinction becomes a much more feasible approach. It has been found possible to eliminate alcoholic drinking by enlisting the aid of the person's drinking companions. Friends have been instructed to emit, at a high rate, all of their usual social behavior (talking, joking, and other behaviors) as long as the person drank soft drinks. They would immediately withdraw all social reinforcers by ignoring the person the moment he began approaching and drinking hard liquor (Frank, 1969).

If a behavior is learned by means of chaining principles, extinction of such a behavior takes place when the reinforcement to the last terminal (S → R) link is omitted. The terminal behavior disappears first, followed by the other chains leading to the terminal behavior. For example, cigarette smoking is an undesirable behavior. The terminal act of inhaling the smoke is the reinforcement for smoking behavior. If inhaling does not bring reinforcement during smoking by giving pleasure or because of an unpleasant taste, then the behavior will soon become extinct, and all the chains leading up to the terminal behavior will also disappear; such as lighting the cigarette, taking the pack out of one's pocket, and so on (Gagne, 1970).

Behaviors that are learned by means of verbal associates are also subject to extinction. Gagne (1970, p. 146) pointed out that "the important event underlying interference is extinction of previously learned connections. In other words, forgetting, as it occurs in verbal chains is a matter of interference, and this in turn is more usefully conceived of as extinction." For example, when students make errors in trying to recall the correct link in a verbal chain, they subject the correct response to extinction. When a correct link suffers extinction, new learning must take place over again to reestablish the correct link (Gagne, 1970, p. 146).

Gagne (1970) also pointed out that extinction is the fundamental cause of interference in multiple-discrimination learning. Extinction of any particular chain in a set that is to be discriminated may be accomplished by omitting the reinforcement, which can take the form of failure of confirmation of the correct response. Extinction is important when an *incorrect* response link is to be unlearned. However, research findings suggest that the occurrence of such errors fosters extinction of correct responses also. Therefore, they must be relearned.

Gagne (1970) noted that concepts, principles, and problem-solving behaviors are very difficult, if not impossible, to extinguish. These behaviors are very resistant to extinction.

One of the famous characteristics of extinction procedure is *spontaneous recovery*. This phenomenon occurs when, after an initial period of extinction, upon presentation of the signal (CS), the conditioned response may appear again after an interval. The connection between the signal and the conditioned response (CR) is weaker and may be reextinguished in a few trials in which the signal is presented alone. Ultimately, under the extinction procedure, the connection will disappear completely. For example, a student's hand-raising response may be extinguished in one day if the teacher ignores the student and does not pay attention to the student; but on the next day the response of hand raising appears again even though it lasts a shorter time. This behavior may occur for several days with the tendency each time for the response to be weaker. Eventually, the hand-raising response will be totally extinguished.

In the foregoing section, we discussed how a behavior that has been previously learned by means of reinforcement is eliminated when the behavior is permitted to occur without reinforcement. This process is referred to as extinction. As mentioned previously, there are other methods of eliminating behavior besides the extinction procedure. These include counter-conditioning, flooding or broncobusting, and punishment.

COUNTER CONDITIONING

Counter conditioning refers to the effect of conditioning the subject to a new stimulus-response connection, which is incompatible with the previous response. The new response, if stronger, will be exhibited in preference to the old response. Counter-conditiong method is also called elimination of maladaptive behaviors by means of *reciprocal inhibition* (Eysench, 1960). Counter-conditioning method can be used with such behaviors as excessive maladaptive emotional responses, such as fear, anger, and others. For example, excessive "fear of needles—injections" can be eliminated by this method. Initially, the maladaptive behavior of "fear of needles" is stronger than the to-be-conditioned response of (candy eating). Eating behavior and fear behavior are incompatible behaviors. By using the stimulus gradient concept, the problem behavior of "fear of needles" is overcome. For example, a needle in proximity to the subject produces a strong conditioned fear, but a needle in the distance produces a much weaker reaction. If we now introduce the candy while the needle is being introduced in the distance, the new pleasant response of eating candy eliminates (counteracts) the weak fear produced by the needle. As this new response grows in strength, the needle can be brought nearer and nearer until the needle itself produces no fear response. Guthrie (1935) called this method of eliminating maladaptive behavior a *method of toleration*—the conditioned stimulus is introduced subliminally.

Bandura and Walters (1967) used this method of counter-conditioning in the gradient reduction of fear in a little boy to the presence of rabbits by feeding the child in the presence of the rabbits. Conditioning of this type is essentially used in reducing emotionally charged feelings and in correcting maladaptive behaviors such as phobias.

FLOODING OR BRONCOBUSTING

The flooding, or broncobusting, method of eliminating behavior is also known as implosive method of eliminating behavior. In this situation the conditioned stimulus is repeated until the subject is not able to respond, in other words, until the subject is fatigued. For example, a person who has no appetite control and has a severe problem of overweight, be made to eat until not able to eat any more, that is, to the point of being sick of eating. Such methods have been used with alcoholics, where they were forced to drink until they got sick. Saturation to this degree eliminates the maladaptive behavior. Other situations where this technique is sometimes used is when a person is afraid of an object. The person is placed in close contact with that object and is not permitted the usual response of avoidance. This method, however, can be quite disturbing to the subject and may yield new behavior responses that are less desirable than the previous avoidance response.

PUNISHMENT

Sometimes the nature of the troublesome behavior is such that elimination by extinction cannot be humanely used. Lovaas and Schaeffer (1967) pointed out that since self-destructive behaviors of autistic children (head banging, biting own hands or arms) are maintained in part by attendant attention, they are amenable to extinction. However, most often these behaviors must be dealt with by punishment because of the physical dangers consequent to the behavior.

The use of punishment as an effective means of eliminating undesirable behaviors has as many proponents as opponents and is an issue that has not been resolved. In the literature there are just as many studies showing how effective the use of punishment is as there are studies showing that the use of punishment does not change the behaviors in the long run and, in fact, increases the behavior in some cases. Punishment, according to some theorists, suppresses old behaviors, and by breaking up an old behavior pattern, punishment can provide the occasion for the positive reinforcement of new operants that are of greater value to the person (Kanfer and Phillips, 1970, p. 359).

It seems to be the opinion of the opponents of using punishment to stamp out behavior that permitting a behavior to die out by not reinforcing it is the appropriate process for breaking habits. Moreover, it is felt that many interventions intended as punishments actually serve as positive reinforcers that maintain undesirable behavior. Skinner's (1950, 1968) opinion is that a response cannot be eliminated from an organism's repertoire by the action of punishment alone because punishment may temporarily suppress the occurrence of maladaptive behavior, but it does not tell the subject what the desirable behavior should be. The combination of positive reinforcement for the occurrence of new adaptive behavior and punishment of the maladaptive behavior appears to be most effective in eliminating behavior. Skinner (1968) also pointed out that the use of punishment in eliminating behavior was maladaptive or had adverse side effects. He stated that,

Whenever punishment is effective it is mainly for one reason. Any aversive stimulus (spanking, criticizing, etc.) is likely to produce emotional side effects as respondents. These respondents are likely to be incompatible with the punished response and thus reduce the probability of its recurrence. For example, criticizing a student for talking about a patient in public may produce feelings of humiliation that are incompatible with the act of speaking out, but once the aversive stimulus is removed, the emotional effect of humiliation soon dissipates and talking out is likely to occur again.

The basic mechanisms underlying extinction — the nature of extinction

In extinction the conditioned response undergoes a progressive decrement when the conditioned stimulus (CS) is repeatedly presented without the reinforcement (unconditioned response). Kimble (1961) pointed out that reduction in strength of the conditioned response is not a spontaneous decay, but diminishes very slightly with passage of time. Many studies (Marquis and Hilgard, 1936; Razran, 1939; Skinner, 1950) have shown that conditioned responses are retained for a long period of time and that only slight decrement is seen because of disuse. Extinction of a behavior is an active process, it is not just forgetting. Many examples of behavior can be shown to exist (be nonextinct) after long periods of disuse. Skinner found that chickens conditioned to peck in response to a specific stimulus would respond appropriately years later without interval practice with the stimulus. Extinction had not taken place as a function of passage of time. Human behavior, although more complex, offers some similar examples of people not forgetting how to swim or to drive after years of nonpractice.

The determination of the basic mechanisms of extinction is very difficult because of its complexity. Kimble (1961) noted that resistance to extinction is a measure of the degree of learning. In order to understand extinction it is necessary first to understand how learning had taken place and under what conditions the contigencies of reinforcement had taken place to establish the conditioned response.

The most crucial variable, which has the greatest significance for extinction of behavior, is the reinforcement conditions. As discussed by DeCecco and Crawford (1974, p. 184), the principle that is of greatest importance both in initiating and eliminating behavior is Thorndike's (1911) law of effect, which states:

Of the several responses made to the same situation, those which are accompanied or closely followed by satisfaction to the animal will, other things being equal, be more firmly connected to the situation, so that when it recurs, they will be more likely to recur; those which are accompanied or closely followed by discomfort to the animal will, other things being equal, have their connection weakened, so that, when it recurs, they will be less likely to recur.

Omission of reinforcement seems to account for the majority of extinction procedures. Kimble (1961, p. 281) stated that omission of reinforcement has the following effects, which describe the mechanism underlying the process of extinction:

1. Inhibition or adaptation of the response mechanism
2. Instigation of interfering responses
3. Generalization decrement, which results from changes in the stimulus situation
4. Decreases in the level of motivation, which occur when extinction involves the omission of the negative reinforcer
5. Frustration, which results when the extinction procedure involves the omission of the positive reinforcer

These five consequences of omission of reinforcement are reviewed by different theorists to be hypotheses accounting for the process of extinction. In the next section a brief description of each hypothesis is given.

INHIBITION THEORY

Inhibition theory proposes that,

Every response elicited during extinction adds to the strength of an inhibitory tendency which opposes that response. Furthermore, it is assumed that inhibition increases with the number of responses and the effortfulness of the response, and that it dissipates or decays with rest (Kimble, 1961, p. 325).

Experimental evidence (Hilgard and Marquis, 1935; Rohrer, 1947; Capehart, Viney, and Hulicka, 1958; Lewis, 1958) based on this theory shows that (1) there is faster extinction with massed than with distributed extinction trials; (2) increasing effortfulness of the response leads to increasingly rapid extinction; and (3) spontaneous recovery occurs as inhibition dissipates with rest.

Experimental studies have also shown some other findings that are outside the requirement or are the opposite of inhibition theory. For example, (1) at times, the widely spaced extinction trials have produced faster extinction than massed trials; (2) spontaneous-recovery phenomenon rarely restores the response strength to the preextinction level; and (3) resistance to extinction is higher following a partial schedule of reinforcement than following continuous reinforcement. Kimble (1961) suggested that these adverse findings imply that other types of explanations besides inhibition theory are necessary to account for the mechanism of extinction.

GENERALIZATION DECREMENT

Kimble (1961, p. 293) described the generalization decrement hypothesis that accounts for the extinction mechanism as:

All extinction procedures involve changes in the experimental situation in that the proprioceptive consequence of reinforcement, and eventually respondings, are eliminated. If the conditioned response is at all under the control of these stimuli, it should lose strength as a result of such changes, and extinction should be hastened to a degree that depends on the magnitude of these differences of stimulation between conditioning and extinction. The generalization decrement hypothesis stresses this interpretation.

The usefulness of this concept, has been shown to occur in situations other than extinction. For example, the study of Fink and Patton (1953) has shown that when the usual environmental cues to drinking are eliminated, the drinking behavior of rats progressively diminished also.

Also, the warm-up phenomenon that is characteristic of the performance of motor skills (Ammons, 1947) and rate of learning (Thune, 1950) are a matter of overcoming the decrement that is produced by the loss, with rest, of response-produced cues that control the learned response to some measure (Kimble, 1961, p. 293).

Experimental evidence (Reynolds, 1945) of this theory indicates that "altering the time between trials in extinction should lead to relatively more rapid extinction that would be obtained had the conditions of distribution used in training been maintained" (Kimble, 1961, p. 325). Again, as in the case of inhibition theory, the studies that are conducted in connection with partial reinforcement and spontaneous regression suggest that the concept of generalization decrement as a hypothesis of extinction mechanism is valuable, but that it does not provide a thorough explanation of extinction.

INTERFERENCE THEORY

Interference theory describes extinction as the situation in which the conditioned stimulus comes to elicit a response other than the conditioned response. The concept of response competition is basic to interference theory. The major proponents of this theory are Guthrie (1935) and Pavlov (1927).

This theory has been criticized for three reasons. The first is the theorists had not specified clearly where the competing response came from. The second is that "even if the source of interfering or competing response were known, it would still be difficult to account for the strengthening of this response during nonreinforced extinction trials" (Kimble, 1961, p. 326). Finally, it is difficult to explain the phenomenon of spontaneous recovery and the effects of distribution of practice by means of interference theory.

In order to answer the criticism of interference theory, Hull developed a two-factor explanation of extinction that combined inhibition theory with interference theory. According to Hull's theory (Kimble, 1961, p. 326):

Unreinforced practice results in the development of reactive inhibition which is a negative drive capable of instigating the response of resting. Resting, however, leads to the dissipation of reactive inhibition. The reduction of inhibition is reinforcing (drive reducing) with the result that a conditioned resting response is acquired during extinction. This conditioned resting response (continued inhibition) interferes with the CR and produces a permanent extinction.

THE FRUSTRATION HYPOTHESIS

The basic assumption of frustration hypothesis is that the omission of positive reinforcement is frustrating. Frustration is conceived to be a drive (motivating force) that (1) energizes behavior and (2) produces interfering responses, which may interfere with the conditioned response. The experiments conducted by Amsel and Roussel (1952) and Adelman and Maatsch (1956) on the role of frustration in extinction determined that frustration is a drive and that the responses produced by this drive are very resistant to extinction. Frustration theory explains very clearly the great resistance to extinction of habits that are learned under conditions of partial reinforcement (Kimble, 1961, p. 326).

EXPECTANCY THEORY

The basic assumption underlying expectancy theory that accounts for the underlying mechanism of extinction is that extinction occurs when the organism develops an expectancy that reinforcement will not follow the conditioned stimulus or the occurrence of the instrumental response.

Expectancy theory of extinction resembles interference theory in that it involves new learning. The variable of perception occupies an important role in this theory. Two hypotheses have emerged from expectancy theory that attempt to explain extinction: discrimination and latent extinction.

1. *Discrimination hypothesis* proposes that "conditions which make it difficult for the organism to recognize that training has ended and extinction begun will lead to great resistance to extinction" (Kimble, 1961, p. 327). Factors that make this discrimination difficult are: partial reinforcement and irregularly patterned reinforcements. These two factors make behaviors that have been learned under these conditions very resistant to extinction. Kimble indicated that changes in the physical situation at the beginning of extinction trials should hasten the extinction.

2. *Latent extinction*—also referred to as indirect extinction, goal extinction, or nonresponse extinction—"refers to a reduction in response strength, achieved without the occurrence of the response itself, by exposing the animal to the goal situation in the absence of reinforcement." (Kimble, 1961, p. 320).

Experiments illustrating latent extinction have been done using mazes. After animals mastered the maze, they were subject to extinction procedures in one of two ways. Animals in the control group underwent normal extinction procedure. Animals in the experimental group received a series of trials in an empty goal box prior to subjecting them to regular extinction trials. Results of these studies (Seward and Levy, 1949; Deese, 1951; Brown and Halas, 1957) have shown that the experimental group of animals extinguished the behavior more rapidly than the control group. These results have been explained by expectancy theorists as "negative expectancies developed through the experience with the empty goal box" (Kimble, 1961, p. 327). The stimulus-response (S→ R) theory explains the latent extinction phenomenon in terms of the extinction of secondary reinforcements.

• • •

As can be seen from these theories, there is not one theory that can explain the mechanism underlying extinction. Kimble (1961) indicated that it is no longer possible to hold a simple one-factor theory of extinction. This issue of explaining the mechanism underlying extinction is resolving. Kimble also stated that there are no longer any proponents of the classical inhibition, expectancy, and interference theories of extinction. This has come about because the lines separating rival theories have become blurred. For example, "S–R theory has assimilated latent extinction with relative ease, reducing it to the extinction of secondary reinforcement and sometimes specifically evoking the $R_G \rightarrow S_G$ mechanism as a part of the explanation. Beyond this, theorists of all schools have tended to increase the number of principles used to explain extinction" (Kimble, 1961, p. 324).

Summary and conclusion of the theoretical framework

Based on the theoretical framework and methods of eliminating behavior, one can safely formulate a specific strategy to eliminate unwanted, undesirable behavior. The strategy follows a specific sequence:

1. Identify the maladaptive behavior to be eliminated

2. Determine how behavior to be eliminated was learned (classical conditioning, operant conditioning, chaining, or other method); in other words, determine the type of learning used

3. Determine the reinforcement that keeps the behavior going doing the following:
   a. Establishing a baseline record of behavior for a period of time (such as 1 day, 1 week, or 2 weeks—the more variable the behavior, the longer period of time necessary to establish an adequate baseline record of behavior)
   b. Determining the consequences of behavior (What goes on with the subject once the behavior is emitted? Who does what? What reinforces? What is the reinforcement?)
   c. Determining the schedule of reinforcement by keeping record of the behavior and the number and occaasion of reinforcement used (continuous level of reinforcement or intermittent)

4. Determine the most appropriate method of eliminating behavior in that specific situation (extinction procedure, counterconditioning methods, flooding technique, or the use of punishment)

5. Eliminate the reinforcement that follows the maladaptive behavior until the behavior is extinguished (The omission of reinforcement depends on the type of the behavior that is being planned for elimination—for example, if it is a behavior that is learned by means of classical conditioning, such as emotional habit like fear, extinction occurs when the conditioned and unconditioned stimuli are unpaired; if it is an operant behavior, then the reinforcement following the behavior has to be eliminated; if it

is a chained behavior, reinforcement of the final stimulus-response link has to be eliminated; and so on).

6. Initiate and reinforce a desirable behavior that is incompatable with the maladaptive behavior by using the techniques and procedures of initiating behavior described in previous modules

Application to nursing education and practice

It is the opinion of most stimulus-response theorists (Skinner, 1968; Bijou and Baer, 1961; Travers, 1967; Gagne, 1970; DeCecco and Crawford, 1974; and many others) that extinction procedures are most appropriate in the majority of situations, especially when teachers encounter maladaptive behaviors in school settings. The other methods are generally used in therapy situations. Eliminations of behaviors through various methods mentioned are very applicable to the practice of nursing and are indeed used in many nursing situations, especially in psychiatric and pediatric settings.

The effectiveness of the use of extinction as an appropriate nursing intervention in eliminating behaviors of psychotic patients has been amply demonstrated. For example, it has been shown that when the nursing staff continuously ignored delusional conversation in psychotic patients, this behavior showed a tremendous decrease. This has also been an effective method in reducing the activity level of some psychotic patients. In another example cited, a patient walked into the nursing stations all day long, and the nurses reprimanded her every time for her behavior. However, when all the staff began to ignore her activity, her trips to the nurses' station dropped off at a tremendous rate (Frank, 1969).

Hermantz and Rassmussen (1969) have utilized behavior-modification technique in eliminating head-banging behavior in mentally retarded patients in mental institutions.

With the use of a protective football helmet they were able to observe the nature of head banging (frequency and other aspects) and were able to conclude that this self-destructive behavior was maintained by "social-attentional" reinforcers that were elicited from the environment (nurses and staff). With knowledge of the maintaining stimuli, Hermantz and Rassmussen were able to extinguish the head-banging response by removing the accompanying social reinforcement. They also developed new, more appropriate social reinforcement (from other retardates) that was effective in maintaining other socially accepted responses that were elicited from the subjects.

In Creer and Yoches' 1971 study on behavioral patterns of asthmatic children, it was shown that absenteeism from asthma was highly correlated with habits that interfered with the learning process. "Nonattending habit patterns" were the specific behaviors that were investigated. In each experimental classroom setting, the children were given 40 points with which to purchase prizes at the end of each session (20 minutes). A child would loose 1 point for each unit (30 seconds) of nonattending behavior (playing with pencil, gazing about, and other such behaviors). The number of points to purchase a prize increased by 2 points each day. It was shown that there was a substantial decrease in nonattending behaviors, which generalized to the normal classroom setting and was still in effect 6 months later. This is an example of an extinction procedure where, in order to eliminate the undesirable behavior of unattending, the incompatible behavior of attending was being initiated.

Other types of patient behaviors can be eliminated by means of extinction procedure; for example, excessive dependency behaviors can be eliminated by first finding out what the reinforcement is for the existing dependency behavior and, second, cutting out reinforcement for this undesirable behavior and making reinforcement contingent on the behaviors of independence, such as doing things for oneself and taking part in one's own care. The dependency behaviors should not be reinforced at all because, if a nurse reinforces the patient by attention or by doing things for the patient that the patient can do alone, then the nurse is placing the patient's undesirable behavior on an intermittent schedule of reinforcement, which is very difficult to extinguish.

Mikilic's (1971) study showed that nursing personnel unconsciously extinguished independent behaviors of patients in an extended-care facility. In this 6-week study, it was shown that the nursing staff socially rewarded dependent patient behaviors by increased attention, praise, and agreement and withheld reinforcement of independent behaviors by ignoring them.

The same principles can be applied in the classroom and in counseling nursing students. For example, a senior nursing student was assigned to her section for pediatric experience. This student had received the following grades during the past two quarters: two "incompletes" and one "F." This student was being considered for discharge from school. The instructor talked to this student about what had happened in the past two quarters: what she did and what her instructors did as a result of her behavior. Then the instructor talked to the student's previous instructors about the type of behaviors they had observed in the student and what they had done about it (data gathering and attempting to establish a baseline). The teacher found out that this student had not submitted her reports (term papers) on time and as a result had ended up having incompletes as a course grades in the two courses the previous quarters. The student admitted that she did not start writing her papers until the last week of the quarter, at which time, the student sought the teachers' help. The teachers

paid attention to her and tried to help her at this time, giving her special sessions of instruction. In spite of all this attention and help the student did not meet the deadlines for submitting the term papers.

Let us now analyze this case and apply the extinction procedure:

1. The maladaptive behavior in this situation that has to be eliminated is the not writing of the term paper until the last week of the quarter.

2. The reinforcement for this behavior is probably the teacher's attention, probably given on a continuous schedule of reinforcement at the end of the quarter.

3. The behavior is an operant.

4. The behavior that needs to be initiated that is incompatible with not writing is to get the student to start writing parts of the paper starting the second week of the quarter and to continue during the rest of the quarter until the paper is completely written.

5. The strategy of implementing the extinction procedure is to cut out attention for "not-writing" behavior and making attention contingent on "writing" behavior. This can be done by first asking the student to write the outline, then setting a target date for submitting it to the teacher; and finally, positively reinforcing the student by giving attention and praise as the student performs this act. (This is what Skinner [1968] would refer to as initiating the first instance of behavior by means of nonduplicative repertoire of imitative behavior, where the teacher instructs or gives direction and the student performs by writing.) Therefore, by causing the incompatible behavior of "writing" to occur, extinction of the undesirable behavior of "not writing" will occur. Until the new behavior becomes a part of the student's repertoire, every writing behavior must be reinforced (continuous schedule of reinforcement). However, once the student has initially mastered the behavior, then an intermittent schedule of rein-

forcement needs to be implemented in order to maintain the desirable behavior.

When this procedure of eliminating behavior was followed exactly, the student responded very positively by dropping the maladaptive behavior. This behavior also generalized to other courses. Eventually, at the end of the program of study, this student graduated from nursing school.

Even though this is an example of one case, the principle of eliminating an undesirable behavior can apply to most maladaptive behaviors in school settings or in patient-care situations.

Researchable questions

1. What is the effect of the use of punishment alone to stop maladaptive behavior versus punishment for maladaptive behavior *and* positive reinforcement for desirable behavior on the number of extinction trials necessary to extinguish the physically self-destructive behavior of an autistic child?
   a. Independent variable: the use of punishment versus the use of punishment and positive reinforcement
   b. Dependent variable: number of extinction trials necessary to extinguish the maladaptive behavior
2. What is the effect of peer pressure from "normal-acting" adolescent patients on the regressive behavior of another adolescent patient who is his roommate?
   a. Independent variable: peer pressure from roommate
   b. Dependent variable: regressive behavior of one of the adolescent patients

ADDITIONAL LEARNING EXPERIENCES—RECOMMENDED READING LIST

Bandura, A., and Walters, R. *Social learning and personality development.* New York: Holt, Rinehart and Winston, Inc., 1967, 224-259.
Gagne, R. *The conditions of learning.* (2nd Ed.) New York: Holt, Rinehart and Winston, Inc., 1970, pp. 100-101, 111-112, 131-132, 143-146, 170.
Kimble, G. A. *Hilgard and Marquis' conditioning and learning.* New York: Appleton-Century-Crofts, 1961, pp. 281-327.

INSTRUCTIONS TO THE LEARNER REGARDING POSTTEST

Now you are ready to take the posttest to determine the extent to which you have achieved the objectives of this module. Return to the pretest of this module and take it again as the posttest. Correct your answers using the answer key found at the end of this module. You need to obtain 50 points to achieve mastery at the 95% level. If your score is less than this, correct your errors, study the content of this module again, and read some of the references in the recommended reading list. Take the posttest again. You need to study in this fasion until you achieve the 95% level of mastery.

ANSWER KEY TO PRETEST AND POSTTEST

1. b (Gagne, 1970, pp. 96-97)
2. c (Bandura and Walters, 1967, pp. 231-238)
3. a and c (Bandura and Walters, 1967, pp. 188-200)
4. a (Lovaas, 1967, pp. 672-678)
5. a (Text, p. 304)
6. b (Kimble, 1961, p. 281)
7. b (DeCecco and Crawford, 1974, p. 191)
8. a (Gagne, 1970, p. 100)
9. a (Gagne, 1970, pp. 103-104)
10. a and b (Gagne, 1970, p. 167)
11. a and b (Gagne, 1970, p. 170)
12. a and b (Gagne, 1970, p. 145)
13. b and c (Gagne, 1970, p. 131)
14. d (DeCecco and Crawford, 1974, pp. 190)
15. a (Gagne, 1970, p. 101)
16. b (Gagne, 1970, p. 101)
17. c (Gagne, 1970, pp. 100-101)
18. d (Gagne, 1970, pp. 111-112)
19. a (Gagne, 1970, pp. 131-132)
20. b (Gagne, 1970, p. 167)
21. a (Bandura and Walters, 1967, pp. 224-259)

22. a (Bandura and Walters, 1967, pp. 224-259)
23. e (Bandura and Walters, 1967, pp. 224-259)
24. a (Bandura and Walters, 1967, pp. 224-259)
25. i (Bandura and Walters, 1967, pp. 224-259)
26. e (Bandura and Walters, 1967, pp. 224-259)
27. e (Bandura and Walters, 1967, pp. 224-259)
28. a (Bandura and Walters, 1967, pp. 224-259)
29. a (Bandura and Walters, 1967, pp. 224-259)
30. i (Bandura and Walters, 1967, pp. 224-259)
31. i (Bandura and Walters, 1967, pp. 224-259)
32. e (Bandura and Walters, 1967, pp. 224-259)
33. a (Bijou and Baer, 1961, pp. 5-9)
34. c (Bijou and Baer, 1961, pp. 5-9)
35. e (Bijou and Baer, 1961, pp. 5-9)
36. f (Bijou and Baer, 1961, pp. 5-9)
37. b (Bijou and Baer, 1961, pp. 5-9)
38. d (Bijou and Baer, 1961, pp. 5-9)
39. After an initial period of extinction, on presentation of the signal (Gagne's type-1 learning), the conditioned response may appear again after an interval. However, the connection is weaker and may be reextinguished in a few trials in which the signal is presented alone. Eliminated behavior may have a "spontaneous recovery," but the behavior will disappear if not again reinforced. (Gagne, 1970, p. 100)
40. a. Practice is used to permit the extinction of residual incorrect connections, rather than to establish new ones. (Gagne, 1970, p. 131).
    b. Similarly, DeCecco stated that distributed practice is beneficial because the intervals allow time for unwanted or erroneous responses to drop out or become extinguished. (DeCecco and Crawford 1974, pp. 222-223)
41. The parents must first know that extinction is the process of weakening a response by *not* following it with reinforcement. They must also realize that when a child has a tantrum and is picked up or talked to, even in a disapproving way, the behavior is inadvertently being reinforced. The process then is to completely and consistently ignore the tantrum behavior. This is much easier to say than to do. The parents whose child has a temper tantrum in the middle of the supermarket may find it difficult indeed to ignore this behavior. They then must realize that if they give in this

one time, they put the child on an intermittent schedule of reinforcement, which makes the behavior even more difficult to eliminate. So then, the success of extinction lies in completely and consistently ignoring the undesired behavior (not yielding or giving in this one time) and then positively reinforcing good behavior when it occurs. (Bandura and Walters, 1967, pp. 224-259; Kimble, 1961, pp. 281-327)

REFERENCES

Adelman, H. M., and Maatsch, J. L. Learning and extinction based upon frustration, food reward, and exploratory tendency. *Journal of Experimental Psychology*, 1965, **52:**311-315.

Ammons, R. B. Acquisition of motor skill: I. Quantitative analysis and theoretical formulation. *Psychology Review*, 1947, **54:**263-281.

Amsel, A., and Roussel, J. Motivational properties of frustration: I. Effect on a running response of the addition of frustration to the motivational complex. *Journal of Experimental Psychology*, 1952, **43:**363-368.

Bandura, A., and Walters, R. *Social learning and personality development.* New York: Holt, Rinehart and Winston, Inc., 1967.

Bijou, S. W., and Baer, D. M. *Child development: I. A systematic and empiral theory.* New York: Appleton-Century-Crofts, 1961.

Brown, W. L., and Halas, E. S. Latent extinction in a multiple T-maze with heterogenous and homogeneous environments. *Journal of Genetic Psychology*, 1957, **90:**259-266.

Capehart, J., Viney, W., and Hulicka, I. M. The effect of effort upon extinction. *Journal of Comprehensive Physiological Psychology*, 1958, **51:**505-507.

Creer, T., and Yoches, C. The modification of an inappropriate behavioral pattern in asthmatic children. *Journal of Chronic Diseases*, 1971, **24:**507-512.

DeCecco, J., and Crawford, W. *The psychology of learning and instruction: educational psychology.* Englewood Cliffs, N.J.: Prentice Hall, 1974.

Deese, J. The extinction of a discrimination without performance of the choice response. *Journal of Comprehensive Physiological Psychology*, 1951, **44:**362-366.

Eysenck, B. *Behavior therapy and neurosis.* Elmsford, N. Y.: Pergammon Press, Inc., 1960.

Fink, J. B., and Patton, R. M. Decrement of a learned drinking response accompanying charges in several stimulus characteristics. *Journal of Comprehensive Physiological Psychology*, 1953, **46:**23-27.

Franks, C. *Behavior therapy*. New York: McGraw-Hill Book Co., 1969.

Gagne, R. *The conditions of learning*. (2nd Ed.) New York: Holt, Rinehart and Winston, Inc., 1970.

Guthrie, E. R., *The psychology of learning*. New York: Harper and Row, Publishers, 1952.

Harmantz, M., and Raussmussen, W. A behavior modification approach to head banging. *Journal of Mental Hygiene*, 1969, **53:**591-593.

Hilgard, E. R., and Marquis, D. G. Acquisition, extinction, and retention of conditioned lid responses to light in dogs. *Journal of Comprehensive Psychology*, 1935, **19:**29-58.

Kanfer, F., and Phillips, J. *Learning foundations of behavior therapy*. New York: John Wiley & Sons, Inc., 1970.

Kimble, G. A. *Hilgard and Marquis' conditioning and learning*. New York: Appleton-Century-Crofts, 1961.

Lewis, D. J. Acquisition, extinction, and spontaneous recovery as a function of percentage of reinforcement and intertrial intervals. *Journal of Experimental Psychology*, 1956, **51:**45-53.

Lovaas, T., and Schaeffer, B. Building social behavior in autistic children by use of electric shock. *Journal of Abnormal and Social Psychology*, 1967, **68:**672-678.

Marquis, D. G., and Hilgard, E. R. Conditioned lid responses to light in dogs after removal of the visual context. *Journal of Comprehensive Psychology*, 1936, **22:**157-178.

Mikilic, M. Reinforcement of independent and dependent patient behaviors by nursing personnel. *Nursing Research*, 1971, **20:**162-165.

Pavlov, I. D. *Conditioned reflexes*. London: Oxford University Press, 1927. (Translated by G. V. Anrep.)

Razran, G. H. S. Studies in configural conditioning. VI. Comparative extinction and forgetting of pattern and of single-stimulus conditioning. *Journal of Experimental Psychology*, 1939, **24:**432-438.

Reynolds, B. Extinction of trace conditioned responses as a function of the spacing of trials during the acquisition and extinction series. *Journal of Experimental Psychology*, 1945, **35:**81-95.

Rohrer, J. H. Experimental extinction as a function of the distribution of extinction trials and response strength. *Journal of Experimental Psychology*, 1947, **37:**473-493.

Seward, J. P., and Levy, N. Sign learning as a factor in extinction. *Journal of Comprehensive Physiological Psychology*, 1949, **39:**660-668.

Skinner, B. F. Are theories of learning necessary? *Psychology Review*, 1950, **57:**193-216.

Skinner, B. F. *The technology of teaching*. New York: Appleton-Century-Crofts, 1968.

Thorndike, E. L. *Animal intelligence*. New York: The Macmillan Co., 1911.

Thune, L. E. The effect of different types of preliminary activites on subsequent learning of paired-associate material. *Journal of Experimental Psychology*, 1950, **40:**423-438.

Travers, R. M. W. *Essentials of learning: an overview for students of education*. (2nd Ed.) New York: The Macmillan Co., 1967.

Williams, C. The elimination of tantrum behavior by extinction procedures. *Journal of Abnormal Social Psychology*, 1959, **59:**269.

Behavior modification: retaining behavior

DESCRIPTION OF MODULE

This unit of instruction deals with retaining or maintaining cognitive or motor behavior. The text of the module covers five major areas: (1) theoretical framework, (2) research studies, (3) issues, (4) application to nursing education and practice, and (5) researchable questions.

In addition to the text, the module contains a diagnostic pretest and evaluative posttest, an answer key, and specific instructions to the learner. The content is presented in sequential order.

MODULE OBJECTIVES

At the completion of this module and having studied the material presented in the recommended reading list, the student will be able to accomplish the following set of objectives at the 95% level of mastery:

1. Describe what maintaining or retaining behavior means
2. Describe the basic theoretical framework that accounts for the retaining of behavior
3. Identify and describe the factors that affect retaining of both cognitive and motor behaviors
4. Cite relevant research studies that sub-

stantiate the theoretical framework and factors influencing retaining of behavior
5. Identify one issue in the area of retaining behavior
6. Select a specific patient- or student-teaching situation and apply the basic principles of retaining behavior and indicate factors influencing it
7. Raise one researchable question and identify both the independent and dependent variables

PRETEST AND POSTTEST

Circle the correct answers. Each question is worth 1 point except the last two questions, which are worth 4 and 10 points respectively. The 95% level of mastery for this test is 38 points. Take the test and correct your answers using the answer key that is found at the end of this module (p. 325).

Multiple choice

1. Which of the following statements are *not* true of retention of learning?
   a. The "entering behavior" of the learner has a significant effect on the amount of practice necessary to ensure effective retention of learning.

b. Rote drills are the very best way of ensuring retention of learning.

c. The greater the meaningfulness, the more rapid the learning is and the longer the material is retained.

d. Continuous reinforcement schedules are the most successful way to ensure optimal retention of learning.

e. Most theorists believe that discovery learning enhances retention.

2. The total learning material equals the amount of material retained plus the amount:
   a. transferred
   b. forgotten
   c. meaningfully learned
   d. saved

3. If you use the method of cramming before an exam, you would expect:
   a. more learning than retention to take place
   b. more retention to take place
   c. both retention and learning to take place in equal proportion

4. Evidence from studies in animal learning indicates that responses resist extinction more when they have been reinforced on:
   a. a delayed schedule
   b. ·a partial schedule
   c. a continuous schedule
   d. an immediate schedule

5. Research studies on the amount of learning accomplished prior to going to sleep indicate that:
   a. there is very little loss of learning during sleep
   b. there is no difference in loss of learning during sleep or wakeful hours
   c. there is more loss of learning during sleep

6. The amount of material remaining over a period of time may be referred to as:
   a. meaningful
   b. retention
   c. savings
   d. mediators

7. The optimal amount of overlearning to produce the most retention for the amount of effort (practice) expended, according to Kreuger's (1929) classic experiment, is:
   a. mastery-level practice
   b. 50% overlearning

c. 150% overlearning
d. 100% overlearning

8. The method of measuring mnemonic behavior (retention) that shows the greatest amount of retention is:
   a. recognition
   b. reproduction
   c. reconstruction
   d. anticipation
   e. relearning (savings)

9. Within the context of the relationship of meaningfulness to retention of cognitive material, how is meaningfulness measured?
   1—By the number of associations the learner can make
   2—By the familiarity of the material
   3—By the speed with which the learner can memorize the content
   4—By the learner's ability to understand what is being read
   5—By the relatedness of the parts of the material
   6—By the length of the material
   a. all of the above
   b. 1, 2, 3, 5
   c. 2, 4
   d. 1, 4, 5, 6

10. Simpler forms of learning, such as chains (skills) and multiple discriminations, are _____ to retain than are more complex forms, such as concepts and rules.
    a. more difficult
    b. easier
    c. equally easy

11. A nursing student who cannot remember the center portion of the procedure to prepare a patient for an upper gastrointestinal diagnostic test is said to be experiencing a phenomenon called:
    a. retroactive inhibition
    b. proactive inhibition
    c. mental block
    d. serial position effect

12. The method of measurement of retention that is the most sensitive is:
    a. recall
    b. recognition
    c. reconstruction

d. anticipation
e. savings

True or false

Within the context of the relationship of practice to retention of behavior, which of the following statements are true?

13. Distributed practice is more useful than massed practice in the learning of psychomotor skills.
14. There are optimal limits to the rest period, with lengthening the practice period being more important than shortening the rest period.
15. Mental practice is much better than no practice and is as beneficial as actual practice.
16. Massed practice is better for learning, and distributed practice is better for retention.
17. When error tendency is high, distributed practice must be used.
18. If the content matter can be organized and divided into logical parts, then the part method should be used instead of the whole method in practicing the task.

Matching

What is the effect of practice on retention in the following conditions of learning? Place an "a" in the blank if it is critical and a "b" if it is minor.

_____19. Problem solving
_____20. Concept learning
_____21. Skill learning
_____22. Multiple discrimination learning
_____23. Verbal learning
_____24. Classical conditioning
_____25. Principle learning
_____26. Operant conditioning

Discussion questions

27. Identify four motivational factors that will affect positively the retention of learned material.
28. Select a specific patient- or student-teaching situation and identify a specific behavior you want to maintain in the student or patient, then briefly describe how you would take into consideration the five factors that affect the retention of that specific behavior.

TEXT
Theoretical framework
Introduction

In a discussion of learning, it is easy to assume that learning tasks seek to develop immediate skills that function at that moment. However, learning is much more than a day-by-day process. No one would be very interested in mastery learning if it did not prove useful at a later date and under different circumstances. It is obvious that no learning is completely permanent, and teachers and students alike must reconcile themselves to the fact that a considerable degree of forgetting is inevitable. By controlling certain aspects within the learning situation, however, forgetting can be controlled and kept within bounds.

Retention can be defined as the process of or capacity for remembering things, through which responses, information, motor skills, or cognitive skills, once acquired, are available for use by the person at a later time. If memory were perfect, or if the loss of learned material proceeded at the same rate irrespective of the material involved or the conditions under which it was learned, retention would not be an important consideration. It is a reality, however, that material is forgotten, and many characteristics of the learning situation, of the material to be learned, and of the other activities of the learning (and remembering) individual will influence the amount retained at any time. Some loss of retention results from simple "forgetting"—a passive process common to all learning in which learned material gradually "fades away" with the passage of time.

Friasse and Piaget (1970) see memory as consisting of three phases. First is the acquisition phase, during which the material is presented and memorized. Next, the material is retained, or stored, for short or long periods of time, and the material remains latent. Third, the material is reactivated in observable behavior. It is important to keep in mind that the retention phase takes place within the individual and cannot be directly observed. It can only be inferred from observations of what they termed "mnemonic behavior."

There are several categories of mnemonic behaviors. The first is *recall*, in which the individual reproduces a response acquired earlier and narrates or describes it. The second type is *recognition*, in which the person identifies a situation as the same, or similar, to one responded to in the past. The third behavior is *relearning*, in which the individual does not at the time recognize consciously that the situation is one that has been responded to in the past, but is nonetheless able to learn the material much more quickly than if in fact it had been new. Therefore, it is assumed that some retention occurred because of the observed behavior (Friasse and Piaget, 1970).

Memory and retention depend largely on the degree of learning that takes place originally. Memory is an effect of learning, and depends on it. In order to ensure retention, the amount of actual learning must be identified. Also, in measuring retention, it is necessary to know the degree of acquisition that was originally present in the learning situation.

Retention develops over time and does not cease immediately following the learning activity. This activity is continued for a short time before it weakens. This explains the interesting phenomenon called reminiscence, in which learning is observed actually to rise after initial learning. This is explained in terms of inhibition, which develops during the learning situation and disappears afterward (Friasse and Piaget, 1970, p. 277). Basically, retention follows a sloping curve that drops rapidly at first and then levels off, but some retention will not follow this curve. Highly meaningful learning is not forgotten rapidly; even when it is, it can be quickly relearned. Retention, therefore, depends on

the learning process, as well as on forgetting. Total learning can be described as the amount retained plus the amount forgotten.

Factors determining the retention of behavior—cognitive and motor

There are several important variables that affect either positively or negatively the retention or maintenance of behavior; For example, rote versus meaningful learning, interference factors, practice or lack of practice, motivation, and schedule of reinforcement used during the acquisition phase. The effect of each of these variables is described in this section.

ROTE VERSUS MEANINGFUL LEARNING

The effectiveness of original learning and, later in time, the retention of what has been learned is greatly influenced by the content of the material presented. Learning of unrelated material, which must usually be learned by rote, is forgotten very rapidly. In fact, about 70% of rote learning is forgotten in a day. Klausmeier and Goodwin (1966) pointed out that the greatest loss of memory among college students occurs with technical information, but little loss in the ability to apply principles to new situations has been demonstrated.

In another study by Guilford (1952), it was shown that when the effects of nonsense syllables are compared to those of meaningful material, the meaningful material not only is retained for longer periods of time, but is learned faster in the first place. This validates Tyler's (1934) study, where he found that retention of factual information (that is, technical terms) is low, while there is usually a gain (or enhancement) on material dealing with conceptual information. Unfortunately, in using this information, some teachers dispense with teaching technical terms and information. What this really showed was that the job of teachers should be to find ways to make the technical material more meaningful.

Meaningfulness of material to be learned, on the other hand, affects retention positively. If the material has relatedness among parts, and the student can see associations between them, then it will be incorporated more readily into the student's own framework. This role of meaning in retention is also related to familiarity: if it is recognized as familiar, it will be identified as more useful and will be retained more effectively (Friasse and Piaget, 1970, p. 224). It must also be kept in mind that while familiarity can facilitate retention, it may also cause interference.

Gagne (1970) divided the knowledge needed for *lifetime retention* into two groups. The first group is *verbalizable information,* which includes general verbal information that must be readily available in order to communicate with others and specialized vocabulary for a special field of work. Outside of this factual information, Gagne believes that the educated adult need only recall broad categories and clues for "how to look it up." The second type includes *Intellectual skills,* which are skills that are useful for many purposes and are necessary for continuing learning and problem solving. Only a few of these are very specialized skills (such as how to find a square root).

With the simpler types of learning, such as motor chains and verbal chains, the most important variable for long-term retention is the amount of practice during initial learning. An example of this is a motor skill, such as swimming, which is quickly remembered even after long periods of disuse.

Ausubel (1968) has an interesting theory. He believes that meaningful new *ideas* are learned by being incorporated into an already existing structure of knowledge. He considers the following factors to be important in the retention of new knowledge: (1) prior existence of relevant *anchoring ideas;* (2)

uniqueness of the new ideas, since new information that is not easily distinguished from the preexisting knowledge will tend to be lost; and (3) the stability and clarity of the anchoring ideas. In his view the differences and similarities between the new ideas and those previously learned should be explicitly pointed out, which requires the student to have mastered the prior information before the new ideas are introduced. The task of retaining what has been learned is more difficult when a multiple set of discriminations is being learned.

Gagne (1970) followed this thinking to some extent when he noted that in the higher steps of learning (concepts and principles) *ideas* are retained better and longer than specific facts. His idea was that if concepts and principles are learned and can be applied to a novel example, then it is possible for additional practice to have no appreciable effect on its retention.

Studies have shown that both guided and unguided discovery learning enhances retention. Some theorists have reasoned that this is because the learning is thus made more meaningful. Kersh (1963) disagreed with this. He did research in this area and found that the big factor is motivation.

INTERFERENCE

Many people think interference is the major cause of forgetting of verbal learning. It is the process where "learning new associations causes one to forget old associations learned earlier in time and to forget the new associations as well" (DeCecco, 1968, p. 351). The old and new associations compete with each other within the learner, causing forgetting. Interference has two distinct forms: proactive inhibition and retroactive inhibition. In *proactive inhibition,* associations that are learned earlier in time interfere (inhibit) the retention of the material that is being learned now. In *retroactive inhibition,* associations learned later in time interfere with associations learned previously. The main difference in proactive and retroactive inhibition is in the sequencing of the interfering material.

As students mature, they bring into new learning situations many past learning experiences. This situation causes some educators to contend that proactive inhibition is inevitable. In fact, many call it the actual cause for forgetting (DeCecco, 1968). "Forgetting is an active process influenced by activities interpolated between original learning and later recall" (Klausmeier and Goodwin, 1966, p. 480).

The study by Jenkins and Dallenbach (1924) demonstrated the effect of interference on retention of nonsense syllables.

These investigators have studied the differences in retention following periods of sleeping and of waking. They have required the two subjects in the experiment to recall lists of ten nonsense syllables after various periods of ordinary waking activity and after sleeping. The waking-sleeping periods were one, two, four, and eight hours in duration. (DeCecco, 1968, p. 351.)

The subjects had learned the list before going to bed, then they were awakened at the specified intervals and were tested for recall of the list. For the waking part of the experiment, the subjects had to return to the laboratory during the day at the specified intervals (the same intervals as for the sleeping segment) and were tested for recall of the list. Results showed that ". . . recall after sleeping was considerably higher than recall after waking. The first two intervals show a similar drop in retention for both sleeping and waking, but the forgetting continues for the waking state in the later intervals" (DeCecco, 1968, p. 351).

The conclusion of this study was that the intervening activity between learning and recalling the lists and not the simple passage of time is considered to be the cause of forgetting (DeCecco, 1968, p. 351).

Klausmeier and Goodwin (1966) proposed another theory to account for forgetting phenomena. They stated that when something is learned but not used in further learning, it is then forgotten. *Disuse* causes deterioration of connections in the brain and results in loss of retention. This is a neurophysiological theory of forgetting, implying that inactivity of the mechanism of memory causes a disappearance of the memory trace as a gradual fading away.

The serial position of the information to be retained is of no little significance. Studies (Jensen, 1962; Hovland, 1938) have verified the following facts. First, as a list is presented over and over again to an individual, information at the beginning and at the end of the list are learned much more rapidly than the material that is right in the middle. The material in the middle is learned slowly, with the segment right after the middle section being learned most slowly. This phenomenon is called the "serial position effect." (Observe this in action in giving several instructions at a time to a patient or to children; see which ones are not remembered. Research could be done here to study the most efficacious order of listing instructions to patients in a particular setting to achieve maximum retention of the most important data.)

Secondly, if a list contains a few items that differ significantly from the bulk of the items, these "isolated" items are learned better and are retained better after the list is learned in toto. Because this was first noted by von Restorff in 1933, it is known as the "von Restorff," or "isolation," effect.

PRACTICE

Practice can be defined as an external condition of learning and is the repetition of a response in the presence of a stimulus (Kimble, 1961). Some practice on the components of a skill is always essential before a series of discrete responses can become an integrated skill. By repeated practice, memory pathways are polished, and interference and misconceptions are reduced to a minimum.

Underwood (1964) has shown that certain kinds of instructional events facilitate retention of learning. For example, simple types of learning such as motor or verbal chains can be retained for longer periods of time if these chains are practiced. Practice is of diminishing importance as a condition as learning moves from the simple to the complex. In classical conditioning, skill learning, and verbal learning, it is of critical importance. In concept learning, principle learning, and problem solving, it is of minor importance if the other learning conditions are properly provided.

The effect of practice on the retention of concepts, rules, and problem-solving skills is not clear. If these higher types of learning are initially learned well (that is, the learner can apply them to novel situations and examples), Gagne (1970) stated that additional practice may have no appreciable effect on its retention.

There are several conditions for practice that affect retention of both motor and cognitive skills; for example, in massed versus distributed practice, part versus whole practice, and amount of overlearning.

Massed versus distributed practice. The learning of skills or cognitive tasks can be concentrated into one time period, or it can be spread out over several time periods. The former is called "massed" learning, and the latter is called "distributed" learning. Research (Underwood, 1961) on massed versus distributed practice has shown that when error tendencies are high, the interval between practice periods must be shorter. Also, when the probability of forgetting is high, massed practice should be used instead of distributed practice. Underwood (1964) has also shown that massed practice is good for learning and very short-term retention,

whereas distributed practice is good for retention. Underwood (1961) explained the superiority of distributed practice in retention by stating that the intervals of rest in distributed practice allow time for the erroneous and unwanted responses to drop out and be extinguished.

Part versus whole practice. Part method is also known as progressive part method. It refers to practicing the segments of the task separately at first, and then combining the segments together. This is commonly practiced, for example, when learning the stanzas in poetry. The whole method refers to studying (memorizing) technique where the entire task is practiced once before any part of it is repeated. The research study of Deese and Hulse (1967) has demonstrated that the relative effectiveness of each method depends on the internal organization of the task to be learned. If dividing the material into parts makes the learning of the task easier, then the part method should be used. However, if the material to be learned cannot be logically divided into parts, and division makes the task difficult to learn, then whole method should be used. Therefore, the choice of part versus whole method depends on the internal organization or structure of the material to be learned. If the task is learned better, then it can be retained longer.

Overlearning. Overlearning refers to practicing the learning task beyond the initial mastery of it. Experiments have shown the value of overlearning. Kreuger (1929) demonstrated that overlearning can reach a point of diminishing returns and that the maximum benefit is acquired with 50% overlearning. Anything above this amount increases retention only slightly, so the effort surpasses the gain.

MOTIVATION

A student's motivation, attitudes, and emotions affect retention, much as they do during learning. A highly motivated student will retain more, and the more actively the student is allowed to participate in the learning process, the more will be recalled later. If, however, the student's emotions or attitudes are in conflict with the learning situation, learning and retention are markedly reduced. On the other hand, if the learning experience is emotionally pleasant and rewarding, the student will be able to recall more of the situation later. It is interesting to note that while pleasant associations with the learning situation increase retention, unpleasant associations are recalled better than neutral ones (Friasse and Piaget, 1970, p. 277). Thus, attitudes and interests do affect retention because they act either to distort the learning act or to act at the moment of memory. Furthermore, learning that (1) has been positively reinforced and (2) has been reviewed later in time and summarized, and does not threaten the learner with failure, is very likely to be retained well.

SCHEDULE OF REINFORCEMENT

The scheduling of reinforcement is an important variable in the retaining of behavior. The four patterns of reinforcement schedules are: (1) *fixed interval* in which reinforcement comes after a specific period of time; (2) *variable interval* where the reinforcement comes after varying periods of time; (3) *fixed ratio* where reinforcement occurs after a specific number of responses; and (4) *variable ratio* in which the number of responses required before reinforcement changes from one trial to another. In general, responses on the variable schedules of reinforcement show more resistance to extinction than responses on the fixed schedules (DeCecco, 1968, p. 257).

Bandura and Walters (1967) accounted for the persistence of deviant behaviors in terms of social-learning principles that are based on the different schedules of reinforcement. They stated that "persistent antisocial be-

havior appears to result from intermittent reinforcement; moreover, the persistence of anxiety-motivated avoidance responses can be primarily attributed to the intermittent occurrence of reinforcement through anxiety reduction" (Bandura and Walters, 1967, p. 223).

The five different factors that affect retention of behavior and attempt to account for the causes of maintaining behavior at a certain level make it apparent that none of these individual factors can account solely for or explain adequately the process of maintaining both cognitive and motor behaviors. A more adequate explanation results when these determinants are integrated to account for the process of maintaining behavior.

Methods of measurement of retention

There are five methods of measurement. They are the following: recall, recognition, reconstruction, anticipation, and savings.

Recall. The recall method involves having the student recreate what has been learned. This method is considered to be the least sensitive and is the measurement used in essay test questions.

Recognition. Recognition requires that the student recognize and pick out the desired material or item from amidst a number of items. This necessitates discrimination. Multiple choice objective examinations are a prime example of recognition methodology. In this method, the cues are there, making it easier for the student to identify the answer; whereas in the recall method, there are no cues available to the student.

Reconstruction. The method that requires the student to make some order out of an unorganized presentation is reconstruction. In other words, the student is presented with the material in scrambled order or sequence and is asked to rearrange them in proper order. For example, the teacher may present a list of concepts and ask the student to rank-order them according to a hierarchy.

Anticipation. Anticipation requires that the student recall the next item or step in a series. The student is usually given cues if an answer is forgotten. For example, the teacher may start the steps of a nursing procedure, and then ask the student to fill in the subsequent steps.

Savings, or relearning. The savings, or relearning, method requires the student to learn a given amount of material to an errorless performance and then, at a later date, to relearn the material. Retention is measured by how much less time it takes for the student to relearn the same material to mastery level than it took for the initial mastery. It has been found that relearning takes less time if the student does not recognize it as being familiar (DeCecco, 1968). This method is considered to be the most sensitive measure of retention, because it is able to demonstrate retention even when the more usual methods indicate that there has been none.

DeCecco (1968, p. 358) also pointed out, "After one or two days, the amount of retention is greatest for the recognition method, and diminishes as we move through the reconstruction, reproduction, relearning, and anticipation methods." Anticipation and relearning methods are considered to be the most demanding, or sensitive, measures of retention.

Application to nursing education and practice

The major concepts and principles of retaining behavior that can be applied to patient- or student-teaching situations revolve around the five key factors that determine the degree of retention of behavior.

It is important to keep in mind that factors that affect acquisition of behavior affect retention; it is the desirable behavior that is to be maintained; and the type of behavior (motor skill or cognitive skill) determines the type of measure that needs to be undertaken to maintain that specific behavior.

Let us take each of the five factors and implement them in specific patient- or student-teaching situations.

1. *Rote versus meaningful learning.* It was pointed out previously that the more meaningful the task to be learned (cognitive skill), the more retention there will be at a later time. Meaningfulness was defined as the number of associations a person can make to the specific concept that has to be kept in mind; that is, word familiarity. Therefore, it is the teacher's or nurse's responsibility to make the task meaningful to the student or patient. This can be done by: (1) showing the student or patient the relevance of what is being learned now and its future usefulness; (2) showing relatedness of the new concept to another one; (3) providing the student with mediators (words, pictures, and others) that the student can recall later, (4) asking the student or patient to describe the new concept or principle and provide an example of it. These are but a few examples that the teacher can use. For further information, the reader is referred to Module 5 on verbal learning, where these techniques are explained, in greater detail.

2. *Interference.* It was pointed out that retroactive and proactive inhibitions adversely affect retention of both motor skills and cognitive skills. It was also pointed out that content in the center of a long chain of material is more often forgotten than content at the beginning or at the end of the verbal or motor chain. Therefore, it is the teacher's task to decrease interferences. There are several ways to do this: (1) focusing on the differences, when two materials are too similar and confusing and the student or patient is required to discriminate between them, by magnifying them with pointing, underlining, and exaggeration, so that the learner can keep the differences in mind (retain them); (2) including events that carefully relate the

new verbal (cognitive) material to previously acquired knowledge in order to integrate the new material into previously learned ideas and keep the new material distinguishable; (3) suggesting that the student or patient learn the material before going to sleep rather than after waking up or in the midst of learning something else; (4) asking the student or patient to practice the center portion more, since content in the center of a verbal or motor chain is forgotten the most because of both retroactive and proactive inhibition. Again, these are but a few examples and suggestions for reducing interferences. For further details, read the module on verbal associates.

3. *Practice.* Research also seems to substantiate the fact that practice is of less importance in the retention of learning as one progresses from the simple to the more complex types of learning. That is to say, classical conditioning benefits remarkably from practice, whereas problem solving benefits little, if at all. This would seem to say to us in nursing that if students or patients are furnished with the basic principles, they will function more efficiently and retain information longer than if they learn by rote methods or blind rituals.

There are three conditions of practice that should be kept in mind in teaching a student or patient: (1) whether to suggest that the learner use distributed or massed practice; (2) whether or not to have the learner overlearn, and if so, how much; (3) whether to have the learner learn on a part or a whole basis. The important research findings in the previous sections were clear-cut in their suggestions to teachers. To reiterate, the teacher can make decisions based on the following:

a. Massed practice is superior for learning and immediate recall of learned material; distributed practice is superior for retention (especially long-term retention). The fact that most patient teaching (such as of diabetic patients) is of the massed-practice variety explains why the teaching effect is of short duration and why it is so subject to failure. Perhaps periodic follow-up teaching sessions, either by a public health nurse or the nurse in the physician's office could change this.

b. Distributed practice is better because it allows erroneously learned behaviors to drop out during the rest period.

c. Massed practice should replace distributed practice if error tendency in the learning task is high.

d. Massed practice should again replace distributed practice if the chance of forgetting is high.

e. Shortening the rest period is more important than lengthening the work period.

In the area of overlearning, research by Krueger (1929) suggested that 50% overlearning produced the most amount of learning and retention. For example, if it takes a student or patient 10 trials to perform the task at the initial mastery level (errorless performance), then ask the learner to practice 5 more times (which is 50% overlearning).

The determination of whether to suggest part or whole learning should be based on the internal organization of the task to be learned. If it can be logically divided into sections, and this division facilitates learning, then the part method should be used; if it cannot, then the whole method is recommended. For example, the task to be learned is the memorization of both the names of the bones in the skeletal system and the names of the arteries and veins in the circulatory system. If the names are all scrambled up to the point where the student cannot put them into orderly fashion, then the "whole" method should be used. However, if the student can divide them into sections (for example, learning all the names of the bone first, then all the names of the arteries and veins, or if the learner can divide them into sections of the body, such as head, trunk, and extremities, and learn the bones, arteries, and veins of the head first, then of the trunk, and then of the extremities), then the "part" method can be very helpful in learning the names faster and retaining them better.

4. *Motivation.* It was pointed out that motivation and retention were positively related with each other. Some of the factors that the teacher can use are: make the learning experience rewarding for the student or patient; let the learner experience success; let the learner be actively involved in the learning and experiencing of success; enable the student to provide own positive reinforcements (intrinsic) for tasks well done, rather than receive external reinforcements (where the teacher gives them all the time). All these factors enhance motivation and thus enhance retention. For further details, refer to Module 28 on motivation.

5. *Schedule of reinforcement.* In order to maintain almost any type of behavior (motor or cognitive), the partial schedules of reinforcement (variable-ratio and variable-interval-schedules) should maintain the desired behavior for long periods of time. It is important to keep in mind that variable schedules of reinforcement should be used after the behavior is initially completely learned or initiated and is within the repertoire of the person. Initially, continuous (100%) schedules of reinforcement should be used until the behavior is acquired. Then, in order to maintain it at a certain level, the partial schedule of reinforcement should be used. Reinforcement can be either primary, such as food, shelter, air, or water, or secondary, such as praise, money, prestige, or "gold stars." The age and the circumstances of the learner should indicate which reinforcement categories should be used. For further details, refer to Module 21 on reinforcement.

Researchable questions

1. What is the effect of massed versus distributed practice of care concepts about diabetes to diabetic patients on (1) the number of errors they will make in the area of care at the end of the first month after teaching and (2) the retention of the concepts about the illness?
   a. Independent variable: massed versus distributed practice of care concepts about diabetes
   b. Dependent variables: the number of errors about care in one month and the retention of concepts about illness
2. What is the effect of meaningfulness of a diet (as measured by the patient identifying the associations made with foods that are allowed, their familiarity, and personal preferences) to a patient on the maintenance of the diet regimen in the prescribed manner?
   a. Independent variable: meaningfulness of the diet
   b. Dependent variable: maintaining the diet regimen

ADDITIONAL LEARNING EXPERIENCES—RECOMMENDED READING LIST

DeCecco, J., and Crawford, W. *The psychology of learning and instruction: educational psychology.* (2nd Ed.) Englewood Cliffs, N.J.: Prentice Hall, Inc., 1974, pp. 184-192, 210-215, 222-234.

Gagne, R. *The conditions of learning.* (2nd Ed.) New York: Holt, Rinehart and Winston, Inc., 1970, pp. 92, 115, 133, 161-162, 201-210, 319.

INSTRUCTIONS TO THE LEARNER REGARDING POSTTEST

Now you are ready to take the posttest to determine the extent to which you have achieved the objectives of this module. Return to the pretest and take it over again as the posttest. Correct your answers using the answer key that is found at the end of this module (p. 325). You need to score 38 correct points to achieve mastery at the 95% level. If your score is less than 38, study the content of this module over again, read the articles in the recommended reading list, and take the posttest again. You need to study in this fashion until you achieve the 95% mastery level or better.

ANSWER KEY TO PRETEST AND POSTTEST

1. b, d (DeCecco, 1968, pp. 257, 333)
2. b (DeCecco, 1968, p. 337)
3. a (DeCecco, 1968, p. 337)
4. b (DeCecco, 1968, p. 257)
5. a (DeCecco, 1968, p. 351)
6. b (DeCecco, 1968, p. 337)
7. b (DeCecco, 1968, pp. 347-348)
8. a (DeCecco, 1968, p. 357)
9. b (Friasse and Piaget, 1970, p. 224)
10. a (Gagne, 1970, p. 210)
11. d (DeCecco, 1968, p. 355)
12. e (DeCecco, 1968, pp. 356-358)
13. True (DeCecco, 1968, pp. 314-317, 346-349)
14. False (DeCecco, 1968, pp. 314-317, 346-349)
15. False (DeCecco, 1968, pp. 314-317, 346-349)
16. True (DeCecco, 1968, pp. 314-317, 346-349)
17. False (DeCecco, 1968, pp. 314-317, 346-349)
18. True (DeCecco, 1968, pp. 314-317, 346-349)
19. b (DeCecco, 1968, p. 250)
20. b (DeCecco, 1968, p. 250)
21. a (DeCecco, 1968, p. 250)
22. a (DeCecco, 1968, p. 250)
23. a (DeCecco, 1968, p. 250)
24. a (DeCecco, 1968, p. 250)
25. b (DeCecco, 1968, p. 250)
26. a (DeCecco, 1968, p. 250)
27. a. Positive emotional experiences with the learning situation
    b. Learning which has been positively reinforced
    c. When students are allowed and encouraged to participate in the learning process
    d. Learning situations which do not threaten the learner with failure
    (Friasse and Piaget, 1970, p. 277)
28. The answer should include the five major points:
    a. Make learning situation more meaningful.
    b. Reduce interference.

c. Provide appropriate practice.
d. Increase motivation.
e. Provide partial schedule of reinforcement. (Text, pp. 322-324)

REFERENCES

Ausubel, D. P. *Educational psychology: a cognitive view*. New York: Holt, Rinehart and Winston, Inc., 1968.

Bandura, A., and Walters, R. *Social learning and personality development*. New York: Holt, Rinehart and Winston, Inc., 1967.

DeCecco, J. *The psychology of learning and instruction: educational psychology*. (1st Ed.) Englewood Cliffs, N.J.: Prentice-Hall, Inc., 1968.

Deese, J., and Steward, H. H. *The psychology of learning*. (3rd Ed.) New York: McGraw-Hill Book Co., 1967.

Fraisse, P., and Piaget, J. *Experimental psychology: its scope and method, Part IV: Learning and memory*. London: Routledge and Kegan Paul Ltd., 1970.

Gagne, R. *The conditions of learning*. (2nd Ed.) New York: Holt, Rinehart and Winston, Inc., 1970.

Guilford, J. P. *General psychology*. (2nd Ed.) Princeton, N.J. Van Nostrand Reinhold Co., 1970.

Hovland, C. I. Experimental studies in rote learning theory: II. Reminiscence with varying speeds of syllable presentation. *Journal of Experimental Psychology*, 1938, **27**:271-284.

Jenkins, J. G., and Dallenback, K. M. Oblivescence during sleep and waking. *American Journal of Psychology*, 1924: **35**:605-612.

Jensen, A. R. Spelling errors and serial position effect. *Journal of Educational Psychology*, 1962: **53**:105-109.

Kersh, B. Y. The motivating effect of learning by discovery. *Journal of Educational Psychology*, 1963: **53**: 65-71.

Kimble, G. A. *Hilgard and Marquis' conditioning and learning*. New York: Appleton-Century-Crofts, 1961.

Klausmeier, H. J. and Goodwin, W. *Learning and human abilities: educational psychology*. New York: Harper and Row, Publishers, 1966.

Kreuger, W. C. I. The effect of overlearning on retention. *Journal of Experimental Psychology*, 1929: **12**:71-78.

Tyler, R. Some findings from studies in the field of college biology. *Science*, **18**:133-142.

Underwood, B. J. Ten years of massed practice on distributed practice. *Psychological Review*, 1961, **68**: 229-247.

Underwood, B. J. The representatives of rote verbal learning. In A. W. Melton (Ed.), *Categories of Human Learning*. New York: Academic Press, Inc., 1964, pp. 48-78.

PART FOUR

Variables influencing learning and instruction

MODULE 21

Reinforcement

DESCRIPTION OF MODULE

This is an independent unit of instruction on the variable of reinforcement. Reinforcement is one of the most important external conditions that affects learning and instruction. The content of this module is presented in an integrated form. The text covers five major areas: (1) theoretical framework, (2) relevant research studies, (3) issues, (4) application to nursing education and practice, and (5) researchable questions. The module also contains the pre- and posttest to gauge and pace learning and an answer key to provide feedback. A list of learning objectives and additional learning experiences are also provided to enable you to achieve each of the objectives.

MODULE OBJECTIVES

At the completion of this module, having studied the text and the recommended reading list, the student will be able to accomplish the objectives at the 95% level of mastery. The student will be able to:

1. State, compare, and discuss three classical, and three contemporary views of reinforcement
2. Define reinforcement in terms of reward and as a procedure
3. Distinguish between positive and negative reinforcers and give illustrations of each

4. Distinguish between primary, secondary, and transsituational (or generalized) reinforcers and give examples of each
5. Define reinforcement in terms of informational feedback and give two examples
6. Identify four conditions of reinforcement and describe the major effects of each condition on learning
7. List the four basic schedules of reinforcement and briefly illustrate each
8. Describe the procedure of extinction in terms of reinforcers and incompatible responses
9. Describe the procedure of shaping in terms of reinforcement
10. Differentiate punishment from positive and negative reinforcement
11. Describe at least three recent, relevant research findings, including the hypothesis and independent and dependent variables of each
12. Draw some extrapolations to nursing from the readings and illustrate how reinforcement theory may be applied to patient care, patient teaching, and nursing education
13. State at least one relevant, current issue regarding the nature of reinforcement, types of reinforcers utilized, and schedules of reinforcement employed, giving support findings if able
14. Identify current and future trends for re-

329

search in reinforcement; propose at least one researchable question in nursing using reinforcement theory as a variable

PRETEST AND POSTTEST

Circle the correct answers. Each question is worth 1 point. The 95% level of mastery for this module is 25 correct points. Take the test and correct your answers utilizing the answer key that is found at the end of this module (p. 345). If your score is 25 or better you need not study this module; proceed directly to the next one.

Multiple choice

1. When a conditioned reinforcer is paired with several unconditioned reinforcers, it becomes a:
   a. secondary reinforcer
   b. transsituational reinforcer
   c. positive reinforcer
2. For reinforcement to occur, the reinforcer must immediately follow the response with a delay of no longer than:
   a. 1 or 2 seconds
   b. 5 seconds
   c. 2 to 3 seconds
   d. 0.5 seconds
3. In an experiment, pigeons are reinforced with food for pecking a key in a standard experimental box. After 10 minutes have elapsed, the key and magazine are connected and the next response is reinforced. Responses during the 10-minute intervals are not reinforced. The schedule described in this experiment is:
   a. fixed ratio
   b. fixed interval
   c. variable ratio
   d. variable interval
4. In the same experiment as in question 3, the experimental equipment is arranged so that a response is reinforced after a period of time, which may vary from a few seconds to 6 minutes, measured from the previous reinforcement. The average time period is 3 minutes. The schedule employed here is:
   a. fixed ratio
   b. fixed interval

c. variable ratio
d. variable interval

5. A man who brings candy to his wife when she is especially agreeable may find that she argues:
   a. less frequently
   b. more frequently
   c. occasionally
   d. as usual
6. A man who brings candy to his wife to end an argument may find later that his wife argues:
   a. less frequently
   b. more frequently
   c. occasionally
   d. as usual
7. Evidence from studies of animal learning indicates that responses resist extinction more when they have been reinforced on:
   a. a delayed schedule
   b. an intermittent schedule
   c. a continuous schedule
   d. a 1:1 ratio schedule
8. The schedules of intermittent reinforcement that are dependent on the amount of response output are:
   1—variable interval
   2—fixed ratio
   3—fixed interval
   4—variable ratio
   a. 1, 2, and 3
   b. all of the above
   c. 2 and 4
   d. 1 and 2
9. The schedules of reinforcement that are dependent on the amount of time passed are:
   1—variable interval
   2—fixed ratio
   3—fixed interval
   4—variable ratio
   a. 1 and 2
   b. 1 and 3
   c. 2 and 4
   d. 2 and 3
10. According to DeCecco (1968) the conditions of reinforcement are:
    1—immediacy
    2—frequency
    3—amount
    4—number
    5—punishment

a. 1, 2, and 5
b. 2 and 3
c. 3, 4, and 5
d. 1, 2, 3, and 4

11. A reinforcement that will serve to enhance more than one learning set is called:
    a. positive
    b. negative
    c. transsituational
    d. feedback

12. In operant conditioning the reinforcer is given:
    a. before the response is emitted
    b. at the same time as the response is emitted
    c. after the response is emitted
    d. contiguously

13. Removal of a positive reinforcer after the occurrence of a behavior is called:
    a. negative reinforcement
    b. punishment
    c. secondary negative reinforcement
    d. aversive stimuli

14. Withholding of a reinforcer after the occurrence of a behavior produces:
    a. suppression of the behavior
    b. increase in the behavior
    c. extinction
    d. spontaneous recovery

15. Reinforcement in the form of kinesthetic and information feedback plays the most important role in:
    a. classical conditioning
    b. operant conditioning
    c. chaining
    d. verbal learning

16. Reinforcement plays the least role in:
    a. classical conditioning
    b. concept learning
    c. problem solving
    d. operant conditioning

Matching

Part A

_____ 17. Punishment
_____ 18. Intermittent reinforcement
_____ 19. Positive reinforcer
_____ 20. Negative reinforcer
_____ 21. Feedback
_____ 22. Primary reinforcer
_____ 23. Incompatible responses

_____ 24. Extinction
_____ 25. Punishment
_____ 26. Reinforcer

Part B

a. Any stimulus that increases the probability of a response
b. A stimulus that when presented strengthens or increases the probability of a response
c. An event or stimulus whose removal strengthens the probability of a response
d. An event or stimulus that only temporarily suppresses the behavior that produces it
e. Providing the student with knowledge of correct responses
f. A stimulus whose reinforcing power does not depend on previous conditioning
g. When two responses cannot be emitted at the same time
h. The procedure designed to weaken and subsequently eliminate a behavior
i. A schedule of reinforcement where the response is reinforced only occassionally
j. Delivery of an aversive stimulus and/or removal of a positive reinforcer

Discussion question

27. In the two-dimensional chart below, show the relationship between punishment and reinforcement.

TEXT
Theoretical framework
The nature of reinforcement

Reinforcement is one of the most important conditions for learning. Kimble (1961, p. 203) defined *reinforcer* as

an event which, employed appropriately, increases the probability of occurrence of a response in a learning situation. Without exception these events are stimulus changes such as accompany presenting food or water, turning a shock on or turning it off, or presenting a stimulus that has a history of being correlated with such happenings.

This definition generalizes that reinforced responses tend to be repeated in given situations, and unreinforced responses tend to be discontinued. An overwhelming amount of evidence supports this generalization. The definition and the generalization are based on the famous law of effect that was proposed by Thorndike (1911), which states:

Of the several responses made to the same situation, those which are accompanied or closely followed by satisfaction to the animal will, other things being equal, be more firmly connected to the situation, so that when it recurs, they will be more likely to recur; those which are accompanied or closely followed by discomfort to the animal will, other things being equal, have their connection weakened, so that, when it recurs, they will be less likely to recur.

In the *procedure* of reinforcement the organism or the individual is presented with a specific stimulus (reinforcer) either before (as in classical conditioning) or after (as in operant conditioning) the response is made. In a given situation the organism or the individual will repeat those responses that are reinforced and discontinue those that are not reinforced. DeCecco and Crawford (1974) pointed out that a reinforcer can be distinguished from other stimuli because it has this particular effect on behavior.

As pointed out, the main difference between classical and operant conditioning or type of learning is in the procedure of reinforcement. In close classical conditioning the reinforcement is given *before* the response is is made. For example, Pavlov placed the meat powder (reinforcer plus unconditioned stimulus) on the dog's tongue before the dog salivated (the response.) In operant conditioning in human learning situations, the reinforcer (praise) is given after the response is

made; for example after the patient has identified (response) the correct choice of food for a low-salt diet.

The problem of defining reinforcement is reflected in diverse and sometimes controversial attempts. It is important to note that reinforcement has several different meanings, and it is doubtful at the present time that these can be conceived as being similar to each other. We have already mentioned Thorndike's classical statement of the law of effect. From the works of Hull (1943), Spence (1956), and Miller (1959) reinforcement became synonymous with reward. The term reward replaced drive reduction. This reward theory considers reinforcement to occur when a motive is directly satisfied, as when a fundamental drive like hunger is reduced in intensity. As conceived by Skinner (1968), reinforcement does not depend entirely on reward. Reinforcement is the name for a particular arrangement of stimulus and response conditions that result in learning. It is Skinner's position that some events that follow responses have the effect of increasing the likelihood of an operant response. Such events are reinforcers in terms of any effect they might have on the probability of a response, not in terms of any effect they might have on the internal mechanisms of the organism. Skinner's theory is appropriately referred to as contingency of reinforcement theory. This theory specifically states that if, in an experiment, a teacher wants students or subjects to learn a response, the response must be made contingent on the occurrence of the certain stimulus conditions, which in turn bring about another response. Therefore, the selection of the conditions of reinforcement is very important in initiating desirable stimulus-response (S_S–R) behaviors. It requires the appropriate arrangement of the contingencies of reinforcement, in such a way that the reinforcement is made contingent on the occurrence of the desired behavior. These techniques are often called *contingency management,* and their effects are referred to as *behavior modification.*

Working with reinforcement contingencies requires careful attention to the *sequence* of events, which reflects the correct contingencies. The reinforcing state of affairs must *follow* the to-be-learned desirable behavior and not precede it. The reinforcement must also have consistency. In other words, reinforcement occurs when the desired behavior occurs, and it is omitted when the desired behavior does not occur (Gagne, 1970, pp. 120-121).

Behavior modification, utilizing the principle of reinforcement contingencies, can be a useful and powerful tool in the management of learning. Such techniques have been used with helping change the undesirable behaviors of emotionally disturbed children in classroom settings (Hewett, 1968) and also in training mentally retarded children (Orlando and Bijou, 1960).

In conclusion, therefore, the different definitions and explanation of reinforcements are far from being unitary in their meanings, but they have something in common in their emphasis on after-effects of the response to be learned. As summed up by Gagne (1970, p. 19):

To Thorndike, the satisfying after-effects strengthened the association. To Hull and his associates, learning was influenced by after-effects of a sort that brought about drive reduction (or motive satisfaction). To Skinner, the activity to be learned must be made to take place in such a way that after-effects are made contingent on its occurrence.

The mechanism of reinforcement

Classically there were three influential theories of reinforcement that dominated early research in psychology of learning. They were formed as contiguity or substitution theory, effect theory, and expectancy theory. Kimble (1961) described these early theories as hypothetical principles of reinforcement and as parts of theories because each position has functioned in combination with other principles.

The more contemporary theories of reinforcement that attempt to describe the mechanism of reward are tension reduction, conservatory behavior, and reinforcing stimuli. The crux of the contemporary theories is based on analyzing each aspect of the reinforcement event. The event or the occasion of reinforcement consists of three distinguishable parts: "(1) the presentation of a *stimulus* to which the organism (2) *responds* in a way which typically contributes to (3) *tension reduction* of some sort" (Kimble 1961, p. 238). The contemporary theorists are attempting to find out if one of these three parts is the critical event in the reinforcement process.

In this section each of the past and present views on the mechanisms of reinforcement will be presented briefly. For more detailed explanation, the reader is referred to Kimble (1961, pp. 203-280).

Contiguity, or substitution, theory. The contiguity theory held that the conditions for learning were simply the occurrence of a response in the presence of a stimulus. The essential condition for learning is the simultaneous, or nearly simultaneous occurrence of a neutral stimulus and the response with which it is to become associated. This theory is more directly applicable to classical conditioning. No additional principle of reinforcement was hypothesized.

Effect theory. Thorndike's classic law of effect proposed that responses that have satisfying consequences are strengthened, and those followed by discomfort or annoyance are weakened. Other definitions of a "satisfying state of affairs" as proposed by Hull (1943), Spence (1956), and Miller (1959) emphasized the tension-reducing character of reinforcement and used the terms reward, reinforcement, and drive reduction. Learning, according to this theory, requires: (1) stimulus-response contiguity and (2) reward in the form of satisfaction, or drive reduction.

Expectancy theory. Tolman's (1932) expectancy theory of learning (also known as sign learning) postulates that in learning a sequence of behaviors or acts leading to a goal, the individual or the organism follows the "signs" that mark out the "behavior route" leading to the goal or "significate." The perceptual and the cognitive capacities of subjects are involved in this type of learning, for when subjects see the sign, they expect the goal to appear if they follow the behavior route. The inference that Tolman draws is that subjects will behave in such a way that is consonant with the anticipated consequence. If the goal is achieved, the expectation is confirmed, which will strengthen that type of behavior to recur again. If the goal is not achieved, the expectancy is weakened, and the behavior will be different on the next trial. Tolman's expectancy theory is often referred to as nonreinforcement theory. For Tolman, learning consists of the acquisition of knowledge and involves intersensory (S–S) associations, rather than the stimulus response (S–R) associations as hypothesized by the previous two positions (Kimble 1961, pp. 208-209).

• • •

There are mainly two issues dividing these three theories (Kimble, 1961, p. 235). First, is reward (effect) necessary for learning to take place, or is mere contiguity (whether S–S or S–R) enough? Second, what is learned—is it knowledge in the form of intersensory associations, or is it stimulus-response connections?

The contemporary views on the nature of reinforcement are somewhat more limited in scope than the previous classical theories. As mentioned previously, these new positions

identify reinforcement in terms of: tension reduction, evocation of a response, or the presentation of a stimulus.

Tension reduction theory. There have been three versions of tension-reduction theory:

1. The need-reduction theory viewed reinforcement as satisfying some biological need. This view was criticized and eventually abandoned because secondary reinforcements (such as saccharine, or the onset of light) were reinforcing, and the need-reduction theory could not explain or incorporate this phenomena. Hull then used the term *drive* reduction in place of *need* reduction, which brought about the second point of view.

2. The drive-reduction theory treats motives abstractly and relates them to appropriate antecedent conditions. Hull considered drive as an intervening variable whose value depends on specific drive conditions (C_D). Kimble (1961) stated that many of these drives correspond closely to need-establishing operations.

3. Drive-stimulus–reduction theory describes drives as strong stimuli that impel action. The reduction of this stimulation is considered to be reinforcing (Kimble, 1961, pp. 238-240, 278).

Evocation of a response theory. A response theory proposes that certain forms of behavior, mostly consummatory behavior, are reinforcing. Evidence (Sheffield, Wulff and Backer, 1951) indicated that there is very high correlation between the vigor of consummatory behavior and the vigor of the instrumental response in certain learning situations. Kimble (1961) pointed out that there is also evidence that activity and manipulation will reinforce learned acts. The reason this theory is not very popular is because of methodological problems. There is difficulty separating the stimulus theory from the drive-reduction theory.

Presentation of the stimulus theory. The

stimulus theory of reinforcement assures that certain forms of stimulation are innately rewarding; for example, sexual stimulation, certain tastes, odors, tactile stimuli, sights, and sounds. Experimental evidence (Ribble, 1944) has shown that human infants respond pleasurably to stimulation. Harlow (1958) demonstrated that tactile stimulation may provide the primary basis by which the infant monkey develops an attachment and affection for its mother. Experiments (Olds and Milner, 1954) have also indicated that stimulation of certain areas (limbic system) of the brain is capable of positively reinforcing many kinds of learning. Stimulation of other parts of the brain also acts as a negative reinforcer. Whether a brain shock is positive or negative is determined by the intensity and the duration of the electrical stimulus and by the drive state of the animal. Kimble (1961) indicated that this last result makes a strong case that brain stimulation is related to the process of reinforcement as it normally occurs in conventional experiments on learning.

Kimble also noted that experimentally the distinction between the reinforcing stimulus theory and the consummatory responses theory is difficult to make because most of the stimuli that are used as reinforcers also elicit behaviors. Whether the reinforcing value is in the stimulus or in the response is difficult to determine. Further experimentation is needed to sort out their differences.

The conditions of reinforcement

There are four conditions of reinforcement that affect the strength of the response or the adequacy of the performance. These are: (1) the immediacy of the reinforcer, (2) amount of the reinforcer, (3) number of reinforcers, and (4) frequency of the reinforcement.

The immediacy of the reinforcer. Experimental evidence has shown that the reinforcer must immediately follow the response with a delay of no more than 1 or 2 seconds, if the organism is to associate the response to the stimulus (DeCecco and Crawford, 1974). This situation is not very clear in human learning because language seems to bridge the gap between the response and the stimulus. The study by Brackhill, Wagner, and Wilson (1964) demonstrated that a delay in feedback and reinforcement was related to the quality of the student's efforts. The importance of the student receiving feedback is not diminished by the uncertainty about the timing of the feedback. The study indicated that unless feedback is planned, the teacher may ignore this important condition of learning. This is why it is important to give immediate feedback before the teacher forgets or ignores it.

The amount of reinforcers. The amount of reinforcers affects behavior. The study by Wolfe and Kaplan (1941) found that chickens ran faster for four quarter-grains of corn than for 1 whole grain of corn. This finding suggests that the additional running activity involved in consuming the four quarter-grains of corn contributed something to the incentive or reward value. DeCecco and Crawford (1974) questioned the applicability of this finding to human learning. They speculated about the possibility that it may help the students to appreciate what they are learning if they expand the maximum effort.

The number of reinforcers. The strength of a response increases until a limit is reached, each additional reinforcement adds smaller and smaller amounts to the strength of the response. DeCecco and Crawford (1974) speculated that this may be the very reason why students report tedium when they are using teaching machines or programmed instruction. This tedium is the result of more reinforcement of correct responses than the students believe is necessary.

The frequency of reinforcement. Reinforcement is continuous when it occurs after every correct response. When it is provided only occasionally according to some schedule, reinforcement is said to be intermittent or partial. Greater emotional upset is involved in extinction after continuous reinforcement as compared to extinction after intermittent reinforcement. The latter is also extremely resistant to extinction. Ferster and Skinner (1957) have conducted extensive studies on various reinforcement procedures that are known as *schedules of reinforcement*. In certain schedules the organism is reinforced for varying amounts of work or varying amounts of time. In certain other schedules the organism is reinforced for a fixed amount of work or after a fixed amount of time. In the next section the different schedules of reinforcement and the characteristics of each will be presented in greater detail.

Schedules of reinforcement

A schedule of reinforcement is a rule that enables the teacher to choose from among the many occurrences of a behavior those few that will be reinforced.

Skinner (1938) has studied extensively the two main classes of intermittent reinforcements that are dependent on either amount of *time passing* (interval reinforcement) or amount of *response output* (ratio reinforcement). These schedules are further classified according to regularity or variability into fixed or variable schedules of reinforcement.

Ferster and Skinner (1957) identified 16 different schedules of reinforcement, but only the four basic varieties of intermittent reinforcement are discussed here, since they are the most frequently used. These four schedules are illustrated in Table 2.

Fixed-interval (FI) reinforcement. In a fixed-interval schedule the subject receives reinforcement after the passage of a standard (fixed) interval of time, such as every 3 minutes, every 10 minutes, or the like. (Technically speaking, if the time elapsed is less than

Table 2: The four basic schedules of intermittent reinforcement

	Time interval	Response-output ratio
Fixed	Fixed-interval (FI)	Fixed-ratio (FR)
Variable	Variable-interval (VI)	Variable-ratio (VR)

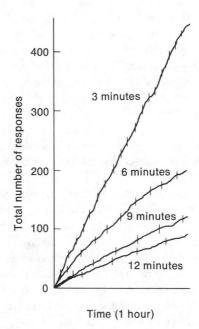

Fig. 21-1. Responses within one session of fixed-interval reinforcement. A pellet was delivered every 3, 6, 9, and 12 minutes respectively. The more frequent the reinforcement, the more rapid the rate of responding, although each rate is relatively uniform. (After Skinner [1938]; from Hilgard, E., and Bower, G. H. *Theories of learning,* New York: Appleton-Century-Crofts, 1966, p. 115.)

5 seconds, the schedule could become continuous.) Schedules of reinforcement that are based on fixed intervals results in careful rates of responding, the rate is proportional to the interval between reinforcements. The shorter intervals yield more rapid rates. Fixed-interval schedules produce a regular performance after reward: pause, acceleration, high rate. This results in minor scalloping of curves in the graph (Fig. 21-1). Skinner (1938) found that under standard conditions of experimentation and drive, the response rate was 18 to 20 times per reinforcement, over a considerable range of intervals. Fig. 21-1 illustrates the uniformity of rates of responding.

The uniform number of responses per reinforcement is also known as the *extinction ratio*. This is the ratio of unreinforced responses. The size of the ratio does not change much from one length of interval to another, provided that drive stays constant (Hilgard, 1956, p. 114).

Variable-interval (VI) reinforcement. Under a variable-interval arrangement, reinforcement is given on the basis of a variable period of time elapsed since the last rein-

forcement, described in terms of the average of the periods of time. A response may be reinforced every 5 minutes on the average, in some cases the second reinforcement immediately follows an earlier schedule, and at other times it is delayed. Under this type of schedule, performance is uniform and stable and very resistant to extinction (Fig. 21-2).

Fixed-ratio reinforcement. In the fixed-ratio situation the organism is given a reinforcement after a standard number of responses; for example, a 2:1 ratio when the subject is rewarded for every second response. A continuous schedule, or 1:1 ratio, is the simplest form of a fixed-ratio schedule. The larger ratio has to be approached gradually, otherwise the phenomenon of *strain* occurs, which increases the likelihood of pauses during performance. Occasional reinforcements as in larger ratios (such as 96:1) can maintain a response only if the organism is already responding at very rapid rates. Once they have reached such high ratios, the less frequent the reinforcement is, the more rapid is the response.

When responses based on fixed-ratio schedules of reinforcement are plotted on a

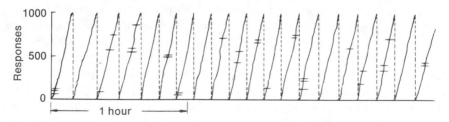

Fig. 21-2. Responses within variable-interval reinforcement. The curves are of the pecking responses of an individual pigeon reinforced at intervals ranging from 10 seconds to 21 minutes, but averaging 5 minutes. Each of the sloping lines represents 1,000 responses; the pen resets to zero after each 1,000. The whole record represents some 20,000 responses in about 3 hours, with an average of 12 reinforcements per hour. Each reinforcement is represented by a horizontal dash. (From Skinner, B. F. "Are theories of learning necessary?", *Psychological Review*, 1950, *57*, p. 208.)

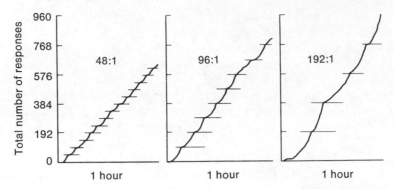

Fig. 21-3. Responses within ratio reinforcement. Responses from individual rats reinforced every 48, 96, and 192 responses, as indicated by the horizontal lines. Under these circumstances very high rates of responding develop, the highest rate being found with the lowest frequency of reinforcement. (After Skinner [1938]; from Hilgard, E. R., and Bower, G. H. *Theories of learning,* New York: Appleton-Century-Crofts, 1966, p. 116.)

graph, they demonstrate a very distinctive steplike character of performance. This is more pronounced with larger fixed ratios (Fig. 21-3). There is a burst of responding just before reinforcement, then a period of very slow responding just after reinforcement. If the ratio is too large, then a long period of no response follows a reinforcement. Skinner (1953) used the analogy of the student's behaviors after an examination or a term paper. Just before the deadline the student is busily engaged in studying or writing the term paper. Once the examination is taken and the term paper submitted, the student finds it difficult to start work again on a new project.

Variable-ratio reinforcement. A variable-ratio schedule of reinforcement employs a range of ratios around a mean value. In other words, the subject is rewarded *on the average* for every certain number of responses, but can never tell exactly when the next reinforcement is going to come because the number of required responses varies ran-

domly. An example would be that the average ratio (mean value) may be 5:1, but the organism actually gets reinforced at a random ratio of 5:1, 7:1, 3:1, 2:1, 4:1, and so on. Variable-ratio schedule maintains an extremely high rate of responding. It also eliminates the scalloping (step-like character) effect that one gets with a fixed-ratio schedule.

Types of reinforcements

Positive reinforcers are events or stimuli whose presentation strengthens the probability of a response. The procedure of presenting stimuli is positive reinforcement. Food, water, and certain lights or tones are positive reinforcers under appropriate states of need.

Negative reinforcers are events or stimuli whose removal strengthens the response that takes it away and also weakens the response that produces it (Keller, 1966). A patient is reinforced by getting rid of stimulation as, for example, (1) the eyes are closed to cut out glaring lights, or the ears are covered to avoid hearing the patient on the next bed retch or cough productively; (2) the oxygen face mask is removed because it makes the patient feel claustrophobic; or (3) the complaints are stopped and an "ideal patient" role is maintained to avoid the nurses' anger and indifference (the "ideal behavior" is a positive reinforcer for the nurse).

Positive reinforcers involve an adding operation, and the behavior producing the stimulus is *strengthened* (Bijou and Baer, 1961). In all cases, the positive reinforcer, when given after a response, tended to lead to the response being repeated (Steinberg, 1967). Negative reinforcers involve a subtracting operation, and the behavior causing this removal is strengthened (Bijou and Baer, 1961). In other words, negative reinforcement is the procedure of terminating stimuli —the stimuli to be terminated are the negative reinforcers (DeCecco and Crawford, 1974).

Positive and negative reinforcers can be either primary, having biological significance, or secondary, being acquired, derived, conditioned, or generalized. Examples of primary positive reinforcers are food, water, air, and sexual contact; secondary positive reinforcers include a smile, money, approval, special privileges, affection, a passing grade, or a promotion (Gardner, 1971). Feedback or knowledge of results is also an example of secondary positive reinforcement. In this procedure the student is given knowledge of correct responses. DeCecco and Crawford (1974) pointed out that the term *reinforcement* connotes the hedonic aspect of reward, whereas, the term *feedback* stresses the informational aspect of the instructor's function. It is very difficult if not impossible to separate the reward function of the feedback from the informational function.

Examples of primary negative reinforcers are the *deprivation* of food, air, water, or sexual contact; also included as primary negative reinforcers are loud noises, shock, and extremes in temperature. Secondary negative reinforcers include a frown, a poor grade, removal of play period, criticism, rejection, nonattention, and a penalty (Gardner, 1971).

Transsituational reinforcers are generalized reinforcers because they strengthen all or most learnable responses in a given species (DeCecco and Crawford, 1974). For example, a reinforcer that is effective in improving performing of one skill (making a bed) will also be effective in improving another skill (washing a patient). An excellent example of a transsituational reinforcer is money, which has acquired its property by being frequently paired with many different reinforcers through buying. Praise or approval is another transsituational reinforcer relevant for students, and attention is one often seen in interactions with patients. Other examples of transsituational reinforcers are status and success.

As noted, both positive and negative reinforcement result in an *increase* in the strength of behavior; these procedures should not be confused with *punishment*. The presentation of a negative reinforcer, or the removal of a positive reinforcer following a behavior constitutes a punishment. According to Hull, punishment does not weaken the stimulus-response connection; its termination strengthens them. Skinner and associates define punishment as an experimental arrangement whose effects remain to be investigated empirically—an arrangement that is opposite to reinforcement (the effects are not). Wilcoxon (1969) stated that the effect of reinforcement is always to increase the probability of response, but this is not true for punishment. Punishment procedures have as their objective the weakening of behavior. To summarize, a schema of the relationship is shown:

	Presentation	**Withdrawal**
Positive reinforcer	Positive reinforcement	Punishment
Negative reinforcer	Punishment	Negative reinforcement

Noncontingent reinforcement and other procedures

In all the procedures previously described, reinforcement was contingent on a specific response. The presentation of a reinforcer, regardless of response, is noncontingent reinforcement. Frequent occurrence of noncontingent reinforcement produces superstitious behavior, which in pidgeons is observed as stereotyped routine behavior. Superstitious behavior is the mechanism (Skinner) that endows on secondary reinforcers the property of enabling the organism to bridge spans of time in between reinforcements (Kimble, 1961, p. 197).

Other procedures involving reinforcement

Withholding a reinforcer to weaken, and subsequently eliminate, a response is the procedure of *extinction*. It is also accomplished by making two responses incompatible.

Shaping is the technique of reinforcing successive approximations toward a desired response.

The role of reinforcement in different conditions of learning

As a basic condition for learning, reinforcement is important in almost all forms of learning. In classical conditioning reinforcement takes the form of an unconditioned stimulus. When the unconditioned stimulus (such as food) is paired with a conditioned stimulus (such as light or a sound) a sufficient number of times, the conditioned stimulus acquires the properties of the unconditioned stimulus. The reinforcement here is given to the subject prior to making the response; whereas in operant conditioning, reinforcement is given after the behavior has occurred.

In operant conditioning the terminating response must be a satisfying one for the learner. Satisfying means that either the learner does the behavior vigorously or that the act must lead to a reward; for example, food, praise, or relief of pain (Gagne 1970).

In skill learning or chaining, reinforcement in the form of kinesthetic and informational feedback plays an important role. The terminal link in a chain must lead to a satisfying state of affairs. If reinforcement is omitted at the end of the last link, the whole chain is subject to extinction. Immediacy of reinforcement is important in order for chain learning to occur most readily. Delay in reinforcement increases the difficulty of learning (Gagne, 1970; DeCecco and Crawford, 1974).

In verbal learning, reinforcement in the form of confirmation of correct responses (feedback) constitutes an essential external condition of verbal learning. Confirmation is given in two ways: (1) if a student is learning a list (such as a list of medical terminology), a copy of the list is presented after the student has reproduced it; and (2) if the student is learning by means of the anticipation method (for example, stating the next step in a procedure), the student must guess the next step and then be presented with the correct step. This exposure to the correct word or step is a form of reinforcement (DeCecco and Crawford, 1974).

In discrimination learning, reinforcement takes the form of feedback or confirmation of the correct response (discrimination). The student matches the responses to the discriminative stimuli (S^D) with those that are known to be correct. This operation is one of reinforcement. The mere act of discrimination learning is based on reinforcement. An S^D is the occasion on which the response is reinforced. In the S^Δ situation, the response is not reinforced. By this mechanism, the subject learns to respond only to the S^D.

In concept learning, reinforcement takes the form of confirmation of correct identification of the concept—the new set of stimuli. Confirmation has to be immediate.

In principle learning, reinforcement in the form of feedback is provided to the learner when the rule is exhibited in its complete form. The teacher may say "right." The student can also receive reinforcement by matching own response (terminal act) with a form remembered from the initial instruction (Gagne, 1970).

The role of reinforcement as an external condition for problem solution generates its own reinforcement or feedback. It can be concluded that the importance of reinforcement diminishes as we move toward the higher types of learning because successful learning at these levels generates its own feedback.

Relevant research studies

The research studies cited in this section are chosen because of their obvious relevance to patient care and learning. Other studies that have been done on the effect of reinforcement on different types of learning, especially in operant conditioning, have been presented in previous modules.

Scott and associates (1973) did a study on the use of shaping and reinforcement in the operant acceleration and deceleration of heart rate, using commercial television programs as the reinforcer with two subjects and money with one subject. One subject showed a heart-rate acceleration of 16 beats per minute from the baseline rate; and another showed an increase of 17 beats per minute

from the baseline. A patient with tachycardia was conditioned to produce a heart rate that averaged 16 beats per minute less than the baseline.

A number of studies (Martin, 1963; Whiting and Mowrer, 1943; Solomon, 1964) have indicated that punishment, alone or in combination with reward, leads to better performance than reward alone. One hypothesis suggests that presentation of the reward may serve to distract the attention and thus retard learning; while another indicates that punishment may increase attention and thus facilitate learning. These two hypotheses involve an attentional mechanism. A third one, which indicates a motivational process, suggests that punishment facilitates learning by increasing level of motivation. Witte and Grossman (1971) dealt with this issue in a study of the effects of reward and punishment on children's attention, motivation, and discrimination learning. Nonverbal reward consisted of tokens to be exchanged for a toy; and punishment was a 98 dB 2,800 cps tone. Sixty kindergarten-aged children were presented with a tactile form-discrimination task and were compared under three reinforcement conditions: (1) reward only, (2) punishment only, and (3) reward and punishment. There was no difference in correct responses for the punishment and reward-punishment groups, and both made more correct responses than the reward group. There was also evidence supporting an attentional hypothesis, although the exact role of punishment and reward is not clear.

Bachrach (1964) treated a patient with anorexia nervosa by operant-conditioning techniques. Since by definition this patient is one who ate with a frequency significantly below her usual and critically below group normal frequency, the eating response and food did not have their expected reinforcing quality. The therapists assessed her to identify what reinforcers would be significant for her. They found that she enjoyed visits from people, music, and television and was accordingly deprived. The availability of these reinforcers was made contingent on eating and weight gain. After over a year of conditioning, she more than doubled her initial experimental weight and continued to gain weight.

To test the hypothesis that reinforcement of imitative responding will result in generalized imitation, Masters and Morris (1971) exposed nursery-school children first to a female model who exhibited a sequence of aggressive behaviors, followed after a short lapse of time by a male model displaying a sequence of neutral behaviors. Contingent reward from the models results in greater subsequent generalized imitation than contingent reward from a mechanical device and noncontingent prepayment of rewards.

Other recent research that was mentioned in previous modules has dealt with the use of tokens in the management of behaviors of institutionalized people, contingency procedures in the control of alcoholism, and behavior therapy in general.

Issues in reinforcement

Earlier research in the psychology of learning revolved around the issues dividing the major classical theories of reinforcement, namely: (1) is reward (effect) necessary for learning or is mere contiguity (whether stimulus-to-stimulus or stimulus-response) enough, and (2) what is learned—stimulus-response connections or knowledge in the form °of stimulus-to-stimulus connections (Kimble, 1961)? Over half a century of extensive work has produced some answers and has generated even more questions. More recent views of reinforcement have variously emphasized one or several attributes common to all conditions in which reinforcement occurs: motivation, stimulus, and response (Tapp, 1969, p. 389). Others subscribe to an

eclectic view. According to Estes (Tapp, 1969), the principle function of reward is to modify the selection of a response. In this light, reward is seen to influence performance only after information about which response brings reward has been acquired. This gives rise to several unanswered questions about what special properties give reward the capacity to facilitate the formation of stimulus-response associations and the subsequent selection of responses. How does an event with such capacity relate to motivational variables in the past history of the patient?

Morse and Kelleher (1970) contended that it is wrong to assume that the reinforcing or punishing effect of an event is specific property of the event itself while overlooking the importance of both antecedent and subsequent behavior. They stated that "the effectiveness of an event in maintaining a sequential pattern of responding depends on the ongoing pattern of responding itself," which in turn depends on the subject's history of reinforcement. A neutral stimulus paired with a reinforcer is said to have become a conditioned reinforcer, but actually it is the behaving subject that changed, not the stimulus. Another issue involves the specificity versus the generality of rewards. Some theorists believe that various rewarding agents have little in common apart from their power to reinforce instrumental responses; while others suggest that all rewards must work through some common mechanisms, so in principle it would be possible to predict how rewarding an event will be (Berlyne, 1969). The specificity issue is linked with the controversy between partisans of a general drive (recent variant, arousal) and those who believe in a list of specific drives. Several issues are beyond this text's scope because they demand detailed treatment. These are issues about the meaning of schedules of reinforcement, concepts of response contingency, and definition of response. The role of reinforcement in maintaining behavior is better understood than its role in producing new behavior. All these must be clarified through investigations at both the macromolar and molecular levels (Tapp, 1969). The reader who wishes to go into greater depth is advised to read the books of Kimble (1961) and Tapp (1969).

Application to nursing education and practice

As a powerful condition for most learning, reinforcement is indispensable to nursing education and practice. Reinforcements abound everywhere—in the ward, in the classroom, and at home. They are an integral part of our lives and are reflected in our patterns of behavior. Hence, for the nurse practitioner, a major task should be *the identification of what events or stimuli reinforce which behaviors under what conditions.* Nursing assessment should include the identification of the patient's sources of rewards; nursing intervention should include the presentation of reinforcers to obtain a desired behavior to maintain a functional behavioral system, as well as to evaluate which reinforcer is most likely to achieve this end. Reinforcement employed purposefully is a basic component of the nursing process and is a powerful tool in the hands of a skilled behavior therapist.

The types of reinforcement—whether they be positive or negative, primary or secondary—and the scheduling of the reinforcement certainly have their implications for the practice of nursing. A primary positive reinforcer paired with a seondary positive reinforcer could most likely be used in a continuous or fixed 1:1 ratio to initially shape self-help skills such as spoon-feeding, dressing, and toileting. As soon as the behavior pattern is well established, the nurse can fade assistance, rely more heavily on secondary positive reinforcers, and give reinforcement on a variable ratio schedule. Negative reinforcement or punishment might be called

for to reduce an inappropriate behavior such as extreme aggression in the play situation, temper tantrums, or throwing food on the floor. Initially, a fixed ratio will be needed; later, a variable ratio may be appropriate.

Some caution, however, should be used with regard to the use of positive and negative reinforcers and punishment. First, the nurse should be aware that what is a reinforcer for one child or one psychiatric patient may not necessarily be a reinforcer for another child or psychiatric patient— reinforcers are *highly individualized.* If the individual has a defective reinforcement history—that is, for example, has been given reinforcement only minimally for motor, social, or intellectual behaviors—and, as a consequence, appropriate social behavior has not developed (Bijou, 1968) the nurse may be required to shape a whole new repertoire of reinforcers. Second, punishment, besides being intrinsically unpleasant, may result in generalized avoidance responses, such as the individual may pair the unpleasant experience with the person giving the punishment and thereby avoid the person altogether (Dushkin, 1970). That is why it is often more advisable to reinforce a response incompatible with the undesired response—for example reinforce eating, which would be incompatible with throwing food—or to use other methods that avoid the necessity of punishing incorrect behavior altogether, ensuring from the start that only correct behavior occurs (Dushkin, 1970).

The token-economy system also represents a major breakthrough in the application of operant reinforcement principles to the hospital or institutional setting (Dushkin, 1970). The system utilizes tokens, which are given contingent on performance of specified desirable behaviors, and has several distinct advantages (Dushkin, 1970):

1. Tokens are generalized reinforcers
2. Tokens encourage delay of gratification

3. Value of the token may be changed to manipulate desired behavior

4. Program develops behaviors that will lead to social reinforcement from others in a natural setting

5. System enhances skills necessary for the individual to take a responsible social role in the institution and eventually to enable the individual to live outside the hospital

Nursing educators should certainly analyze their roles in the dispensing of reinforcement in order that their students may more effectively learn, for this variable is not only applicable to the simple stimulus-response situation but also is highly relevant to chaining, verbal association, discrimination, concept, role, and problem solving (Gagne, 1970). The nurse-educator should specify expected behaviors that earn positive reinforcement and should reinforce appropriate behaviors instead of only pointing out incorrect learning. Individual reinforcers can only be discovered by knowing the students.

Researchable questions

Current research is focused on the neurophysiological, neurochemical, and neuroanatomical bases of reinforcement. Many investigations are concerned with the consequences of rewards on behavior in order to specify the limits of their operations and identify the variables that predispose organisms to be responsive to the consequences of rewards. A possible nursing research project would be to investigate the effects of different types of rewards on the self image of patients. This is concerned with identifying specific rewards to bring about desired outcomes in specific types of patients, such as patients with organ loss, or threat of loss, with dominant dependency or dominant achievement subsystems. Conceivably, one hypothesis might be: chronic hemodialysis patients with dominant achievement subsystems will show a higher increase in self image

when praised on their task performance as compared to those patients with dominant dependency subsystems. Another hypothesis might be: patients with dominant dependency subsystems will show an increase in self image when given person-oriented praise as compared to task-oriented praise.

Further research is also needed in the following areas: (1) the discovery of new, highly individualized reinforcers, (2) the decrease of the unwarranted effects of punishment, (3) the further systematic application of the schedules of reinforcement to human situations, and (4) the use of reinforcement in producing long-term effects.

ADDITIONAL LEARNING EXPERIENCES—RECOMMENDED READING LIST

DeCecco, J., and Crawford, W. *The psychology of learning and instruction: educational psychology.* (2nd Ed.) Englewood Cliffs, N.J.: Prentice Hall, Inc., 1974, pp. 184-195.

Gagne, R., *The Conditions of learning.* (2nd Ed.) New York: Holt, Rinehart & Winston, Inc., 1970, pp. 17-19, 109, 131, 167-168, 142, 181, 202.

Kimble, G. A. *Hilgard and Marquis' conditioning and learning.* New York: Appleton-Century-Crofts, 1961, pp. 203-280.

INSTRUCTIONS TO THE LEARNER REGARDING POSTTEST

At this stage of your learning process you are ready to take the posttest to determine the extent to which you have achieved the objectives of this module. Return to the pretest and take it over again as the posttest. Correct your answers using the answer key at the end of this module (p. 345). You need to achieve 25 correct points for 95% mastery. If your score is less than this, study the contents of this module over again and read some of the articles in the recommended reading list. Then take the posttest again. You need to study in this fashion until you achieve the 95% mastery level.

ANSWER KEY TO PRETEST AND POSTTEST

1. b (DeCecco and Crawford, 1974, p. 187)
2. a (DeCecco and Crawford, 1974, pp. 190-191)
3. b (Kimble, 1961, pp. 160-164)
4. d (Kimble, 1961, pp. 160-164)
5. a (DeCecco and Crawford, 1974, p. 190)
6. b (DeCecco and Crawford, 1974, p. 190)
7. b (DeCecco and Crawford, 1974, p. 190)
8. c (Kimble, 1961, pp. 160-164)
9. b (Kimble, 1961, pp. 160-164)
10. d (DeCecco and Crawford, 1974, pp. 190-192)
11. c (DeCecco and Crawford, 1974, p. 187)
12. c (Gagne, 1970, p. 109)
13. b (DeCecco and Crawford, 1974, pp. 192-195)
14. c (DeCecco and Crawford, 1974, p. 190)
15. c (DeCecco and Crawford, 1974, pp. 194-195)
16. c (DeCecco and Crawford, 1974, pp. 194-195)
17. j (DeCecco and Crawford, 1974, p. 192)
18. i (Kimble, 1961, pp. 160-164)
19. b (DeCecco and Crawford, 1974, pp. 186-187)
20. c (DeCecco and Crawford, 1974, pp. 186-187)
21. e (DeCecco and Crawford, 1974, p. 187)
22. f (DeCecco and Crawford, 1974, pp. 186-187)
23. g (DeCecco and Crawford, 1974, p. 190)
24. h (DeCecco and Crawford, 1974, p. 190)
25. d (DeCecco and Crawford, 1974, p. 192)
26. a (DeCecco and Crawford, 1974, pp. 184-187)

27.

	Presentation	**Withdrawal**
Positive Reinforcer	Positive Reinforcement	Punishment
Negative Reinforcer	Punishment	Negative Reinforcement

(DeCecco and Crawford, 1974, pp. 186, 192)

REFERENCES

Bachrach, A. Some applications of operant conditioning to behavior therapy. In J. Wolpe, A. Salter, and L. J. Reyna (Eds.), *The conditioning therapies.* New York; Holt, Rinehart and Winston, Inc., 1964.

Bijou, S. W. Behavior modification in the mentally retarded. *Pediatric Clinics of North America*, 1968, **15**(4):969-987.

Bijou, S. W., and Baur, D. M. *Child development, Vol. 1: A systematic empirical theory.* New York: Appleton-Century-Crofts, 1961.

Brackhill, Y., Wagner, J. E., and Wilson, D. Feedback delay and the teaching machine. *Psychology in the Schools*, 1964, **1**:148-156.

DeCecco, J., and Crawford, W. *The psychology of learning and instruction: educational psychology.* (2nd Ed.) Englewood Cliffs, N.J.: Prentice Hall, Inc., 1974.

Ferster, C. B., and Skinner, B. F. *Schedules of reinforcement.* New York: Appleton-Century-Crofts, 1957.

Gagne, R. *The conditions of learning.* (2nd Ed.) New York: Holt, Rinehart and Winston, Inc., 1970.

Gardner, W. I. *Behavior modifications in mental retardation.* Chicago: Aldine-Atherton, Inc., 1971.

Harlow, H. F. The nature of love. *American Psychologist*, 1958, **13**:673-685.

Hewett, F. M. *The emotionally disturbed child in the classroom.* Boston: Allyn & Bacon, Inc., 1968.

Hilgard, E. R. *Theories of learning.* New York: Appleton-Century-Crofts, 1956.

Hull, C. L. *Principles of behavior.* New York: Appleton-Century-Crofts, 1943.

Keller, F. S. *Learning: reinforcement theory.* New York: Random House, Inc., 1966.

Kimble, G. A. *Hilgard and Marquis' conditioning and learning.* New York: Appleton-Century-Crofts, 1961.

Martin, B. Reward and punishment associated with the same goal response: a factor in the learning of motives. *Psychological Bulletin*, 1963, **60**:441-451.

Masters, John, and Morris, R. Effects of contingent and noncontingent reinforcement upon generalized imitation. *Child Development*, 1971, **42**:385-397.

Miller, N. E. Liberalization of basic S—R concepts: extension to conflict behavior, motivation, and social learning. In S. Koch (Ed.), *Psychology, a study of a science*, Vol. 2. New York: McGraw-Hill Book Co., 1959.

Morse, W. H., and Kelleher, R. T. Schedules as fundamental determinants of behavior. In W. N. Schoenfeld (Ed.), *The theory of reinforcement schedules.* New York: Appleton-Century-Crofts, 1970, pp. 139-183.

Olds, J., and Milner, P. Positive reinforcement produced by electrical stimulation of septal area and other regions of rat brain. *Journal of Comparative Physiology Psychology*, 1954, **47**:419-427.

Orlando, R., and Bijou, S. W. Single and multiple schedules of reinforcement in developmentally retarded children. *Journal of Experimental Analysis of Behavior*, 1960, **3**:339-348.

Ribble, M. A. Infantile experience in relation to personality development. In J. McV. Hunt (Ed.), *Personality and the behavior disorders.* New York: The Ronald Press Co., 1944.

Scott, R. and others. The use of shaping and reinforcement in the operant acceleration and deceleration of heart rate. *Behavior Research and Therapy*, 1972, **11**:179-185.

Sheffield, F. D., Wulff, J. J., and Backer, R. Reward value of copulation without sex drive reduction. *Journal of Comparative Physiological Psychology* 1951, **44**:3-8.

Skinner, B. F. *The behavior of organisms: an experimental analysis*. New York: Appleton-Century-Crofts, 1938.

Skinner, B. F. *Science and human behavior*. New York: The Macmillan Co., 1953.

Skinner, B. F. *The technology of teaching*. New York: Appleton-Century-Crofts, 1968.

Soloman, R. L. Punishment. *American Psychologist*, 1964, **19**:239-253.

Spencer, K. W. *Behavior theory and conditioning*. New Haven, Conn.: Yale University Press, 1956.

Tapp, J. T. Current status and future directions. In Tapp, J. T. (Ed.), *Reinforcement and behavior*. New York: Academic Press, Inc., 1969, pp. 387-416.

Thorndike, E. L. *Animal intelligence*. New York: The Macmillan Co., 1911.

Tolman, E. C. *Purposive behavior in animals and men*. New York: Appleton-Century-Crofts, 1932.

Whiting, J. W. M., and Mowrer, O. H. Habit progression and regression—a laboratory study of some factors relevant to human socialization. *Journal of Comparative Psychology*, 1943, **36**:229-253.

Wilcoxon, H. Historical introduction to the problem of reinforcement. In J. Tapp (Ed.), *Reinforcement and behavior*. New York: Academic Press, Inc., 1969, pp. 2-44.

Witte, K. L., and Grossman, E. The effects of reward and punishment upon children's attention, motivation and discrimination learning. *Child Development*, 1971, **42**:537-542.

Wolfe, J. B., and Kaplan, M. D. Effect of amount of reward and consummating activity on learning with chickens. *Journal of Comparative Psychology*, 1941, **31**:353-361.

Feedback

DESCRIPTION OF MODULE

This is a self-contained unit of instruction on the variable of "feedback" as it affects learning and instruction. The main text of the module covers five major areas that are presented in an integrated form: (1) theoretical framework, (2) relevant research studies, (3) issues, (4) application to nursing education, practice, and the development of other social behaviors, (5) researchable questions.

In addition to the main text, the module contains instruction to the learner, list of a specific objectives to be achieved by the learner, and a pretest and posttest to determine the extent of the accomplishment of objectives.

MODULE OBJECTIVES

At the completion of this module on feedback, having studied the content presented and the recommended reading list, the student will be able to accomplish the objectives at the 95% level of mastery. The student will be able to:
1. Describe in writing the theoretical framework of the role of feedback in learning and instruction, including the following:
   a. Defining feedback
   b. Identifying and defining the different types of feedback
   c. Describing the different functions of feedback

d. Describing the theoretical account of the nature of feedback
   e. Specifying how feedback should be given in different conditions of learning
2. Cite relevant research studies that test the effect of feedback on learning, performance
3. Apply the principles of feedback to nursing education and practice and specify how the student can use them in specific learning or social-learning situations
4. Identify at least one issue in feedback
5. Raise one researchable question and identify the inependent and dependent variables

PRETEST AND POSTTEST

Circle the correct answers. Each question is worth 1 point. The 95% level of mastery for this unit is 19 points. Take the test and correct your answers by using the answer key that is found at the end of this module (p. 361). If you score 19 correct points or better you need not study this module, but should move to the next one.

Multiple choice

1. Feedback can best be defined as:
   a. that part of reinforcement theory pertaining to rewards and punishment
   b. the information available to the person that makes possible the comparison of actual

performance with some standard of performance

c. an incentive measure to increase student motivation

2. Knowledge of results as a demonstrable form of feedback serves which of the following major functions:
   a. goal attainment, grading, determination of the degree of progress made
   b. informative, reinforcing, incentive, prompting, and motivational functions
   c. drive reduction, drive increase, effort increase

3. Feedback can act as a form of prompting or cueing. Which of the following best illustrates this statement?
   a. The teacher is nodding in an approving manner as the student is verbally answering a question.
   b. The teacher gives hints pertaining to the correct answer before the student verbally answers or as the student makes the response.
   c. The teacher waits until the student is finished verbally answering and then gives immediate feedback (without any delay).

4. In skill learning, the effect of delaying feedback causes:
   a. such confusion that it becomes impossible to learn the skill
   b. a decrease in the rate of learning the skill
   c. no major difficulties in the rate of learning the skill

5. In early skill learning, which types of feedback are relied on most:
   1—extrinsic
   2—intrinsic
   3—external
   4—internal
   a. 1 and 4
   b. 1 and 3
   c. 2 and 4
   d. 2 and 3

6. Positive reinforcement stresses the reward effect of learning; feedback emphasizes:
   a. internal control or motivation
   b. knowledge of results and informational aspects of learning

c. need for practice
d. only what the student is doing wrong

7. Lack of feedback in any learning procedure will tend to result in:
   a. loss in student motivation and decrease in performance
   b. no difference in motivation or learning
   c. the student trying harder
   d. the student being frustrated

You are faced with the task of teaching beginning nursing students fundamental nursing skills. You decide that a good place to start would be with how to give a bed-bath. The students are in a simulated hospital ward with training dummies for practice. You have demonstrated the procedure step by step to the students, and it is now time for them to practice. (Use this situation in answering questions 8-9.)

8. Utilizing your knowledge of feedback principles, it is necessary for you to:
   a. let the students rely on intrinsic feedback in this initial phase of giving a bed-bath
   b. make sure the students follow each step in its proper sequence so that they will experience success in their first attempts
   c. supervise the students closely, offer them frequent extrinsic feedback, and draw their attention to external cues and to their own movements

9. As the students move into the autonomous phase of learning to give a bed-bath you would expect them:
   a. to utilize intrinsic feedback and assuming responsibility for their own evaluation
   b. to still rely on you for cueing and prompting
   c. to rely more heavily on extrinsic feedback

10. The situation that provides the least feedback to the instructor is:
    a. recitation
    b. discussion
    c. programmed instruction
    d. homework assignments

11. In verbal and discrimination learning, feedback takes the form of:
    a. verbal expression
    b. confirmation of correct responses
    c. extrinsic feedback
    d. internal feedback

Fill in the blank

12. Giving the student advance information on the performance of a skill may be _____ efficient than using only feedback for information.
    a. equally
    b. less
    c. more

Matching

Part A

____ 13. Intrinsic feedback
____ 14. Internal feedback
____ 15. Augmented feedback
____ 16. Action feedback
____ 17. Learning feedback
____ 18. Extrinsic feedback
____ 19. External feedback

Part B

a. Information supplied by another concerning the effectiveness of action
b. Information received through the sensory organs
c. Feedback that arrives and can be utilized by the subject during a response
d. Information obtained through one's own actions
e. Information obtained from the internal receptor organs
f. Feedback that comes after the completion of the response, such that information cannot be used to control the response being measured but can only be used by the subject for subsequent responses
g. Additional feedback added by the experimenter to the situation, such as a nod of the head in approval

Discussion question

20. Diagram a TOTE unit on a nursing procedure of your choice.

TEST
Theoretical framework
Introduction

Feedback is also known as *knowledge of results*. Feedback is operationally defined as the information the learners receive about their own performances that enables them to compare actual performance with that of a standard performance. In other words, it is the information by which learners determine what is going on and how well they are doing. They gather clues and indications from what the teacher says and does, from the behavior of others, from readings, and from their own reflections on the events taking place.

Feedback acts as a form of prompting for the student by giving information before or at the same time the response is being made. The basic intention of feedback is to motivate learning. For this end, as pointed out by Gagne (1970, p. 315), "Some means or other must be provided during instruction for him to perceive the results of his activity, to receive from the learning environment some feedback that enables him to realize that his performance is 'correct.' "

Knowledge of results motivates learning by rewarding the learners through recognizing their contributions, through validating that they are on the right track, through helping to identify the additional knowledge or skill that might be needed. For this end the learning situation must be constructed with liberal opportunities for feedback; for example, formative evaluations provide frequent opportunities for feedback. The teacher has the critical responsibility for developing these opportunities. The teacher must point out discrepancies in the student's performance of the skill. In reporting their observations, teachers should direct attention to external clues and discrimination in movements that the student tends to ignore. Feedback should be positive and encouraging; sarcasm and ridicule are virtually always fatal to effective learning.

There are very few actions that have no perceptible results. Knowledge of the results of actions are important to the performer and usually have a definite effect on future behavior. Feedback has a wide range of manifestations—visual, auditory, and kinesthetic. Feedback can appear as a numerical score, a financial reward, a nod from the instructor, or even a flashing light on an experimentation panel. Feedback, or knowledge of results, constitutes one of the most general features of all learning situations (Annet, 1969, pp. 11-12).

Types and modes of feedback

There are various types of feedback specific to the way in which knowledge of results is obtained (DeCecco and Crawford, 1974, pp. 260-261; Annet, 1969, pp. 26-29):

intrinsic feedback obtained through own actions; normally present and not often subject to experimenter manipulation

extrinsic feedback supplied by another concerning the effectiveness of the subject's actions (as between teacher and student)

external feedback received through the external sensory organs (vision, hearing, touch, smell, and taste)

internal feedback obtained from internal receptor organs (kinesthetic feedback)

augmented feedback obtained when an experimenter adds additional feedback (such as a nod of the head in approval)

learning feedback received after the completion of the response, such that the information cannot be used to control the response being measured but can only be used by the subject for subsequent responses

action feedback arrives and can be utilized by the subject during a response

The role of feedback in the different types of learning

In simple forms of learning, such as operant conditioning, feedback from the performance of desired responses needs to occur immediately—within a few seconds—if learning is to progress rapidly. In animal learning, feedback is obtained if the animal obtains a reward (such as a food pellet after pressing the correct lever). If the delay of re-

ward is more than 30 seconds, learning takes place more slowly, though Gagne (1970) pointed out that it is possible for animals to learn behaviors even when the reward is delayed for a minute or longer. Gagne (1970) and Kimble (1961, pp. 196-198) proposed that observations of learning under such feedback conditions have suggested that animals actually learn chains that are made up of links that they themselves provide and that fill the gap between their correct performance and the occurrence of reinforcement. This kind of event stresses the importance of immediate feedback.

In skill learning feedback constitutes one of the basic conditions of learning. *Intrinsic feedback* in skill learning is obtained by the learner's own action. For example, when the student nurse correctly performs the procedure of catheterization and obtains the urine from the patient's bladder and relieves the patient's distension, the effects of the actions (obtaining the urine and relieving distension) become intrinsic feedback.

Extrinsic feedback is the information the teacher gives the student about the effectiveness and correctness of the actions. For example, in the above example, the nursing instructor may point out to the student that the receptacle (curve basin) where the urine is being emptied should be below the patient's bladder level so that urine will not syphon back into the patient's bladder and cause infection.

Annet (1964) further stated that, as the student moves from the fixation stage of skill learning to the autonomous stage, the student relies more on intrinsic feedback and less on extrinsic feedback. In this way, skill learning becomes self-evaluative.

The two modes of feedback in skill learning are internal and external feedback (Robb, 1966). The *internal* feedback in skill learning is the information the student receives by means of internal receptor organs, such as in kinesthetic feedback. For example, in putting on sterile gloves, the feeling that the glove on the hand feels right would be kinesthetic feedback. The *external* feedback in skill learning is the information the student receives about the performance by means of external sensory organs, such as vision, hearing, touch, smell, and taste. For example, in putting on the gloves, when the student looks and see that the left glove is on the left hand and the thumb of the glove is toward the body, this provides external feedback by means of vision. Fitts (1951) pointed out that the more accomplished the student is in performing a specific skill, the more the student will rely on internal feedback. Gagne and Fleishman (1959) further proposed that not until the learner is able to sort out the internal feedback dependably is the specific skill performed consistently performed.

Extrinsic and external feedback are important in the early stages of learning, whereas intrinsic and internal feedback are important in the later stages of learning. Since the motivational aspects of feedback may affect performance in terms of the amount of effort the student will invest in practicing the skill, feedback should be given immediately, or very nearly immediately. In some instances, giving the student advance information on the performance of a skill may be more efficient than using feedback alone for information.

Two major sources of evidence that feedback is important in skill learning are: experiments in which feedback has been withheld and experiments in which feedback has been delayed. The following is a discussion of research experiments that were done to prove the importance of feedback.

Elwell and Grindley (1938) did an experiment where feedback was withheld. The skill that they taught the students was a coordinated movement with both hands, by which the students could direct a spot of light on a specific target (bull's-eye). The amount of error in the movement of either hand was indicated by the degree of deviation of the spot of light from the target—a form of intrinsic feedback. At a specific point in the experiment, feedback was withdrawn, that is, the students could no longer see the target. The withdrawal of feedback led to a drastic drop in performance, which adversely affected motivation. The students became bored, lost their keenness, and even began coming late to the experiment. Results of this experiment demonstrated that feedback not only has an effect on skill learning but also affects the conscious attitude of the student to want to perform the task with accuracy.

The effect of delaying feedback on skill learning was tested by Lorge and Thorndike (1935). The skill to be learned in this experiment was for the students to throw two wooden balls over their heads at an unseen target of concentric circles. They had eight groups of students:

Group 1—the informational and motivational aspects of the feedback were not separated; feedback was extrinsic, that is, students were told about the accuracy of their throws
Group 2—received no feedback
Group 3—received immediate feedback
Group 4—received feedback after 1 second
Group 5—received feedback after 2 seconds
Group 6—received feedback after 4 seconds
Group 7—received feedback after 6 seconds
Group 8—received feedback for a previous throw after making an intervening throw.

Results of this experiment showed that groups 2 and 8 showed no improvement. Also, less improvement was observed in groups 6 and 7, which received four- to six-second delays, than in groups 4 and 5, which received one- to four-second delays.

In another experiment Greenspoon and Foreman (1956) tested the effects of an extended period of delay of feedback on skill learning. The task was for the students to draw 3-inch straight line while blindfolded, with hands and arms off the table. The extrinsic feedback provided was: if the line was more than $3^1/2$ inches long, they were told "long"; if less than 2 inches long, they were told "short"; and if between $2^1/2$ and 3 inches long, they were told "right." There were five groups of subjects:

Group 1—given immediate feedback
Group 2—given no feedback
Group 3—given feedback after a delay of 10 seconds
Group 4—given feedback after a delay of 20 seconds
Group 5—given feedback after a delay of 30 seconds

Results of this experiment showed that increasing the length of delay of feedback reduced the rate of learning. When delay of feedback was 10 seconds or less, it had little effect on performance. After 10 seconds, performance dropped sharply.

DeCecco and Crawford (1974) pointed out further that feedback also acts as a form of *prompting*. In this role, feedback provides information to the learner at the same time that the response is being made. Annet (1964) stressed that feedback really comes between responses. He stated that the fact that information comes before the next response in a series of responses may be as important as information that comes after the preceding response. In one study Annet (1964) demonstrated that advance information was more effective than feedback given after the response. Both Annet (1964) and DeCecco and Crawford (1974) stressed the fact that providing advance instructional guidance to enable the students to avoid making mistakes in the first place may be as important as feedback after the response. This, of course, is the major concern of programmed instruction. Feedback after the performance is only one way to provide the students with neces-

sary information to achieve desired actions. It may not always be the most effective and efficient instructional method (DeCecco and Crawford, 1974, p. 263).

From these experiments on the effects of withholding and delaying feedback on learning, it can be concluded that:

1. Feedback is a form of reinforcement affecting motivation and learning
2. The informational aspect of feedback is important in learning, and the motivational aspect is important in performance
3. Both reward and punishment act as emphasizers because individuals tend to remember responses that are rewarded or punished
4. Emphasis (pleasant and unpleasant) on the right responses is more effective than that on the wrong responses
5. Feedback directs the student's attention and increases efforts in learning
6. Reward and punishment affects, either adversely or beneficially, the way a student learns a skill
7. Success or failure that is reported to the student can both increase and decrease efforts

Annet (1969) further stressed the role of feedback on the development of perceptual skills. Perceptual skills are divided into the three categories: (1) detection, (2) discrimination, and (3) magnitude judgments.

Detection is the simplest form of perceptual task. Feedback functions in perceptual tasks as a simple confirmation of the "yes" or "no" response and can change the proportion of right and wrong responses in succeeding practice sessions, but at the expense of lowering the response criterion. In other words, many more "yes" responses will be given, therefore, a larger number of detections will be produced (Annet, 1969, pp. 62-68).

In detection tasks, feedback in the form of giving advance information instead of knowledge of results can be termed cueing. Cueing in perceptual tasks is related to guidance or action feedback in motor tasks and prompting in verbal tasks. Thus, the main function of feedback becomes an informative one in perceptual skill learning (Annet 1969, pp. 62-68).

In a discrimination task, the subject is usually presented two stimuli, a standard and a variable. The task is to say if there is a difference or in what way the one stimului differ from each other. Various studies reveal a lack of improvement with practice, either with or without feedback (Annet, 1969, pp. 68-70).

In a magnitude judgment task, the subject is usually asked to examine the stimulus and make an estimation of the magnitude of some property of the stimulus. The evidence gathered from experimentation with feedback and magnitude judgments suggests that perceptual learning can take place without explicit knowledge of results and that learning does seem to be greatly assisted by giving the subject frequent pairings of the stimuli to be judged with the appropriate scale values (Annet, 1969, pp. 70-72).

To summarize, in a variety of perceptual tasks various forms of feedback have been found to be effective. It appears that the most important effect of feedback in perceptual learning is to increase the subject's readiness to respond, rather than to increase sensitivity to the signal. This increased sensitivity is the result of the information provided in the cue or feedback signal (Annet, 1969, pp. 74-75).

In summarizing the effects of feedback on overall skill learning DeCecco and Crawford (1974, pp. 263-264) further concluded that:

1. Feedback is the most important variable that governs the learning of skills
2. Extrinsic and external feedback are important in the early stages of skill learning, and intrinsic and internal feedback are important in the later stages of skill learning

3. Feedback should be immediate in order to be effective
4. Giving the student advance information on performance expected may be more important and efficient than using it as feedback for information after it has been performed
5. The motivational aspect of feedback is both the student's performance and perseverance, or the amount of effort the student will invest in learning a skill

In *verbal learning*, feedback, confirmation of correct responses, is one of the external conditions of learning. This is mostly done by exhibiting in print the correct response to the learner after the response has been made. If the response is correct, this exposure enables the learner to confirm the link by matching what was just said with what is seen. Learning theorists consider this method of giving feedback as a form of reinforcement because it gives the learner a feeling of satisfaction about responding correctly (Gagne, 1970, p. 142).

Most of the experiments done to test the effect of feedback on verbal learning has been with serial list learning. Annet (1969, pp. 77-95), in summarizing the results of experiments dealing with errors and the type of feedback provided to correct the errors, stated that errors are valuable and that the making of errors subsequently corrected by feedback is a necessary and desirable part of verbal learning. The ways in which subjects are permitted to respond and obtain feedback information does have some effect on verbal learning.

The role of feedback in *discrimination* learning is similar to that in verbal learning. Knowledge of results, in the form of *confirmation* given to the learner either in terms of extrinsic or intrinsic feedback, constitutes one of the essential external conditions of discrimination learning. Gagne (1970, p. 167) stated that in order for multiple discrimination to be learned, the learner must obtain confirmation, that is, "the matching of the responses with those that are known to be correct. When the learner reinstates a chain, he must have a way of knowing that it contains a correct terminal response." This can be done by showing the learner the word that is correct, soon after a response is made. As in the case of verbal learning, most learning theorists perceive this operation as one of reinforcement.

The role of feedback in the learning of concepts, rules, or a set of interrelated rules (as in problem solving) is also very important. Gagne (1972) stated that, in concept or rule learning, the learner making a response that reflects a newly acquired capability and then being told whether it is "right" or "wrong" constitutes feedback that is of reinforcing value also. In the teaching situation, supplying acknowledgement of correct responses to the student can be accomplished by many other means, such as a nod, smile, or glance; proceeding to the next point, or formative evaluations in the form of appraisal tests at the end of small units of instruction.

The frequency of supplying feedback in rule learning is also very important. Gagne noted that the designers of programmed instruction stress the importance of supplying confirming responses each step of the way. When lengthy topics are to be learned, feedback for the correct accomplishment of each subtopic is of considerable value in efficient learning of concepts and rules. Gagne also stated that feedback need not always come from external sources, the learner may provide it by being able to recall concepts and rules. Often the learner knows whether a response is right or wrong because of an internal check that can be applied to the responses produced. This internal checking may be interpreted as a reinforcing state of affairs that facilitates the learning of rules and hierarchies of rules.

Gagne further stressed that if immediacy of feedback is important in learning concepts and rules, as is true for simple forms of learning, self-checking may be the best way to achieve it. Even though at times "knowledge that one is right" may be incorrect, when the learner further verifies the answers with an external standard, the effect of self-checking provides some immediate satisfaction and facilitates and speeds learning (Gagne, 1970, p. 317).

In problem solving, the student will be able to solve the problem faster when verbal instructions (advance feedback) are given about the nature of the performance expected because this enables the student to recall certain subordinate rules and helps guide thinking. This concept was tested with college students to enable them to solve Maier's pendulum problem (Gagne, 1970, pp. 220-221).

Theoretical explanation of the nature of feedback

Different schools of thought have different explanations about the nature and function of feedback. A classical view is that all forms of feedback can be regarded as either rewarding or punishing. On this basis, a rewarding result preserves the behavior that preceded it by some as yet unexplained mechanism. Thus, a stimulus-response-result pattern becomes normally related in a coherent behavior.

According to reinforcement theory, learning is viewed as an adaptation to the exigencies of the real world. Behavior is adapted or modified by the beneficial and detrimental effects of individual responses. This leads to the principle that behavior is subject to selection by results. The idea that behavior is preserved by desirable effects and is altered by undesirable effects becomes extremely compelling. Unfortunately, this idea has proved difficult for experimenters to work out in detail (Annet, 1969, pp. 29-33).

E. L. Thorndike did extensive research relating feedback to reinforcement theory. He formulated a systematical learning theory that attributed the selection of behavior to the consequences or effects of action. Basically, Thorndike claimed that stimulus-response connections can be strengthened or weakened by feedback and that learning is a process of changing the strength of these connections and of acquiring new connections. Thorndike's view can be diagrammatically represented:

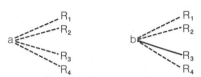

In the diagram, a is the representation of the connection before any reinforcement; whereas b is the representation of the connection after reinforcement of response R_3.

Thorndike was mainly concerned with two possible reasons for the strengthening or reinforcement of these connections: (1) the frequency of repetition has the possibility of strengthening the connection (law of exercise), and (2) the after-effects have the possibility of strengthening the connection (law of effect). Thorndike produced substantial evidence that repetition alone could not strengthen the the connection and that some positive after-effect was required. The point that Thorndike stressed, and the one that constitutes the major source of dissatisfaction among his critics, is that the function of reinforcers is automatic and inevitable. He described the function of reinforcers as a "biological" force that acts in a direct and irresistible fashion (Annet, 1969, pp. 32-33, 39).

The theory of servomechanisms can offer an integration of consequences and results with antecedent stimuli. A simple servomechanism is essentially a machine that is controlled by the consequences of its own behavior. It will maintain a uniform output despite variations in load conditions. A diagramatical representation of a simple servomechanism is shown at bottom of this page. Information about the motor output is turned into appropriate instructions to the power-supply control and, thereby, a relationship is established between the power-supply control and the motor speed. When the feedback loop of a servomechanism is interrupted the equilibrium of the system is disrupted (Annet, 1969, pp. 16-18).

In terms of feedback loops, behavior as a whole is capable of description in terms of hierarchies of feedback loops. Miller, Galanter, and Pribram (1960) developed a systematical description of a behavior unit, called a TOTE (an acronym for "test, operate, test, exit"). The "test" is an inspection of sensory data that detects any incongruity between the desired and the actual state of affairs. On detection of an incongruity, the "operate" action is initiated and is followed by a further "test." This cycle continues until the incongruity disappears, and the activity is then switched off, or to "exit." The following diagram of a surgical skin preparation illustrates a recurrent TOTE cycle:

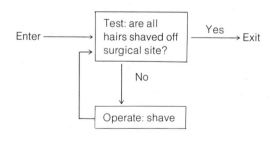

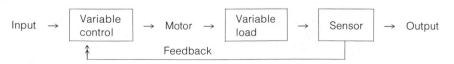

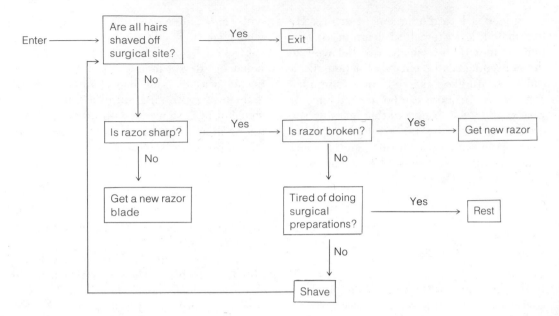

Surgical skin preparation can constitute an entire plan (for surgical skin preparations) by linking TOTE units together in a hierarchial structure:

Descriptions of behavioral plans represented in this way are called algorithms. They have been used with success in describing the activities a person must engage in to achieve a given objective (in this case, surgical skin preparation) (Annet, 1979, pp. 21-25).

Relevant issues

Issues regarding feedback are mainly concerned with feedback's function. There are those who believe feedback serves only a motivational or incentive function; others believe feedback's function is merely that of reinforcement; and still others claim feedback serves only an informational function.

Among those who believe feedback's function is motivational are the cognitive theorists. They tend to emphasize the intellectual, rational, or information processing aspects of behavior. They run the risk of leaving the organism "rapt in thought" with no apparent motive to do anything at all.

On the other hand, those who emphasize drives, motives, and needs tend to paint a picture of the organism or the learner at the mercy of biological urges, stumbling irrationally from one deprivation state to another without thinking.

There appear to be two motivational functions of feedback: the incentive effect and the reinforcing effect. The incentive effect induces a temporary change in behavior and constitutes a promise along with changed behavior before any reward is given. The reinforcing effect induces a permanent change in behavior; however, physical rewards must have incentive value to be satisfying.

In summary, motivation could be described as feedback in action. The feedback model fits the data on incentives but the implication is that incentive effects are not basically different from informational effects (Annet, 1969, pp. 105-121).

Explanation of feedback purely in terms of reinforcement is subject to criticism. According to stimulus-response theorists, learning usually occurs when subjects are given "right" or "wrong" feedback. If the reinforcement principle is extended to secondary or symbolical reinforcement, it appears to have a fairly direct analogy with primary and secondary reinforcement in animal learning. However, the theory breakdown arrives when one tries to directly apply the law of effects. There seems to be no evidence for the operation of drive reduction (Williams, 1973, pp. 85-86).

The information hypothesis regarding feedback's function has been proposed by several psychologists (Bilodeau, Fitts, and Posner), as cited by Williams (1973), who have mainly been concerned with human learning. These investigators claim that "knowledge of results," or "response feedback," is reinforcing for an individual in terms of whether or not the appropriate response was performed. Thus, saying "that's right" to a person after a correct response has been made appears to be functionally similar to presenting an organism with a secondary reinforcer following an instrumental response (Williams, 1973, pp. 85-86).

In conclusion, behavior can be described in terms of hierarchies of feedback loops, as was suggested by Miller, Galanter, and Pribram. Emphasis is placed on the crucial importance of results at all levels of behavior. A survey of motor, perceptual, and verbal tasks has shown that feedback has different functions in each. Various forms of prompting, cueing, and guiding are efficient teaching techniques (Annet, 1969, pp. 168-170).

Application to nursing education and practice

Feedback, or knowledge of results, serves many functions; and the principles of giving and receiving feedback can be applied and used in teaching, communicating, counseling, and T-groups (small group interactions).

Within the realm of instruction the major functions or uses of feedback that are obtained by means of performance assessment that facilitates learning and increases the efficiency of instruction are that it enables the teacher to determine (1) how well the learner has achieved the instructional objectives, (2) the adequacy of the student's entering behavior, and (3) the adequacy of the teacher's instructional procedures (DeCecco and Crawford, 1974, p. 410).

As mentioned previously, feedback should be immediate and frequent to facilitate learning and motivate students. Frequently giving formative tests (Bloom, 1968) is one method that the nursing teacher can utilize to provide feedback to the students about the extent of the objective that they have achieved. The teacher must arrange instructional procedures in ways that permit students to develop checkpoints and standards for assessing their own achievements. de Tornyay (1971) suggested that another method by which to see if student have achieved the objective is to ask for examples that illustrate the main point. This feedback mechanism allows the teacher to ascertain the level of understanding students have and also the adequacy of the instructional procedure. Furthermore, asking students to share experiences that exemplify the concept under consideration not only helps other students to broaden their understanding but also reinforces learning and promotes transfer.

Another area where the teacher must be alert to the utilization of feedback is in the realm of sensitivity in interpreting nonverbal cues from the students. Some of their nonverbal cues may indicate lack of understanding, boredom, or daydreaming.

There has been extensive research in the area of feedback, and the knowledge of the importance of supplying feedback has sparked several technological innovations, including programmed instruction and computer-assisted instruction.

Frequent and immediate knowledge of results is a central feature in programmed learning and instruction. In addition to immediate feedback, all programming methods emphasize that the student should be active rather than passive in learning.

Skinner regards the knowledge of results in programmed learning as providing immediate reinforcement. The learner is induced to make correct responses, and these are reinforced by immediate confirmation. Learning is better when feedback is made contingent on responding.

Skinner's idea of a good unit of programmed instruction approximates a good tutor by:

1. Beginning where the pupil is and not insisting on moving beyond what the pupil can comprehend
2. Moving at a rate consistent with the pupil's ability to learn
3. Not permitting inaccurate answers to remain uncorrected
4. Not lecturing, but instead using hints and questioning to help the pupil find and state answers

Furthermore, programmed learning does not allow mistakes to be perpetuated while waiting for feedback. Findings of experiments with teaching machines suggest that a delay of knowledge of results usually, but not always, causes less adequate performance (Williams, 1973, pp. 202-205).

Extensive use of the feedback concept has been made in the social sciences—in particular the study of communication. Students of social sciences have put great stress on achievement of insight about themselves from their observation of what others say and do. Kurt Lewin (1951), in the training of individuals in human relationships, extended the idea to practically every social situation; for instance, to action researchers trying to improve the operations of organizations, to businesses or social-work agencies, to supervisors learning to improve their managerial skills and relationships, to parents trying to improve their relationship with their children, and so on. The role of feedback in communication within an organization was well illustrated by McMurry. He stated that chief executives repeatedly fail to recognize that in order for communication to be effective it must be a two-way system. There must be feedback to ascertain the extent to which the message has actually been understood, assimilated, and accepted. This is a step few organizations ever take. This may be because they are afraid to find out how little of the message has actually been transmitted (Brown, 1967, pp. 226-227).

Brown (1967, p. 226) further pointed out that almost all learning is based on the idea of obtaining information about our performance, then determining to what extent have the behaviors approximate the desired goal. This is why there are report cards in schools, advice columns, performance appraisals, person-to-person talks, evaluations, and other more covert ways to obtain some notion about how we are doing.

Feedback is also used in sensitivity-training groups and in T-groups. In these groups members acquaint one another with their own ways of feeling and reacting in a dilemma-invention situation. Feedback also helps in evaluating the consequences of actions that have been taken as a result of the dilemma situation. What is meant by effective feedback, according to Chris Argyris (1964), is that, it is the type of feedback that minimizes the probability of either the sender or receiver of the feedback being defensive and maximizes their opportunity to express their own values, feelings, and attitudes. Within this context, own refers to being aware of and accepting responsibility for their own behavior (Brown, 1967, pp. 226-227).

Bradford further pointed out the importance of feedback both to the group as well as to the group member. He stated that individuals and groups need a feedback process. They need to get accurate information about the difference between the attempt to achieve a skill and how well they actually are doing it. This information is important because it will enable them to correct or change actions. By so doing they steer themselves (Brown, 1967, pp. 226-227).

Such claims for feedback suggest that knowledge of the use of feedback is important to individuals not only in understanding social processes, but in learning their own part in it. Smith and Smith (1966, p. 177) stated that feedback is adequate for the task at hand; that is, if it is immediate, frequent, detailed, and accurate, the task can be performed more effectively and behavior or performance can be improved more through practice than if feedback is delayed, infrequent, incomplete, misleading, or distorted.

To help develop and use the techniques of feedback for personal growth, Lehner (1972) formulated some aids for giving and receiving feedback:

1. *Focus feedback on the behavior rather than on the person;* for example, saying that a person talked for quite a long time in a meeting, rather than that this person is a loudmouth. Focusing on *behavior* implies that it is related to a specific situation that might be changed. Furthermore, to the person who is receiving the feedback, it is less threatening to hear comments on behavior than personal traits.

2. *Focus feedback on observations rather than inferences.* Inferences are interpretations of what has been seen or heard about the behavior of the other person. They contaminate observation, which is a report of what is seen or heard in the behavior of another person.

3. *Focus feedback on description rather than judgment.* Description represents neutral reporting, whereas judgments refer to an evaluation in terms of good or bad, right or wrong. Judgments arise from an individual's personal frame of reference and values.

4. *Focus feedback on descriptions of behavior in terms of more or less rather than in terms of either-or.* The more-or-less terminology implies a continuum on which any behavior may fall. It stresses quantity, which is objective and measurable, rather than quality, which is judgmental and subjective. For example, an individual's participation may be classified as low to high rather than good or bad.

5. *Focus feedback on behavior related to a specific situation, preferably to the here-and-now rather than to behavior in the abstract, placing it in the there-and-then.* Lehner suggested that to increase understanding of a behavior, it should be associated to the time and place where it occurred. Feedback is more meaningful when it is given immediately after the behavior has occurred because it is more free of distortions that come with the lapse of time.

6. *Focus feedback on the sharing of ideas and information rather than on giving advice.* When ideas are shared, each person is free to use them in the light of personal goals in a particular situation and at the appropriate time. When people are told what to do or even are given advice, it takes away their freedom to determine for themselves what is the most appropriate course of action.

7. *Focus feedback on exploration of alternatives rather than on answers or solutions.* The more we focus on the variety of procedures and means for attaining goals, the less likely we are to accept prematurely a particular answer or solution.

8. *Focus feedback on the value it may have to the recipient, not on the value, or the "release," that it provides the person giving the feedback.* Feedback should serve the

needs of the recipient rather than the needs of the giver. Feedback and help should be given and heard by the recipient as an offer rather than an imposition.

9. *Focus feedback on the amount of information the recipient can use, rather than on the amount you may have or may like to give.* To overload the recipient with feedback reduces the possibility of the recipient effectively using what is received.

10. *Focus feedback on time and place so that personal data can be shared at appropriate times.* Feedback about one's own behavior may cause an emotional reaction. It is, therefore, important to be sensitive to when it is appropriate to give the feedback. Good feedback given at an inappropriate time may cause more harm than good.

11. *Focus feedback on what is said rather than why it is said.* The aspects of feedback that relate to what, how, where, and when are observable characteristics. In concentrating on why a person said something, one may not hear *what* the person says. Furthermore, why implies an inference and judgment and brings up the questions of motive and intent.

Lehner concluded by saying that the giving and receiving of feedback require courage, skill, understanding, and respect for oneself and for others (Lehner, 1972, pp. 1-3).

Researchable questions

In sensitivity, or encounter groups, feedback about the person's behavior is given for maybe one to four sessions. It is expected that such a "treatment" should change that specific person's behavior in a specific area (such as relationship with others). How long do the effects of feedback received in sensitivity groups last? Should the person return periodically to these sensitivity groups to receive booster doses of feedback? Are there effective ways of giving feedback to one's own self, like self-checking?

Also, within a school system or during instruction, what is the effect of feedback given to the student in the presence of peers versus when alone on the utilization of feedback and on learning?

Are there individual differences in accepting and utilizing different modes of feedback; for example, verbal versus nonverbal, written versus oral, external versus internal?

Since programmed instruction is one method of instruction that provides immediate feedback to the learners, the question arises as to the appropriateness of the use of programmed instruction in all learning situations. It would be worthwhile to identify and classify the type of cognitive and motor learning tasks in nursing that could be effectively taught by the use of programmed instruction.

ADDITIONAL LEARNING EXPERIENCES-RECOMMENDED READING LIST

DeCecco, J., and Crawford, W. *The psychology of learning and instruction: educational psychology.* (2nd Ed.) Englewood Cliffs, N.J.: Prentice-Hall, Inc., 1974, pp. 187-188, 259-264, 282-283, 410-411.

Gagne, R. M. *The conditions of learning.* (2nd Ed.) New York: Holt, Rinehart and Winston, Inc., 1970, pp. 142, 167-168, 220-221, 315-317.

INSTRUCTIONS TO THE LEARNER REGARDING POSTTEST

At this stage of your learning process you are now ready to take the posttest to determine the extent to which you have achieved the objectives of this module. Return to the pretest and take it over again as the posttest. Correct your answers by utilizing the answer key that is found at the end of this module (p. 361). You need to score 19 correct points to achieve mastery at the 95% level. If you score less than 19 points, study the content of this module again and read the articles in the recommended reading list. Take the posttest again. You need to study in this fashion until you achieve the 95% mastery level or better.

ANSWER KEY TO PRETEST AND POSTTEST

1. b (DeCecco and Crawford, 1974, p. 260)
2. b (DeCecco and Crawford, 1974, pp. 260-264)
3. b (DeCecco and Crawford, 1974, p. 262)
4. b (DeCecco and Crawford, 1974, p. 263)
5. b(DeCecco and Crawford, 1974, p. 264)
6. b (DeCecco and Crawford, 1974, p. 260)
7. a (DeCecco and Crawford, 1974, p. 263)
8. c (DeCecco and Crawford, 1974, p. 264)
9. a (DeCecco and Crawford, 1974, p. 264)
10. a (DeCecco and Crawford, 1974, pp. 239-240)
11. b (Gagne, 1970, pp. 142, 167)
12. c (DeCecco and Crawford, 1974, p. 264)
13. d (DeCecco and Crawford, 1974, pp. 260-261; Annet, 1969, pp. 26-29)
14. e (DeCecco and Crawford, 1974, pp. 260-261; Annet, 1969, pp. 26-29)
15. g (DeCecco and Crawford, 1974, pp. 260-261; Annet, 1969, pp. 26-29)
16. c (DeCecco and Crawford, 1974, pp. 260-261; Annet, 1969, pp. 26-29)
17. f (DeCecco and Crawford, 1974, pp. 260-261; Annet, 1969, pp. 26-29)
18. a (DeCecco and Crawford, 1974, pp. 260-261; Annet, 1969, pp. 26-29)
19. b (DeCecco and Crawford, 1974, pp. 260-261; Annet, 1969, pp. 26-29)
20. Answers will vary. (Text, p. 355-356)

REFERENCES

Argyris, C. T-groups for organizational effectiveness. *Harvard Business Review*, 1964, **42**:60-74.

Annet, J. *The role of knowledge of results in learning: a survey.* Port Washington, New York: U.S. Naval Training Service Center, 1964.

Annet, J. *Feedback and human behavior.* Baltimore: Penguin Books Inc., 1969.

Bloom., B., Learning for mastery. *Evaluation Comment*, 1968, 1(2):1-12.

Brown, D. Some feedback on feedback. *Adult Leadership*, 1967, **15**(7):226-228, 251-252.

DeCecco, J., and Crawford, W. *The psychology of learning and instruction: education psychology.* (2nd Ed.) Englewood Cliffs, N.J. Prentice-Hall, Inc., 1974.

de Tornyay, R. *Strategies for teaching nursing.* New York: John Wiley & Sons, Inc., 1971.

Elwell, J. L., and Grindley, G. C. The effect of knowledge of results on learning and performance. I: A coordinated movement of the two hands. *British Journal of Psychology*, 1938, **29**:39-53.

Fitts, P. Engineering psychology and equipment design. In S. S. Stevens (Ed.), *Handbook of experimental psychology.* New York: John Wiley & Sons, Inc. 1951, pp. 1237-1240.

Gagne, R. M. *The conditions of learning.* (2nd Ed.) New York: Holt, Rinehart and Winston, Inc., 1970.

Gagne, R. M., and Fleishman, E. A. *Psychology and human performance.* New York: Holt, Rinehart and Winston, Inc., 1959.

Greenspoon, J., and Foreman, S. Effect of delay of knowledge of results on learning a motor task. *Journal of Experimental Psychology*, 1956, **51**:226-228.

Kimble, G. A. *Hilgard and Marquis' Conditioning and Learning (2nd Ed.).* New York: Appleton-Century-Crofts, 1961.

Lehner, G. F. Aids for giving and receiving feedback. Unpublished manuscript, Department of Psychology, University of California, Los Angeles, 1972.

Lewin, K. *Field theory in social science.* New York: Harper & Row, Publishers, 1951.

Lorge, I., and Thorndike, E. L. The influence of delay in the after-effect of a connection. *Journal of Experimental Psychology*, 1935, **18**:186-194.

McMurry, R. N. Clear communication for chief executives. *Harvard Business Review*, 1945, **23**:132.

Miller, G. A., Galanter, E., and Pribram, K. H. *Plans and the structure of behavior.* New York: Holt, Rinehart and Winston, Inc., 1960.

Robb, M. Feedback. *Quest,* Monograph VI, 1966, pp. 38-43.

Smith, K., and Smith, M. *Cybernetic principles of learning and educational design.* New York.: Holt, Rinehart and Winston, Inc., 1966.

Williams, J. *Operant learning: procedure for changing behavior.* Monterey, Calif.: Brooks/Cole Publishing Co., 1973.

MODULE 23

Practice

DESCRIPTION OF MODULE

This is a complete unit of instruction on the variable of practice and how it influences learning, and modifies instruction. The content is presented in an integrated form. Five basic areas are covered: (1) theoretical framework, (2) issues, (3) relevant research, (4) application to nursing education and practice, and (5) researchable questions. In order for students to assess their own entering behavior with regard to the level of knowledge about the role of practice in learning and instruction and the extent of the accomplishments of set objectives, a pretest and posttest is provided with appropriate answers to guide the student in self-evaluation. Supplementary learning experiences in the form of reading assignments are also suggested.

MODULE OBJECTIVES

At the completion of this module, having studied the content provided and the recommended reading list, the student will be able to accomplish the following objectives at the 95% level of mastery. Upon completion of this module the student will be able to:
1. Define explicitly the term practice
2. Identify and describe the different types of practice conditions
3. Explain the theoretical framework of the role of practice and its effect on learning and instruction

4. Identify the main issues
5. Cite relevant research studies
6. State specifically and give examples on how to apply the principles of practice conditions
7. Determine when and how to apply the different kinds of practice conditions
9. Identify a researchable question

PRETEST AND POSTTEST

Circle the correct answers. Each question is worth 1 point except the last question, which is worth 10 points. The 95% level of mastery for this test is 26 points. Take the test and correct your answers using the answer key found at the end of this module (p. 374). If you score 26 correct points, you need not study this module.

Multiple choice
1. The repetition of a response in the presence of a stimulus is called:
   a. contiguity
   b. practice
   c. reinforcement
   d. feedback
2. Provision for student practice should be based on:
   a. the learning task
   b. the level of overlearning, which should be 50%

362

c. the student's need for practice to achieve instructional goals

d. the time allowed by the school's schedule

3. Practice is:
   a. an internal condition of learning
   b. a condition inherent in the learning task
   c. an external condition of learning
   d. a form of feedback

4. The type of learning that is likely to require less practice if other learning conditions are properly provided is:
   a. classical conditioning
   b. concept learning
   c. skill learning
   d. operant conditioning

5. Studying and cramming for an exam the day before is an example of:
   a. whole learning
   b. massed practice
   c. overlearning
   d. distributed practice

6. A learning situation where the nursing student repeats the list of medical terminology for 1 hour every day for 7 days, is an example of:
   a. part learning
   b. overlearning
   c. mastery learning
   d. distributed practice
   e. massed practice

7. Massed practice is better than distributed practice because the student:
   a. learns more when the time allowed for learning is limited
   b. retains more
   c. can get a higher grade in the test than with distributed practice
   d. can perform the task in a hurry; therefore, making it more motivating

8. Practice is necessary in skill learning in order to:
   a. prevent forgetting
   b. act as reinforcement
   c. ensure learning of skills by smoothing out any rough spots in the sequence
   d. a and c

9. Kientzle's (1946) study on the effects of the length of the rest period on learning and performance showed that:

a. the most gain in performance was made in 1 minute

b. after 45 seconds of rest the performance increased very little

c. between 0 and 10 seconds of rest the sharpest gains in performance were experienced

d. the more the student rested, the better the performance

10. Which of the following statements is true for skill learning:
    a. Lengthening the rest period is more important than shortening the work period.
    b. Shortening the rest period is more important than lengthening the work period.
    c. The rest period should be nearly as long as the work period.
    d. The length of the rest period must depend on the length of the work period.

11. In verbal learning, such as learning medical terminology and abbreviations, if the error tendency in learning such material is high, the type of practice condition that should prevail is:
    a. part method
    b. whole method
    c. shorter intervals between practice periods in distributed practice
    d. more frequent rest periods

12. In a verbal learning situation, if the probability of forgetting is very high, the type of practice condition that the teacher should recommend is:
    a. distributed practice
    b. massed practice
    c. part method
    d. whole method
    e. overlearning

13. The factor that should determine whether a verbal learning material should be learned by means of part or whole method of practice is:
    a. the length of the material
    b. the time allowed for learning
    c. the internal organization or the structure of the material
    d. if the segments or the units of the learning material can be divided equally

14. When a teacher requires the nursing student to practice a nursing procedure beyond the in-

itial mastery level, the situation is referred to as:

a. mastery
b. overlearning
c. mental practice
d. massed practice

15. According to Kreuger's (1929) experiment on the effectiveness of overlearning, in order to be reassured that the material has been learned and will be retained, the student should practice:

a. to mastery level
b. 50 more times than it took to learn it at the initial mastery level
c. to 100% overlearning
d. to 50% overlearning

16. When the school schedule does not allow the nursing student to practice a skill as many times as is necessary for mastery, the best advice the teacher can give is:

a. to read the assignment
b. to practice the assignment mentally
c. to read some related articles

17. In learning skills in which *speed* is the predominant factor in successful performance, the most efficient results are obtained by:

a. retarding the speed until the student has obtained a reasonable level of accuracy, and then increasing the speed gradually
b. putting emphasis on speed initially
c. emphasizing both speed and accuracy equally

Discussion question

18. Select a specific patient- or student-teaching situation and determine how and why you would implement the different conditions of practice.

TEXT
Theoretical framework
The nature of practice

Practice is one of the important components of external conditions of learning. It is especially important for the simpler conditions of learning, such as classical conditioning, operant conditioning, chaining (also known as skill learning), verbal associates, and multiple discrimination. Practice is not found to be as essential for the higher types of learning, such as concept learning, principle learning, and problem solving.

The rationale for the need for practice is based on the law of exercise. Kimble and Garmezy (1963, p. 133) defined learning as "a relatively permanent change in behavioral tendency and is the result of reinforced practice."

Practice is the repetition of a response in the presence of a stimulus. It is necessary to practice stimulus-response associations if they are to be retained for long periods of time. De Cecco and Crawford (1974) pointed out that, currently, educational systems are emphasizing cognitive and meaningful learning. The term practice is becoming a very highly and negatively valenced word and a very unpopular learning condition. It is important for teachers to keep in mind that provisions for student practice should be based on the student's need for practice to achieve the instructional goals and objectives. This is specifically important in nursing education because there are a variety of students, having different educational backgrounds and experiences. For example, an undergraduate freshman student may be a registered nurse returning to school to get a baccalaureate degree, a practical nurse, a nurses' aide, or a recent high-school graduate who knows nothing about nursing and has never been in contact with patients. Therefore, how do nursing educators differentiate the amount and quality of practice needed for the registered nurse as a student versus the basic student? What provisions are needed to meet each student's needs? What are the criteria needed to set up specific objectives for practice in each area for each student?

The role of practice or repetition in different conditions of learning

As mentioned in the previous modules on conditions of learning, the role of practice, or repetition, is very important as an external condition in simpler forms of learning. In the next section, the role of practice in each of the simple forms of learning is presented. Issues and research studies relevant to each are presented. The teacher's role in providing practice and extrapolations to nursing education and practice are made.

CLASSICAL CONDITIONING

In *classical conditioning* repetition of the paired stimuli (conditioned and unconditioned) is necessary. The amount of repetition varies depending on the response involved and on the intensity of the unconditioned stimulus with which it is evoked. As pointed out by Gagne (1970), the connection between the conditioned and unconditioned stimuli increases in strength as the number of repetitions of paired stimuli is increased.

OPERANT CONDITIONING

In operant conditioning, repetition of the stimulus situation is also a necessary external condition of type-2 learning. The amount of repetition necessary varies depending on the difficulty of the discrimination involved and the degree to which it conforms with responding that is either previously learned or innately determined. Repetition serves the function of *selection* of stimuli to be discriminated (Estes, 1959). In successive repetitions of the learning situations, the specific samples of the total stimulus situation are associated with specific responses. Some of these associations are more successful in producing reinforcement than are others. The successful associations are selected, and the unsuccessful ones drop out. Thus the desired behavior is shaped by means of this selective process. Gagne (1970) pointed out that, according to this concept, the total learned connection is composed of a number of individual stimulus-response units, and learning is considered to be the gradual recruitment of the "bundle" of individual connections that result in reinforcement, rather than strength-ening of individual stimulus-response connections (Gagne, 1970, pp. 109-110).

CHAINING, OR SKILL LEARNING

In chaining, or skill learning, practice is a necessary external condition for the attainment of a high level of performance in complex skills. Repetition of the sequence of a chain serves the function of "smoothing out" the rough spots. Practice also enables the student to rehearse those particular subtasks that are only partially learned. Practice prevents extinction and forgetting of the subtasks. In the learning of skills, practice is a way of coordinating the subtasks so that they are performed in the proper sequence and with appropriate timing. It also facilitates the development of the skill to the autonomous stage of learning.

Several issues have been raised with regard to the necessity of practice and the type of practice needed in skill learning. In this next section, these specific issues are presented.

Issues in skill learning with regard to the need and type of practice necessary

Massed practice versus distributed practice. Is it better to practice a task with as little interruption for rest as possible, or is rest beneficial to the learning and performance of skills? In other words, which is more useful—massed practice or distributed practice?

Massed practice is the learning situation where the student repeats or performs the task over and over again with no or little interruption or rest period. An example of massed practice would be cramming and studying for an examination the night before.

Distributed practice refers to those learning situations where the student repeats or performs a task several times then takes a rest period. Another example may be the nursing student learning a list of medical terminology 1 hour per day for several days or learning how to perform a procedure (such as cathe-

Groups	Trials	Rest period between trials	Performance results (amount of time required to complete drawing on each trial)
Group 1 (massed practice)	20	No rest	No drop in time per trial
Group 2 (distributed practice)	20	1 minute rest between trials	On trials 3 and 4, rapid drop in amount of time per trial
Group 3 (distributed practice)	20	1 day rest between trials	On trials 3 and 4, rapid drop in amount of time per trial

terization) once or twice a day for a week or more until mastering the task. Distributed practice allows for rest periods.

The classical experiment of Irving Lorge (1930) demonstrated the different effects of massed and distributed practices. He had three groups of students. Among other tasks, these students had to learn to draw a figure, using only a mirror image of the figure they were drawing. The students had very little previous practice on this task. The experiment could be summarized as shown in the table.

As can be seen, results are in favor of the distributed practice. Lorge's findings are typical of experiments that have compared the effects of massed and distributed practice. This experiment raises another very important question: length of the rest period, which is the second issue.

Length of rest period. Does the length of the rest period make an important difference in the learning and performance of the skill? In Lorge's (1930) experiment a rest period of 1 minute and a rest period of 1 day had about the same effects. To test at what point in time the rest period no longer pays off, Mary Kientzle (1946) performed an experiment. Her task for the students was to print the alphabet upside down so that when the paper was turned 180 degrees the alphabet could be read in the usual manner. The rest period varied from 0 seconds (massed practice) to 7 days (distributed practice). Results of this ex-

periment showed that after 45 seconds there were very few increases in performance. The most gain was made between 0 and 10 seconds. This experiment confirmed Lorge's findings and also demonstrated clearly that a rest period of a few seconds produces the maximum gains in distributed practice (De-Cecco, 1968). This experiment also raises another question, which brings up the third issue.

Rest period versus work period. Which is more important, the rest period or the practice, or work, period? Kimble and Bilodeau (1949) performed an experiment to answer this question. They asked the students to perform a simple task—to overturn cylindrical blocks in a large board containing circular holes. The experimental conditions were as follows:

Groups	Work period (in seconds)	Rest period (in seconds)
Group 1	10	10
Group 2	10	30
Group 3	30	10
Group 4	30	30

Results of this experiment showed that shortening the rest period is much more important than lengthening the work period. They also found out that the length of the rest period must depend on the length of the work period. DeCecco (1968) and Deese (1958) also pointed out that one cannot arbitrarily decide how long the work period must be without taking into consideration the nature of the task. Deese suggested that it would be unwise to interrupt someone solving a puzzle before it is solved (DeCecco, 1968, p. 288).

In summarizing the findings of these studies DeCecco (1968) arrived at the following conclusions:

1. For performance of motor skills, distributed practice or some rest period is better than none at all. The effect of rest periods varies with different skills.

2. The effects of massed practice are not as detrimental in verbal learning as they are in skill learning, and they do not occur as consistently in verbal learning as in skill learning. In verbal learning, the findings are more complex and may indicate no significant difference in the effects of massed versus distributed practice. On the other hand, in skill learning, experiments have consistently demonstrated that distributed practice is superior to massed practice (DeCecco, 1968, p. 290).

PRACTICE CONDITIONS IN VERBAL LEARNING (VERBAL ASSOCIATION)

Gagne (1970, p. 145) stated, "But by all odds the most important condition for the prevention of forgetting of verbal sequences is *repetition* . . . the longer the sequence, the greater the interference and the more repetition is needed for adequate recall." Gagne also indicated that the function that repetition or practice serves in retaining the learned verbal chains. He stated that, "One good possibility is that repetition is needed to overcome the effects of errors and error tendencies" (Gagne 1970. p. 145).

De Cecco (1968), in making reference to overall verbal learning, noted that research on the effects of practice on verbal learning has not resulted in the same degree of certainty as it has with skill learning. The value of practice in knowledge acquisition has been questioned by students and teachers. He pointed out that it is not practice itself but the conditions of practice that pose problems for the teacher and the experimenter. DeCecco (1968) discussed three conditions of practice that have drawn a lot of attention. They are: (1) massed versus distributed practice in verbal learning, (2) the effects of overlearning, and (3) the effects of part versus whole practice. In the next section, these three practice conditions are presented.

Massed versus distributed practice. Many conditions influence how much and how fast individuals learn. Practice is one of the external conditions of verbal learning. Underwood (1961) conducted many research studies on the effects of massed versus distributed practice on verbal learning. Based on 10 years of research on this subject, he arrived at the following conclusions:

1. When the error tendency in the subject matter is high, then the interval between practice periods (in distributed practice) must be shorter than if the error tendency is low. For example, in learning verbal associations, such as medical terminology and abbreviations, if the student tends to forget the response (terms), the intervals of practice should be shortened; long intervals will result in forgetting.

2. Both DeCecco (1968) and Underwood (1961) also pointed out that if the probability of forgetting is very high, massed practice should be used instead of distributed practice.

3. Evidence (Underwood, 1964) also demonstrated that distributed practice is better for retention and that massed practice is better for learning. This point is well exemplified in students who cram their studies just before the examination. These students usually obtain high test performance, but they forget what they have learned very rapidly. Both Underwood (1961) and DeCecco (1968)

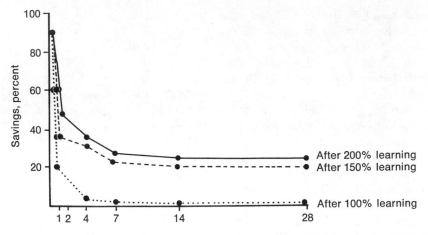

Fig. 23-1. Three degrees of overlearning and their effects on retention. (From Kreuger, W. C. F. The effect of overlearning on retention. *Journal of Experimental Psychology,* 1929, **12**:76.

stated that, theoretically, distributed practice is superior and more beneficial than massed practice in this situation because the intervals allow time for the unwanted or erroneous responses to drop out or to become extinguished.

Overlearning. Overlearning refers to the practice situation where the teacher requires the student to practice or repeat the task beyond the initial mastery level. Overlearning is a form of massed practice. Krueger (1929) demonstrated that overlearning can reach a point of diminishing returns. At this point, further practice adds very little toward retention of material. The effort surpasses the gain. Krueger proved this point by the following experiment. He had three groups of students and had three degrees of overlearning.

Group 1—assigned to 0% overlearning (initial mastery) of a list of nonsense syllables, until subjects could recite them without error

Group 2—assigned to 50% overlearning; for instance, a subject requiring 10 trials for original mastery would recite the list 50% more, that is, 5 more times

Group 3—assigned to 100% overlearning; for

example, a subject requiring 10 trials for initial mastery would recite the list 10 more times.

Results of this experiment (Fig. 23-1) show that the gains for the 50% overlearning are are very striking and that 100% overlearning adds very little to these gains.

Part versus whole practice. *Part practice* refers to the situation when the verbal material is learned by parts or segments, each part being learned separately before they are combined. One such method is the *progressive-part method.* It requires that the student practice the material by combining several units into fewer (McGeoch, 1942). In this method the student learns unit 1 first, then unit 2, then combines units 1 and 2. Later unit 3 is learned separately and is practiced with units 1 and 2, and so on. An example of this would be when the nursing student starts to memorize all the names of the bones of the body. It is almost impossible to memorize all the names of the bones of the body from head to toes in one whole lump. The student first may start memorizing the names of the skull with the bones of the upper extremities, and then may put the names of the bones of the skull with the bones of the upper extremities. Then the student might memorize the vertebrae and practice them with the previous two groups, and so on, until all the names of the bones of the body have been memorized. This method is time consuming, but often very effective.

Whole practice refers to the situation when the entire verbal material is practiced once before any part of it is repeated. An example of whole method would be when the teacher assigns the students to read the whole chapter on the physiology of the heart. The student who reads the whole chapter once before reviewing each page or reading separately is said to have practiced the whole method.

DeCecco (1968) pointed out that studying the relative effectiveness of the part and the whole methods focuses our attention on their relative efficiency. Their efficiency is determined by finding out which method requires less time for gaining mastery.

The study by Deese and Hulse (1967) demonstrated that the relative effectiveness of the part versus whole method of practice in verbal learning depends on the internal organization of the material to be learned. If dividing the material into parts makes learning of the material easier and simpler, then part method of practice should be used. On the other hand, if dividing it makes the learning more difficult then whole method of practice should be used (DeCecco, 1968, p. 348-349).

PRACTICE (OR REPETITION) CONDITIONS IN DISCRIMINATION LEARNING

Gagne (1970, pp. 166-167) stated that,

The arrangement of repetition to accomplish learning of the entire set of discriminations best is a question that has not yet received a clear experimental answer. Whether one should learn two chains, or three, or four, or ten, before repeating those previously learned is not known. It may not even make much difference.

Gagne further noted that the role of repetition in multiple-discrimination learning is not to strengthen the individual components, but rather is to overcome the effects of forgetting brought about by interference. Also, the amount of repetition required to learn a multiple-discrimination task is directly related to the number of chains to be discriminated. In other words, the more the chains, the more the practice or repetition is required.

Practice or repetition in the higher forms of learning, such as concept learning, principle learning, and problem solving, does not appear to be necessary when all the other internal and external conditions are optimal (Gagne, 1970, pp. 182, 202, 224).

Application to nursing education and practice

In nursing education and practice the need for practice seems mostly centered and used in situations where a skill or verbal learning is concerned. Of course in modifying the behaviors of patients or students the role of repetition in implementing classical or operant conditioning or discrimination learning is also very important. In this section how the principles of practice condition can be applied in the learning of psychomotor skills and verbal learning is stressed.

The teacher's role in providing practice in skill learning

The major principles that DeCecco (1968) and Underwood (1961, 1964) brought out in relation to the learning of skills that the nurse-teacher must be aware of and must implement in teaching are the following:

1. Distributed practice is superior and more useful than massed practice in the learning of psychomotor skills, as in the case of learning a procedure, such as making a bed, giving an injection, or others

2. Learning is retained longer when achieved by distributed practice than by massed practice
3. Effects of distribution are powerful and reliable
4. Rest periods have optimal limits
5. Shortening the rest period is more important than lengthening the work period
6. Massed practice may adversely affect performance but not learning (DeCecco [1968, p. 290] stated that after a rest period of a suitable amount of time following massed practice, whatever was originally lost in performance due to inhibitions may be regained.)

Very little is known about the effects of distribution of practice on learning skills of varying difficulty or on constancy, complexity, coherence, and continuity.

DeCecco identified the problem of *scheduling* the practice and rest periods that are consistent with the above findings to be one of the major teaching problems. He has recommended some practical guidelines that the nurse-teacher can use in determining the number and length of practice and rest periods.

1. The nature of the learning task or the procedure should determine to some degree the length of the practice period. For example, a very physically involved psychomotor skill, such as making an occupied bed or giving passive exercises to the lower extremities of the patient, is physically very tiring to the nurse, so the practice period should be shorter than for a procedure where the student nurse is learning how to put on sterile gloves.

2. During the rest periods, students can practice tasks they have already learned in preparation for tasks they are beginning to learn. Of course, when the task involves gross body movements and is very tiring, then rest period means really to rest, with no other physical activity being done. Provisions can be made for students to practice the task on their own, at their own pace, at various times that are appropriate for them, like after school hours. DeCecco pointed out that most complex physical and manipulatory skills require more practice time than is provided within the structure of formal instruction.

3. When the choice is massed practice or no practice at all, massed practice is better. Even though retention of the learned task is not as good in massed practice as in distributed practice, as far as learning is concerned, massed practice may be equal in effect to distributed practice. DeCecco again indicated that when the school schedule does not permit time for distributed practice, the teacher may have to provide periods of massed practice. He further asserted that, "Unless the instructor allows the student to develop a skill to the autonomous phase of learning, the necessary expenditure of time, effort and energy may well deter the student from continued practice of skill" (1968, p. 316).

When there is no time available for massed practice or for distributed practice within the formal instructional period, the teacher can recommend that students practice a procedure mentally while they are at home or any other place. A respectable amount of research has been conducted that supports the beneficial effects of mental practice. Twining (1949) compared three types of practice conditions. The task was for students to learn to throw rope rings over wooden pegs. He had three groups of students:

Group 1—the no-practice group, threw 210 rings on the first day and on the twenty second day

Group 2—the live-practice group, threw 210 rings on the first day and 20 rings each day up to and including the twenty second day

Group 3—the mental practice group, threw 210 rings on the first day, then mentally rehearsed their first day's activity for 15 minutes daily until the twenty second day, when they again threw 210 rings

Results of this experiment showed that no significant learning had occurred in group 1. Group 2 showed a 137% improvement. Group 3 showed a 36% improvement. The conclusion that is derived from this study is that mental practice is much better than no practice, but not as beneficial as actual physical practice.

Other studies conducted by Clark (1960) and Jones (1965) lend further support to these findings. Lawther (1966) and DeCecco (1968, p. 316) further claimed some other advantages of mental practice that he derived from reviewing studies of mental practice. They are that mental practice:

1. Provides the means for reviewing previous performance and planning the next trials
2. Is a means of planning the order of movements in simple skills
3. Reduces the amount of extinction in the next performance
4. Preserves the student's mental alertness and mental set for a quicker start at the next practice session

DeCecco further concluded that mental practice is a form of student verbalization. Most of the benefits of mental practice are derived in the early phases.

DeCecco cited three other aspects of practice that are also very important to the nurse-teacher.

1. Poppelreuter's law of practice states that in skill learning the best results are obtained when speed is retarded until the student has obtained a reasonable level of accuracy, then the speed is increased gradually. Solley (1952) tested this law and found that in skills in which speed is the predominant factor for successful performance, the most efficient results are obtained by putting the emphasis on speed early. In skills in which both accuracy and speed are equally important, then equal emphasis on accuracy and speed yields the optimal results (DeCecco, 1968, p. 316).

2. Slow practice should not be used in skills in which the timing requirements are important. Robb (1966) tested this by studying the effects of slow practice in which students go through the movement pattern of a skill slowly before practicing at the standard rate. She found that this method hindered the student's learning of a simple skill (DeCecco, 1968, p. 317).

3. DeCecco (1968, p. 317) pointed out that, "In the use of mechanical guidance with the student's cooperative effort, the teacher, in the practice of skills, guides the student through a rough approximation of the movement pattern he must learn." Research shows that mechanical guidance should be used only during the early stages of practice, also in teaching very young children or very old people or with students who are having great difficulty in learning the skill.

The teacher's role in providing practice in verbal learning

To provide the a appropriate practice conditions for verbal learning the teacher must provide opportunities for student responses and practice.

PROVIDING OPPORTUNITIES TO MAKE NECESSARY RESPONSES

DeCecco (1968) cited three ways by which the teacher can provide students with opportunities to make the responses—recitation, discussion, and programmed instruction. Recitation is the traditional method. It is characterized by assignment, study, and report. Recitation allows the student to practice overt responses. Choral recitation is an example of this. It's main disadvantage is there is little opportunity to monitor individual student's responses, and some students may hide their ignorance behind the impressive roar of classmates.

Most studies (Wallen and Travers, 1963, p. 481) find no significant difference between discussion method and lecture method. De-Cecco (1968) pointed out that the effect of discussion method on retention of learning has rarely been investigated. One study that was conducted by Ward (1956) showed greater retention of material for student of high academic ability with discussion procedures, while students with low ability retained more with the lecture method. The disadvantage of discussion method is the same as with choral recitation in that there is little opportunity to monitor individual student responses. Furthermore, discussion method has another disadvantage—it provides only limited opportunity for students to make overt responses. When one student talks, all others must listen.

DeCecco (1968, p. 365) stated,

Unless the teacher provides oral instruction on a one-to-one basis, programmed instruction is one of the few instructional procedures that provides each student in a group of students with the opportunity to respond and to obtain knowledge of results for each response.

SCHEDULING PRACTICE ON A MASSED OR A DISTRIBUTED BASIS

The teacher must decide how to schedule the student's practice, whether to provide massed or distributed practice.

The criteria for providing the best schedule of practice is the one that utilizes the student's and the teacher's time in the most efficient way and produces the most amount of learning and the longest period of retention. As pointed out by DeCecco, the criteria are very clear, but the procedure for accom-, plishing them is not clear. He has, however, provided some helpful hints that the nurse-teacher can utilize. They are as follows:

1. When there is very little time for learn-ing of the new material, massed practice is more efficient than distributed practice because massed practice does not allow for rest periods. For distributed practice, the teacher must allow for both learning time and interval time.

2. When the teacher is interested in having the students learn large amounts of material and have it retained for long periods of time, distributed practice is the schedule of choice. It is important to remember that inherent in the use of distributed practice is the rest period. The teacher must provide for this and decide what the students will do during the practice interval—rest period. DeCecco indicated that if the intervals are to be effective, the students should not be occupied with learning related material, because it will interfere with the retention of the previously practiced material. He suggested that students can be given relatively unrelated material to learn or can be occupied with some recreational activity.

3. DeCecco cautioned teachers that practice should not be left to chance. If teachers do not arrange for practice to occur, there will not be practice. He stated that is seems wise to teach a few things well with practice, rather than a lot of things poorly, without practice.

DETERMINING THE DEGREE OF MASTERY THE STUDENT MUST ATTAIN

The teacher must decide which instructional tasks should be overlearned and must then allow the student to practice these tasks beyond the initial mastery level. DeCecco recommended that the task schedules for overlearning must be those that are mandatory entering behaviors for a learning of a wide variety of future tasks. For example, in nursing, this could be the basic skills, concepts, and fundamentals of nursing. Certain skills and concepts must be overlearned so that they can be automatically applied in more advanced learning. In using this text on conditions of learning and instruction in nursing, it is mandatory to overlearn the components of the basic conditions of learning and instruction and the teaching models. If students do not, understanding of the course organization and transfer to other tasks and to patient teaching will be poor.

DeCecco also suggested one other method of overlearning. Overlearning can sometimes be provided by a spiral treatment of the particular learning task. In other words, the student can return to the same task several times and practice it in continuously changing contexts.

PROVIDING EITHER PART OR WHOLE PRACTICE

The decision whether to require part or whole practice must be based on the internal organization and the structure of the material to be learned. Students learn faster by part practice that material which logically divides into parts and recombines into wholes. For material that cannot be divided into meaningful parts or segments, whole practice should be used. The criterion again is learning the most in the least amount of time (DeCecco, 1968, p. 366-367).

Researchable questions

When registered nurses return to school to get their baccalaureate degree, they are often placed in practice situations where they overlearn skills and concepts that they have already mastered at the initial mastery level. Nurse-educators and evaluators have not identified the specific areas where these registered nursing students do not need any more practice. Neither have they identified those areas that need practice and categorized them according to deficiencies in psychomotor skills or verbal-cognitive skills to determine what type of practice condition is most applicable.

The area of mental practice has never been investigated in nursing. The specific question that can be asked is what effect mental practice has on the retention of the steps of a nursing procedure (such as bathing a patient).

Also, many patient-teaching sessions in out-patient clinics and physician's offices occur on massed-teaching and massed-practice bases. No studies have been done to measure the degree of learning or retention that occurs in patients. Often these patients do the return demonstration of the learning task (such as applying Ace bandages to the lower extremities) only once. If they do it correctly the first time—which may happen—the nurse lets the patient go. This is the initial mastery level. No overlearning has occurred. What are the chances that this patient will retain what has been learned until the next day or week. A study could be done to compare the performance of a patient who applies the Ace bandage correctly once (0% overlearning) with a patient who applies it 50% more (50% overlearning). Recommendations from this study would be applicable to most patient- and student-teaching situations.

ADDITIONAL LEARNING EXPERIENCES—RECOMMENDED READING LIST

DeCecco, J. P., and Crawford, W. *The psychology of learning and instruction: educational psychology.* (2nd Ed.) Englewood Cliffs, N. J.: Prentice-Hall, Inc., 1974, pp. 183-184, 222-225, 239-241, 256-259, 279-282.

Gagne, R. *The conditions of learning.* New York: Holt, Rinehart and Winston, Inc., 1972, pp. 98-99, 109-110, 130-131, 145, 166-167, 182, 202, 224.

INSTRUCTIONS TO THE LEARNER REGARDING POSTTEST

Now you are ready to take the posttest to determine the extent to which you have achieved the objectives of this module. Return to the pretest and take it over again as the posttest. Correct your answers in a similar fashion by using the answer key that is found on this page of the module. You need to score 26 correct points to have mastered it at the 95% level. If your score is less than this, correct your errors, study the content of this module over again more carefully, and read the articles in the recommended reading list. You need to study in this fashion until you achieve the 95% mastery level.

ANSWER KEY TO PRETEST AND POSTTEST

1. b (DeCecco, 1968, p. 249)
2. c (DeCecco, 1968, p. 249)
3. c (Gagne, 1970, pp. 105-110)
4. b (DeCecco, 1968, p. 250)
5. b (DeCecco, 1968, pp. 287-288)
6. d (DeCecco, 1968, pp. 287-288)
7. a (DeCecco, 1968, pp. 365-366)
8. d (Gagne, 1970, pp. 130-131)
9. b and c (DeCecco, 1968, p. 288)
10. b (DeCecco, 1968, p. 288)
11. c (DeCecco, 1968, p. 347)
12. b (DeCecco, 1968, p. 347)
13. c (DeCecco, 1968, p. 348-349)
14. b (DeCecco, 1968, p. 347-348)
15. d (DeCecco, 1968, pp. 347-348; Kreuger, 1929, pp. 76-77)
16. b (DeCecco, 1968, p. 316)
17. b (DeCecco, 1968, pp. 316-317)
18. Answer should include:
    a. Identification of the task to be learned—what kind of learning it is
    b. Reason why practice is important in this specific situation
    c. Type of practice needed—massed or distributed—and why; other factors to take into consideration—speed, accuracy, or others
    d. Amount of overlearning necessary and why
    e. Method of evaluating the degree of learning

REFERENCES

Clark, L. V. Effect of mental practice on the development of a certain motor skill. *Research Quarterly,* 1960, **31**:560-569.

DeCecco, J. P. *The psychology of learning and instruction: educational psychology.* (1st Ed.) Englewood Cliffs, N.J.: Prentice-Hall, Inc., 1974.

DeCecco, J. P. and Crawford, W. *The Psychology of learning and instruction: educational psychology.* (2nd Ed.) Englewood Cliffs, N.J.: Prentice-Hall, Inc., 1974.

Deese, J. *The psychology of learning.* (2nd Ed.) New York: McGraw-Hill Book Co., 1958.

Deese, J., and Hulse, S. H. *The psychology of learning.* (3rd Ed.) New York: McGraw-Hill Book Co., 1967.

Estes, W. K. The statistical approach to learning theory. In S. Koch (Ed.), *Psychology: a study of a science,* vol. 2. New York: McGraw-Hill Book Co., 1959.

Gagne, R. *The conditions of learning.* (2nd Ed.) New York: Holt, Rinehart and Winston, Inc., 1972.

Jones, J. G. Motor learning without demonstration under two conditions of mental practice. *Research Quarterly,* 1965, **36**:270-281.

Kientzle, J. J. Properties of learning curves under varied distribution of practice. *Journal of Experimental Psychology,* 1946, **36**:187-211.

Kimble, G. A., and Bilodeau, E. A. Work and rest as variables in cyclical motor learning. *Journal of Experimental Psychology,* 1949, **39**:150-157.

Kimble, G. A., and Garmezy, N. *Principles of general psychology.* (2nd Ed.) New York: The Ronald Press Co., 1963.

Kreuger, W. C. F. The effect of over-learning on retention. *Journal of Experimental Psychology,* 1929, **12**:71-78.

Lawther, J. D. Directing motor skill learning. *Quest,* Monograph VI, 1966, pp. 68-76.

Lorge, I. *Influence of regularly interpolated time intervals upon subsequent learning.* Teachers College Contributions to Education, No. 438. New York: Teachers College Press, 1930.

McGeoch, J. A. *The psychology of human learning.* New York: David McKay Co., Inc., 1942.

Robb, M. Feedback. *Quest,* Monograph VI, 1966, pp. 38-43.

Solley, W. H. "The effects of verbal instructions of speed and accuracy upon the learning of a motor skill. *Research Quarterly,* 1952, **23**:231-240.

Twining, W. E. Mental practice and physical practice in learning a motor skill. *Research Quarterly,* 1949, **20**:432-435.

Underwood, B. J. Ten years of massed practice on distributed practice. *Psychological Review,* 1961, **68**: 229-247.

Underwood, B. J. Laboratory studies of verbal learning. In E. R. Hilgard (Ed.), *Theories of learning and instruction,* Part I of the 63rd Yearbook of the N.S.S.E. Chicago: University of Chicago Press, 1964, pp. 133-152.

Wallen, N. E., and Travers, M. W. Analysis and investigation of teaching methods. In N. L., Gage (Ed.), *Handbook of Research on Teaching.* Chicago: Rand McNally & Co., 1963, pp. 448-505.

Ward, J. N. Group versus lecture-demonstration method in physical science instruction for general education college students. *Journal of Experimental Education,* 1956, **24:**197-210.

MODULE 24

Sequence of instruction

DESCRIPTION OF MODULE

This is a complete unit of instruction on the variable of sequencing of instruction. The content is presented in a systematically organized and sequential order. The test of this module covers five major areas that are presented in an integrated form. They are: (1) theoretical framework, (2) relevant research studies, (3) application to nursing education and practice, (4) issues, and (5) researchable questions. The module is self-paced. It also contains instructions to the learner, module objectives, a pre- and posttest, and an answer key to give immediate feedback to the learner.

MODULE OBJECTIVES

At the completion of this module, having studied the content and the recommended reading list, the student will be able to accomplish the following objectives at the 95% level of mastery. The student will be able to:

1. Define sequencing of instruction
2. Describe how different theorists view sequencing of instruction
3. Describe the theoretical framework of sequencing
4. Cite relevant research studies that have been done in sequencing of instruction
5. Select a specific lesson plan and apply the principles of sequencing to design a strategy for effective sequencing of instruction

6. Identify the essential criteria of sequencing that need to be implemented in planning a curriculum
7. Raise at least one researchable question and identify the independent and dependent variables

PRETEST AND POSTTEST

Circle the correct answers. Each question is worth 1 point except the last question, which is worth 10 points. The 95% level of mastery for this test is 25 correct points. Take the test and correct your answers using the answer key found at the end of this module (p. 391). If you score 95% mastery, you need not study this module.

Multiple choice

1. The definition of the concept of sequencing includes:
   a. a succession of information
   b. chaining
   c. an order in which things follow one another
   d. commonalities in a curriculum
2. The purpose of mapping the sequence of learning is:
   a. to provide organization when teaching
   b. to avoid mistakes arising from omitting essential steps
   c. to permit the student to anticipate future learning

d. to follow the student's capabilities in instructional techniques

3. The major criteria for building an effectively organized learning experience are:
   a. continuity, sequence, evaluation
   b. continuity, sequence, integration
   c. sequence, integration, evaluation
   d. sequence, integration, reinforcement

4. The important components of sequencing are that:
   1—steps in a segment must be arranged in order
   2—steps must be of proper size
   3—steps must be accompanied by reinforcement
   4—segments must be arranged so that the student is properly prepared for each when it is reached
   a. 1, 2, 3, and 4
   b. 1 and 2
   c. 1 and 4
   d. 2, 3, and 4

5. Proper organization and sequencing of instruction has the effect:
   a. that its major benefit is the efficiency of instruction and the ease with which the instructor can relay the material to the student
   b. of increasing the efficiency of instruction and the degree to which major changes are brought about in learners
   c. of making the curriculum so specific that anyone with the proper teaching background could teach any phase of it without difficulty

6. According to Skinner (1968), sequencing is best accomplished when material is presented:
   a. from the simplest to the most complex
   b. in order of relevancy
   c. in order of difficulty
   d. in small steps, arranged in order, so that the student is prepared for each step when it is reached

7. According to Tyler (1970), sequencing (one of the three major criteria for organizing learning experiences) refers to:
   a. the increasing breadth and depth of the learner's development
   b. the increasing unity of behavior in relating to the elements involved
   c. the recurring emphasis in the learner's experience on the particular elements to be learned

8. According to Gagne (1966, 1970), learning hierarchies refer to:
   1—prerequisite capabilities
   2—internal conditions of learning
   3—a route for learning the subject
   4—the same thing as Harow's "learning sets"
   a. 1, 2, and 4
   b. 1, 2, and 3
   c. . 1, 2, 3, and 4
   d. 3 and 4

9. Gagne's (1966, 1970) hierarchy of learning sets demands a specific sequence. Choose the item below that reflects this:
   a. may start at either end of the hierarchy, as long as each step is in sequence
   b. must start with the lowest-level set and proceed in sequence to the highest-level one
   c. immaterial which set is learned first, as long as the learner knows the connectedness to the next set

10. The essential prerequisite in preparing precise sequencing for a course or lesson plan is:
    a. knowledge of the sequence of the curriculum
    b. development of a precise instructional objectives
    c. provision of conditions that reduce interference
    d. examination of the material for its meaningfulness and relevancy

11. The purpose of pretesting in learning a higher-order principle is:
    a. to determine the en-route behavior necessary to achieve the goal
    b. to determine the entry behavior of the student
    c. to determine which subordinate concepts may be eliminated
    d. to determine which subordinate concepts are missing, which will cause decreased understanding of the higher-order rule

12. In verbal learning, the most difficult parts of a sequence to learn are the:
    a. beginning parts
    b. middle parts
    c. end parts
    d. no difference between the parts
13. When teachers make sure that relevant lower-order skills are mastered before the learning of the related higher-order skill is undertaken, they are ensuring the proper _____ of instruction.
    a. external conditions
    b. sequencing
    c. integration
    d. continuity
14. In rule learning, the most appropriate series of instructional tasks is:
    1—questioning to help the student recall relevant concepts
    2—asking students to demonstrate an instance of the rule
    3—cueing to chain concepts
    4—having the learner state the rule
    a. 1, 2, 3, 4
    b. 2, 1, 3, 4
    c. 2, 3, 1, 4
    d. 1, 3, 2, 4
15. In problem solving, the correct sequence of behaviors is:
    1—providing verbal direction to student thinking
    2—recalling relevant concepts and principles
    3—defining the problem
    4—formulating the hypotheses
    a. 3, 2, 4, 1
    b. 3, 1, 2, 4
    c. 3, 2, 1, 4
    d. 1, 3, 2, 4
16. According to Bruner (1964), to present and sequence material ranging from simple to complex the teacher should arrange it in order:
    a. from symbolic to ikonic to enactive representations
    b. from ikonic to enactive to symbolic representations
    c. from enactive to ikonic to symbolic representations
    d. whichever way the student and the teacher prefer

Discussion question

17. Select a specific unit of instruction (one lesson plan) of your choice and design an efficient instructional sequence.

TEXT
Theoretical framework
Overview of sequencing as perceived by different theorists

Throughout the literature, discussions of sequencing have come under such headings as sequential learning, hierarchies of learning, order of instruction, sequences of instruction, programmed learning, and organizing. However, all these viewpoints infer similar operational definitions that are consistent with the definition in Webster's Dictionary. For example, they all imply that sequencing entails:

1. A succession of information
2. An order in which things follow one another
3. A related series
4. Consequences of resulting events
5. One thing coming after another

To illustrate these commonalities let us look at different author's views of sequencing of instruction.

Block (1971) discussed sequential learning through mastery-learning strategies. He described those subjects using these strategies as consisting of a number of well-defined unit whose learning is cumulative in that each unit builds on the learning of all prior units. If at each stage in the sequence the student learns the material on which the next unit builds, learning throughout the sequence is likely to be adequate. Block suggested as good candidates for sequential learning, subjects such as arithmetic reading, science, algebra, and chemistry, and physics.

In Carroll's (1963) model of instruction, effective sequencing of instruction is said to have occurred when the learner has adequate sensory contact with the material to be learned and is allowed adequate time for learning. The various aspects of the learning task are presented in such an order and with such detail that, as far as possible, every step of the learning is adequately prepared for by a previous step.

For Skinner (1968) arranging effective sequences is a good part of the art of teaching. The typical Skinnerian program moves in small steps, arranged in order so that students are properly prepared for each step as they reach it. The five most salient points of Skinner's model of instruction are (1) identification of the terminal behavior (that is, state the objective), (2) initiation of the first instance, (3) prompting behavior, (4) programming complex behavior, and (5) sequencing. It is important to note here that sequencing is listed as one of the five steps, but that the five steps of this model, collectively, may serve as a guide for a sequence of instruction. The students learn through a sequence of planned instruction, and the teacher uses the guidelines in planning instruction sequentially. Skinner has utilized this framework of sequencing in preparing learning material for programmed instruction. He has developed linear programs, in which there is a single path for students to follow. There are also branched programs, where the student proceeds to the next frame until an error is made. The errors branch to provide supplementary material designed to give the student remedial instruction. The third type is adjunct programs in which programmed and testing materials are inserted into conventional instructional materials such as textbooks and laboratory manuals. Skinner pointed out that the crux of constructing programmed materials is in designing effective sequences. Effective sequencing specifies where the student stands

and in what direction the student should move.

Effective sequencing is one of the essential elements of Bruner's (1964, 1967) model of instruction. According to Bruner, instruction should lead the learner through a sequence of statements and restatements of a problem or body of knowledge that increases the learner's ability to understand, grasp, transform, and transfer (apply) what is being learned. The sequence in which cognitive material is presented will determine the level of difficulty the student will have in mastering it (Bruner, 1967, p. 49). Bruner asserted that there is no one sequence for all learners, for much depends on such factors as stage of development, nature of the material, past learning, individual differences, and the learner's capacity to process information. He suggested (Bruner 1964, p. 314) that sequencing should depend on such criteria as:

(a) speed of learning, (b) resistance to forgetting, (c) transferability of what has to be learned to new instances, (d) form of representation in terms of which what has been learned is to be expressed, (e) economy of what has been learned in terms of cognitive strain imposed. (f) effective power of what has been learned in terms of its generativeness for new hypotheses and combinations.

In his model of instruction Bruner (1964, p. 313) further proposed that the usual course of intellectual development moves from "enactive through ikonic to symbolic representative of the world." If this is true, then the sequence of instruction should move in the same direction. Bruner (1966) is also an advocate of discovery learning. He pointed out that in guided discovery learning, the teacher is said to "arrange" the learning environment and learning so that students can see the connectedness between the facts learned and other data and situations. Learning is also "arranged" so that students can fit material into their own organizational systems and can recognize when they have information and can go beyond this information.

Bloom and his associates (1956) developed a method of classifying educational objectives by means of task analysis. It is referred to as taxonomy of educational objectives. As in Gagne's method, the different classes of behavior are arranged in hierarchical order, ranging from the simple to the complex. Each class of behavior utilizes the one before it and is also built on behaviors in the preceeding classes. Bloom and his associates sequenced the instructional objectives in the areas of cognitive and affective domain.

The cognitive domain includes two main categories: knowledge and intellectual abilities and skills. These are in turn subdivided into hierarchical sequencing producing six classes of behaviors: (1) knowledge, (2) comprehension, (3) application, (4) analysis, (5) synthesis, and (6) evaluation. As summarized by DeCecco and Crawford (1974, pp. 40-41), a brief explanation of each class of behavior is presented.

1. *Knowledge.* Knowledge involves the *recall* of specifics, terminology, generalizations, methods and processes, patterns, structure, or setting. An example of an objective that falls under knowledge is alienation. The detailed itemization of classes of behavior that fall into this category is provided in the box (p. 381). The next five classes of behaviors are categorized as intellectual abilities and skills.

2. *Comprehension.* The objectives that fall under the category of comprehension belong to the lowest level of understanding. The student may communicate and use the material without realizing its full implications and may not necessarily relate it to other material; for example, given the formula for transforming centigrade temperature into Farenheit, the student may translate the centigrade temperature into Farenheit.

3. *Application.* The intellectual behavior of application requires the student to use abstractions, such as principles, procedures, theories, and concepts, in concrete situations. An example of an educational objective that falls under this category would be that given a specific patient situation (case study) the nursing student would be able to apply the principles of assessment of the nursing process in making a nursing diagnosis.

4. *Analysis.* Analysis requires the student to be able to relate ideas and specify the relative hierarchy of ideas in a given content matter. The role of analysis is to clarify material and indicate how content is organized and how it can vary its effects. An example of educational objectives under this category is that in writing a proposal of a research study, the student will be able to recognize the unstated assumptions and check the consistency of the hypothesis with the given theoretical framework and assumptions.

5. *Synthesis.* Synthesis requires the student to assemble parts into a whole. It involves the process of organizing and combining the parts and deriving a pattern or structure that was not there before. For instance, in inductive thinking, the student gathers the specific information and attempts to make generalizations by identifying the commonalities and differences to derive the underlying principle. An example of an educational objective that falls under the synthesis category is that in designing a proposal of a research study, the student will be able to propose ways of testing the hypothesis.

6. *Evaluation.* The type of cognitive behavior that requires the student to make judgments about the worth of the material and the value of the methods used for particular purposes is evaluation. The judgments may be qualitattive or quantitative. They may include the application of criteria of acceptability that is either determined by the student or set forth by the teacher. Educational objectives that fall under this category

BLOOM'S TAXONOMIES OF COGNITIVE AND AFFECTIVE DOMAIN

COGNITIVE DOMAIN

Knowledge

1.10 Knowledge of specifics
1.11 Knowledge of terminology
1.12 Knowledge of specific facts
1.20 Knowledge of ways and means of dealing with specifics
1.21 Knowledge of conventions
1.22 Knowledge of trends and sequences

Knowledge of the processes, directions, and movements of phenomena with respect to time

1.23 Knowledge of classifications and categories
1.24 Knowledge of criteria
1.25 Knowledge of methodology
1.30 Knowledge of universals and abstractions in a field
1.31 Knowledge of principles and generalizations
1.32 Knowledge of theories and structures

Intellectual abilities and skills

2.00 Comprehension
2.10 Translation
2.22 Interpretation
2.30 Extropolations
3.00 Application
4.00 Analysis

4.10 Analysis of elements
4.20 Analysis of relationships
4.30 Analysis of organization principles
5.00 Synthesis
5.10 Production of a unique communication
5.20 Production of a plan or proposed set of operations
5.30 Derivation of a set of abstract relations
6.00 Evaluation
6.10 Judgment in terms of internal evidence
6.20 Judgment in terms of external criteria

AFFECTIVE DOMAIN

1.0 Receiving (attending)
   1.1 Awareness
   1.2 Willingness to receive
   1.3 Controlled or selected attention
2.0 Responding
   2.1 Acquiesence in responding
   2.2 Willingness to respond
   2.3 Willingness in response
3.0 Valuing
   3.1 Acceptance of a value
   3.2 Preference for a value
   3.3 Commitment (conviction)
4.0 Organization
   4.1 Conceptualization of a value
   4.2 Organization of a value system
5.0 Characterization by a value or value complex

are that given several related research studies that have been conducted, the student will be able to: critique, compare and relate the findings of each study to one another, and indicate any logical fallacies in arguments relative to the problem area.

The taxonomy as proposed by Bloom and his associates includes test questions that apply to each of their cognitive classes of behaviors (sequences). They illustrate both the behavior expected of each class, and the type of test items that can measure the achieve-ment of the objectives in each class (DeCecco and Crawford, 1974, p. 41).

Bloom and associates (1956) also developed objectives in sequential order in the area of affective domain. There are five categories: (1) receiving (attending), (2) responding, (3) valuing, (4) organizing, and (5) characterizing by a value or value complex. For details of each of these refer to the boxed material above.

Whenever sequencing of instruction is discussed in literature or by educators and educational psychologists, emphasis has been given to the content aspect of the curriculum to the exclusion of the affective domain. This is why most articles on sequencing have dealt mostly with content or subject matter. Bloom has been one of the most verbal advocates of the importance of affective learning in instruction.

DeCecco and Crawford (1974, pp. 41-42) pointed out that, "The test of any system for classifying behavior is in its usefulness for task analysis, which, in turn, should enable the teacher to distinguish various performances and to establish the necessary learning conditions for achieving these performances." In comparing Bloom and associate's (1956) taxonomy of educational objectives with Gagne's (1965, 1970) classes of behaviors, DeCecco and Crawford prefer Gagne's classification to that of Bloom's taxonomy in spite of the fact that the objectives in the taxonomy have greater breadth and variety. The taxonomy presents two difficulties for task analysis: (1) the educational objectives that are cited do not meet Mager's (1962) requirements for task description, and they lack clarification as to the conditions under which the desired performance must occur; and (2) each of the formal characteristics listed in Bloom's taxonomy does not clearly fall into one distinct class of behavior, which creates difficulty in classifying instructional objectives and determining their appropriate learning conditions.

DeCecco and Crawford believe that Gagne's classification of behaviors is more explicit and the statements of instructional objectives more clear. Gagne's classes of behaviors are products of research on conditions of learning, they are very useful for task analysis and provide greater precision in the design and sequencing of instruction.

Gagne's (1970) hierarchy of learning can be described as a "route" for the learning of a subject matter in the sense that it represents what is expected to be a general pattern to be followed for all the students in the group. The pattern must also be "routed," or sequenced, so that the lower-order skills (learning sets or subordinate capabilities) are mastered before the learning of higher-order learning sets. Gagne further pointed out that in using the learning hierarchy as a guide to establishing a learning "route," the proper procedure is, first, to find out what the student already knows (entering behaviors) and second, to begin the instruction at that point.

To elaborate a little further, when a teacher begins with the performance of a specific class of tasks as a criterion of terminal behavior, it is possible to identify the subordinate categories of knowledge required by means of asking Gagne's (1970, p. 122) basic question, "What would the individual have to be able to do in order that he can attain successful performance on this task, provided he is given only instructions?" This question is then applied successively to the subordinate learning sets identified by the answer. By means of this systematical approach or analysis, it is possible to identify all the entities of subordinate knowledge arranged in hierarchical fashion. By this mechanism, Gagne identified eight categories, or types, of learning that are arranged in hierarchical order, ranging from the simple to the complex. They are: classical conditioning, or signal learning; operant conditioning; chaining, or skill learning; verbal associates; discrimination learning; concept learning; principle learning; and problem solving.

Gagne has demonstrated through his research that specific transfer from one learning set to another immediately above it in the hierarchy is zero if the individual cannot recall the lower one; transfer will range up to 100% if the student can recall the subordinate learning set. Gagne perceived the function of learning sets to be mediators of positive transfer from lower-level learning sets to higher-level tasks. Within a hierarchy of learning sets, attainment of each new learning set depends on a process of positive transfer, which is dependent on (1) the student's ability to recall the relevant subordinate learning set, and (2) the effects of instruction (Gagne, 1970, p. 122).

Integrated approach to sequencing — a synthesis

In the previous section principles and concepts of sequencing were presented as perceived by different theorists. In this section an eclectic approach will be taken in synthesizing the strong points of each theorist and applying them in sequencing of educational objectives at the macrolevel (curriculum development) and microlevel (instructional level).

SEQUENCING EDUCATIONAL OBJECTIVES AT THE CURRICULUM DEVELOPMENT LEVEL—MACROLEVEL

In order for educational objectives and learning experiences to produce a cumulative effect, they must be put together to form some kind of coherent program, they must be so organized as to reinforce each other. Organization and sequencing are thus seen as important aspects of curriculum development because they greatly influence the efficiency of instruction and the extent to which major educational changes are brought about in learners (Tyler, 1970, p. 83).

In considering the organization and sequencing of educational objectives and learning experiences, their relationship can be examined over time and from one area to another. Tyler (1970) referred to these two kinds of relationships as vertical and horizontal relations, respectively. They determine the cumulative effect of educational experiences. For example, examining the relationship between freshman-class anatomy and physiology courses and junior-class patho-

physiology is considering the vertical relation. Examining the relationship between a freshman-level cultural anthropology course and freshman-level "sociocultural variables in illness" course is considering horizontal relations. When educational objectives and learning experiences are appropriately arranged, they reinforce each other and provide for greater unity of view and become more effective. However, if they are in conflict, they will nullify each other, or if courses and educational objectives and experiences are not related and connected, the student develops compartmentalized learning that is not related, and the ability to apply this learning in daily living is hindered (Tyler, 1970).

Criteria to organize objectives and learning experiences. Tyler (1970) suggested three major criteria to organize educational objectives and learning experiences: (1) continuity, (2) sequence, and (3) integration.

Continuity. Continuity refers to the vertical reiteration of major elements in the curriculum. For example, in nursing education if the development of skills in application of the nursing process is an important objective, then there should be recurring and continuing opportunity for these skills to be practiced and developed. Continuity is a major factor in effective vertical organization and sequencing.

Sequence. Those criteria where educational objectives and learning experiences are so arranged that each successive objective and experience builds on the preceding one, but goes more broadly and deeply into the matters involved are the sequence. For example, if a nursing student is assigned to take care of one patient with only one type of problem (such as a hygienic problem) during the first week, the second week the educational objective and learning experience may include care of three patients with several problems (such as hygienic, nutritional, and

others). Sequence does not emphasize duplication, but rather higher levels of treatments,
with successive objectives and learning experiences (Tyler, 1970).

Integration. The horizontal relationship of
curriculum objectives and experiences is referred to as integration. These relationships
should be organized and sequenced in such a
fashion that they enable the student to see
and perceive the unified view of the curriculum or the course and to unify behavior
in relation to the elements dealt with. For
example, in developing skill in problem solving in nursing (nursing process), it is also important to consider the ways in which the
problem-solving skill can be utilized in other
courses and in daily living. Therefore, when
objectives and learning experiences are
planned in an integrated form, they provide
the student with a unified view of the curriculum, and there is also unity in the student's outlook, skills, and attitudes (Tyler,
1970).

**Methods of achieving continuity,
sequence, and integration in a curriculum.**
There are several important considerations
and factors that enable the building of an effective curriculum, program of study, or
course that meets the criteria of continuity,
sequence, and integration. These are: (1) elements to be organized, (2) organizing principles, and (3) organizing structure.

Elements to be organized. Identification of
the elements of a curriculum is of utmost importance in making a plan of organization for
a curriculum. These elements also act as the
organizing threads; for example, in nursing,
such organizing elements or threads can be
used for nursing model, nursing process, research, and so on. In planning the nursing
curriculum, or in any other school or field, it
is necessary to decide on the types of elements that most effectively serve as threads
to use in the curriculum. They have to be
elements that are relevant to and significant

matters for that field and also for the total
curriculum. Once the basic elements are decided, they have to appear throughout the
length and breadth of the instructional program, and they have to provide for continuity, sequence, and integration.

Organizing principles. Organizing principles provide the framework or the method by
which the elements or the threads of the curriculum are woven together. Tyler (1970)
identified several commonly used organizing
principles. For example, chronology is one of
the most common principles used in organizing curricula. Chronology enables the student to see the development of events over
time. History courses are commonly organized on this basis. In nursing curriculum,
chronology can be used in organizing and effectively sequencing such courses as nursing
trends, nursing history, child development
(age being the major variable that changes
over time), and other nursing courses that
deal with the entire life span of the human
being. Tyler cautions us and recommends
that faculty carefully check to see whether
chronology as an organizing principle really
provides the psychological organization that
broadens and deepens the student's command of the elements involved. Chronological organization has frequently been found
not to be satisfactory from this point of view.

Other commonly used organizing principles cited by Tyler (1970, p.97) are

increasing breadth of application, increasing
range of activities included, the use of description
followed by analysis, the development of specific
illustrations followed by broader and broader
principles to explain these illustrations, and the attempt to build an increasingly unified world picture from specific parts which are first built into
larger and larger wholes.

In applying any one of these organizing principles in the development of a curriculum, it
is important to check the results by actual
tryout of material to determine how far these

principles prove to be satisfactory in developing continuity, sequence, and integration.

Organizing structure. Organizing structure deals with the main structural elements into which the learning experiences are to be organized. Tyler (1970) cited structural elements that exist at several levels.

At the largest level, structural elements may consist of (1) specific subjects, such as pain, adaptation, trends, nursing history, and others; (2) broad fields, such as nursing sciences, social sciences, and others; (3) a core curriculum for general education combined with specific subjects or broad fields; or (4) a completely undifferentiated structure in which the total program is treated as a unit. Such curricula are adopted by less formal educational institutions, such as the Boy Scouts Of America, YMCA groups, and others (Tyler, 1970, p. 98).

At the intermediate level, organizing structures can be as courses organized as sequences; for example, Research I, Research II, Research III or Nursing Science I, II, or III. Such courses are planned as a unifying sequence. Organizing structures can also be courses that are a single semester or 1-year units without being planned or considered as part of a longer time sequence; for example, an anatomy or physiology course in freshman year, pharmacology in junior year, and pathology in senior year. These courses do not build on each other. They are discrete units rather than sequentially organized courses.

At the smallest level of organization, structure can take several forms. The most widely used structure in this category is the *lesson*, in which a single day's lesson plan (content) is treated as a discrete unit and may not be related to other lesson plans that are to follow. The *topic* is another common structure, it may last for several days or weeks. The *unit* includes experiences covering several weeks and may be organized around problems or

major student purposes (Tyler, 1970, pp. 98-99).

Evidence to date points to some of the advantages and disadvantages of each organizing structure. Tyler indicated that from the standpoint of achievement of continuity and sequence the discrete subjects, courses, and lessons all cause difficulty in making vertical relationship and organization less likely to occur. Vertical transfer and relationship is enhanced when courses are organized over a longer period of time, in larger units and a larger general framework.

When organizing structure is composed of many specific pieces, it is difficult to integrate. The more discrete the pieces (courses), the harder it is to integrate. A core curriculum causes less difficulty in achieving integration, as far as the interposition of boundaries between courses is concerned.

Tyler suggested that in order to achieve desirable organization, it is advisable to have a structural arrangement that provides for (1) larger blocks of time under which planning may occur and (2) broad fields or core programs rather than very narrow units or many small units. The broader fields of study promote better relationships between what is learned in the school setting and what the student experiences or will encounter in life outside school (Tyler, 1970, p. 100).

Process of planning a unit of organization. Planning involves five basic steps (Tyler, 1970, p. 101):

1. Agreement by the faculty as a whole as to the general scheme of organization, that is, whether core programs, specific subjects, or broad fields are to be utilized.

2. Agreement on the general organizing principles that are to be followed within each of the fields that are chosen

3. Agreement on the low-level units to be used, whether a daily lesson plan, teaching units, or sequential topics.

4. Development of flexible plans, also

called "source units," which will be in the hands of the teacher when working with a specific group of students

5. Use of teacher-student planning for particular activities to be carried on by a particular class

In conclusion, it can be seen that planning the organization and sequencing of curriculum objectives and experiences involves a great deal of preplanning and also planning while the curriculum is being implemented. It is only in this way that it is possible to obtain the greatest cumulative effect from the various learning objectives and experiences used.

SEQUENCING OF EDUCATIONAL OBJECTIVES AT THE INSTRUCTIONAL LEVEL—MICROLEVEL

The major purpose of this section is to present a strategy for analyzing and sequencing instruction. Among the main concerns facing instructors is the decision as to what to do to enable students to achieve the desired objectives. Teachers must have some way of identifying and ordering the activities to optimize student learning and to achieve their own objectives. Teachers also need to consider the students' background—their ages, past instructional history, past experiences with success or failure, level of motivation—and their own teaching style. Popham and Baker (1970) suggested a simple strategy that is easy to apply but is comprehensive. It also utilizes most of the concepts on sequencing of instruction that are proposed by different educators and theorists. It includes five steps for analyzing and sequencing instruction.

Identifying the instructional objectives. Specific and precise objectives are prerequisite to planning an instructional sequence. Instructional objectives must be stated in terms of precise behaviors (responses) expected of the learner under given conditions. The criterion of acceptable performance

must also be mentioned so that the student can pace learning and will know when the objective has been achieved. An example of a precise objective may be that upon completion of instruction, given a patient with the diagnosis of diabetes mellitus, the student nurse will be able to develop a nursing-care plan utilizing the nursing-process approach and will be able to implement it.

Identifying entering behavior relevant to the specific objective. Entering behavior refers to the level of knowledge the student has about that specific objective prior to instruction. It is at this level that instruction begins. The strategy for identifying the prerequisite (entering) behaviors for a specific instructional objective is to ask Gagne's basic question about what the student would have to know in order to perform the task successfully, given only instruction. The answer to this question should constitute the entering behavior necessary to accomplish the task. For example, if this question were applied to the above objective, there would be several prerequisite behaviors that the student should have; for instance, the student should know, among other things, what is meant by diagnosis, diabetes mellitus, nursing-care plan, nursing process, and implementation. Knowledge about each of these concepts constitutes essential entering behaviors the student should possess in order to accomplish the objective.

Identifying component tasks of a given objective. The teacher has to analyze a given objective into its components. The process is similar to that of identifying the entering behavior. Popham and Baker referred to it as identifying the "en route" behaviors. These are the in-between behaviors (component learnings) that enable the learner to reach the specified goal, or the objective. For example, if the student is to progress from point A to point B, the *entering behaviors* are those behaviors that the student should possess prior to point A. They are the very basic skills. In order to proceed from point A to point B, the essential behaviors that enable the student to progress from one point to the next are the *en-route behaviors.*

In order for a teacher to identify or analyze the component tasks (en-route behaviors) of a given objective, the teacher should again ask the basic question, "What does the learner need to be able to do before he can successfully perform the desired behavior?" (Popham and Baker, 1970, p. 49). This question enables the teacher to identify the subobjectives that are essential for the student to achieve in order to achieve the final objective. By this process, the basic components of a given objective can be identified.

Let us take the above-mentioned objective and identify the component tasks (en-route behaviors) that the student should be able to do in order to achieve the objective, that is develop and implement a nursing-care plan for a diabetic patient using the nursing-process approach. The student's entering behavior was identified as including basic knowledge about diagnosis, diabetes mellitus, nursing-care plans, and nursing process. Let us assume that the level of knowledge ascertained places the student at point A. The charge to the student (that is, the objective to be achieved by the student) is: (1) to develop a care plan for a diabetic patient, (2) to implement it, and (3) to use the nursing-process approach. This then is the level of knowledge expected of the student at point B.

Now, what should the student be able to do to get from point A to point B? The answer to the basic question about what skill the learner needs will identify the component tasks of the given objective. For example, some of the component tasks (en-route behaviors) that have been identified may be that the student should be able to describe what each of the major concepts (diabetes, diagnosis, nursing care, nursing process) en-

tail or what steps are included in the nursing process and how each step can be implemented. Other examples are to identify what relationships exist between the major concepts and what principles can be used.

These are the component tasks that the student should be able to do to achieve the objective. Popham and Baker (1970) pointed out that not every teacher will analyze a given objective into the same components because not every teacher will agree that all the en-route behaviors that are listed are prerequisite to the terminal objectives. But instructors can infer from their student's postinstructional performance if critical subtasks have been omitted. Also, verification of en-route behaviors through empirical research will enable the teacher to identify the necessary prerequisite skills. But such verification is not usually done in the real world because teachers have other tasks and deadlines to meet.

Popham and Baker also indicated that in analyzing objectives there are limits in using the strategy of asking the basic question. How far does a teacher go in analyzing the objectives into subobjectives and subtasks? One can carry the strategy to the extreme, to the point of having the student identify the letters within the concept. Therefore, all prerequisites are not the teacher's responsibility. When designing instructional materials or sequences, the teacher must set a cutoff point with respect to prerequisites. The student must have with certain basic skills, that is, certain definite entering behaviors.

Providing instructional economy. Instructional economy constitutes an essential strategy in analyzing and sequencing instruction. Instructional economy refers to the elements of efficiency and simplicity of instruction. For example, it is possible to identify more en-route behaviors than are necessary for the accomplishment of the objectives. After delineating all the possible en-route behaviors, the teacher can delete some of them and observe the resulting student behavior on the terminal objective and derive a more efficient set of en-route behaviors. The important point to remember is that choices do exist for the actual component behaviors that are selected for teaching. The teacher should be able to look at the objective and recognize that there are many options in the design of a particular sequence (Popham and Baker, 1970).

Sometimes more en-route behaviors could have been identified in order for the nursing student to accomplish the objective; for instance, specific and detailed information about each of the major concepts (diagnosis, nursing process, and the like) could have been identified as en-route behaviors. However, all these en-route behaviors may not be absolutely necessary to accomplish the terminal objective. Therefore, in order to make instruction more economical—efficient, simple, and fast—some of these subcomponents (en-route behaviors) can be deleted.

Devising the sequence in which instruction takes place. Devising the sequence of instruction deals with determining the order in which the learner is expected to demonstrate the en-route behaviors. The teacher has to determine what order best helps the student to achieve the objective with the least expenditure of instructional resources. It is related to efficiency.

There are some theorists who propose that there is no best order in which a task should be encountered by given students because the sequence, or the order, is psychological rather than logical. They believe that it is more important to ensure that every necessary component behavior is elicited from the student, rather than to omit some and have an optional order (Popham and Baker, 1970, p. 57).

However, there are others who think that instruction does proceed in some order, and

that tasks have to be sequenced properly (Bloom and others, 1956; Gagne, 1970; Popham and Baker, 1970). Different educators have developed schemes for categorizing the tasks that students perform; for example, Bloom's taxonomy and Gagne's hierarchy of learning are prominent among these schemes. En-route behaviors can be sequenced by either of these schemes so that the least complex is taught first, that is subobjectives, learning experiences, and en-route behaviors could be sequenced from the simple to the complex.

The sequencing of en-route behaviors can be accomplished or generated by asking the same basic question: "What skills must the student possess in order to accomplish the objective?" Popham and Baker (1970) suggested that sequencing of en-route behaviors should be subjected to empirical verification.

The strategy of devising the sequence of instruction can be applied to the objective. Since Gagne's hierarchy is more precise than Bloom's, it is applied to the objective mentioned previously. First, it is necessary to ask the basic question of what skills must the student possess to be able to develop and implement a nursing care plan to a diabetic patient utilizing the nursing-process approach. The en-route behaviors that were identified that need to be sequenced are:

1. Describing the major concepts of diabetes mellitus, diagnosis, nursing care, and nursing process (concept learning)
2. Making a diagnosis (concept learning)
3. Making a nursing-care plan (concept learning)
4. Implementing a nursing-care plan (problem solving)
5. Describing a nursing process (concept learning)
6. Implementing the process (problem solving)

7. Integrating the major concepts (principle learning)
8. Generating and using principles (problem solving)

Once the teacher identifies all the components (en-route behaviors) of the objective, then the teacher can start classifying them using Gagne's hierarchy of learning to determine which of these skills are of higher order and which are of lower order and then to order them in proper sequence. Some of the identified en-route behaviors are concepts that the student should learn and be able to do. Some are principles, and others are higher-order cognitive skills that may be classified as problem solving. Implementation and transfer of concepts and principles to actual situations require deductive type of thinking on the part of the student; which is higher-order thinking. Following Gagne's (1970) hierarchy of learning, learning of concepts should preceed learning of principles. Learning principles should be prerequisite to problem solving and implementation; therefore, utilizing this strategy, the teacher can identify and sequence of component tasks and subobjectives to enable the student to achieve the terminal objective.

In summary, the use of this strategy should enable the teacher to design an effective and efficient instructional sequence. The main steps of the sequencing strategy are:

1. Identify the terminal objective
2. Identify the entering behaviors
3. Identify and analyze the component tasks (en-route behaviors) of a given objective
4. Provide for instructional economy
5. Devise the sequence in which instruction takes place

Research studies

Studies in the area of sequencing have been sparse. Most literature dealing with sequencing has been theoretical in nature.

Gagne's (1966) studies on his hierarchy of learning have been among the most outstanding ones on the subject. His model of instruction and his identification of the eight conditions of learning were based on research in which he demonstrated that the eight conditions of learning progress from the simple to the complex, that is, from signal learning to problem solving. Gagne also did a series of other studies that support his framework of the hierarchy of learning (Gagne and Brown, 1961; Gagne and Paradise, 1961).

Additional studies in the area of sequencing have been in programmed instruction, serial positioning, and mathematics. Uprichard (1970), in his doctorial dissertation, discovered that three set mathematical relations can be learned by preschooler if presented in the following manner: equivalent, greater than, lesser than. This is significant in the development of structured mathematical programs in the preschool area. It can also be useful for generating new ideas for exploring the development of mathematical concepts in young children.

Skinner (1968) believes that the teacher who is working with the student is in the best position to evaluate where the student stands and in what direction the student is able to move. This type of situation is lost through programmed instruction. However, programmed instruction does allow for bad items to be spotted and studied to determine why they are bad and what can be done to remove them. In this way, the student essentially writes the program. de Tornyay (1971, p. 120) stated that computer-assisted instruction "in conjunction with autotutorial laboratories in nursing education will revolutionize nursing education." A study was conducted by Bitzer and Boudreaux (1969) in which they designed the computerized system known as PLATO (Programmed Logic for Automatic Teaching Operations). They used this system to test the effect of students learning maternity nursing via a computer-based education system. The control group was exposed to the course content in the conventional classroom manner. A comparison of final examination grades of both control and experimental groups did not indicate a significant difference, however, the PLATO students learned the same amount of material in from one-third to one-half the time required in the classroom.

Issues in sequencing

There are several issues concerning the sequencing process. In nursing education there is constant debate as to how nursing and liberal arts courses can be coordinated and presented in a logical sequence. Many schools maintain that the best order begins with fundamentals and ends with psychiatry and advanced medical-surgical nursing. Some schools make use of the levels concept, where the student moves from the relatively simple to the more complex. Other issues present questions as to the use of a logical order. Skinner (1968, p. 222) stated that "a logical order is not the order in which most behavior is acquired and is therefore not necessarily the best order in which it is to be taught."

There is much controversy over the use of programmed instruction. Skinner (1968) noted the objections made by many: the student does not get an overall view of the material, there is a lack of teacher-student contact, and questions cannot be answered. He believes, however, that the student becomes more deeply involved with the subject matter, that a program can teach a student to ask questions, and that the teacher can be more useful as a guide than as an inducer of behavior.

Researchable questions

What is urgently needed in nursing is the determination of the optimal sequencing of the body of knowledge (cognitive and skill) called "nursing," ranging from the simple (very basic motor skills) to the most complex learning situations (problem solving at the cognitive level). This would enable students to move up the career ladder more easily because their level of knowledge (entering behavior) could be determined by spotting where in the sequence they fall. Evaluation can be done once the sequence of knowledge has been identified. Preliminary work on this subject has already started by Wood (1972).

Another very important area that needs investigating is the graduate nursing curriculum. Two schools of thought prevail: one proposing that all courses be offered in smorgasbord fashion, so there is not a set sequence of courses; the second proposing that there should be a sequence to the type of courses that are offered in the school.

1. A researchable question that can be raised is what the effect of sequencing of courses in a curriculum (smorgasbord versus a set sequence) is on the cognitive and affective behaviors of students.
   a. Independent variable: sequence of curriculum
   b. Dependent variable: cognitive and affective behaviors

ADDITIONAL LEARNING EXPERIENCES—RECOMMENDED READING LIST

Popham, W. J., and Baker, E. L. *Planning an instructional sequence.* Englewood Cliffs, N. J.: Prentice-Hall, Inc., 1970, pp. 43-61.
Tyler, R. W. *Basic principles of curriculum and instruction.* Chicago: University of Chicago Press, 1970, pp. 83-103.

INSTRUCTIONS TO THE LEARNER REGARDING POSTTEST

At this stage of your learning process, you are ready to take the posttest to determine the extent to which you have achieved the objectives of this module. Return to the pretest and take it over again as the posttest. Correct it by using the answer key that is found on this page of the module. You need to score 25 correct points to achieve mastery at the 95% level. If you score less than this, correct your errors and study the content of this module again more carefully and read some of the articles in the recommended reading list. Study in this fashion until you achieve the 95% mastery level.

ANSWER KEY TO PRETEST AND POSTTEST

1. a and c (Webster's Dictionary)
2. b (Gagne, 1970, p. 243)
3. b (Tyler, 1970, p. 84)
4. c (Skinner, 1968, p. 221)
5. b (Tyler, 1970, p. 83)
6. d (Skinner, 1968, pp. 221-222)
7. a (Tyler, 1970, p. 63)
8. b (Gagne, 1970, p. 241)
9. b (Gagne, 1970, pp. 118-119)
10. b (Popham and Baker, 1970, p. 47)
11. a and b (Gagne, 1970, pp. 240-241)
12. b (DeCecco and Crawford, 1974, pp. 230-231)
13. b (Gagne, 1970, p. 240)
14. d (Gagne, 1970, p. 203)
15. c (Gagne, 1970, p. 215)
16. c (Bruner, 1964, p. 313)
17. Answers should include the following steps:
    a. Identify the terminal objective
    b. Identify the entering behaviors
    c. Identify and analyze the component tasks (en-route behaviors) of the given objective
    d. Provide for instructional economy
    e. Devise the sequence in which instruction takes place
    (Popham and Baker, 1970, pp. 44-61)

REFERENCES

Bitzer, M. D., and Boudreaux, M. C. Using a computer to teach nursing. *Nursing Forum*, 1969, **8**(3):234-254.

Block, J. H. (Ed.) *Mastery learning: theory and practice.* New York: Holt, Rinehart and Winston, Inc., 1971.

Bloom, B. S., Englehart, M. D., Furst, E. J., Hill, W. H., and Krathwohl, D. R. (Eds.) *Taxonomy of educational objectives. Handbook 1: Cognitive domain.* New York: David McKay Co., Inc. 1956.

Bruner, J. Some theorems on instruction illustrated with reference to mathematics. In E. R. Hilgard (Ed.), *Theories of learning and instruction.* Chicago: University of Chicago Press, 1964, pp. 306-335.

Bruner, J. The act of discovery. In R. C. Anderson and D. P. Ausubel (Eds.), *Readings in the psychology of cognition.* New York: Holt, Rinehart and Winston, Inc., 1966, pp. 606-620.

Bruner, J. *Toward a theory of instruction.* Cambridge, Mass.: Harvard University Press, 1967.

Carroll, J. A model of school learning. *Teachers College Record*, 1963, **64**:723-733.

DeCecco, J. P., and Crawford, W. *The psychology of learning and instruction: educational psychology.* (2nd Ed.) Englewood Cliffs, N. J.: Prentice-Hall, Inc., 1974.

de Tornyay, R. *Strategies for teaching nursing.* New York: John Wiley & Sons, Inc., 1971.

Gagne, R. M. The analysis of instructional objectives for the design of instruction. In R. Glaser (Eds.), *Teaching machines and programmed learning. II: Data and directions.* Washington, D.C.: National Education Association, 1965, pp. 21-65.

Gagne, R. M. The acquisition of knowledge. In R. C. Anderson and D. P. Ausubel (Eds.), *Readings in the psychology of cognition.* New York: Holt, Rinehart and Winston, Inc., 1966, pp. 116-132.

Gagne, R. M. *The conditions of learning.* New York: Holt, Rinehart and Winston, Inc., 1970.

Gagne, R. M., and Brown, L. T. Some factors in the programming of conceptual learning. *Journal of Experimental Psychology*, 1961, **62**:313-321.

Gagne, R. M., and Paradise, N. E. Abilities and learning sets in knowledge acquisition. *Psychological Monograph*, 1961, **75**:(14): (whole no. 518).

Mager, R. F. *Preparing objectives for programmed instruction*, Belmont, Calif.: Fearon Publishers, Inc., 1962.

Popham, W. J., and Baker, E. I. *Planning an instructional sequence.* Englewood Cliffs, N. J.: Prentice-Hall, Inc., 1970.

Skinner, B. F. *The technology of teaching.* New York: Appleton-Century-Crofts, 1968.

Tyler, R. W. *Basic principles of curriculum and instruction.* Chicago: University of Chicago Press, 1970.

Uprichard, A. E. An experimental study design to determine the most effective learning sequence in three set relations in the preschool years. *Dissertation Abstracts International*, 1970, **30**(12, part 1):5304.

Webster's new collegiate dictionary. Springfield, Mass.: G. & C. Merriam Co., 1961.

Wood, L. (Ed.) *Nursing skills for allied health services.* Philadelphia: W. B. Saunders Co., 1972.

Individual differences

DESCRIPTION OF MODULE

This is an independent unit of instructions that is concerned with the variable of individual differences and how they affect learning and instruction. The module contains instructions to the learner, objectives, pretest and posttest, answer key, and the main text.

The main text covers five major areas that are pertinent to understanding of individual differences in learning and instruction. They are: (1) theoretical framework, (2) research studies, (3) issues, (4) application to nursing education and practice, and (5) researchable questions.

MODULE OBJECTIVES

At the completion of this module, having studied the content and the recommended reading list, the student will be able to accomplish the following objectives at the 95% level of mastery:

1. Identify the important variables around which individuals differ
2. Discuss orally or in writing how each of the main variables influence learning and how they account for individual differences
3. Demonstrate knowledge of the different theoretical frameworks that explain the variables accounting for individual difference

4. Cite relevant research studies that demonstrate how individuals differ in learning
5. Describe and implement a teaching strategy that takes into consideration individual differences in learning
6. Identify at least one issue in the area of individual differences
7. Raise at least one researchable question and identify both the independent and dependent variables
8. Select a patient- or student-teaching situation and apply the principles of individual differences

PRETEST AND POSTTEST

Circle the correct answers. Each question is worth 1 point except the last one, which is worth 10 points. The 95% level of mastery for this test in 24 points. Take the test and correct your errors using the answer key that is found at the end of this module (pp. 410-411). If you score 24 points or better, you need not study this module.

Multiple choice

1. Select the statement(s) that are correct.
   a. Intelligence is synonomous with individual differences.
   b. Intelligence and learning ability will differ among individuals.
   c. The most accurate way to assess individual

differences in the process of learning is by the measurement of intelligence.

2. The concept of individual differences refers to:
   a. physical characteristics
   b. environmental characteristics
   c. motivation and achievement
   d. intellectual strengths and weaknesses
   e. all of the above

3. According to Gagne (1970), the main variable that is responsible for individual differences in learning is:
   a. internal conditions of learning
   b. reinforcement
   c. external conditions of learning
   d. mental ability

4. According to Skinner (1953, 1968), the factor that accounts for individual differences in any type of learning is:
   a. ease of conditionability
   b. the individual's past experiences with regard to reinforcement pattern
   c. schedule of reinforcement
   d. innate capability

5. The success probability of behavior therapy is higher for:
   a. introverted persons
   b. extroverted persons
   c. persons who are highly motivated
   d. persons who have high inhibitory potential

6. The type or condition of learning that is known to be affected by individual differences is:
   a. problem solving
   b. mostly with conditions of learning that have to do with verbal learning
   c. all conditions of learning
   d. transfer of learning

7. According to Jensen (1967), extrinsic individual difference variables are which of the following:
   a. environmental variables
   b. instructions
   c. age, I.Q., sex, and other personality characteristics
   d. learning process

8. According to Jensen (1967), the intrinsic variables that account for individual differences are:

1—those individual differences that are inherent in learning
2—those differences that do not exist independent of learning
3—types of learning
4—content and modality
5—procedural variables
   a. 1, 2, and 3
   b. all of the above
   c. all except 5
   d. 2, 4, and 5

9. One factor that accounts for individual differences in verbal learning, according to Gagne (1970), is:
   a. availability of verbal coding links or mediators
   b. meaningfulness of the verbal task that is to be learned
   c. ability to formulate a hypothesis
   d. learning set

10. According to Carroll (1963) and Bloom (1968), the variables with which individual differences occur are:
    a. aptitude
    b. quality of instruction
    c. ability to understand instruction
    d. perseverance
    e. opportunity

11. The individual difference variables that affect the problem-solving process are:
    1—store of rules the individual has available
    2—ease of recall of relevant rules
    3—ability to recognize concept distinctiveness
    4—maturational age of the child
    5—ability to combine rules into a hypothesis
    6—ability to match specific instances to a general class
    a. 1, 2, and 5
    b. all except 4
    c. all of the above
    d. all except 3

12. The teaching strategies that are appropriate for (1) constructively motivated students and (2) defensively motivated students are:
    a. providing them with problems of moderate risks

    b. spelling out short-term goals
    c. not making intermediate goals too explicit
    d. providing feedback at intervals
    e. giving maximum explanation and guidance
    f. arranging feedback at short intervals
    g. providing for learning by discovery
    h. being very supportive

13. According to Cronbach (1967), what are the personality characteristics of "constructively" motivated people? Differentiate them from others. They have:
    a. high achievement motivation and high anxiety
    b. high achievement motivation and low anxiety
    c. low achievement motivation and high anxiety
    d. low achievement motivation and low anxiety

14. The personality characteristics of a defensively motivated person are:
    a. high achievement motivation and high anxiety
    b. high achievement motivation and low anxiety
    c. low achievement motivation and high anxiety
    d. low achievement motivation and low anxiety

Discussion question

15. Select a patient- or student-teaching situation and implement the principle of individual differences. Identify the specific steps you would follow.

TEXT
Theoretical framework
Introduction

The fact that no two things are exactly alike is so universally recognized as to be a truism. If any two organisms of the same species are compared, it is noted that there are differences between them. This is true of all animals, from the simplest to the most complex. Biologists have found that even the one-celled amebas, although very similar in form and structure, still differ one from another (Gilliland and Clark, 1939). Variations are the deviations among the members of any species of living organisms.

On any given measure, the observed scores of individuals tend to disperse, or spread themselves out, along a continuum. Teachers with heterogeneous classes have to find a way to meet this wide range of differences if they are to provide effective instruction for learning.

Perhaps the most significant variable accounting for the conditions under which learning takes place is the amount of individualized differences that the learner brings to the situation. The importance cannot be overemphasized, since the successful implementation of any instructional model or any learning itself cannot be undertaken without due respect to this enormous variable.

Historical perspective

Before the 1900's, there existed in U.S. schools a largely fixed curriculum with common branches of knowledge, from the academic high school program to the college liberal arts program. Individual differences in students were taken into account mainly by eliminating students. Less successful students merely dropped out.

Ability tests became available and were used by schools to predict success. Some students identified by the use of these tests were allowed to drop, others to remain, gathering mold in slow classrooms. Still others identified were encouraged to proceed at a rapid pace, encouraged to have high aspirations and to continue their education in a collegiate setting. These ability tests thrived, since they had predictive validity for success in the predetermined curriculum.

The prevailing social theory of the time was that "every child should go as far in school as his abilities warrant." On face value, this seems innocuous. Looking deeper, however, one can see the basic assumption is that the abilities of the student can be identified, labeled, and typed, and that beyond these abilities, a point of diminishing return exists. This kind of assumption supported a periodic weeding out of those students who were less responsive to the predetermined curriculum.

The opposite position held that there are certain common learnings that should be attained, and that everyone should stay in school until mastering them. This kind of procedure has not been followed in a pure form, since it would extend the education of some until they were old. As a humane philosophy, it has more value than the keep-pace-or-fall-out policy and is widely practiced in a modified form.

Classification of individual differences variables

In recent years, many studies have been conducted in the area of individual differences that have advanced our knowledge about human differences. It would be convenient if all of these studies could be classified into a logical system, but unfortunately, it is very difficult to arrange them in any such classification.

The following is a representative sample of classifications that have identified variables around which people differ. Educators dealing with children have classified individual differences into a framework of seven categories that have proved useful in accounting for an individual learner's progression through the learning process. These educators look at factors relating to: "(1) family, home, and neighborhood, (2) physical development and health, (3) social development and status, (4) emotional development and mental health, (5) mental development, (6) motivation and (7) achievement" (Cutts and Mosely, 1960, p. 15). Placed along a con-

tinuum and systematically applied to either an educational setting or a potential patient population, implications affecting learning can readily be visualized.

Goodlad (1965, p. 5) talked about individual differences in terms of "academics, past attainment, readiness to learn, in expectations for self, and in energy expenditures." He further discussed a systematical method for handling these differences through the use of "diagnoses, prescriptions, and filling of prescriptions" (Goodlad, 1965, p. 6)—interestingly, his notions are primarily for educators.

Others have classified individual differences into the subheadings: "(1) physical characteristics, (2) intellectual strengths and weakness, (3) social adjustments, (4) home and family background, and (5) cultural background" (Dolan, Price, and Sowden, 1965, p. 97).

Therefore, one school of thought classifies individual differences in terms of the biological (including placement on the health-illness continuum), psychological, and sociocultural. These variables around which individuals differ can be explained more specifically.

Franks (1966) discussed individual differences in relation to behavior-therapy techniques, primarily of the classical-conditioning type. He pointed out that factors such as the modality of the conditioned stimulus, the intensities and relationships of the various stimuli, and the instructions given are directly dependent not only on the subject's motivation and attitude, but also on factors inherent in the subject's biological and neurological system. Furthermore, it is pointed out that wide relationships and variations between conditioning and sex, age, or intelligence have not been consistently demonstrated—the differences rather lying in the circumstances under which conditioning and the variables occurred (Franks, 1966, pp. 155-166). Franks pointed out that this is indeed an area in which there are implications for further research.

Neurologically, some refer to the clue to individual differences as lying in the properties of two central processes, identified as excitation and inhibition, which they believe underlie all higher nervous activity.

Excitation and inhibition, and especially the delicate balance of the two, are viewed as constitutional features of the individual which, in their simplest forms, predispose him to develop either excitatory potentials particularly strongly and inhibitory potentials particularly weakly (the extroverted individual), or else to develop inhibition potentials particularly strongly and excitation ones rather weakly (the introverted individual) (Franks, 1966, p. 158).

Based on this type of theoretical framework, many implications for behavior—at all levels of learning—can be readily conceptualized, especially in relationship to the success probabilities of behavior-therapy techniques for individual patients. As a direct outcome, the theorists envision the day when appropriate laboratory tests will predict beforehand the outcome of behavior therapy by the individual's position on the introversion-extroversion continuum. They postulate that persons in whom inhibitory potentials predominate will condition more poorly and extinguish more rapidly than those that are extroverted in nature. They also point out that increased anxiety levels in each type of individual will contribute toward their conditioning behavior (Franks, 1966; Eysenek, 1957).

Sociocultural aspects of individual differences have long stressed that "conformity to a cultural pattern ensures a large measure of predictability in behavior" (Reed, 1966, p. 53), which in turn affects learning and the learning process. The types of individual differences inherent in this variable especially hold implications for nursing practice, which occurs cross-culturally as well as across social strata. Miller and Dollard spoke of cultural influences as a "recipe for learning" that influences individual responses as well as the value of individual rewards (Miller and Dollard, 1941, p. 5).

Bloom indicated that psychological research seems to indicate that qualities such as self-confidence, self-image, sex identification, self-aspiration, as well as behavioral qualities of future-time orientation and motivation, are more often related to life circumstances and socioeconomic-cultural factors (Bloom, 1965, pp. 72-77). Skinner also ascribed emotional differences of learners primarily to individual conditioned reinforcement . . . and thus found them to be subject to the principles of behavioral modification (Skinner, 1953, p. 241).

Jensen's view (1967) of individual differences is different from those given previously. He recommended looking at individual differences rather than at meager group mean differences. He stated that, if one finds meager group mean differences, one must ask if the effects of the independent variables have been buried in the error term. The error term contains the interaction between the independent variable and the subject. He stated that averaging the individual performance scores could result in false conclusions. Jensen is convinced that the interaction between the subject and the independent variable is the proper place to look for individual differences if one wants to assess the potency of the experimental variable. He also pointed out that experimental psychology of learning considers individual differences to be the very heart of its subject matter.

Jensen (1967) classified individual differences into two main categories: intrinsic and extrinsic. The essence of the difference is illustrated by his two statements, "(a) individual differences *in* learning, and (b) the effects of individual differences *on* learning."

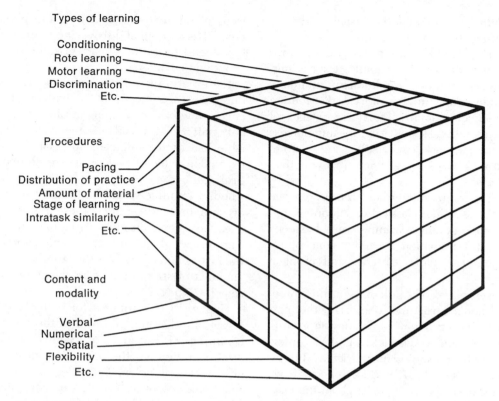

Types of learning

Conditioning
Rote learning
Motor learning
Discrimination
Etc.

Procedures

Pacing
Distribution of practice
Amount of material
Stage of learning
Intratask similarity
Etc.

Content and
modality

Verbal
Numerical
Spatial
Flexibility
Etc.

Fig. 25-1. A representation of the classes of variables in learning tasks. (From Jensen, A. R. Varieties of individual differences in learning. In Gagne, R. (Ed.), *Learning and individual differences.* Columbus, Ohio: Charles E. Merrill Publishing Co., Jensen, 1967, p. 123).

Jensen viewed *extrinsic* individual differences as referring to those subject variables that do not operationally resemble the learning process as it is traditionally conceived. Yet they affect the individual's performance in the learning situation. Examples of extrinsic variables are those variables that ordinarily one attempts to control in laboratory experimentation; for example, chronological age, mental age, I.Q., sex, and other personal characteristics.

Intrinsic individual differences refer to "those individual differences which are inherent in learning and which do not exist independent of learning phenomena. In other words, intrinsic individual differences consist of intersubject variability in the learning process itself" (Jensen, 1967, p. 122). Jensen described the domain of intrinsic individual differences in learning by using the analogy of a large, three-dimensional cube, made up of many small cubes (Fig. 25-1). The three dimensions of the cube and the enclosed cells represent three major classes of variables in which any learning task may be located and individuals differ.

1. The horizontal dimension represents the content and modality variables. This refers to the stimulus classes of the material that is to be learned by the individual. This variable includes such content (or stimulus classes) as verbal, numerical, spatial, and

flexibility classes and the visual, auditory, and others sensory modalities.

2. The vertical axis deals with the procedural variables; for example, task pacing, stimulus duration, conditioned stimulus–unconditioned stimulus interval, distribution of practice, amount of material, stages of learning, intratask similarity, meaningfulness of material, task complexity, and instructional variables such as differentially motivating sets.

3. The third dimension represents the types of learning: classical conditioning, operant conditioning, chaining, verbal associations, discrimination learning, concept attainment, principle learning, and problem solving.

Jensen noted that in looking at this three-dimensional structure, one faces the possibility that each row or column on each of the dimensions could yield significant interaction between subject and variables. For instance, Jensen (1967, p. 124) stated, "If we run a group of subjects through all the tasks and conditions represented in this cube, there is the possibility that as we go from cell to cell the rank order of the subjects' learning performance will continually be changing." He further pointed out that just how much shifting of rank order to expect in this situation is not known. Nor is it known which variable will produce the most interaction with subjects. This is, then, the task that future researchers on individual differences in learning have to tackle. They have "to delineate the basic dimensions or genotypes of all the between-subjects variation associated with all the phenotypes of learning depicted in this 3 dimensional scheme. And then some!" (Jensen, 1967, p. 125).

Jensen described phenotypes in terms of task characteristics, that is the location of the learning task on the three-dimensional structure. Genotypes refer to the underlying factors, or basic processes, that cause the patterns of intercorrelation among the phenotypes. He stated that discovering these genotypes constitutes the primary task of research on individual differences.

Jensen also placed some personality traits under intrinsic types of individual differences, when the development of the personality trait itself is based on some essential variable in learning's domain; for example, extroversion, which develops as a result of cortical inhibition, plays a role in learning. Another example would be the trait of anxiety or neuroticism. Both of these traits would affect learning through variations in task complexity, along with the manipulation of the instructional variables that arouse varying amounts of stress or ego involvement (Jensen, 1967, p. 122).

Gagne (1970) accounted for individual differences in learning in terms of the *internal conditions* of learning. For example, in classical conditioning, the individual must possess a natural reflex. Examples of reflexive emotional responses are startle, fear, anger, pleasure, and the like. Furthermore, an unconditioned stimulus should be able to evoke an unconditioned response. Individual differences occur in this area. For instance, there are marked individual differences in the rapidity with which individuals acquire stimulus-response connections. Such differences are not significantly related to intelligence or to academic learning. But they are related to the level of *anxiety* the individual experiences when faced with life's problems and decisions. Many studies (Taylor, 1951; Franks, 1966) have shown that anxious people condition more rapidly than nonanxious people, and individuals differ in level of anxiety.

In operant conditioning, the individual must be able to perform a terminating (or consummatory) act that provides satisfaction or reinforcement. For instance, the child should be able to suck on the nipple in order to fill the mouth with milk. This consummatory act produces a satisfying state of affairs. Such responses are either innately present or are learned. Individuals differ with regard to the availability of such responses. Skinner (1968) further determined that the individual's past experiences with regard to reinforcement patterns accounts for individual differences in operant conditioning.

In chaining, or skill learning, it is necessary that each individual stimulus-response connection be *previously learned*. Individual differences occur in this area, that is, individuals differ in the extent to which they have previously learned the individual stimulus-response links. If learners lack this necessary prerequisite knowledge of individual stimulus-response links, then external cues need to be provided in order for these learners to discriminate the individual links and perform the skills. The speed of learning of chains is dependent on the minimum amount of cueing necessary and the number of previously learned individual links available to the learner. This is where individuals differ.

In verbal associations, individual differences occur in the areas of (1) availability of previously learned discriminated verbal stimulus-response units or links within the learner and (2) availability of previously learned mediating connections between each verbal unit and the next. Gagne (1970) pointed out that the greater the number of "coding links" the learner has, the more rapidly learning takes place. Noble (1963) supported this hypothesis. Noble found that verbal associations are learned more rapidly when learners possess a greater number of verbal "free associates" that can be chained to syllables or words. In addition to verbal "codes," the availability of other types of mediators could enhance the learning of verbal associates where individuals seem to differ; for example, in availability of visual or auditory images, as in pictures or rhythms.

In discrimination learning, the areas within which individual differences occur are similar to those of verbal associations, in that: (1) the learner must have previously learned, *in isolation,* each link or chain that is to be learned and discriminated and (2) the learner must have previously learned and discriminated the initial stimulus links from each other, and the response links also must have been learned previously as discriminated stimulus-response connections. For example, let us take the case of the student nurse trying to discriminate between a plus three (+3) and a plus four (+4) in testing urine for sugar. Discrimination learning will occur more readily if the student (1) can identify the color of each specimen, (2) is able to name or label them when on sight, and (3) has available a mediating link. For example, the student can associate the actual sample with the calibrated picture of a +3 or +4 sugar test. The availability of such links will vary with individuals. Evidence (Deese, 1961) suggests that those people who have greater supplies of coding links acquire a set of chains and discriminate more rapidly than those who have fewer available links.

In concept learning, individual differences occur in the area of prerequisite capabilities that the student must possess prior to the learning of concepts, especially those that are established by means of multiple discrimination, chaining, operant conditioning, and classical conditioning. Gagne (1970, p. 180) pointed out that "a set of verbal (or other) chains must have previously been acquired to *representative* stimulus situations that exhibit the characteristics of the class that describes the concept, and that distinguish these stimuli from others not included in the class."

In rule learning, the prerequisite knowledge that the person must possess is knowledge of chains of concepts that constitute the rule and their ability to see relationships between the concepts that formulate the rule. Furthermore, in order to learn upper-level rules, the learner must posses as entering behavior a reservoir of related lower-level rules. Individuals also differ in the amount of stored up lower-level rules they have.

Gagne (1970, p. 223) discussed the individual differences that affect the problem-solving process and spoke of them in terms of abilities inherent in the learner. Problem solving, it seems, takes place more rapidly and has a higher instance of being correct in those individuals who have:

(1) a great variety of stores of rules, (2) ease of recall of relevant rules, (3) ability for concept distinctiveness or ability to readily define the problem, (4) facility to combine rules into hypotheses, and (5) ability to match specific instances into a general class in order to verify the problem solution.

The individual differences that occur in social learning are similar to those classical conditioning. operant conditioning, chaining, discrimination learning, and verbal learning. If the social behavior that is to be acquired is an instrumental response, then the individual differences that occur are similar to those that occur in operant conditioning. Therefore, the type of behavior that is to be acquired determines what type of individual differences to expect.

Gagne also perceived individual differences to occur in transfer of learning. His theory of transfer states that in order for an individual to transfer knowledge acquired at the subordinate levels of learning sets to higher levels, the individual must have acquired *all* relevant subordinate sets prior to expecting much transfer. Individuals differ in the amount of knowledge they have acquired at the subordinate level that is relevant for transfer to the upper level.

Ellis discussed the characteristics of the learner that are known to influence the trans-

fer of learning; namely, intelligence and motivational factors, especially anxiety. Studies have indicated that intelligence is directly proportional to the learner's ability to see relationships as well as to the learner's "set" for transfer. While it is not difficult to see that the poorly motivated student will learn less, it is interesting to note that studies by Spence (1964) and Gaier (1952) suggested that heightened anxiety, although it increases the probability of a correct response when dealing with a relatively few choices, lowers the probability for correct response to complex behaviors, such as synthesis and application (Ellis, 1965, pp. 67-68; Gaier, 1952, pp. 404-411; Spence, 1964, pp. 120-139).

Bloom (1968) and Carroll (1963) pointed out that regardless of the individual differences, students of average aptitude can achieve mastery of learning, although there may be a wide variation in the time required to do so. According to this theoretical framework, achievement is possible for 95% of the student population, given enough time and appropriate types of help. The variables influencing this type of developmental mastery are: (1) aptitude, (2) quality of instruction, (3) ability to understand instruction, (4) perseverance, and (5) time allowed for learning. Of these five variables, those that reside within the individual—namely, aptitude, ability to understand instruction, and perseverance—account for the variations in individuals.

How to adapt instruction to individual differences

Gagne (1970, pp. 22-24) stated that the internal and external conditions under which learning takes place are very interdependent. His view is under which learning takes place are very interdependent. His view is that the "initial capabilities of the learner" are crucial for subsequent learning to transpire and that for learning to be effective, the external conditions must be altered to take into consideration the individual differences of the learner.

Skinner (1970, p. 240) likewise pointed out that individual sensory capacities, such as preference for auditory versus visual learning, can be made contingent on environmental factors in order to reduce learning differences of this kind. He noted that his model, as an effective "technology of teaching," will design environmental contingencies dependent on individual reinforcement patterns.

Cronbach (1967) pointed out that adapting education to meet the individual's need has meant many things to many people in education. Several different methods of adapation have been utilized that are not necessarily mutually exclusive. They can combine in various forms. There are four methods of adaptation.

USING A PREDETERMINED PROGRAM

In the early part of this century, the educational curriculum was fixed, progressing from common branches of knowledge and proceeded through high school programs and then to a college liberal arts program. Individual differences were taken into consideration by eliminating unsuccessful students. Later, with the advancement of ability tests, educators used these tests to decide which students should be dropped off, which needed to follow "slow" classes, and which had to proceed more swiftly and be indoctrinated with high aspirations for higher education. These mental tests have shown some predictive validity for success in the predetermined curriculum. Cronbach has noted that some of these old educational practices are still in use. For example, children in the first grade were kept there until they could read the primer. In today's nongraded primary unit, there are some children who complete it in 2 years, others in 4 years. Proponents of this form of adaptation claim that by using linear programmed instruction, they can bring all learners to criterion on its fixed

content, but at the students pace. Homogenous groupings of students have also been utilized to adjust the pace of instruction. Adjusting pace or time refers to changing the amount of exercise given to a particular connection or subskill. It is Cronbach's hypothesis that "the person's learning rate will vary, depending on the nature of instruction; I therefore expect that adapting instructional *technique* will in the long run be more important than merely altering the duration of exposure" (Cronbach, 1967, p. 26).

MATCHING GOALS TO THE INDIVIDUAL

Fifty years ago, when educational institutions were dropping off unsuccessful students and were considering the dropouts as undesirable, the big influx of unwanted students created a radical alteration in the educational program. Margaret Cobb, working in Thorndike's lab in 1922, found that there was a considerable risk of failure if a pupil with a mental age below 15 years 6 months enrolled in high school algebra. She wrote that the average or less intelligent should be encouraged to try some other type of training. Schools introduced vocational and homemaking curricula, and other new courses were designed. Algebra was replaced by a course in general mathematics.

Danger existed in setting differentiated goals. Differentiation of mathematics courses meant that the discipline of math was kept as the possession of a selected class, while the lower classes drilled in formulas useful to shopkeepers and tradesmen. Today, the theme in math teaching and other areas is to give every pupil an understanding of the same basic disciplines, even though some pupils go farther and deeper. An example of the new approach to the teaching of mathematics can be seen on early morning television, as preschool children are making games of basic algebraic concepts.

Goals are also modified when students are allowed to select their own major field of study and select their elective courses. This is necessary and will continue.

ERASING INDIVIDUAL DIFFERENCES

Individual differences can be erased by using remedial instruction, which adds onto the common program rather than redesigning it. Remedial work, according to Cronbach, takes for granted that classroom work is largely a fixed program.

Some remedial treatments are developed by breaking the subject matter into component processes, classifying pupil errors, and providing special explanations and drills. The Thorndikean view is to take an inventory of combinations mastered and not mastered and direct practice to weak areas. Gagne (1962) had similar thinking in describing the hierarchies that exist in the individual in relation to information and skill.

Other treatments include a branched programmed instruction, where there is a continuous diagnosis of misconceptions or gaps in recall, followed by an appropriate remedial loop as each error occurs.

Also seen is the assignment of a short linear program covering a single topic or subskill for independent study when the teacher finds the pupil weak in that area.

Cronbach (1967) believed all of the above methods to be of limited value. What is monitored in a branched program is subject-matter mastering in the narrowest sense. The programs check on the learner's ability to give the response as taught. The goal of education is aimed at developing transferable responses, both cognitive and affective, rather than emphasizing the learner's ability to give the response as taught. Unless the broader outcomes are monitored, the remedial programs do more harm than good.

Cronbach also pointed out that compensatory education, such as in Head Start programs, is remedial. The hopes of such programs are that with appropriate stimulation, they will develop the intellectual skills and attitudes that constitute normal readiness for primary school. There is knowledge about readiness for reading and its development on which these activities can draw. Cronbach further indicated that what is needed is a theory about information intake and study. The study of Bloom and associates (1965) on encoding, mediation, and feedback is a good start in the right direction.

Cronbach's views on remedial education have been criticized by Carroll (1967). Carroll believes that remedial instruction is necessary, and its role is more than that of "hole patching." For example, remedial instruction is good when a teacher is confronted with problems of distorted attitudes of an individual pupil or with problems of perception about some aspect of subject matter or specific disability in perception.

ALTERING INSTRUCTIONAL METHOD

Teachers adapt instructional methods according to the needs of the individual pupil, both on the macro- and microlevel. Cronbach (1967) noted that teachers often use intuitive cues from students to direct differential teaching methods. This method of adaptation may be misleading, if not harmful. He stated that teachers are likely to overdifferentiate. They tend to expect too much from the persons who test high on aptitude tests and too little from those who test low.

Evidence exists that modifying treatment too much produces a worse result than treating everyone alike. Cronbach further asserted that the poorer the differential information, the less the teacher should depart from the teaching methodology that works best for the average. Aptitude information is not useful in adapting instruction unless aptitude and treatment (instructional methodology) interact (Cronbach, 1955, 1967; Cronbach and Glaser, 1965).

Jensen (1962) concluded by stating that to

systematize the process of adaptation to reduce errors calls for a theory whose propositions indicate the conditions of instruction best suited for certain types of students. Both the conditions of instruction and the types of pupils should be described in broad dimensions.

Cronbach (1967) mentioned three variables that educators seem to take into consideration in providing differential methodology to different students. These are general ability, modes of presentation, and constructive versus defensive motivation.

General ability. General ability seems to be considered one of the first variables that should give the teacher indications as to how to modify instruction. In general, educators think that teaching very bright students calls for a different method of instruction than used for average students. Cronbach (1967) pointed out that interactions of instructional method with mental age are not well established within any age group. One reason for this is that general aptitude would correlate with performance no matter what the instructional methodology used.

Aptitude is defined in this context as:

. . . a complex of personal characteristics that accounts for an individual's end state after a particular educational treatment, i.e., that determines what he learns, how much he learns, or how rapidly he learns . . . Aptitude, pragmatically, includes whatever promotes the pupil's survival in a particular educational environment, and it may have as much to do with styles of thought and personality variables as with the abilities covered in conventional tests (Cronbach, 1967, pp. 23-24).

The studies of Stolurow (1964), Schramm (1964), Osler and Fivel (1961), and Osler and Trautman (1961) have found contradictory and inconsistent results when they have related teaching methodology to mental ability. Findings about the interaction between the two were inconsistent.

Modes of presentation. Cronbach (1967,

p. 32) recommended that researchers invent interactions. He stated, more specifically, "we ought to take a differential variable we think promising and design alternative treatments to interact with that variable." He also commented that it is time that institutions specify only the criterion, not the treatment, and let each psychologist select an aptitude variable and design treatments that are expected to interact with it.

One place to begin is to start with the abilities that are suggested by the factor analysis, such as spatial ability, numerical ability, verbal ability, and the others. Cronbach stated that by defining the distinct tasks and sorting persons on differential aptitudes rather than general aptitude, a larger proportion of the students will be able to succeed. A proposal like this was suggested by Gagne (1960) for eighth grade math classes. However, his study has not been carried out.

Constructive versus defensive motivation. Cronbach (1967) pointed out that the interaction that has been studied most in the area of motivation involves attitudes about confidence, willingness to risk failure, and motivation for self-directed achievement.

Subjects (students) in most studies on motivation have been classified as what Cronbach calls (1) "constructively" motivated subjects, who are high on achievement motivation and low on anxiety, and (2) "defensively" motivated subjects, who are low on achievement motivation and high on anxiety. Intermediates have intermediate results. Stated differently:

Constructives = ↑ achievement motivation and ↓ anxiety

Defensives = ↓ achievement motivation and ↑ anxiety

Results of several studies that have shown an interaction between motivational variables and instructional methodology are as follows;

and these guidelines have been used to adapt to individual differences.

1. Constructives show most persistence when dealing with problems of moderate risk.

2. Defensives are most persistent when the chance of success is very low (Feather, 1961).

3. Defensives are rigid when in difficulty and will not withdraw from blind-alley situations (Kogan and Wallach, 1964).

4. Constructives achieve well when given simple instruction to get the work done, but adding pressure lowers their scores. The same pressure and a cash prize or pacing and stern supervision improves the work of the defensives (Atkinson and Reitman, 1956).

5. Constructives improve their work when told they have done poorly, while defensives improve with favorable comment (Mandler and Jarason, 1952).

6. Homogeneous groups facilitate the school learning of constructives; however, it has no appreciable effect on the defensives (Atkinson and O'Connor, 1963).

Cornbach (1967, p. 35) concluded from these studies the following hypothesis: that defensive students will benefit most when the teacher:

1. Spells out the short-term goals
2. Gives maximum explanation and guidance
3. Arranges feedback at short intervals to keep the students from going astray
4. Maximizes the opportunity for dependence

and that constructives will benefit most when:

1. The task they need to learn is moderately difficult
2. Intermediate goals are not too explicit
3. Feedback is provided at intervals for purposes of teaching them to judge themselves, rather than for motivational purposes
4. There is a shift from didactic teaching to learning by discovery

Cronbach (1967) pointed out that if further work confirms the findings of the foregoing research, then these findings will be applied to educational situations. Some part of the school program should be designed to help defensives increase their self-assurance rather than allowing them to remain the same. A fundamental question is raised of whether we want to reduce individual differences. Benjamin (1949), writing at Harvard, made a plea for the cultivation of idiosyncrasy.

Cronbach (1967, p. 37) concluded his speculations on adaptation of the instruction to individual differences by stating, "As I see it, our greatest hope for fitting the school to the individual lies in the development of theory that marries the differential and experimental approaches to learning."

SUMMARY AND CONCLUSION

The different conceptual approaches to classification of variables around which individuals differ are very disintegrated. Each approach has its strengths and weaknesses. Three major approaches to the taxonomy of individual differences were presented: (1) the biopsychosociocultural approach, (2) Jensen's intrinsic- and extrinsic-variable approach, and (3) Gagne's approach by means of differences in internal conditions of learning. The three approaches focus on individual differences from different perspectives. The approach used by each school of thought overlaps the others. It is like cutting the same pie of individual differences differently.

It is the opinion of this writer that these three different approaches can be integrated into a more cohesive whole that explains the variables around which individuals differ more clearly, logically, and systematically.

Since we are concerned mostly with conditions of learning and instruction in human beings, then the most useful framework to use is the modified version of Gagne's basic approach within this framework Jensen's intrinsic and extrinsic variables are accounted for. Stated more explicitly:

1. The conditions *within* the person under which learning takes place will be the areas where individuals differ the most.

2. The basic conditions of learning are those in Gagne's (1970) hierarchy of learning and social learning.

3. The internal conditions of learning are affected by the student's biological, psychological, sociocultural, and developmental variables.

In order to meet the educational needs of each individual, the external conditions of learning and models of instruction, which are the instructional methodology, must adapt to the individual differences. Furthermore, depending on the policy of the educational institution and the theoretical framework of the teacher, instructions can be adapted to meet individual differences.

From the previous presentation of the theoretical background of individual differences, it is evident that many issues have not been resolved. For example, there are still tremendous variations in ideas about what the best way is to account for individual differences, what the real dimensions or variables are around which individuals differ, how to measure these differences accurately, what methodology to use in research studies, what the best method is to adapt instruction to individual differences and others. The resolution of these issues awaits further experimentation and a more systematical integration of the different schools of thought that identify the variables influencing individual differences in learning and instruction.

Relevant research studies
Relationship of I.Q. to instructional method

To determine the relationship of intelligence to instructional method, Stolurow (1964), in a typical study, set up two different program sequences. He developed two programs to teach fractions. In the first, he ordered the fractions consecutively, so that the students could anticipate what fractions would come next. In the second program he presented the fractions in mixed or scrambled sequences. Stolurow then compared the achievement of high and low ability groups on both programs. Findings in several such studies have been consistent. With the first program, achievement between high and low ability groups differed little. With the second program, the high ability group obtained scores much higher than those of the low ability group.

Eigen and Feldhusen (1964) studied normal ninth-, tenth-, and eleventh-grade students using a programmed text and machine instruction on sets, relations, and functions. Also measured was how much of the material students could transfer, or apply, to novel test situations. The study was concerned with three variables; I.Q., acquisition, and transfer. Acquisition refers to achievement, that is, how much of the material is learned; transfer refers to the application of what is learned. From the study, the trend is clear: in programmed instruction, I.Q. may be a much less reliable predictor of achievement than the previous achievement level of what the student in those areas directly related to the content of the instruction. This study suggests that a direct assessment of entering behavior under optimal instructional conditions is more useful than a general assessment of intelligence. Also, the ability to transfer what has been learned by programmed instruction is determined more by how much the student has learned than by I.Q. (DeCecco, 1963).

I.Q. and problem solving

Koyanagi (1953) and Corman (1957) compared groups of students of high and low mental ability. Koyanagi's bright children learned to cover a hole in a path so that a ball they were rolling along the path would not drop through. The dull children's set for rolling the ball seemed to prevent their learning the anticipatory response of covering the hole. Corman's brighter high-school students benefited from large amounts of information on how to attack Katona's matchstick problems, but less bright students were able to utilize only small amounts of such guidance (Duncan, 1959, p. 415).

I.Q. and creativity

Another challenge to the concept of general intelligence comes from the studies on creativity. Guilford (1950) raised the question concerning the relationship between I.Q. and creativity when she predicted that the highly intelligent would probably not be highly creative and the highly creative would not be highly intelligent.

Getzels and Jackson (1962) administered creativity tests to 533 students with an average I.Q. of 130. Highly creative students were compared with students with high I.Q. scores on total scholastic achievement. It was found that creativity was equal to or more important than intelligence in determining scholastic achievement.

Individual differences in concept attainment

Of interest, particularly as it holds implications for nursing education, is the effect of individual variables on concept attainment. Two such individual differences are researched in relationship to concept attainment in the following studies.

In a study by Osler and Fivel, the role of age and intelligence in concept attainment was studied by the induction method. The induction method does not necessarily require verbalization on the part of the subject, but rather tests concept attainment by requiring like responses to different stimuli belonging to a common category. In this exper-iment, 180 elementary-school and junior-high-school students—half of whom were of average intelligence (mean WISC I.Q., 101.6) and half of whom were of high intelligence (mean WISC I.Q. 121.3)—were studied in relationship to one of the following concepts: bird, animal, or living thing. Research design required the correct matching of like concept–correct pictures on a metal frame cube from two card stimuli (one concept-correct, the other similar in area, color, and brightness but unrelated to the concept) offered the students, with subsequent rewards for correct responses. The students were given 150 trials to achieve 10 consecutive responses for indication of successful understanding of the concept. Results indicated the following conclusions (Osler and Fivel 1961, pp. 1-7):

1. Age and intelligence were associated with significant differences in errors in concept and number of successful subjects.

2. The effect of concept hierarchy had no effect on errors to individual concepts, but did produce significant differences in the number of subjects of normal intelligence who achieved the criterion of success.

3. When subjects were divided into sudden and gradual learners, the frequency of sudden learners was a function of intelligence rather than age.

The object of the research study by Osler and Trautman, which also dealt with concept attainment, was to further study the implication from the above findings of the relationship between intelligence and the specific learning mechanism involved in concept attainment. It was postulated that a mediated symbolical process or set of stimulus-response associations played a crucial role in concept attainment. Research design was similar to the previous experiment, with the exception of the differentiated stimuli-response patterns. Results concluded that subjects of normal intelligence attain concepts through stimulus–stimulus (S–S) associative learning, while subjects of superior intelligence obtain concepts by testing hypotheses (Osler and Trautman, 1962, pp. 9-13).

Individual differences in attention

Individual differences in attention point to physiological responses. The initial condition for attending is stimulus change. This has been called the orienting reflex. It is defined as a concept with observable antecedents and consequent conditions. Gagne (1967) described several studies where the orienting reflex was measured in cephalic vasodilation, peripheral constriction, pupillary dilation, increased cerebral temperature, and increased blood volume. In summary, subjects high in orienting reflex were found to be more sensitive to their environment than those low in orienting reflex.

This has importance when considered with the several studies of Zeaman and House (1967). These researchers found that with retardates, when teaching focused on a dimension to which the students were attending (paying attention), their I.Q. differences did not affect learning capability. When brighter and slower students were mixed in a group, of course the brighter students learned more quickly; but the I.Q. differences could be diminished if one could engineer the instruction to the attention of the retardates.

Sex differences

Not infrequently, men have been found to be better problem solvers than women, but close examination of the literature reveals some qualifications of this finding. Van de Geer (1957) reported two experiments showing that 12-year-old girls were both more susceptible to set and less able to surmount set than were boys of the same age. Van de Geer also showed that girls developed no more set from two training problems than did

boys, but that with six training problems, girls developed so much set that unsolvable problems or speed instructions did not further increase their set. Rhine (1957) reported no sex differences in set on text anagrams (Duncan, 1959, p. 412).

In studies with other complex problems, sex differences have been mentioned occasionally. Hilgard and associates (1954) found high school boys superior to girls on Katona's card-trick problems. Saugstad (1952) used five complex problems to test his hypothesis that incidental memory should correlate negatively with ability to solve such difficult problems. Significant negative correlations were found for boys, but not for girls (Duncan, 1959, p. 413).

Application to nursing education and practice

In general, the subject of individual differences is one that should be given major study and consideration by the nursing profession, for nursing is a profession that deals with many types of people from all walks of life. Each person is different and has many varied ways of interacting and coping with illness and the many problems of daily living.

For these reasons, nursing education should plan programs that include theory on the individual differences of patients and how they relate to the many ways patients cope with illness. By possessing knowledge about the individual differences of patients, nurses will be better prepared to give nursing care and teaching based on theory instead of intuition. Nurses would then give more humanized and individualized care instead of treating patients like objects.

Not only should nursing programs consider the individual differences among patients, they should also consider the individual differences among students. Individual differences are the source of creative contributions to our society. Thus, curricula and teaching methods should be designed so that students can learn to the maximum of their abilities. The major weakness of many of the traditional forms of instruction is that slow and rapid learners are, in effect, penalized by academic routines designed for "average" students. DeCecco (1963, p. 491) stated that "Inadequate educational stimulation may mean not only that students learn less than they should, but also that they become less able to acquire further thinking skills." A program designed toward individualization would take this and other variables into consideration.

The provision of high-quality learning opportunities for personnel in the health care fields is shifting rapidly from option to necessity. Since change is the idiom of our times, nursing schools' major purpose should be to create innovative curricula that reflect the relevance and futuristic styling demanded in today's world, to meet the varied needs of heterogenous groups of learners, and to enable both students and teachers to grow professionally (Beyers, Dickelmann, and Thompson, 1972). Thus, nursing schools should experiment with and utilize many of the new concepts and methods available on individualization of instruction; such as computer-assisted instruction, self-instruction programs, or any innovative methods that advance the concept of individualization. It is only through use of innovative methods and techniques that consider the total student and individual differences that well-qualified nurses can be produced.

Also of interest in nursing education is the seeming implication of respecting individual differences for the fostering of creative students. According to Aichlmayr (1969, p. 21), "Research demonstrates that intelligent, nonconforming students—characteristically creative—drop out of nursing," thus perpetuating in the nursing profession the more docile convergent thinker. Aichlmayr identified the creative student's differences as being the degree of intelligence, originality, independence, rebelliousness, perceptiveness, intuitiveness, doctrinairism, and estheticism that the student exhibits. Furthermore, "Nursing educators can cultivate students' creative talents by respecting imaginative and unusual ideas and questions, by demonstrating that students' ideas have value, by providing unevaluated experimentation, and by stimulating self-initiated learning" (Aichlmayr, 1969, p. 26).

On the more specific side, recognizing learning differences in nursing education and practice would seem to lie in the choice of learning approaches as well as the appropriate implementation of an instructional model geared to the differences of a particular student or patient population.

The following is a list of principles that can be implemented to handle individual differences. A specific example of a learning situation is given, and the principles are applied to it.

1. Determine what you will teach the student or the patient; that is, identify the objectives. Assuming that you want to teach the four basic foods, at the completion of instruction the student or the patient will be able to identify or select from a variety of food items those foods that represent the four basic foods.

2. Determine what type of learning it is; in other words, is it skill learning, operant conditioning, problem solving, or another type. In this specific situation, the task to be learned is a concept: the concept of four basic foods.

3. Determine what the internal condition for concept learning is. In this example, the student or patient must have the capability of multiple discrimination in that the subject must have the capability of identifying the individual food items (stimulus situations) that exhibit the characteristics of the class (carbohydrate, protein, and the others) that describes the concept and that distinguishes

these stimuli (food items) from others not included in the class. Stated more specifically, can the student identify and label fruits or meats and differentiate them from other food items?

4. Assess the entering behavior of the student or the patient to see whether the internal conditions specified in item 3 exist.

5. Assess the student's or patient's biopsychosociocultural background and determine in what capacity each of these variables affect learning. For example, for biological variables, consider the student's age, health status, and so on. For psychological variables, consider the level of motivation, that is, how interested the student is, whether constructively motivated or defensively motivated; use Cronbach's guidelines in determining approximately the nature and status of the subject's motivation. This is very important, because it determines whether to give a very structured presentation, as for defensives, or simple instructions with minimum guidelines, as for constructives. For sociocultural variables, consider the nationality and ethnic background of the subject. The food habits and food choices they have developed may not be what you would have experienced, and you, as their teacher, may not be aware of some of their low-cost, nutritious food choices.

6. Determine what method of instruction to use and how to provide the external conditions of learning that are essential for concept learning. This instructional methodology will determine whether the method of teaching is adapted to the needs of the student or patient. The external conditions for concept learning are embodied in a set of verbal instructions, involving the following:

a. The specific stimulus objects are presented simultaneously or in close time succession; for example, the foods of the protein group (fish, poultry, meat, eggs, lentils, dried pinto beans, peanuts, and others) are presented to the subject either all together or one at a time in close succession. Correct labels are given by the subject. The teacher may ask: "What is this?" for three to five different food items that belong to the same or different food categories, and expect the answer "protein" to those that are appropriate. This would then be done for the other food groups.

b. Instruction then goes on to elicit the same link (that is, the concept of protein) to a stimulus situation (specific food item that is new) belong to the proper food category but to which the learner has not previously responded. Instruction may again include the question: "What is this?" directed to the new food items, or the teacher may alter the question by requesting: "Show me a food that belongs to the protein group."

c. Once these events have occurred, the new capability (whether the patient or the student has acquired the concept of the four basic foods) may be verified by asking for the identification of several additional new instances of each class to which the learner has not been previously exposed. If the learner identifies them correctly, then one may conclude that the concept of the four basic foods has been learned.

d. The final external condition is the *positive reinforcement* that should be present in the concept-learning situation. This positive reinforcement can be in the form of praise, confirmation, or feedback. It should follow the correct response immediately; in other words, it should be contingent on the utterance of the correct response by the learner.

Therefore, utilizing the strategy enumerated, any type of instruction can and should be individualized to meet the needs of the learner. Other forms of commercially prepared materials can be used in conjunction with didactic teaching methodology.

Individualized instruction in nursing education seems to be gaining impetus, examples of which are programs stressing independent study as well as the utilization of programmed materials. de Tornyay (1971) projected that nursing education would provide for differences in learners through the use of autotutorial laboratories, mechanized libraries, computerized instruction, and increased utilization of television. The reports of a Russian research study that compared computer-assisted instruction with traditional instruction indicated a statistically higher level of performance among students in the computer-based program as well as a much lower drop-out rate among these students (de Tornyay, 1971, pp. 121-122). "There is no question that the increasing available technology will change the role of the teacher from conveyor of information . . . to that of learning diagnostician, guider, and motivator" (de Tornyay, 1971, p. 123).

Researchable questions

1. What is the effect of individualized instruction on the drop-out rate of baccalaureate nursing students and on their grade-point average?
   a. Independent variable: individualized instruction
   b. Dependent variables: (1) drop-out rate and (2) grade-point average
2. What is the effect of mastery-learning methods of instruction on the students' cognitive ability in relation to whether they are "constructively" or "defensively" motivated?
   a. Independent variables: (1) the mastery-learning teaching technique and (2) "constructively" or "defensively" motivated students
   b. Dependent variable: cognitive ability (the amount learned by the students)

3. What tools can be developed that will measure the personality characteristics ("constructive" or "defensive") of motivation?

ADDITIONAL LEARNING EXPERIENCES—RECOMMENDED READING LIST

Cronbach, L. J. How can instruction be adapted to individual differences? In R. M. Gagne (Ed.), *Learning and individual differences*. Columbus, Ohio: Charles E. Merrill Publishing Co., 1967, pp. 23-39.

Gagne, R. M. (Ed.) *Learning and individual differences*. Columbus, Ohio: Charles E. Merrill Publishing Co., 1967.

Jensen, A. R. Varieties of individual differences in learning. In R. M. Gagne (Ed.), *Learning and individual differences*. Columbus, Ohio: Charles E. Merrill Publishing Co., 1967, pp. 117-135.

INSTRUCTIONS TO THE LEARNER REGARDING POSTTEST

At this stage of the learning process you are ready to take the posttest to determine the extent to which you have achieved the objectives of this module. Return to the pretest and take it over again as the posttest. Correct your answers using the answer key that is found on pp. 410-411 of this module. You need to obtain 24 correct points to have achieved mastery at the 95% level. If your score is less than 24 points, correct your errors, and study the content of this module over again more carefully, and read some of the articles in the recommended reading list. You need to study in this fashion until you achieve the 95% mastery level on the posttest.

ANSWER KEY TO PRETEST AND POSTTEST

1. b (Cronbach, 1967, pp. 23-39)
2. a, c, and d (Dolan, Price, and Sawden, 1965, p. 97)
3. a (Gagne, 1970, pp. 97, 108, 128-129, 141, 166, 180, 200, 223)
4. b (Skinner, 1953, p. 240)
5. b (Franks, 1966, p. 158)

6. c (Gagne, 1970, pp. 97, 108, 128, 141, 166, 180, 200, 223)
7. c (Jensen, 1967, p. 121)
8. b (Jensen, 1967, p. 122)
9. a (Gagne, 1970, p. 141)
10. a, c, and d (Bloom, 1968)
11. b (Gagne, 1970, p. 223)
12. (1) a, c, d, and g
    (2) b, e, f, and h
    (Cronbach, 1967, pp. 34-37)
13. b (Cronbach, 1967, pp. 34-37)
14. c (Cronbach, 1967, pp. 34-37)
15. Answers should include the following steps:
    a. Identify the objective
    b. Determine what type of learning it is
    c. Determine the internal conditions for the specific task
    d. Assess the student's entering behavior
    e. Assess the student's biopsychosociocultural background
    f. Determine the method of instruction best suited for that specific student
    g. Implement the plan
    h. Evaluate the instruction
    (Gagne, 1970, pp. 97-223)

REFERENCES

Aichlmayr, R. H. Creative nursing: a need to develop the creative student. *Journal of Nursing Education,* 1969, 8(4):19-26.

Atkinson, J. W., and O'Connor, P. Effects of ability grouping in schools related to individual differences in achievement related motivation. Final Report, Office of Education, Cooperative Research Program, Project No. 1283, University of Michigan, 1963. (Available in microfilm from Photoduplication Center, Library of Congress, Washington, D.C.)

Atkinson, J. W., and Reitman, W. Performance as a function of motive strength and expectancy of goal attainment. *Journal of Abnormal Social Psychology,* 1956, 53:361-366.

Beyers, M., Dickelmann, N., and Thompson, M. Developing a modular curriculum. *Nursing Outlook,* 20(10):643-647.

Bloom, B. S. Learning for mastery. *Evaluation Comment,* 1968, 1(2):1-12.

Bloom, B. S., Davis, A., and Hess, R. *Compensatory education for cultural deprivation,* New York: Holt, Rinehart and Winston, Inc., 1965.

Carroll, J. A model for school learning. *Teachers College Record,* 1963, 64:723-733.

Carroll, J. Instructional methods and individual differences: discussion of Dr. Cronbach's paper. In R. M. Gagne (Ed.), *Learning and individual differences.* Columbus, Ohio: Charles E. Merrill Publishing Co., 1967, pp. 40-44.

Corman, B. R. The effect of varying amounts and kinds of information as guidance in problem solving. *Psychological Monographs,* 1957, 71(2):(whole no. 431).

Cronbach, L. J. Processes affecting scores on 'understanding of others', and 'assumed similarity.' *Psychological Bulletin,* 1955, 52:177:194.

Cronbach, L. J. How can instruction be adapted to individual differences? In R. M. Gagne *Learning and individual differences.* Columbus, Ohio: Charles E. Merrill Publishing Co. 1967, pp. 23-39.

Cronbach, L. J., and Glaser, G. C. *Psychological tests and personnel decisions.* (2nd Ed.) Urbana, Ill.: University of Illinois Press, 1965.

Cutts, N., and Mosely, N. *Providing for individual differences in the elementary school.* Englewood Cliffs, N.J.: Prentice-Hall, Inc., 1960.

DeCecco, J. P. *Human learning in the school.* Chicago: Holt, Rinehart and Winston, Inc., 1963.

Deese, J. From the isolated verbal unit to connected discourse. In C. N. Cofer (Ed.), *Verbal learning and verbal behavior.* New York: McGraw-Hill Book Co., 1961.

de Tornyay, R. *Strategies for teaching nursing.* New York: John Wiley & Sons, Inc., 1971.

Dolan, D., Price, W., and Sowden, J. Human diagnosis of an individualized program. Presented at the 4th Annual Conference on Grouping and Individualized Instruction, Fountain Valley, Calif., 1965.

Duncan, C. P. Recent research on human problem solving. *Psychological Bulletin,* 1959, 56:397-429.

Eigen, L. D., and Feldhusen, J. Interrelationships among attitude, achievement, reading, intelligence, and transfer variables in programmed instruction. In J. P. DeCecco (Ed.), *Educational technology.* New York: Holt, Rinehart and Winston, Inc., 1964, pp. 376-386.

Ellis, H. *The transfer of learning.* New York: The Macmillan Co., 1965.

Eysenck, H. J. *The dynamics of anxiety and hysteria.* London: Routledge, 1957.

Feather, N. The relationship of persistence at a task to expectations of success and achievement related motives. *Journal of Abnormal Social Psychology,* 1961, 63:552-561.

Franks, C. Individual differences in conditioning and associated techniques. In Wolpe J. (Ed.), *The conditioning therapies.* Holt, Rinehart and Winston, Inc., 1966.

Gagne, R. M. Ability differences in the learning of concepts governing directed numbers. In *Research problems in mathematics education,* Cooperative Research Monographs, No. 3, 1960, pp. 112-113.

Gagne, R. M. The acquisition of knowledge. *Psychological Review,* 1962, **4:**355-365.

Gagne, R. M. (Ed.) *Learning and individual differences.* A Symposium of the Learning Research and Development Center, University of Pittsburgh. Columbus, Ohio: Charles E. Merrill Publishing Co., 1967.

Gagne, R. M. *The conditions of learning.* (2nd Ed.) Holt, Rinehart and Winston, Inc., 1970.

Gaier, E. L. The relationship between selected personality variables and the thinking of students in discussion classes. *Scholastic Review,* 1952, **40:**404-411.

Getzels, J. W., and Jackson, P. W. *Creativity and intelligence.* New York: John Wiley & Sons, Inc., 1962.

Gilliland, A. R., and Clark, E. L. *Psychology of individual differences.* New York: Prentice-Hall, Inc., 1939, 15-21.

Goodlad, J. Human variability demands alternatives. Presented at the 4th Annual Conference on Grouping and Individualized Instruction, Fountain Valley, Calif., 1965.

Guilford, J. P. Creativity. *American Psychologist,* 1950, **5:**444-454.

Hilgard, E. R., Edgrin, R. D., and Irvine, R. P. Errors in transfer following learning with understanding: further studies with Katona's cardstack experiments. Journal of Experimental Psychology, 1954, **47:**457-467.

Jensen, A. R. Reinforcement psychology and individual differences. *California Journal of Educational Research,* 1962, **4:**174-178.

Jensen, A. R. Varieties of individual differences in learning. In R. M. Gagne (Ed.), *Learning and individual differences.* Columbus, Ohio: Charles E. Merrill Publishing Co., 1967, pp. 117-135.

Kogan N., and Wallach, M. *Risk taking.* New York: Holt, Rinehart and Winston, Inc., 1964.

Koyanagi, K. An experimental study on relations between the intellectual cognition and the intellectual activity in children. *Tohoku Psychological Follow,* 1953, **13:**100-113.

Mandler, G., and Aarason, S. B. A study of anxiety and learning. *Journal of Abnormal Social Psychology,* 1952, **47:**166-173.

Miller, N. E., and Dollard, J. *Social learning and imitation.* New Haven, Conn.: Yale University Press, 1941.

Noble, C. E. Meaningfulness and familiarity. In C. N. Cofer and B. S. Musgrave (Eds.), *Verbal behavior and learning.* New York: McGraw-Hill Book Co., 1963.

Osler, S. F., and Fivel, M. W. Concept attainment: I. The role of age and intelligence in concept attainment by induction. *Journal of Experimental Psychology,* 1961, **62**(1): 1-7.

Osler, S. F., and Trautman, G. E. Concept attainment: II. Effect of stimulus complexity upon concept attainment. *Journal of Experimental Psychology,* 1961, **62**(1):9-13.

Read, M. *Culture, health, and disease.* Philadelphia: J. B. Lippincott Co., 1966.

Saugtad, P. An analysis of Maier's pendulum problem. *Journal of Experimental Psychology,* 1957, **54:**168-179.

Schramm, W. *Four case studies of programmed instruction.* New York: Fund for the Achievement of education, 1964.

Skinner, B. F. *Science and human behavior.* New York: The Macmillan Co., 1953.

Skinner, B. F. *The technology of teaching.* New York: Appleton-Century-Crofts, 1968.

Spence, K. W. Anxiety (drive) level on performance in eyelid conditioning. *Psychology Bulletin,* 1964, **61:**129-139.

Stolurow, L. M. Social impact of programmed instruction: aptitudes and abilities revisited. In J. P. DeCecco (Ed.), *Educational technology.* New York: Holt, Rinehart and Winston, Inc., 1964, pp. 348-355.

Taylor, J. A. The relationship of anxiety to the conditioned eyelid response. *Journal of Experimental Psychology,* 1951, **41:**81-92.

Van der Geer, J. P. *A psychological study of problem solving.* Haarlen: Uitgeverij De Toorts, 1957.

Zeaman, D., and House, B. J. The relation of I.Q. and learning. In R. M. Gagne (Ed.), *Learning and individual differences.* Columbus, Ohio: Charles E. Merrill Publishing Co., 1967, pp. 192-212.

MODULE 26

Environmental variables

DESCRIPTION OF THE MODULE

This is an independent unit of instruction on the effects of environmental variables on learning and instruction. The main text of the module covers five major areas: (1) theoretical framework, (2) research studies, (3) issues, (4) application to nursing education and practice, and (5) researchable questions. These five areas are presented in an integrated form. In addition to the main text, the module contains student objectives, instructions to the learner, a pre- and posttest, an answer key, and additional learning experiences in the form of a recommended reading list.

Full understanding of the contents of this module is dependent on the student's entering behavior, which should include knowledge of: (1) Gagne's (1970) conditions of learning, (2) models of instruction, and (3) behavior-modification techniques.

MODULE OBJECTIVES

On completion of this module and having studied the recommended reading list, the learner will be able to accomplish the following objectives at the 95% level of achievement:

1. Describe the theoretical framework (concepts, principles, and different authors' views) of environmental variables as they influence learning and instruction

2. Cite research studies that demonstrate the effect of environmental variables on learning and instruction
3. Identify one issue relevant to environmental variables
4. Apply the principles and concepts of environmental variables to nursing education and practice
5. Raise one researchable question and identify the independent and dependent variables

PRETEST AND POSTTEST

Circle the correct answers. Each question is worth 1 point except the last three questions, which are worth 10 points each. The 95% level of mastery for this test is 42 points. Take the test and correct your answers using the answer key found at the end of this module (pp. 430-431). If your score is 42 points or better, you may proceed to the next module.

Multiple choice

1. The effects of sensory deprivation on a child result in:
   a. the child overreacting to learning, that is, learning much quicker at a later date as compared to an ordinary student
   b. possible irreparable cumulative deficit in ability to learn
   c. no difference in the ability to learn between children experiencing and those not experiencing sensory deprivation

2. An unwed mother has identical twins. She has decided not to keep the children, but wants some direction as to a choice of alternatives. She has a close friend who lives in a backward mountain town in the South with an illiterate husband who wants to care for the babies. She also knows a family in a larger southern city who are both school teachers, who also want to care for the babies. An effective way a nurse can counsel this unwed mother would be to
   1—discuss moral responsibility
   2—discuss issues of wed and unwed mothers
   3—point out the effects of environment on child-rearing techniques
   4—explain the effects of initial stimulus deprivation on a child's cognitive growth and development
   5—convince the mother that it is better for her to keep the babies
   a. 1, 3, and 5
   b. all of the above
   c. 4 and 5
   d. 3 and 4

3. The period when deprivation is the most serious is:
   a. the first 4 years of life
   b. from 8 to 17 years of age
   c. from 6 to 13 years of age

4. Environmental variables that affect learning are those factors that:
   a. deal with the mutual interaction between the organism and the environment
   b. are only physical in nature
   c. are physical, social, disciplinary, and type of management
   d. deal mostly with heat, noise, and seating arrangements

5. Sensory deprivation refers to the situation where:
   a. the person is blind
   b. there is an insufficient amount of or reduction in stimulation to one or more sensory modalities from the environment
   c. the child is not provided with play books
   d. the person does not talk to others for long periods of time

6. According to Coleman and Provence (1957), the syndrome of "hospitalism" refers to:

a. the situation where the child is hospitalized without the mother being present
b. the situation where the hospitalized infant experiences environmental retardation from insufficient stimulation
c. fear of hospital equipment and personnel
d. mental retardation resulting from isolation

7. According to Jensen (1966, 1968), what proportion, or percent of growth of intelligence is attributed to the role of the environment?
   a. 80%
   b. 50%
   c. 20%
   d. 10%

8. The areas in which environmental variables influence learning and instruction are:
   a. the ability to discriminate and generalize
   b. perception, language, and cognitive development
   c. ease of conditioning
   d. skill learning

9. According to Gagne (1970), the physical environmental variables that affect learning are:
   a. the immediate physical environment of the learner
   b. objects within the environment and the modes of instruction
   c. heat, light, and humidity
   d. the number of pupils in the classroom

10. The aspect of the learning environment that deals with the particular arrangements of the communication media that is manipulated to interact with the student is referred to as:
    a. instructional media
    b. modes of instruction
    c. organization of media
    d. audiovisual media

11. The components that are aspects of the psychosocial environment that affects learning and instruction are:
    1—affective relationships among students and teachers
    2—the teacher
    3—student-to-student relationships
    4—discipline, class management, and mental hygiene
    5—the instructional media
    6—the number of homework problems assigned to students

a. 1, 2, 5, and 6
b. 1, 2, 3, and 4
c. 1, 3, 4, 5, and 6
d. all of the above

Listing

12. Identify five examples of instructional media:
    a. _____
    b. _____
    c. _____
    d. _____
    e. _____
13. Identify five examples of instructional modes:
    a. _____
    b. _____
    c. _____
    d. _____
    e. _____

Discussion questions

14. Identify one issue in the area of environmental variables that affects learning and instruction.
15. What effect does sensory deprivation have on a child's cognitive, perceptual, lingual, and affective development?
16. What should the role of the nurse be with regard to the prevention and treatment of sensory deprivation of the child during the first years of life?
17. Select a specific-patient or student-learning situation and determine how you would take into consideration the various environmental variables

TEXT
Theoretical framework

Environmental variables are those variables dealing with the mutual relationship and interaction between an organism and its physical environment. Education seeks to communicate knowledge in several ways, and among them, theorists have stressed human cognitive and perceptual abilities, perhaps to the exclusion of a most important external variable, the environment. The influence that the environment exercises over learning can be evaluated on two levels. First, the individual's early environment bears a relationship on the development of genetic potential, influencing perception, language development, and cognitive development. Secondly, the immediate environment of any learning situation influences attention, motivation, perception, and efficiency. Recognizing the significance of such nonmanipulatable variables as age, maturational level, genetic constitution, and sensory functionality, it is the purpose of this module to explore the influence of the environmental variables on learning and instruction.

Effect of early environment on learning

The majority of individuals begin life equipped with five central sense organs and a kinesthetic awareness. The function of these are to recognize, explain, and interpret the surrounding environment. Thereafter, genetic equality is shaped and molded by the environmental complex that the individual experiences. Through the course of his research, Bloom has demonstrated that half of the development of a child's intelligence occurs within the first 4 years of life, and that one-third of the child's potential for school achievement is determined before entering school (DeCecco, 1968, p. 213). Clearly, then, the effect of early environmental variables directs the course of the child's ability to learn.

Sensory deprivation is an insufficiency or a reduction in stimulation to one or more sensory modalities from environmental resources. This deprivation can assume many forms, however, and its effects on learning operate in one of the following three ways. (1) Perceptual monotony is a decrease in, or a lack of, variability of stimulation, and is frequently the effect one sees demonstrated in institutionalized people.

(2) Perceptual deprivation can take on two

forms: a lack of meaningfulness of congruent information in the environment (richness, novelty) or (3) a lack of patterning in the environment, which lends order, continuity, and predictability to cues. Such an environment, "which lacks optimal stimulation and a variety of new and interesting things and events to see, to hear, and to talk about" will produce a cumulative deficit in a deprived child and irreparably damage the ability to learn (DeCecco, 1968, p. 214). Coleman and Provence (1957) described a syndrome of "hospitalism" in a set of noninstitutionalized infants who experienced environmental retardation from insufficient stimulation (Coleman and Provence, 1957, pp. 285-292). Goldfarb described in detail the effects of institutional privation in infancy on later learning abilities and found evidence verifying that "inferior intellectual performance is characteristic of the institution children at all ages studied," that they demonstrated an "unusually defective level of conceptualization," and that "all learning based on insight or the sizing up of a situation was difficult" (Goldfarb, 1945, p. 247-294). His conclusion was that "institution children show a primary thinking defect characterized particularly by extremely limited capacity for abstract performance" (Goldfarb, 1945, p. 254). A third study compared the environments of institutionalized, lower-class home, and middle-class home children and attributes the differences between the three types in developmental abilities to the results of the range and variety of environmental stimuli that they were exposed to and allowed to explore and manipulate either alone or with others (Collard, 1971, pp. 1003-1015).

Jensen (1966, 1968) hypothesized a model for the growth of intelligence that attributes 80% of intelligence to genetic endowment and 20% to the environment, yet the scope of that 20% can equate to 20 to 30 IQ points, depending on the level of enrichment in the environment. He stated more specifically:

But even this difference of twenty or thirty IQ points that can be effected through the environment can mean the difference between functional illiteracy, between educational attainments equivalent to less than an eighth grade education and college education, between an unskilled job and a skilled job, between employment and gainful occupation, and in some cases it can even mean the difference between the designation "mentally retarded" and "normal" (DeCecco, 1968, p. 210).

In Jensen's theoretical model (1968), perceptual learning and a class of future learning comprise the two types of elements in the environment. Perceptual learning represents specialized achievement knowledge, while the future learning is a cumulative type of knowledge that builds on previous levels of knowledge. Jensen's model illustrates "how an impoverished environment may retard intellectual development and eventually produce cumulative deficits" (DeCecco, 1968, p. 211).

Furthermore, some of the adverse effects of an impoverished environment are irreversible, because the organism's plasticity decreases with age (DeCecco, 1968, p. 209). This is why the importance of early home environment, nursery school, and kindergarten should be emphasized. Head Start programs were created to fulfill this need and provide an enriched environment to children of disadvantaged families. These programs have been successful in attempting to overcome some of the handicaps of early deprivation. In the education of the disadvantaged child, environment plays a vital role. Three areas in which environmental variables influence learning and instruction are perception, language development, and cognitive development.

People constantly use visual and auditory senses to learn. We are exposed to many objects and sounds to which we respond. Through perception, we learn to distinguish different characteristics of various objects and people so that we can recognize their individuality. The disadvantaged child is sometimes deprived of an enriched environment; therefore, perceptual learning is hampered. Perception and gaining the attention of a child are closely aligned. Gagne (1970, pp. 280-281) stated:

The child needs to learn to notice many aspects of his environment. As an attentional set, this capacity expands upon simpler observations by encompassing attention to a number of properties of the environment at once and perhaps through multi-sensory channels. Acquiring such behavior may be carried out with reinforcement emphasizing variety and novelty of stimulation as the child is encouraged to make broader and more intensive exploration of his environment.

A classroom that provides the necessary objects and experiences will enhance perceptual learning. A quiet environment in which the child can explore and develop good learning habits is of great help to the disadvantaged child.

Environment also plays a crucial role in language development. In an analysis of the language of a disadvantaged child, Bernstein (1961) distinguished between the restricted code (language of the disadvantaged child) and the elaborated code (language of those of higher socioeconomic status). "The restricted code seriously limits the scope of expression and thought . . . and has far reaching consequences for the disadvantaged child" (Bernstein, 1961, pp. 171, 174). When a disadvantaged child attends school knowing only the restricted code and the teacher uses the elaborated code, the child is seriously handicapped. If this deficit is not overcome at an early age, the loss may be irreversible. Here again, the Head Start program can be of great service to the child.

In discussing the cognitive development of a child, Bruner (1961) stated "that the disadvantaged child lacks both the richness of environment for developing models and strategies of thought and the corrective feedback necessary for their maintenance" (De-

Cecco, 1968, p. 221). In an experiment by John and Goldstein (1964), a study was made of the use of labels as mediators. The performance of black children of high and low socioeconomic status was studied. The results showed that the children from the high socioeconomic background produced the appropriate name or label, while the children from the low socioeconomic background were involved in the nonessential details. There are other studies that also support the contention that those children deprived of an enriched environment perform poorly. John and Goldstein (1964) suggested there are two reasons for this: "Low SES homes do not provide the stable conditions which keep object and name properly tied together and the low SES child is given little or no correction when he misapplies a label to an object" (DeCecco, 1968, p. 220).

Effect of immediate environment on learning

The immediate environment for learning can be viewed as having these components: (1) physical, (2) conceptual (psychosocial), (3) classroom management, and (4) discipline. Different authors categorize environmental variables that affect learning and instruction differently, depending on their research interests and theoretical orientation.

PHYSICAL ENVIRONMENT

Wittrock (1970) looked at the learning environment from the evaluation point of view. He stated that evaluation studies have concentrated on making explicit the physical and human characteristics of the learner's environment. They consider such characteristics as the number of books in the libraries, the school budget per student, hours spent in instruction in the classroom, number of homework problems or assignments made to the students, intellectual qualifications of the teachers, teacher credentials, and others. These, Wittrock (1970, p. 9) stated, "are examples that measure environmental characteristics commonly used by teachers and administrators to index learning." Wittrock criticized such an approach. He stated that evaluation of such environmental characteristics alone are not sufficient to enable one to make objective inferences about their effect on learners. Such an approach to evaluation of instructors is futile. Measures of intellectual and social processes in the learners, which affect the outcome of learning, are needed. In order to evaluate instruction, measures of the interaction between the environment, the learner, and the learning are needed. In making reference to the importance of the instructional environment, Wittrock (1970, p. 9) specifically stated that the primary function of the teacher is:

. . . to provide environments best suited to the learner to enhance his learning and development as an individual. To do this, a teacher obviously must make decisions and inferences about the educational value of environments and their probable effects upon individuals. He needs to characterize and describe those crucial qualities of environment he can manipulate; but he also needs to be able to relate them objectively to individual learners and to change in the behavior of learners.

For Gagne (1970), the physical variables are composed of the objects within the environment and the techniques of the setting that encourage or stimulate learning. He described these modalities as coming within two categories: instructional media and modes of instruction.

Instructional media. Instructional media refers to the different types of components of the learning environment that generate stimulation in the learner. Instructional media consist of the following:

1. *Objects for instruction* may be common things that have been learned because they have been seen during the day. They may be, however, the initial stimuli for instruction of a child. The objects chosen must be selected carefully. If multiple discrimination among various objects of the same series is to be established, then care must be taken to select the samples so that the differential features will be emphasized.

2. *Demonstration* consists of objects displaying an interaction to illustrate an event or a cause-and-effect sequence.

3. *Human models* are the main factor involved in social learning. Imitation is a prime example where the learner imitates the behaviors of a model (most often parents, teachers, and peers). Gagne pointed out that patterns of interaction with other people, the combined total of which constitute the personality of the person, are learned in situations involving another human being, often an adult.

4. *Oral communication* by the teacher can provide *all* the required instructional functions in many situations, but not in every situation. Oral communication can be used to gain the pupils' attention and stimulate the recall of prerequisite capabilities.

5. *Printed language media* includes such things as books, pamphlets, and leaflets.

6. *Pictures* serve the purpose of displaying the stimulus situation. They can also be used for prompting and identifying cues.

7. *Audiovisual aids* in the form of motion pictures and television add another dimension to still pictures. They can display events and sequences of events rather than just objects. They can extend the range of stimulus situations that can be brought to the classroom. Audiovisual aids also provide external prompting needed to learn chains and procedures. They can inform the learner about the terminal behavior expected, especially when complex motor behavior is to be learned, and can provide feedback to the learner about performance. Such aids are often used in simulated microteaching situations.

8. *Teaching machines* represent a combi-

nation of media rather than a single medium. A typical teaching machine contains printed material with still pictures, as in programmed instruction. Gagne pointed out that self-instructional programs attempt faster transfer of knowledge.

Several studies have been done to determine which media to use for which instructional purpose. The studies of Campeau (1967), Lumsdaine and May (1965), and Briggs and associates (1967) have concluded that no single medium has the properties that make it best for all purposes, most instructional functions can be performed by most media, and media generally have not been found to be differentially effective for different learners.

In designing instruction with media, Gagne (1970) has suggested a sequential stage-by-stage approach:

1. To answer the question, "Which media are to be selected for a learning task?" Gagne suggested that one ought to look at the properly defined set of objectives. They ought to provide information about the nature of stimuli to which the learner is expected to respond after learning the task. Such stimuli are the ones that are inherent to the learning task. For example, if the objective states that a student demonstrate how to bathe a baby, then the medium for instruction might include the actual objects (an actual baby in a home or hospital setting and all the bathing equipment, or a doll baby in a simulated laboratory setting with all the bathing equipment). A motion picture demonstrating bathing of a baby would be appropriate also.

2. Stage two of the designing includes the following: having determined which medium is the most appropriate for the task to be learned, one can proceed to check the characteristics various media may have in performing other instructional functions. For example, if prompting is necessary in this specific baby-bathing situation, oral communication by the teacher can help prompt the student or enable the student to recall the previously learned capability.

3. The third stage deals with synthesizing, or integrating, the chosen media into a reasonable instructional sequence. Good media decisions are made by matching instructional functions to media, followed by cost-conscious synthesis into a total instructional sequence. In designing instruction using media, the teacher first needs to decide "what media can best be used for the various events of an instructional sequence and then proceed to make practical decisions about what medium or combination of media to employ—whether this turns out to be a motion picture, a tape recorder, or a laboratory demonstration" (Gagne, 1970, p. 367).

Mode of instruction. Mode of instruction refers to the particular arrangements the various communication media may have in relation to the learner. It is the learning environment that is manipulated to interact with the student. Modes of instruction include the following:

1. *Tutoring sessions* entail one-to-one interaction between the student and the teacher, where most of the work or the learning and reading is to be done by the student. The teacher's role is:

   a. To guide the student's thinking by answering questions

   b. To assess the student's performance in terms of determining what the student has learned from the readings

   c. To provide feedback to the student based on assessment

   d. To recommend direction for further learning.

2. The *lecture method* is the traditional method of instruction, where the teacher can attempt to stimulate achievement, relate expected outcomes of learning, and provide prompting and guidance to learning.

3. *Recitation* is a mode of instruction de-

voted to assessment and feedback of the material learned by the student.

4. *Discussion* creates the opportunity to explore new ideas, analogies, similarities, and differences among various branches of knowledge and general hypotheses with the students. In order for a discussion session to be successful, the participants must have a certain minimum amount of prerequisite knowledge.

5. The *laboratory* is an instructional mode where the main aim is to present a stimulus situation that brings the student into contact with actual objects and events. It is most useful in science courses and other courses where other types of skills (cognitive and motor) are to be learned. It is also useful where experimentation and testing of hypotheses needs to take place.

6. *Homework* is utilized to practice the new material to be learned. It can take the form of self-instruction on a prescribed topic, writing a term paper, practice of a variety of examples, or others.

All these modes of instruction are organizations of media to accomplish specific instructional purposes. Other educators have discussed these various techniques within the framework of educational technology (De-Cecco, 1968; Sielber, 1972).

Up until the twentieth century, teachers relied on the traditional methods of instruction, but with the advances in business and industry, innovations have taken place within the school environment to augment the learning process. DeCecco cited two definitions: one is the detailed application of the psychology of learning to practical teaching problems, termed software; and the other applies to the engineering principles in the development of electromechanical equipment, or hardware. He believes that both areas are connected by the stimulus elicited from the material and by the mode of presentation.

DeCecco stated that the instructional procedures and materials utilized should provide the best performance in terms of achievement, money, and time. Also, in deciding the appropriate method, the availability of the instrument, the analysis and design of the instructional systems, and the research on the effectiveness of the media should be included before employment within the learning set. By observing behavior in students before and after use, one should be able to ascertain the practicality of the innovation.

This evolves into the means of communication introduced by the stimulus of the new technique. Gagne formulated nine components of instruction that should result. They are: gaining and controlling attention; providing a model for expected learning outcomes; stimulating recall of prerequisite capabilities; presenting the stimuli for learning; offering guidance for learning; appraising learned performances; providing feedback; transferring learned concepts and rules; employing means for ensuring retention.

Different devices will fulfill the characteristics expected in a variety of ways, and it is up to the judgment and creativity of the teacher to recognize which combination of media will synthesize the desired learned behavior.

The actual physical setting where students gather to learn is also very important. Such things as lighting, temperature, seating arrangements, and presence of irrelevant stimuli (such as distracting pictures) all affect learning.

CONCEPTUAL/PSYCHOSOCIAL ENVIRONMENT

The term conceptual environment was coined by Arndt and Huckabay (1975). It refers to the abstract, cognitive component of a milieu that deals with the human element. It fosters thinking and effective relationships among people. It is that aspect of abstract environment that deals with people's feelings, attitudes, spirits, emotions, and psychosocial needs. Arndt and Huckabay also pointed out that in the conceptual environment, the individual seeks satisfaction, achievement, and responsibility—the attainment of which fosters growth, stability, and interaction. The means by which the individual achieves these aims are through cooperation, integration and communication, and commitment and reward.

Furthermore, human relations help make up the social environment and play a vital part in learning and instruction. The idea of human relations implies an extremely complex process of human interplay of one personality with another. Because this human process affects learning and instruction, it is the role of the teacher to maintain control of the social environment (Heidgerken, 1965).

A matter of great concern to the teacher who wishes to increase teaching effectiveness is the group climate, or group atmosphere (sometimes referred to as emotional climate), which should be positive and conducive to learning because it will have greater influence on the amount and type of learning that takes place. Shaffer, Indorato, and Deneselya (1972, p. 37) defined a positive classroom climate as "one in which the students and teacher interact freely to discuss appropriate educational material." They also defined the negative classroom climate as one in which "there is minimal classroom interaction and in which teacher and students do not interact; there is only lecturing and occasional negative reinforcement." Educators agree that an effective learning climate reflects the respect that the teacher has for the individuality of the students, posits a warm working relationship between the teacher and the group being taught, enables the students to see the group experience as contributing to or maintaining a sense of personal worth and importance, and contributes to healthy per-

sonal and social as well as intellectual development (Heidgerken, 1965). Carl Rogers supported the theory that in order to accomplish the aims of the learning process, it is necessary to have the acceptable group climate.

Variables affecting the group climate of the classroom are: (1) the teacher, (2) the student-teacher relationship, (3) student-student relationships, and (4) discipline and mental hygiene as they affect the emotions in the classroom. These variables are discussed under these headings.

The teacher. Palmer (1908) referred to the touch of the teacher as being formative. McKenney (1910) stated " . . . We may rightly measure our education not by the number of years we have spent in school, but by the number of stimulating, suggestive, and inspiring teachers it has been our good fortune to have known." Spaulding (1971) wrote " . . . the teacher is the school; what the soul is to the body, what the mind is to man, that the teacher is to the school." Many writers believe that the teacher and the teacher's relationship with the students is the most important variable in the learning and instruction process. Personality has been described by one author as the result of all the traits possessed by one individual. Personal traits of the teacher, as recognized through many studies, that are known to bring about social environments conducive to effective learning are: personal goodness, love, cheerfulness and a sense of humor, sympathy, enthusiasm, confidence, justice, neat personal appearance, and knowledge. Bernard (1972, p. 5) stated that "experience attests to the fact that such problems as motivation, discipline, social behavior, pupil achievement, and above all, the continuing desire to learn, all center around the personality of the teacher." McClelland, in a study in 1971 on the importance of teacher personality and environment, wrote, "We really do not know how great human potential is until consistent effort is made to develop it" (Bernard, 1972, p. 266). Flanders conducted a study in 1965 of the effect of teacher behavior on pupil behavior and achievement and found superiority in many ways for what he called "indirect" behaviors of teachers. *Indirect influence* means that the teachers accept pupils' feelings, praise them, use pupil's ideas, and ask them questions. These students made better achievement scores, produced higher levels of critical thinking, and gave more active manifestations of curiosity than did pupils of direct teachers. *Direct influence* consists of lecturing, giving directions, and criticizing. Direct teachers, more frequently than indirect ones, have confused and apathetic pupils (Bernard, 1972, p. 8). Bernard also noted that pupil behavior reflects teacher behavior in many ways. He commented (p. 8), "Acting like the teacher is not simply a matter of modeling oneself after an idol, it is also a matter of identifying with the teacher. Rejection is illustrated in the pupils' determination never to be a teacher."

Heidgerken viewed the function of the teacher as arranging the environment, as much as possible, so that the extent of the field of stimuli filters out the irrelevant through the use of different media and teacher instructions. Surely, as teachers fulfill their role and function, they will arrive at a goal described by Jerome S. Bruner (1965, p. 17); "The first object of any act of learning, over and beyond the pleasure it may give, is that it should serve us in the future. Learning should not only take us somewhere, it should allow us later to go further more easily."

Teacher-student relationships. The group climate should consist of a combination of properties that will produce a group mood of interdependence, where members will communicate easily and well. Groups can develop hostility and passivity, which inhibit learning; or they can develop cooperation,

flexibility, and creativity, which enhance learning. Group climate can either help or hinder the building of relationships between the teacher and the students and among the students in the group.

Classroom management. Heidgerken (1953, p. 163) stated that "a vital and positive force in successful teaching is successful classroom management." Reference was made to working conditions, both teaching and learning, in that only when such conditions are favorable can the routine procedures and activities be carried on economically and efficiently. Poor management on the part of the teacher can cause wasted time in a classroom, and again the effective way for students to learn the value of time is by the teacher's example. Heidgerkin's (1953, p. 164) attitude on this subject is expressed thusly: "The teacher can transmit no greater heritage to her students than a wholesome appreciation of the value of time." Efficient classroom management can provide a living pattern for the students to follow.

Other variables in efficient classroom management involve good methods of instruction, a desirability that the routine leave the students and teachers free for the major activities of the class period, promptness, good methods of distribution of instructional materials, and classroom courtesy.

Discipline. Social regulations are designed to make it possible for people to live together harmoniously and, in contemporary society, to enhance the living conditions of individuals. This basic social phenomenon can also be applied to the classroom—to enhance learning and instruction. William Glasser, in his book *Schools Without Failure* (1969), spoke of reasonable rules as being a part of a thoughtful, problem-solving education and noted that a school cannot function without an effective administration that develops reasonable rules and enforces them. Discipline in the classroom is a way in which social interaction may be facilitated or retarded by teacher activities. The teacher is responsible for establishing the framework within which the society of the classroom functions. The teacher protects the rights of each of the students and at the same time helps them grow in ability to assume responsibility for their own actions. The rules appropriate to a classroom are the rules of normal civilized behavior of individuals in a social setting. They involve courtesy and a consideration for others (Biehler, 1971). The aims of discipline, according to Heidgerken (1953, p. 180) are: "(1) the creation and maintenance of a wholesome atmosphere for learning and (2) the development and stimulation of the right motives and appreciations, as well as proper habits for student conduct." Teacher qualities that contribute to maintenance of good discipline are: (1) using proper methods of teaching, (2) recognizing individual differences, (3) having a pleasant personality, and (4) having a good attitude toward the students.

Mental hygiene. Mental health and discipline are not synonymous, but they are intimately related. Both are central focuses in day-to-day classroom procedures. Both call for ego strength and an ever-shifting balance between freedom and responsibility. Bernard believes that for the classroom teacher, mental health involves being the kind of person and using the kinds of approaches that will help pupils realize a greater amount of their potential for well-rounded and constant growth and efficient living. Mental helath is a particular way of looking at classroom control. It involves the teacher's attitude toward the task and the pupils, use of methods, choice of objectives, use of materials, and the teacher's influence on the personality development of the pupils (Bernard, 1972).

Relevant research studies

To promote maximum attention and retention of learning, an instructor must assume as much control of exteroceptive stimuli as is possible. In three sequential studies done by Vernon and Hoffman (1956), Vernon and McGill (1957), and Arnhoff and Leon (1962), the effects of sensory deprivation on the learning rate in human beings was tested, and it was initially found that experience improved the learning rate. Later studies failed to support this data on a significant level of analysis; however, the test situations were slightly altered, and a considerable amount of data has been accumulated that demonstrates marked changes in perceptual and cognitive functioning during periods of sensory deprivation. Grissom, Sudefelt, and Vernon (1962, p. 430) analyzed the effects of sensory deprivation on memory retention and found that "sensory deprivation as the intervening experience in a retroaction design facilitates retention of verbal material."

The effect of media on the students' perception has been studied by Nengen (1970). Since the influx of instructional media relies on adequate visual interpretation, Nengen (1970) was emphasizing the necessity of uncovering how pictures are read and how they are structured to achieve meanings. In his study with school-age children. Nengen demonstrated the multiplicity of responses to one still picture that depicted an action scene. He postulated that if individuals translate different meanings from pictures, how can the teacher hope that pupils will derive the correct information from a collection of printed matter. Other educators lend their support to Nengen's theory and concur that not enough data is known about how people respond to visual aides (Gropper, 1963). Also, what are the basic elements involved in learning from pictures, and how is visual literacy in learners developed? Another view is that illustrations are usually interpreted according to the viewer's past experience, age, intelligence, and educational level (Spaulding, 1971). Since our culture is mainly heterogeneous, even within the elementary school, it seems inevitable that there are discrepancies in how different children react to the same stimuli. The researcher believes a sensitivity to these problems of deriving meanings from nonverbal communication must be investigated further.

Current research in nursing is investigating the learning climate in multiple ways: for classroom education of the baccalaureate student and for education of the patients by nurses.

Research (Rubin, Allan, and Leak, 1971) was done in the bachelor of science degree program at the University of California (San Francisco) to determine attributes of a learning climate in seminars for nursing students. Researchers could identify students with high grade point averages by their highly verbal and creative behaviors and their immediate grasp of leadership in the seminar. Students with low grade point averages took longer to express ideas and were generally quiet. Some recommendations from this study were that quieter members of the high group be transferred to the low group to quietly stimulate interest and discussion. Researchable questions could be raised to find out:

1. Do students with a low grade point average (or nonverbal students) merely need more episodes of seminar experience to attain mastery of the communication techniques required?

2. Given motivation in discussion of patient problems (as this seminar group did) and more exposure to the seminar, would the low students participate more fully?

3. What makes homogeneity; can students be separated by areas of greatest interest rather than grade point average to enable a low student who has great interest in rehabilitation, for example, to contribute motivation and enthusiasm in a heterogeneous group?

The long-known difficulty of educating a cardiac patient or a post-operative patient (recuperating from extensive surgery) in an intensive care unit has been given a new focus in terms of environment. The impersonal or even hostile environment found by Taylor (1971) to exist in many intensive care units produces the intensive care syndrome: apathy, loss of judgment and concentration, progressing to psychotic signs and symptoms. This apathy and loss of judgment from the alien environment preclude any successful health teaching until the environment is manipulated. The author suggested improved design to keep machines out of sight and hearing of the patient, varying the continuous illumination to resemble night and day, and allowing the patient to have a certain amount of continuity from home through presence of personal belongings.

Carl Rogers (1969) found that pupils' viewpoint of a good teacher consisted of those teachers who are democratic, cooperative, kindly, patient, fair, consistent, open-minded, helpful, and companionable. Pupils' preferences are for teachers who have: a sense of humor, varied interests, knowledge of subject matter, flexibility, and an interest in pupils. Pupils prefer to avoid teachers who are sarcastic and nagging (Bernard, 1972, p. 13).

Allport's study (1969) dealt with the influences of teachers on pupils. Subjects consisted of 100 successful pupils and 4632 teachers. Results showed that 8% had strong influence on pupils, 15% had a well-remembered but not strong influence, and 77% were remembered vaguely if at all (Bernard, 1972, p. 7).

Clements (1968) studied the teacher's influence on pupil self-concept. Results showed that more important than grade-equivalent index is the pupils' belief in their own worth and capability. Teachers do influence that concept, and that self-concept should be a focal concern for the really professional teacher (Bernard, 1972, p. 7).

Cronbach (1963) studied teacher personality patterns and identified them as impersonal or supportive. Impersonal teachers may like their pupils, but see themselves as work directors and the classroom as a work laboratory, not a place for social interaction. Frequently, this atmosphere degenerates into a critical attitude and conflict between teachers and pupils, who do not understand each other. Supportive teachers, on the other hand, are interested in children and frequently have a need for loyalty, affection, and trust, often giving children more help than is needed. They like the students to lean on them, pupils like them, and they may have a strong influence in the development of attitudes. The classroom atmosphere is likely to be cohesive and warm and suited to the child with strong affection needs, but the achievement-oriented child may be less happy (Mouly, 1968, p. 530).

Levine (1970) studied the teacher's acceptance of the student. He concluded that teacher rejection of a student can lead to a dropout. Emphasis is placed on accepting pupil differences and trying to make pupils appreciate their own abilities and worth. Such acceptance is more a matter of what the teacher is than what the teacher does (Bernard, 1972, pp. 8-9).

Maslow (1954) studied children's safety needs as related to discipline. He concluded that an indication of the safety needs is the children's preference for some kind of undisrupted routine or rhythm. They seem to want a predictable, orderly world and seem to thrive better under a system that has at least a skeletal outline of rigidity, in which there is a schedule of a kind, something that can be counted on, not only for the present, but also for the future (Bernard, 1972, pp. 340-341).

Tenenbaum's study (1944) dealt with mental health in relation to the teacher's ability to generate warm pupil-teacher and pupil-pupil relationships based on understandings, mutual acceptance, and respect. The study revealed that 20% of the children disliked their teachers, 28% hoped that when they went to work they would not have a boss like their teacher, and 6% disliked all teachers. The conclusion was that "when a student dislikes school, it is largely because of the teacher" (Mouly, 1968, p. 527).

Jersild and Lazar (1962) performed a study that revealed that lack of friendliness in the classroom was traced to teacher sarcasm and criticism by administrators. Harrison (1970) also traced lack of friendliness to grades, ability grouping, nonpromotion, competition between unequals, imposed discipline, and nonstructure (Bernard, 1972, pp. 352-353).

Ryans' study (1960) found that greater pupil initiative was evident with teachers who tend to be democratic, understanding of pupils, and original, but less responsible and less organized. Docile students tend to be found in the class of the teacher who was more systematical, inflexible, constant and predictable, responsible, and autocratic. His conclusion was that it seems that the more dominant the part played by the teacher, the less responsibility students accepted. Perhaps if teachers want to encourage pupil initiative, they need to refrain from exercising excessive leadership (Mouly, 1968, p. 530).

Heil's study (1960) found that pupil responsibility was lowest under an orderly teacher and highest under a spontaneous teacher. Pupil achievement was found to be a function of the interaction between teacher and pupil personality: the strivers did about as well under all kinds of teachers; conformers did badly under the spontaneous teacher (who was less democratic and supportive); the opposers did best under the firm hand of orderly teachers but badly under the spontaneous and the fearful teacher (Mouly, 1968, p. 530).

Issues in environmental variables

In gathering data in the area of educational technology, it seems that there is a dilemma occurring between two schools of thought (Sielber, and others, 1972). One position suspects the power of a subtle force to reduce human beings to standardized components that can readily be assimilated to whatever system is being served. It absorbs them into her man-machine systems by robbing them of their humanity and making them human machines. This is analogous to a robot, and seems to make the individual devoid of human qualities. Another group counteracts this notion by believing that technology will lead to greater centralization and freedom, making technology malleable to human needs. It is easy to observe the fast pace at which technology is progressing, and one person stated that more study is needed in the philosophical, psychological, and social implications of technology in order to cope with the changes and to facilitate learning (Sielber, 1972). Emphasis should be balanced by realizing the benefits of employing a broad range of resources.

One other issue arising from the media revolution is the change in the role of the teacher. Previously, the instructor was a dictator in the classroom, but now, with industry and technology in the room, the teacher is forced to alter the traditional methods of teaching. The role presently calls for a person who can manipulate the media within the instructional system to assure that each student's learning style is being responded to in a manner that will allow the individual to progress smoothly and rapidly toward the stated objectives (Fruehling, 1972). According to one educator, teachers are required to participate in a new level which, he called a "sensorium"* (Pratte, 1970). He stated that

*Sensorium: the sensing-emotional-intellectual process by which individuals take in perspective and organize new stimuli.

instructors are urged to explore new ways of communication, as well as to understand the attraction of the new media for youth. The instructor needs to enjoy the new sensorium and must be able to help youth intelligently assess the choices they can make for sensory contact.

Application to nursing education and practice

The applications of environmental variables and their relationships to nursing education and practice are numerous. Public health nurses face challenges along these lines almost every day. In visits to homes for whatever reason—be it making a postnatal visit, teaching family planning, or providing nutritional guidance—they may encounter an environment completely foreign to them. The success of these missions to a great degree depends on how well they relate with the families, speaking in terms they understand and guiding them within the framework of their life-styles. If nurses are accepted and understood, they can broaden the horizons of the culturally deprived tremendously. They can instruct parents how to enrich their infant's environment by having colored pictures in the room or on the crib, playing the radio or other music, talking to the child, taking the child places, and labeling objects. For, older children (3 to 4 years old or older) who can watch television, nurses could suggest having them watch the *Sesame Street* program, which is geared to enriching children's vocabulary and environment. Also, if there are schools for Head Start programs in the community, nurses can suggest that parents take younger children there. Of course, the parents have to be educated and informed why and how an enriched environment helps the young child's intellectual, as well as psychosocial, development.

Since learning and teaching are a predominate activity within nursing, both for students and patients, the use of technological paraphernalia is also widely used and accepted. The settings are multisituational; therefore, different instruments and modes of instruction are beneficial and conducive within the nursing field. Past issues of journals illustrate the utilization of various techniques. Instructors and nurses, when introducing new knowledge to the student or patient, can implement teaching aides. These vary from direct demonstration of the use of certain equipment, such as the syringe, sphygmomanometer, catheterization tray, and others, to the use of videotapes, programmed instruction, and study groups to augment the desired learning.

The effect of multimedia has been documented in literature as allowing the students to progress at their own rate without any significant differences in achievement and anxiety between a control and an experimental group (Stein, and others, 1972). Students were shown to develop more positive attitudes toward instructors who placed more emphasis on learning than on evaluation, reducing the pressure of grades. The study provided supportive data for the idea that by the use of various stimuli—visual, auditory, tactile, kinesthetic, and feedback —the student is capable of studying independently, without the traditional teaching methods (Langford, 1972).

One primary expectation of multimedia is the anticipation of instructing a large number of students. The previously mentioned study demonstrated that the approach was not satisfactory in the large group setting. Students were found to require personal contact along with audiovisual materials in order to derive the maximum benefit from the learning process (Mentzer, 1970).

The use of self-instruction frees the teacher to guide students in analyzing, evaluating, and using the information they have obtained, and it allows the students to proceed at their own pace and in their own way (Reed, 1970). As an outcome, a higher level of proficiency and self-confidence was reflected in the students' clinical situations.

Microteaching, utilizing videotapes, has proved to be an effective vehicle for feedback, and the general consensus of the students was there should be more use of television (Beyer, Dickelmann, and Thompson, 1972). In comparing videotapes to live demonstrations, the amount of material learned from the film was significant. Also, it provided uniform content to all students and was conducive to large groups of students (Langhoff, 1972).

The use of media in assessing the patient situation has been practiced in different nursing settings (Curtis and Rother, 1972). These instruments are available, convenient, easy to use, and have the potential of ameliorating the quality of nursing practice by providing increased instructional material and making these materials available to practitioners in the health care settings as well as in the educational environment.

As mentioned previously, the teacher of nursing is concerned with three environmental situations for learning and instruction: the classroom, the laboratory, and the clinical situation. The environmental variables influencing learning and instruction are much the same as those previously stated as being applicable to the age and growth development of the nursing student.

In nursing, the atmosphere for learning and instruction becomes more complex than in ordinary situations, since the instructor is concerned with the three categories of environmental situations that involve more people in different personal interactions. The role of the nursing instructor in classroom management should consist of effective planning and judicious direction. The classrooms of today and tomorrow may well consist of one group looking at slides, another using programmed materials, while still another having a group session, all at the same time, within the confines of one classroom. This will call for careful classroom management to ensure a favorable environment for learning, one that will have some order, yet permit flexible, creative student learning activities. The nursing instructor should be aware of the assets and benefits of proper management of attendance, activities, and movement of students during class, handling of instructional materials and equipment, and improvement of working conditions. For example:

1. *Regulation of physical conditions.* Cool, well-lighted, adequately ventilated classrooms do not distract the students' attention to the environment.

2. *Regulations concerning attendance and seating.* If the class is large, it is helpful to have a set routine to determine attendance and make wise use of time.

3. *Handling of instructional materials and equipment.* All necessary equipment (such as overhead projectors and others) should be ready and in working order. To prevent distraction, each student should have a copy of hand-out materials before the discussion begins.

4. *Improvement of working conditions.* Provide favorable working conditions to facilitate learning and teaching. The primary purposes of routine in the classroom are:

  a. Economy of time and effort

  b. Prevention and decrease of confusion

  c. Teaching of good habits of study and ideals of workmanship.

The nursing instructor and the students constitute a small social system in which persons influence one another as they are drawn together by similar concerns, goals, and values for the purpose of learning and instruction. All groups have certain characteristics in common; the instructional group comes together for the purpose of learning. Control and leadership are vested in the teacher. Informal lines of authority are among the students, but they cannot occur unless delegated or permitted by the teacher, either explicitly or implicitly.

Groups can develop hostility and passivity, which inhibit learning; or they can develop cooperation, flexibility, and creativity, which enhance learning.

Group climate will determine to some degree the standards or norms for participation, for shared problem solving, and for goal setting. In an atmosphere of interdependence, the members will communicate easily and well. The climate will have much to do with whether the organization of the work is efficient for growth and learning by the individuals.

For inservice education, the learning climate must meet the needs of an adult staff to keep up with the young (Ferguson, 1971). The nurse-leader must be motivated to help the staff to catch up, keep up, and stay ahead. In the proper climate, the nursing staff is inspired to augment and transfer knowledge, competencies, and skills into viable forms as they practice.

The *physical structure of a group* can facilitate communication. Leavitt (1951) determined that face-to-face contact facilitates feedback, so circular or around-the-table seating arrangements are more satisfactory than row-by-row seating.

The instructor facilitates communications by setting a friendly environment and by helping students know one another (de Tornyay, 1971). The introductory phase of group process may take several meetings, depending on the size of the group. The role of the teacher is not necessarily to be the group leader, but to assume the needed roles to keep the group goals in sight.

Shaffer, Indorato, and Deneselya (1972) wrote that the method in which nursing education is conducted today provides the nursing instructor with unique opportunities for interacting with students, so there is an increased probability of the instructor having a significant influence on students. The personality of the nursing instructor should include those traits already mentioned as desirable for the effective teacher to establish a good social environment. Among the traits mentioned, love is the particular one considered for the moment, for it influences much success of learning and instruction in nursing. Heidgerken (1965, p. 208) gave an eloquent account of this process as she stated, ". . . to be a good teacher in the fullest sense of the word, the teacher of nursing must be filled with the love of nursing . . . if she does not herself feel this love of nursing, she will not be able to inspire this feeling in her students." Charles McKenney (1910, p. 69) wrote, "A true teacher lives to teach, while others teach to live." Educational aims the instructor may wish to utilize are: (1) creating an active, participant set toward learning; (2) stimulating initiative, creativity and independence of spirit; (3) creating an atmosphere of shared problem solving (Heidgerken, 1965, p. 205). Favorable student-student relationships are necessary to the development and maintenance of a good social environment. Since most nursing classes are made up of adolescents, it is good to look at the psychosocial needs of this age group. Peer-group attitudes transfer readily and are powerful in setting the climate. There is a need for conformity and acceptance, a desire to belong to the group, and a desire to be accepted (Rogers, 1961).

A nursing instructor can utilize this knowledge in acting as a catalytic agent to bring about group "togetherness" with a cooperative and tolerant attitude among members. A variable influencing the behavior of the students is the unique relationship with patients, with hospital personnel, with physicians, and with others in a real-life work situation (Heidgerken, 1965).

Discipline has been considered a variable influencing learning and instruction. This is true for nursing; as expressed in the words of Heidgerken (1965, p. 177):

. . . this applies to nursing where life and death are so vitally affected by good or poor nursing, by the carrying out of certain orders to the letter of the law, there must be rules and regulations to guide young nursing students. However, the teacher of nursing, should seize all other less vital occasions to give the student an opportunity for developing the qualities of independence, self-control, and self-reliance that she may mature into an integrated personality.

William F. Cunningham (1940) called ideal discipline ". . . liberty under the law" and said that the first thing a teacher can do to facilitate this is to understand that discipline can be accomplished on different levels. One of the levels that could pertain to nursing is the social-discipline level, which is centered in the group, as opposed to the individual level. It is the discipline of democracy, that is, self-control exercised by the larger group through common consensus (Heidgerken, 1965, pp. 177-178). Mental hygiene is considered here in relation to the democratic principles as they are applied to nursing. This application begins in the classroom with respect for the individual and belief in the dignity and value of people and is incorporated into our philosophy of nursing (Guinee, 1966, p. 83). Mental hygiene is reflected in the instructor who finds teaching a pleasure, is capable, and promotes emotional growth in students.

Researchable questions

A few topics for further study have been alluded to within the preceeding discussion. In reading the literature, educators are realistic enough to admit that the area of educational technology is still new, and much more substantive data is needed concerning machines and their contribution to learning.

One significant area is the person's attitude towards mechanized learning. It is possible that this may be one factor involved with the group of educational technologists who view technical learning as a threat to humaneness. For individuals who possess an insecure self-concept, the introduction of physical learning devices may act as a hindrance rather than an aide. If pretesting were created to indicate students who would do better with the modified learning, this may circumvent problems and avoid delays in the instructional process.

One other point is the amount of stimulation that instructional media produces within the situation. Everyone has a certain threshold of receiving input; and if the stimuli are out of proportion, learning may be deterred. Knowing the limits of effectiveness is important.

1. What is the effect of a teacher's or nurse's attributes (for example, rushed versus time giving, abrupt versus accepting of conversation, educative versus dictative) on the learning climate? From this study one could identify those attributes that contribute to a warm learning climate.

    a. Independent variables: the nurse's attributes

    b. Dependent variable: the learning climate

2. In inservice education, which kinds of learning experiences (the planned group class or the more direct, on the ward application of principles for a few staff members) provide the best learning climate for adult staff members?

    a. Independent variables: the kinds of learning experiences

    b. Dependent variable: the learning climate

ADDITIONAL LEARNING EXPERIENCES—RECOMMENDED READING LIST

DeCecco, J. The Education of the disadvantaged child. In *The psychology of learning and instruction: educational psychology*. (1st Ed.) Englewood Cliffs, N.J.: Prentice-Hall, Inc., 1968, pp. 182-223.

DeCecco, J., and Crawford, W. *The psychology of learning and instruction: educational psychology*. (2nd Ed.) Englewood Cliffs, N.J.: Prentice-Hall, Inc., 1974, pp. 70-135.

Gagne, R. M. *The conditions of learning*. (2nd Ed.) New York: Holt, Rinehart and Winston, Inc., 1970, pp. 345-380.

INSTRUCTIONS TO THE LEARNER REGARDING POSTTEST

Having completed the text of this module, you are now ready to take the posttest to determine the extent to which you have achieved the objectives of this module. Return to the pretest and take it over again as the posttest. Correct your answers using the answer key found on this page and the following. You need to score 42 points to achieve the 95% mastery level. If your score is less than 42 points, correct your errors, study the text of the module again more carefully, and read some of the articles in the recommended reading list. Study in this fashion until you achieve the 95% level or better in the posttest.

ANSWER KEY TO PRETEST AND POSTTEST

1. b (DeCecco, 1968; p. 214)
2. d (DeCecco, 1968; p.213)
3. a (DeCecco, 1968; p. 213)
4. a and c (DeCecco, 1968; p. 213)
5. a and b (DeCecco, 1968; p. 214)
6. b (Coleman and Provener, 1957; pp. 285-292)
7. c (DeCecco, 1968; p. 210)
8. b (DeCecco, 1968; p. 211)
9. b (Gagne, 1970, pp. 245-380)
10. b (Gagne, 1970, p. 367)
11. b (Bernard, 1972, pp. 5-17)
12. The examples can be any five from this list:
    a. Objects for instruction
    b. Demonstration
    c. Human model
    d. Oral communication by the teacher
    e. Printed language

f. Pictures
g. Motion pictures and television
h. Teaching machines
(Gagne, 1970, pp. 350-363)
13. The examples should be from this list:
    a. Tutoring session
    b. Lecture
    c. Recitation
    d. Discussion
    e. Laboratory
    f. Homework
    (Gagne, 1970, pp. 367-380)
14. The issue can be either a. or b.
    a. The use of educational media (teaching machines) treating students as machines versus the view that educational technology individualizes instruction (Sielber, and others, 1972, pp. 39-44)
    b. Issue of the change of the role of the teacher from that of dispenser of information to teacher as facilitator (which came about as a result of educational technology replacing the teacher) (Fruehling, 1972, pp. 45-47; Pratt, 1970, p. 207)
15. The answer should include content presented under the heading "Effect of early environment on learning." (Text, pp. 415-417).
16. The answer should include content presented under "Application to nursing education and practice." (Text, pp. 426-429)
17. Answer should include aspects of both the physical environment and the conceptual environment—discipline, management, mental health, teacher-student interaction. For details, see "Application to nursing education and practice." (Text, pp. 426-429)

REFERENCES

Allport, G. W. Psychological models for guidance. *Harvard Educational Review*, 1963, **32**:373-381.

Arndt, C., and Huckabay, L. M. D. *Nursing administration: theory for practice with a systems approach.* St. Louis: The C. V. Mosby Co., 1975.

Arnhoff, F., and Leon, H. Sensory deprivation: its effects on human learning. *Science*, 1962, **23**:899-900.

Bernard, H. W. *Psychology of learning and teaching.* (3rd Ed.) New York: McGraw-Hill Book Co., 1972.

Bernskin, B. Social structure, language, and learning. *Educational Research*, 1961, **3**:163-176.

Beyer, M., Dickelmann, N., and Thompson, M. Developing a modular curriculum. *Nursing Outlook*, 1972, **20**(10):643-647.

Biehler, R. F. *Psychology applied to teaching.* Boston: Houghton Mifflin Co., 1971.

Briggs, L. G., Campeau, P. L., Gagne, R. M., and May, M. A. *Instructional media.* Monograph No. 2. Pittsburgh: American Institute for Research, 1967.

Bruner, J. S. The cognitive consequences of early sensory deprivation. In P. Solomon (Ed.), *Sensory deprivation.* New York: Wiley & Sons, Inc., 1961.

Bruner, J. S. *The process of education.* Cambridge, Mass.: Harvard University Press, 1965.

Campeau, P. L. Selective review of literature on audiovisual media of instruction. In L. G. Briggs, P. L. Campeau, R. M. Gagne, and M. A. May (Eds.), *Instructional media.* Monograph No. 2. Pittsburgh: American Institute for Research, 1967.

Clements, M. Research and incantation: a comment. *Phi Delta Kappan*, 1968, **50**:107.

Coleman, R., and Provence, S. Environmental retardation (hospitalism) in infants living in families. *Pediatrics*, 1957, **19**(2):285-292.

Collard, R. Explanatory and play behaviors of infants reared in an institution and in lower-middle class homes. *Child Development*, 1971, **42**:1003-1015.

Cronbach, L. J. *Educational psychology.* (2nd Ed.) New York: Harcourt Brace Jovanovich, Inc., 1963.

Cunningham, W. F. *The pivotal problems of education.* New York: The Macmillan Co., 1940.

Curtis, J., and Rothert, M. An instructional stimulation system offering practice in assessment of patient needs. *Journal of Nursing Education*, 1972, **11**(1):23-28.

DeCecco, J. *The psychology of learning and instruction: educational psychology.* (1st Ed.) Englewood Cliffs, N.J.: Prentice-Hall, Inc., 1968.

de Tornyay, R. *Strategies for teaching nursing.* New York: John Wiley & Sons, Inc., 1971.

Ferguson, V. D. The learning climate. *Journal of Continuing Education in Nursing*, 1971, **2**:23-28.

Flanders, N. A. *Teacher influence, pupil attitudes and achievement.* Office of Education, Department of Health, Education and Welfare, Washington, D.C., 1965.

Fruehling, D. L. Beyond hardware and software. *American Vocational Journal*, 1972, **47**:45-47.

Gagne, R. M. (ed.) *Learning and individual differences.* Columbus, Ohio: Charles E. Merrill Publishing Co. 1967.

Gagne, R. M. *The conditions of learning.* (2nd Ed.) New York: Holt, Rinehart and Winston, Inc., 1970.

Glasser, W. *Schools without failure.* New York: Harper and Row Publishers, 1969.

Goldfarb, W. Psychological privation in infancy and subsequent adjustment. *American Journal of Orthopsychology*, 1945, **15**:247-255.

Grissom, R. J., Sudefelt, P., and Vernon, J. Memory for verbal materials effects of sensory deprivation. *Science*, 1962, **138**:429-430.

Gropper, G. Why is a picture worth a thousand words? *AV Communication Review*, 1963, **11**:75-95.

Guinee, K. *The aims and methods of nursing education.* New York: The Macmillan Co., 1966.

Harrison, C. H. South Brunswick, N.J.: schools put a town on the map. *Saturday Review*, 1970, **53**(8): 66-68.

Heidgerken, L. E. *Teaching in schools of nursing, principles and methods.* 2nd Ed.) Philadelphia: J. B. Lippincott Co., 1953.

Heidgerken, L. E. *Teaching and learning in schools of nursing.* (3rd Ed.) Philadelphia: J. B. Lippincott Co., 1965.

Heil, L. M., and others. *Characteristics of teacher behavior related to the achievement of children— several elementary grades.* Cooperative Research Project, U.S. Office of Education, Washington, D.C., 1960.

Jensen, A. R. Individual differences in concept learning. In H. J. Klausmeier and W. Harris (Eds.), *Analyses of concept learning.* New York: Academic Press, Inc., 1966, pp. 139-154.

Jensen, A. R. Social class and verbal learning. In M. Deutsch A. R. Jensen, and I. Katz (Eds.), *Social class, race, and psychological development.* New York: Holt, Rinehart and Winston, Inc., 1968.

Jersild, A. T., and Lazar, E. A. *The meaning of psychotherapy in the teacher's life work.* New York: Teacher's College Press, 1962.

John, V. P., and Goldstein, L. S. The social content of language acquisition. *Merrill-Palmer Quarterly*, 1964, **10**:265-275.

Langford, T. Self-directed learning. *Nursing Outlook*, 1972, **20**(10):648-651.

Langhoff, H. F. Audiovisual equipment. *American Journal of Nursing*, 1972, **72**(11):2029-2031.

Leavitt, H. J. Some effects of certain communication patterns on group performance. *Journal of Abnormal Social Psychology*, 1951, **46**:38-50.

Lumsdaine, A. A., and May, M. A. Mass communication and educational media. *Annotated Review of Psychology*, 1965, **16**:475-534.

Maslow, A. H. *Motivation and personality.* New York: Harper & Row, Publishers, 1954, pp. 63-122.

McClelland, D. To know why men do what they do. *Psychology Today*, 1971, **4**(8):35-39.

McKinney, C. *The personality of the teacher.* Chicago: Row, Peterson & Co., 1910.

Mentzer, D. S. Audiotutorial lab. *Audio-Visual Instruction*, 1970, **15**(4): 29-31.

Mouly, G. J. *Psychology for effective teaching.* (2nd Ed.) New York: Holt, Rinehart and Winston, Inc., 1968.

Nengen, R. Categories of instructional media research. *Viewpoint*, 1970, **46**(5):1.

Palmer, G. T. *The ideal teacher.* New York: Houghton Mifflin Co., 1908.

Pratte, R. Media revolution. *Clearing House*, 1970, **45**(4):207-211.

Reed, C., Collart, M. E., and Ertel, P. Y. Computer-assisted-instrument. *American Journal of Nursing*, 1972, **72**:2035-2039.

Rogers, C. *On becoming a person.* Boston: Houghton Mifflin Co., 1961.

Rubin, F., Allan, J. D., and Leak, A. G. The seminar process—an aid to learning. *Nursing Outlook*, 1971, **19**(1):37-39.

Ryan, D. G. *Characteristics of teachers.* Washington, D.C.: American Council on Education, 1960.

Shaffer, S. M., Indorato, K. L., and Deneselya, J. A. *Teaching in schools of nursing.* St. Louis: The C. V. Mosby Co., 1972.

Sielber, and others. Educational technology. *Educational Technology*, 1971, **11**:39-44.

Spaulding, R. Categories of instructional media resources. *Viewpoint*, 1971, **46**(5):1.

Stein, R. F., Steele, L., Fuller, M., and Langhoff, H. Multi-media independent approach: for improving the teaching-learning process in nursing. *Nursing Research*, 1972, **21**(5):436-477.

Taylor, D. E. M. Problems of patients in an intensive care unit. *International Journal of Nursing Studies*, 1971, **8**:47-59.

Tenenbaum, S. Attitudes of elementary school children to school teachers, and classmates. *Journal of Applied Psychology*, 1944, **28**:134-141.

Vernon, J., and Hoffman, J. Effect of sensory deprivation on learning rate in human beings. *Science*, 1956, **125**:1074-1075.

Vernon, J., and McGill, T. The effect of sensory deprivation upon rote learning. *American Journal of Psychology*, 1957, **70**:637-639.

Wittrock, M. C. The evaluation of instruction: cause and effect relations in naturalistic data, in M. C. Wittrock and D. E. Wiley (Eds.), *The evaluation of instruction: issues and problems.* New York: Holt, Rinehart and Winston, Inc., 1970, pp. 3-21.

Attention

DESCRIPTION OF MODULE

This module on attention is an independent unit of instruction. Attention is a variable that affects both learning and instruction. The content of the module is presented in sequential order. The text of the module covers five areas: (1) theoretical framework, (2) relevant research studies, (3) issues (4) application to nursing education and practice, and (5) researchable questions. The module also contains instructional objectives, a pre- and posttest, answer key, to determine the extent of the student's accomplishment of the set objectives.

MODULE OBJECTIVES

At the completion of this module and having studied the recommended reading list, the student will be able to accomplish the objectives at the 95% level of mastery. The student will be able to:

1. Define:
   a. Attention
   b. Attentional set
   c. Apprehending phase
2. Describe the mechanism by which attention influences perceptual development and problem-solving behavior
3. Cite relevant research studies that support the different theoretical framework of the role of attention in learning
4. Identify variables that affect perception, attention, and problem-solving behavior
5. Cite one issue in the area of attention as it affects learning and perception
6. Describe methods by which the nurse-teacher can attract the learner's (student or patient) attention
7. Identify different methods of focusing
8. Raise one researchable question, using attention as a variable

PRETEST AND POSTTEST

Circle the correct answers. Each question is worth 1 point. The 95% level of mastery for this module is 16 correct answers. Take the test and correct your answers using the answer key that is found at the end of this module (pp. 442-443). If you achieve 16 points, you need not study this module.

Multiple choice

1. The process of the brain that directs, selects, and screens the information received from the senses is:
   a. feedback
   b. motivation
   c. attention
   d. discriminant selection
2. Every act of learning requires an apprehending phase, which is critically dependent on:
   a. perception of the learning event

    b. age of the child attending to the learning event

    c. attention to the learning event

    d. maturational level of the child attending to the learning event

3. Attention means which of the following:

    a. emphasizing the relationship of two concepts

    b. directing senses toward the source of stimulation

    c. recalling knowledge of previous learning

    d. discriminating the essential features of the stimulation

4. Attention, response, order, and exploration are categories of:

    a. motivational sets

    b. sequential sets

    c. attentional sets

    d. learning sets

5. Attentional sets:

    a. are preconditions to learning

    b. are innate to all organisms

    c. must be carefully developed

    d. cannot be learned as a person grows older

6. Attentional sets may also be referred to as:

    a. cognitive strategies

    b. mathemagenic behavior

    c. self-management behaviors

    d. all of the above

7. Attention is a state that can often be detected by:

    a. observing what the learner is looking at

    b. observing what the learner is listening to

    c. watching the teacher

    d. cannot be detected

8. Repetitious or excessive stimulation causes the organism to:

    a. become very attentive

    b. discriminate better

    c. become inattentive

    d. become very curious

9. A means of directing attention is through:

    a. verbal statements

    b. speaking in a loud tone

    c. gestures made by the teacher

    d. sudden movement of object

    e. all except b

10. You are preparing a booklet for the adolescents on the ward to describe pre- and post-surgical care given to patients of open-heart surgery. To direct their attention to the important concepts in the booklet:

    a. give verbal instructions: "Read p. 5 carefully, it's important."

    b. utilize simple sentence structure when explaining important concepts

    c. italicize or underline important concepts

    d. reward those patients that read the booklet

11. The "attentional phase" in learning, according to Trabasso (1968), is when the learner:

    a. attaches correct responses to those features the learner selects as relevant

    b. evaluates the correctness of own responses to the relevant cues

    c. searches among stimulus possibilities until finding those that are relevant

12. According to Trabasso (1968), the difference between fast and slow learners is:

    a. the length of the attentional phase

    b. the length of the associational phase

    c. the length of the evaluative phase

13. The arousal function of the teacher's effort involves the responsibility of:

    1—winning the student's attention

    2—continuing regulation of the student's level of attention

    3—providing for modification of student's expectations

    4—being a resource person

    a. 1 and 3

    b. 2 and 4

    c. 1 and 4

    d. 1 and 2

14. In order for a stimulus to be registered and comprehended it must be:

    a. attended

    b. perceived

    c. coded

    d. all of the above

15. Focusing is a method of getting the learner's attention to a specific point. The following examples that illustrate focusing techniques are:

    a. providing a feedback

    b. making a statement such as: "Look at this."

    c. making gestures

d. underlining the word
e. pointing with an arrow

16. The best method of teaching a nursing student about anatomy of a human heart is by:
    a. providing the student with illustrations (pictures) of a human heart
    b. suggesting reading an excellent book on anatomy of the heart
    c. providing the student with a replica (model) of the heart
    d. showing a movie about the heart

17. The method that does *not* vary the stimuli is:
    a. providing feedback
    b. pausing
    c. changing interaction style
    d. changing sensory channels

TEXT
Theoretical framework
Introduction

Attention was defined by William James (1890, pp. 403-404) as

the taking possession by the mind, in clear and vivid form, of one out of what seems several simultaneously possible objects or trains of thought. Focalization, concentration, of consciousness are of its essence. It implies withdrawal from some things in order to deal effectively with others.

According to Gagne (1970), attention plays an important role in the first phase of the learning sequence, namely the *apprehending phase*. He stated that in order to respond to a stimulation and learn, the student must first *register* the stimulation. The initial event of learning is *attending* to the stimulus. Attending can be thought of as a state that can be detected by observing what the student is looking at or listening to. There is still active debate whether such attending is looking at or listening to. There is still active debate whether such attending is a process itself consisting of one, two, or three stages. Gagne also viewed attending as being a prerequisite event to *perception* of the stimulus. How an individual attends to a stimulus and

perceives it depends on the temporary *mental set* (Hebb, 1966, pp. 82-101) that the individual adopts to is stimulated to adopt by means of verbal instruction (Gagne, 1970, p. 72).

Gagne further pointed out that the act of perceiving implies the learner is differentiating one stimulus from another, or one aspect of the stimulus from another aspect. The limits of what the learner is able to do in this regard is dependent on previous discrimination learning. The prior learning, which determines what the learner can perceive, is referred to as *perceptual learning* (Gagne, 1970, pp. 72-73).

Are attending and perceiving the only events that are necessary in order for an individual to register a stimulation? There is still active debate about this issue too. Some would answer that attending and perceiving is all one needs to register a stimulation. Others insist that a third element, which is hard to detect, is also essential—namely, that a stimulus not only must be perceived but also must be *coded*. Gagne (1970, p. 73) defined this operationally as "the learner apprehends any given stimulus in an idiosyncratic way, in a way that makes it easy for him to 'use' the stimulus." For example, on perceiving the printed term G-11, one student may code it as a brand of antiseptic soap, while another may think of it as a serial number of a machine, and still another student may code it as an inscription. These students may *perceive* the word equally well, but their coding is different.

Gagne (1970, p. 73) in summarizing the different view points on the initial phase of the learning sequence, still holds to the position that the apprehending phase of learning "is concerned with the events that 'register' the stimulus situation for the learner and includes attending, perceiving and coding."

Gagne (1970) further asserted that as a precondition for learning, learners (especially children) need to have certain *attentional sets*. Attentional sets are cognitive strategies, or "intellectual skills that govern the individual's own information-getting behavior, in this case his attentional behavior" (p. 281). Rothkopf (1968) referred to it as "mathemagenic behaviors"; Skinner (1968) called it "self-management behaviors."

According to Gagne (1970, p. 279), attentional sets include such behaviors as:

1. Learning certain stimulus-response units and chains (skills) that govern learner behavior in observing the stimuli that are part of the external condition of learning
2. Learning to continue to direct sense organs toward the source of stimulation
3. Discriminating the essential features of that stimulation
4. Maintaining the internal cues that determine sequences of action
5. Continuing activities that have been started in spite of distraction

Hewett (1968) has also identified some categories of attentional sets. These are:

1. *Attention*, that is learner (child) must observe the stimuli, which is an essential part of a learning event
2. *Response*, in which the learner must be able to respond properly to observation of a stimulus
3. *Order*, in which the learner must be able to carry out a sequence of action (chain) by following verbal directions
4. *Exploration*, that is, the learner must learn to explore and notice many aspects of the environment

It is very important to establish these types of attentional sets in young children as preconditions for further learning.

Jeffrey's (1968 b, c) view of attention and its role in problem-solving behavior of humans is similar to Gagne's, but he emphasized the role of the orienting reflex as an essential element in attention. According to

Jeffrey, the behavior to which the word attention is commonly applied has an alerting or arousal component, a receptor-orienting component, and an internal cue-selection component. Perception, attention, and curiosity are inseparable aspects of the process of obtaining information. One does not perceive without attending, nor attend without curiosity. Orienting reflex (OR) is one observable aspect of attention. It is defined by Sokolov (1963) as a pattern of physiological responses that occurs to novel stimulation. Maltzman and Raskin (1965) considered orienting reflex as a defined concept. Its antecedent condition is change in stimulation, while objective measures include depression of cortical alpha rhythm, the galvanic skin response (GSR), pupilary dilatation, and a complex vasomotor response consisting of cephalic vasodilatation, and a complex vasomotor response consisting of cephalic vasodilatation and peripheral vasoconstriction. Qualitative, intensive, or temporal changes in stimulation all may evoke the orienting reflex as their initial response.

A variety of explanations have been proposed for the stimulus-seeking behavior of organisms (Berlyne 1960; Hunt 1963). Jeffrey (1968) proposed: (1) that cues can be ordered in terms of their salience; for example, the magnitude of the orienting reflex or the likelihood that a cue will elicit an orienting reflex; (2) that when a cue elicits an orienting reflex, attentional responses follow that tend to optimize the perception of that cue; and (3) that as orienting reflexes habituate, attention also declines. If the orienting reflex is a reinforcing state of affairs, as Maltzman and Raskin (1965) suggested, then one could propose that attending behaviors are shaped by the occurrence of the orienting reflex.

The purpose of this module is to present concisely the role of attention in learning. Special emphasis is given to the role of attention in the perceptual development and problem-solving behavior of individuals. The first part of this module covers the means, or the mechanism, by which attention influences problem-solving behavior and perceptual development. The variables that affect attention and perception are also discussed; for example, individual differences, age, sex, I.Q., motivation, and child-rearing practices. Evidence in each of these cases will be drawn from animal and human research studies. The issue of whether the human ability to perceive the form of objects is inborn or must be learned is also presented. Finally, extrapolations to nursing education and practice are made whenever possible.

Mechanism by which attention influences perceptual development and problem-solving behavior

Several different approaches have been taken in explaining the role of attention in cognitive development. Some ways it has been explained have been in terms of discrimination learning (Zeaman and House, 1963), transfer (Spiker and Norcross, 1962; Jeffrey, 1968), acquired distinctiveness of cues (Stevenson and McBee, 1958), and serial habituation (Jeffrey, 1968c).

The study by Stevenson and McBee (1958) compared differences in learning rate in young children (mean ages 4 and 6 years) when the stimuli for discrimination were solid objects (cubes), planometric objects, and patterns. Results showed that the subjects trained with the solid objects performed significantly better than those in the other two groups. The reason for the better discrimination of the solid objects was that they provided more redundancy of stimulus information and drew more attention. It is asserted by Jeffrey (1968b) that the control of selective learning and problem solving is primarily a matter of controlling attention.

Acquired distinctiveness of cues has been

attributed to the learning of orienting reflexes instead of the effect of verbal mediation (Kurtz, 1955). In an article on the role of attention in learning, Trabasso (1968) discussed the findings of the Zeaman and House (1963) study with retarded children who had to learn a discrimination task. Trabasso pointed out that in backward learning curves there are two distinctive portions; an initial phase, which was quite flat, with performance near a chance level of success, and a second phase, which showed a sharp rise from change responding to perfect performance. These two phases were identified as two subprocesses. The first is an *attentional* phase where the learner is viewed as searching among possible features of the stimulus patterns until those features that are relevant are attended. Second is the *associational* phase where the learner attaches correct responses to those features selected as relevant. The main difference between the fast and slow learners. Trabasso stated, was in the length of the initial attentional phase. The associational phases for both fast and slow learners were approximately the same. Zeaman and House's identification of two phases of learning implied that deficits in learning by children, normal or otherwise, might not be in their intellectual ability to form associations or to solve problems, but in their inability to attend to the critical features of the task (Trabasso, 1968).

In subsequent studies (Bower and Trabasso, 1968) found that the attentional phase of the learning curve could be shortened by many stimulus factors that are known to affect the salience of a cue. Furthermore, they showed that the overall learning rate of these problems seems to depend on the ease with which the subject comes to attend to and use whatever attribute the experimenter has chosen to be relevant; for example, markers, arrows, or underlined letters that direct the learner's attention to attributes.

Another way of explaining the role of attention in perception is in terms of learning to detect the distinctive features. It was suggested by Gibson (1963) that the increasing differentiation of the child's world—objects, sounds, pictures—is at least in part a result of learning to respond to the distinctive features of objects, phonemes, graphemes, and so on. An example is in considering letter discrimination; with respect to this issue, Gibson stated that it seems less likely that descrimination is accomplished by developing a concept or image (Piagetian explanation), but rather by discovering the ways in which each letter is unique, that is different from the other members of the set.

A study by Wagner and associates (1968) provided strong evidence for an attentional explanation. They found that a cue element that was only partially correlated with reinforcement tended to be utilized only if no other available cue element was more highly correlated with reinforcement, rather than in proportion to its correlation with reinforcement, as would be predicted from stimulus-response theory.

Labels have been demonstrated to be helpful to the hearing child of 4½ to 5 years of age (Canter, 1965), but as Tighe and Tighe (1966) pointed out, whether labels make stimuli more distinctive through the addition of cues, or whether they function to call attention to the distinctive aspects of stimuli is unclear. It is proposed that a more satisfactory explanation of human problem-solving behavior will be found with a more adequate understanding of the development of attention.

Other studies by Murphy and Miller (1958) and Jeffrey and Cohen (1964) have demonstrated that young children have difficulty utilizing cues that are not integrated with responses in such a way as to ensure receptor orientation. It has also been demonstrated that in the absence of obvious cues children show a strong tendency to respond on the basis of positional cues. Although naive adults may respond to position cues following the first reinforcement, they shift quickly among cues after nonreinforced responses. Such flexibility in adult problem-solving behavior probably reflects hierarchies of both cue-utilization strategies and cue salience. It is proposed that the latter, a hierarchy of cue salience, is more fundamental, and that in order to understand the development of problem-solving ability, it is necessary to learn more about the variable controlling the development of cue salience (Jeffrey, 1968c).

A series of other studies by Canter (1965) and Spiker and Norcross (1962) represented a concerted effort to demonstrate that transfer is the result of acquired distinctiveness of cues rather than predifferentiation.

Finally, a mechanism for the control of attention and the formation of schemata was postulated by Jeffrey (1968b) in his serial-habituation hypotheses. It was proposed that a consequence of the orienting reflex is attending responses, which optimize the reception of stimuli. With repeated stimulation the orienting reflex habituates to a specific cue, and the subject shifts attention. As a result of such serial habituation, chains of attending responses (schemata) are formed to cue sets in which the habituation of the orienting reflex to two or more cues takes place in constant order. Furthermore, if stimuli producing rapidly habituating orienting reflexes are paired with stimuli that produce orienting reflexes that habituate more slowly, the habituation of the orienting reflexes to the first stimuli will be retarded. This notion is primarily a restatement of the secondary-reinforcement paradigm, with emphasis on the orienting reflex rather than the reinforcing stimulus. It has been noted that a virtue of what is typically called reinforcement is the strength of the orienting reflex associated with it.

The serial-habituation model has practical implications for the manipulation of attention in certain problem-solving situations; for example, as the orienting reflex habituates to the more salient cue, the child shifts attention to previously less salient cues; then in order to obtain a response to a cue of low salience, the experimenter may add to that cue a cue that is minimally sufficient to assure an attending response. Given a generally impoverished environment, this more salient cue should elicit appropriate attention, but as the orienting reflex and attention wane to the more salient cue, the subject should attend to the next most salient cue. If only the critical cue remains, and if reinforcement occurs while the subject attends to this cue, then the low-salience cue becomes a conditioned stimulus for those internal events consequent to the delivery of a reinforcer, or at least a discriminative stimulus for the delivery of a reinforcer. Such a mechanism is particularly appropriate for explaining how a so-called color-dominant child may come to use form as a cue in a simple selective learning experiment (Corah, 1965; Jeffrey, 1968c, p. 328).

Variables affecting perception, attention, and problem-solving behavior

The variables that influence perception, attention, and problem-solving behavior are: individual differences, such as age, sex, I.Q., and motivation and the variable of child-rearing practices.

Age. In their study Kagan and associates (1966) found differential reactions with age that were interpreted as indicating the development of schema. It is a frequent observation that infants have difficulty disengaging their attention from a stimulus, whereas older babies are more capable of active exploration of their environment. Lewis (1967) found that the rate of habituation of both fixation time and cardiac deceleration increase with age. Kuenne (1946) and Alberts and Ehrenfreund (1951) each found that ability to respond to relationships correlates positively with age and the ability to verbalize the relationship. Finally, Ghent (1960) found that a child's span of attention is brief, and that, up to a point, it increases with age.

Sex. A study by Kagan (1965) showed that girls display more sustained attention to visual stimulation and prefer more novel auditory patterns than boys at about 6 to 13 months of age. The 6-month data suggests greater cardiac deceleration to the matrix of lights among girls and longer fixation times. Girls attend preferentially to music, boys to tone.

I.Q. A study by Leibowitz and associates (1959) on shape constancy and intelligence level showed that more intelligent subjects tended to produce a geometrical match. The mental defectives, on the other hand, produced matches closest to shape constancy. They concluded that with increasing intelligence level, shape matching exhibits a decreasing tendency toward shape constancy.

Motivation. Motives and personal attitudes interact with age in influencing perception. The study by Dukes and Bevan (1952) showed that when children compared the weight of a jar visibly filled with candy to one filled with sand, they overestimated the candy-filled jar. But more interesting, the precision of judgment was greater when candy was compared with candy. The authors interpreted this improvement in precision to be explained in terms of some attentional concepts.

Child-rearing practices. Lewis' (1967) study showed that cognitive growth (measured in terms of faster habituation) is facilitated by mother-infant interaction, that is, rate of habituation was related to the proportion of times the mothers responded to the infant relative to the number of opportunities to respond.

Issue of nature versus nurture, or maturation versus learning, controversy of perception of forms

One extreme suggests that perceptual organization comes only as the result of the infant's interaction with the environment (empiricism), where as the other extreme assumes that perceptual organization is innate and is either present at birth or appears with subsequent maturation (nativism).

Experiments (Fantz, 1961) with newly hatched chicks showed that the chicks have an innate ability to perceive shape, three-dimensionality, and size. Fantz furthermore showed that newborns prefer inhomogeneities of pattern and texture. Gibson and Walk's (1960) study on "visual cliff" showed that normal human infants, by the time they locomote on their own, can perceive a drop-off and tend to avoid it. This study also showed that research with other animals also confirms the potential innateness of the discrimination of depth.

From the empiricist point of view—the extraction of information from the environment represents interaction between attention, perception, curiosity, and learning, whether the subject is child or adult. Jeffrey (1968b) indicated that even though perception is essential to learning, it is also modified by learning. Even though there is considerable evidence that learning may not play as a major a role in development of perception as once assumed, many subtleties of perceptual development must depend on the types of interactions with the environment that are typified by learning situations. Speech, writing, and facial expressions are examples of perceptual situations where meaning is an obvious part of the percept and in which perception depends on learned relationships. Furthermore, Gibson (1963) showed the significance of certain differentiating features in letters that may have to be learned. Gibson stated that at least three kinds of perceptual learning can be pointed out in developmental studies: (1) increase in specificity, (2) detection of distinctive features, and (3) development of constant error.

There appears to be a complex interplay of innate ability, maturation, and learning in the molding of perceptual behavior of adaptive significance. Further research is necessary to pin down this and other implications more concretely, but the results to date require the rejection of the view that the newborn human or animal must start from scratch in learning to see and to organize patterned stimulation.

In summarizing the theoretical aspect of the role of attention in learning—specifically as it relates to perceptual development and problem-solving behavior—it can be concluded that the available evidence suggesting that perceptual development progresses by both maturation and learning is a truism and that the role of attention is basic to the development of discrimination learning, transfer, perceptual development, and problem-solving behavior. The author furthermore believes that very little is known about those stimulus attributes that are most salient for the infant and how the hierarchy of cue salience changes with maturation and experience. Also, considerable advances in the development of research methodology and in the field of adequate test construction must be made before it will be possible to determine to what extent each of the variables is responsible for differential cognitive development.

Application to nursing education and practice

The importance of attention in learning has been amply demonstrated in the previous sections. The teacher's or the nurse's main function is to get the learner's attention to ensure that what is to be taught will be perceived and coded correctly by the students or patients.

Jeffrey (1968b,c) proposed that cues can be

perceived in terms of their saliency. The teacher's function then is to make the important cues or aspects of the learning task very obvious (salient) to draw the learner's attention. Cues, or specific characteristics of the learning task, can be made more obvious by making them *distinctive*. For example, to teach students how to discriminate afferent nerve and efferent nerve, between insulin shock and insulin coma, or between rubella and roseola, the teacher has to demonstrate the distinctive features of each element of the task that have to be discriminated. For instance, in the first example of discriminating between afferent and efferent nerves, the teacher *focuses* on the main feature of these two words—namely, the *a*fferent and *e*fferent—the first letter of each word. Focusing is a term that refers to drawing the learner's attention to a specific point. Gagne (1970) and de Tornyay (1971) suggested several focusing methods that the teacher can utilize to make the cues salient and to stress the distinctive features of the learning task. The nurse-teacher may use such terms as "look at this" or "remember this" or may use large printed words, underlines, arrows, contrasting colors, or slides that magnify the main difference. All these focusing methods help direct the learner's attention to the relevant stimuli.

Bower and Trabasso's (1968) illustrations of Zeaman and House's (1963) study with mentally retarded children showed that perceiving—learning takes place in two stages: attentional phase and association phase—by using focusing methods can reduce the time of the attentional phase; thus, the learner can perceive the relevant stimulus faster and learn more quickly.

Stevenson and McBee's (1958) study showed that discrimination learning was better when the learners learned by using three-dimensional objects instead of two dimensional objects or pictures. This was because the three-dimensional objects provided

for *redundancy of stimuli*, thus drawing more attention to the task to be learned. The implication of this study is that, to teach a concept to a group of students or to patients, the nurse should utilize three-dimensional objects; for example, if the students are to learn the three bones of the inner ear, it is preferable that they see a replica-model of an inner ear. Since it is three-dimensional, it will provide for redundancy of stimuli and, therefore, will attract the students' attention more. Consequently, they will perceive the relevant stimuli (the three bones) better than if they saw it in a picture.

Similarly, if a clinic nurse is to teach a patient how to apply the diaphragm as a contraceptive measure, letting the patient see and practice on the replica-model of female reproductive organs, then on herself, is better than having her see it in a picture because the patient not only sees it, but also manipulates it. The more one appeals to the different sense organs (eyes, ears, touch, and so on) the more redundant the relevant stimulus becomes, and the more attention is paid to that specific stimulus.

Jeffrey (1968b,c) pointed out that when the orienting reflex habituates, attention declines. Therefore, another function of the teacher is to make sure that the orienting reflex does not habituate before the relevant stimuli are perceived. In other words, the teacher should prolong the learner's attention span. One method for prolonging the attention span is by changing the stimulus to which the learner is attending. For example, if the teacher is showing a group of students slides on how to apply Ace bandages to the patient's lower extremities, it is advisable for the teacher to change the slides every 20 to 30 seconds rather than talking for 5 minutes on each slide. It is preferable that the same type of slide be flashed repeatedly, instead of showing one stationery slide, since each change of slide is a change in stimulation and, therefore, prolongs the time for habituation.

De Tornyay (1971) suggested other methods for varying the stimuli to maintain the student's attention. One of these is to change interaction style. For instance, instead of the teacher lecturing (teacher-to-student interaction) to the students all of the time, the interaction might be changed at frequent intervals to student-to-student interaction style and to teacher-to-group style. The utilization of these three interaction styles provides change in stimulation and thus attracts attention.

Pausing is another method of varying the stimuli. When the teacher pauses (keeps quiet) for awhile, it creates lack of structure thus, the students will strain to hear what the next statement is going to be. Pausing is analogous to a period in a written statement; it serves the function of punctuation in a verbal dialogue. Pausing enables the student to assimmilate what has already been said and prepares them to hear and perceive what is to come next.

Changing the stimulus situation is another way of changing the stimuli. For instance, when the teacher changes the sensory channel—that is, changes from talking (oral-hearing) to writing on the board (seeing) to letting students touch (for example; the bandage or syringe) (kinesthetic)—it makes the relevant stimulus more redundant by appealing to more than one sensory channel, therefore, students will pay more attention.

In this section, samples of how a nurse-teacher can utilize different methods and teaching strategies in attracting the learner's attention and facilitating learning has been presented. Many more examples can be given; the reader is advised to take each of the previous situations and principles and apply them to other nursing examples.

Researchable questions

Research is needed in determining the factors that shorten the attentional phase of learning. For example, what is the effect of different verbal mediators on the attentional phase of learning.

Since motives and personal attitudes influence perception, what would be the effect of having studies select their own patients to care for (that is, making their own assignment) as opposed to the teacher assigning patients to students on the accurate observation and perception of significant signs and symptoms in making a nursing diagnosis (assessment of the patient's needs).

ADDITIONAL LEARNING EXPERIENCES—RECOMMENDED READING LIST

Bower, G., and Trabasso, T. *Attention and learning.* New York: Wiley and Sons, Inc., 1968.

Gagne, R. *The Conditions of learning.* (2nd Ed.) New York: Holt, Rinehart and Winston, Inc., 1970, pp. 72-3, 157, 279-281, 305-306.

Jeffrey, W. E. The orienting reflex and attention in cognitive development. *Psychological Review*, 1968, **75**(4):323-334.

INSTRUCTIONS TO THE LEARNER REGARDING POSTTEST

Having completed your study, you are now ready to take the posttest to determine the extent to which you have achieved the objectives of this module. Return to the pretest and take it over again as the posttest. Correct your answers using the answer key that is found on this page and the next. You need to score 16 correct points to achieve mastery at the 95% level. If your score is less than 16 points, correct your errors, study the content of this module again more carefully, and read some of the articles in the recommended reading list. Study in this fashion until you achieve the 95% mastery level.

ANSWER KEY TO PRETEST AND POSTTEST

1. c (DeCecco, 1968, p. 215)
2. c (Gagne, 1970, pp. 72-73)
3. b and d (Gagne, 1970, p. 279)

4. c (Gagne, 1970, p. 280)
5. a (Gagne, 1970, p. 281)
6. d (Gagne, 1970, p. 281)
7. a and b (DeCecco, 1968, p. 72)
8. c (DeCecco, 1968, p. 215)
9. e (Gagne, 1970, p. 306)
10. c (Gagne, 1970, p. 306)
11. c (Trabasso, 1968, pp. 31-36)
12. a (Trabasso, 1968, p. 32)
13. d (DeCecco, 1968, p. 162)
14. d (Gagne 1970, p. 73)
15. b, d, and e (Gagne, 1970, p. 306; de Tornyay, 1971, pp. 104-106)
16. c (Stevenson and McBee, 1958, pp. 753-754)
17. a (de Tornyay, 1971, pp. 66-68, 70, 73)

REFERENCES

Alberts, E., and Ehrenfreund, D. Transposition in children as a function of age. *Journal of Experimental Psychology*, 1951, **41**:30-38.

Berlyne, D. E. *Conflict, arousal and curiosity.* New York: McGraw-Hill Book Co., 1960.

Bower, G., and Trabasso, T. *Attention and learning.* New York: John Wiley and Sons, Inc., 1968.

Canter, J. H. Transfer of stimulus pretraining to motor and paired-associated and discrimination learning tasks. In Lipsitt, L. P., and Spiker, C. C. (Eds.), *Advances in child development and behavior, Vol. 2.* New York. Academic Press, Inc., 1965, pp. 75-97.

Corah, N. L. The influence of some stimulus characteristics on color and form perception in nursery-school children. *Child Development*, 1966, **37**:205-212.

de Tornyay, R. *Strategies for teaching nursing.* New York: John Wiley and Sons, Inc., 1971.

Dukes, W. F., and Bevan, N. Accentuation and response variability in the perception of personally related objects. *Journal of Personality*, 1952, **20**:457-465.

Fantz, R. L. The origin of form perception. *Scientific American*, 1961, **204**(5):66-72.

Gagne, R. *The conditions of learning.* (2nd Ed.) New York: Holt, Rinehart and Winston, Inc., 1970.

Ghent, L. Recognition by children of realistic figures presented in various orientations. *Canadian Journal of Psychology* 1960, **14**:249-256.

Gibson, E. J. Perceptual development. In H. W. Stevenson (Ed.), *Child psychology.* The 62nd yearbook of NSSE, Chicago: University of Chicago Press, 1963, pp. 144-195.

Gibson, E. J., and Walk, R. D. The "visual cliff." *Scientific American*, 1960, **202**:64-71.

Hebb, D. O. *A textbook of psychology.* (2nd Ed.) Philadelphia: W. B. Saunders Co., 1966.

Hewett, F. M. *The emotionally disturbed child in the classroom.* Boston: Allyn & Bacon, Inc., 1968.

Hunt, J. McV. Motivation inherent in information processing action. In C. J. Harvey (Ed.), *Motivation and social interaction.* New York: The Ronald Press Co., 1963.

James, W. *The principles of psychology, Vol. 1.* New York: Henry Holt & Co., 1890.

Jeffrey, W. E. Transfer. (Mimeograph copy), University of California, Los Angeles 1968a. (To appear in Reese, H. W. and Lipsit, L. P. (Eds.), *The scientific study of child behavior and development.*

Jeffrey, W. E. Perception, attention, and curiosity. In Spenser, T. D. and Kass, N. (Eds.), *Perspectives in child psychology: research and review.* New York: McGraw-Hill Book Co., 1970, pp. 75-97.

Jeffrey, W. E. The orienting reflex and attention in cognitive development. *Psychological Review*, 1968c, **75**(4):323-334.

Jeffrey, W. E., and Cohen, L. B. Effect of spatial separation of stimulus, response, and reinforcement on selective learning in children. *Journal of Experimental Psychology*, 1964, **67**:577-580.

Kagan, J. Studies of attention in human infants. *Merrill-Palmer Quarterly*, 1965, (**2**):95-127.

Kagan, J., and others. Infants' differential reactions to familiar and distorted faces. *Child Development*, 1966, **37**:519-532.

Kuenne, M. R. Experimental investigation of relation of language to transposition behavior in young children. *Journal of Experimental Psychology*, 1946, **36**:271-290.

Kurtz, K. H. Discrimination of complex stimuli: the relationship of training and test stimuli in transfer of discrimination. *Journal of Experimental Psychology*, 1955, **50**:283-292.

Leibowitz, H., Waskow, I., Loeffler, N., Glaser, F. Intelligence level as a variable in the perception of shape. *Quarterly Journal of Experimental Psychology*, 1960, **14**:249-256.

Lewis, M. Infant attention: response decrement as a measure of cognitive processes, or what's new Baby Jane? Paper presented at the Society for Research in Child Development, New York, 1967.

Maltzman, I., and Raskin, D. C. Effects of individual differences in the orienting reflex on conditioning and complex processes. *Journal of Experimental Research in Personality*, 1965, **1**:1-16.

Murphy, J. V., and Miller, R. E. The effects of spatial relationship between the cue, reward, and response in simple discrimination learning. *Journal of Experimental Psychology*, 1958, **56**:26-31.

Rothkopf, E. Z. Two scientific approaches to the management of instruction. In R. M. Gagne and W. R. Gephart (Eds.), *Learning research and school subjects*. Itasca, Ill.: F. E. Peacock Publishers, Inc., 1968.

Skinner, B. F. *The technology of teaching*. New York: Appleton-Century-Crofts, 1968.

Sokolov, Y. N. *Perception and conditioned reflex*. New York: Macmillan Co., 1963.

Spiker, C. C., and Norcross, K. J. Effects of previously acquired stimulus names on discrimination performance. *Child Development*, 1962, 33:859-864.

Stevenson, H. W., and McBee, G. The learning of object and pattern discrimination by children. *Journal of Comparative Physiological Psychology*, 1958, 51:753-754.

Tighe, L. S., and Tighe, T. J. Discrimination learning: two views in historical perspectives. *Psychological Bulletin* 1966, 66:353-370.

Trabasso, T. Pay attention. *Psychology Today*, 1968, 2:(5):32-36.

Wagner, A. R., Logan, R. A., Haberlandt, K., and Price. Stimulus selection in animal discrimination learning. *Journal of Experimental Psychology*, 1968, 76:171-180.

Zeaman, D., and House, B. J. The role of attention in retardate discrimination learning. In N. R. Ellis (Eds.), *Handbook of mental deficiency: psychological theory and research*. New York: McGraw-Hill Book Co., 1963, pp. 159-223.

Motivation

DESCRIPTION OF MODULE

The content of this module is concerned with the variable of motivation as it affects learning and instruction. The content is presented in sequential order. It covers five major areas that are presented in an integrated form: (1) theoretical framework, (2) relevant research studies, (3) issues, (4) application to nursing education and practice and (5) researchable questions. The module also contains a set of student objectives, a pre- and posttest, and an answer key to determine the degree of accomplishment of the objectives by the student. References for additional learning experiences are given in the form of a recommended reading list.

MODULE OBJECTIVES

At the completion of this module, having studied the content presented in it and in the recommended reading list, the student will be able to accomplish the following objectives on motivation at the 95% level of mastery. The student will be able to:

1. Give the historical background of the theory of motivation
2. Describe and give examples of the four basic concepts or factors that account for motivation of the learner
3. Cite relevant research studies to support each conceptual framework
4. Identify two issues in motivation

5. Give specific examples illustrating how the principles and concept of motivation can be applied to nursing education and practice
6. Raise one researchable question using motivation as a variable

PRETEST AND POSTTEST

Circle the correct answers. Each question is worth 1 point except the last question, which is worth 9 points. The 95% level of mastery for this test is 38 points. Take the test and correct your answers using the answer key that is found at the end of this module (pp. 462-463). If you score at least 38 points, you need not study this module.

Multiple choice

1. Select the best explanation or definition of motivation:
   a. verbal reprimands that ensure optional student behavior
   b. praise of students for work well done
   c. factors that increase and decrease the vigor of an individual's activity
   d. performance that increases mastery
2. A motive is best defined as:
   a. those factors that increase and decrease the vigor of an individual's activity
   b. the only causative factor that impels action
   c. an impetus to action directed toward a goal

3. Which of the following are determinants of behaviors:

    1—genes

    2—motives

    3—habits

    4—I.Q.

    5—ability to manipulate and adapt to external stimuli and cues

    a. 2

    b. 3 and 5

    c. 1 and 4

    d. all of the above

4. According to DeCecco and Crawford (1974) the basic factors that account for motivation are:

    a. motives, vigor, and valence

    b. arousal, expectancy, incentives, and punishment

    c. curiosity, boredom, anxiety, and frustration

    d. achievement, mastery, and social and ego integration

5. When a student daydreams during a class session, it is because the student:

    a. is receiving excessive stimulation and is trying to block it off

    b. lacks the appropriate cognitive entering behavior

    c. wants to keep aroused in a monotonous and boring environment by utilizing an internal source of arousal

    d. lacks competence in the subject area discussed in class

6. Factors that affect a student's level of arousal are:

    a. the student liking the course and the teacher, who is the "model"

    b. the student having a clear picture of goals and objectives

    c. curiosity, boredom, anxiety, and frustration

    d. the student having the desire to achieve

7. When teaching senior nursing students, the nurse-instructor should implement the motivational concept of:

    a. eliminating frustration and anxiety so that the student can concentrate on learning

    b. having all students experience the same amount of anxiety to motivate them to learn

    c. creating some degree of discrepancy between what the students expect and what is experienced

    d. introducing the same amount of novelty, adventure, and stimulation to all students

8. In which of the following ways, might an instructor create a state of expectancy for the student:

    a. engaging the student's behavior in learning

    b. providing rewards for learning

    c. describing the instructional objective to the student

9. An underachiever is a student who:

    a. lacks the necessary cognitive entering behaviors

    b. has a low I.Q. in specific areas

    c. expects little satisfaction in academic achievement, even though possesses the ability to succeed

    d. does not have the ability to master the subject matter or the task

10. A teacher spent considerable time developing behavioral objectives and explaining to students the desired outcome of taking the class. By so doing which of the four motivational functions was the teacher most concerned about?

    a. arousal function

    b. expectancy function

    c. incentive function

    d. disciplinary function

11. A student who plans to study vigorously in order to get an "A" on an examination is utilizing the motivational factor of:

    a. arousal

    b. expectancy

    c. incentive

    d. valence

12. The following that are examples of incentives are:

    a. anxiety

    b. positive reinforcer

    c. negative reinforcer

    d. punishment

13. A stimulus an individual seeks to avoid is called:

a. frustration
b. anxiety
c. punishment
d. ripple effect

14. Brainstorming sessions and learning-by-discovery techniques serve the motivational function of:
a. incentive
b. arousal
c. expectancy
d. ripple effect

15. A nursing instructor who attempts to relate what students do today to what they desire to do later in life is performing the motivational function of:
a. incentive
b. arousal
c. expectancy
d. positive reinforcement

16. When a nurse-teacher utilizes feedback of test results, grades, and spoken or written praise, the motivational function being performed is:
a. incentive
b. arousal
c. expectancy
d. reinforcement

17. The nursing instructor who utilizes the disciplinary technique of having the student perform properly what was originally performed improperly and of combining the suppression of one response (deviant) with the substitution of another (desirable response) is using:
a. punishment
b. restitution
c. ripple effect
d. negative reinforcement

18. When a student witnesses a disciplinary action that is taken against a classmate, and the effects are felt by the witnessing student, this phenomenon is referred to as:
a. punishment
b. restitution
c. ripple effect
d. implicit negative reinforcement

Matching

Part A

_____ 19. Level of arousal
_____ 20. Vigor
_____ 21. Expectancy
_____ 22. Valence
_____ 23. Incentives
_____ 24. Achievement motivation
_____ 25. Punishment

Part B

a. A stimulus the individual seeks to avoid and that may effectively suppress undesirable responses
b. An individual's level of activity, wakefulness, vigilance, alertness, and responsiveness
c. The expectancy of finding satisfaction in mastering challenging and difficult performances
d. A momentary belief that a particular outcome will occur that may be a source of arousal
e. Actual goal objects, concrete or symbolical rewards, that incite, arouse, and move to action when they are associated with certain stimuli that signal their presence
f. The individual's anticipated satisfaction or emotional preference for certain outcomes
g. The effect of amount of effort invested on how the student performs

Match theory (part A), theorist (part B), and theory's statement of the nature of motivation (part C).

Part A

	Theory	Theorist	Statement
26.	Drive-reduction	_____	_____
27.	Psychoanalytical	_____	_____
28.	Hedonistic	_____	_____
29.	Effectance	_____	_____
30.	Self-actualization	_____	_____
31.	Curiosity and exploratory	_____	_____

Part B

a. White
b. Maslow
c. Berlyne
d. McClelland
e. Freud
f. Woodworth

Part C Statement of Motivation

a. Human behavior is motivated by innate sexual and aggressive instincts, with resultant action from energy released directly or indirectly.

b. Behavior tends to maximize delight and minimize distress.

c. Motivation comes from the human urge for competence.

d. Human behavior is motivated by drives arising out of homeostatic imbalance or tension.

e. Motivation comes from drive for stimulation.

f. Human behavior derives from a hierarchy of primary, instinctual motives.

Discussion question

32. Utilizing McClelland's propositions on achievement motivation, briefly discuss their relevance to one of the following groups: Weight Watchers, Alcoholics Anonymous, or a behavior modification program with parents of children with "brat" behavior.

TEXT
Theoretical framework
Introduction

Motivation is one of the most popular topics in educational, psychological, and business circles. The main concern of this module is to present those varieties of human motivation that are relevant to the process of learning and instruction.

"Education is a process of changing the behavior patterns of people" (Tyler, 1971, p. 5). But how do behavior patterns change? As students, we want to understand how painlessly and efficiently to change behavior patterns to meet our goals; as nurse-teachers, we want to know how to enable clients, patients, and students to change behavior patterns to meet their desired goals. Looking at motivation as a variable influencing learning and instruction, one realizes that the behavior of the teacher as well as the learner is motivated by internal and external sources. The teacher must be aware of variables that influence own behavior as well as those variables that may influence the learner's behavior.

DeCecco and Crawford (1974, p. 137) defined motivation as "those factors which increase and decrease the vigor of an individual's activity." Sears (1967, p. 35) defined a motive as "an impetus to action directed towards a goal." Risk (1941, p. 41) defined a motive as "a force or drive within the individual· which causes sustained activity in some direction."

Motives are grouped into two classes: (1) intrinsic, which orginate within the individual; for example, desires, purposes, goals, and interests; and (2) extrinsic, which originate with the environment; for example, praise, reproof, reward, punishment, and pain. Extrinsic motives are also called incentives.

The term motivation is also used with reference to the function and the activity of the teacher in directing learning. Within this framework, Risk (1941, p. 499) defined motivation as "the conscious effort on the part of the teachers to establish in pupils motives leading to sustained activity toward the learning of goals." It is, therefore, the role of the teacher to provide the most favorable type of environment and learning activities to enable the student to establish the most desirable goals and to sustain activity until the set goals are attained (Heidgerken, 1953).

The study of motivation is concerned with why individuals behave as they do; it is assumed that there is an explanation, a cause, a reason for everything an individual does. Since behavior may be caused by physiological, psychological, or social stimuli, there is no reason to suppose that a single motive or theory can explain behavior. There are other determinants of behavior besides motives that stimulate, control, and direct behavior. Examples are: (1) the innate structures (genes), which influence the direction and the level of development; (2) the learner's abilities (intelligence), which affect a wide range of behaviors; (3) the individual's ability to manipulate and adapt to external stimuli and the environment; and (4) the individual's habits, which are the acts that have been learned that then control the learner to a certain extent (DeCecco and Crawford, 1974).

Historical background

The drive-reduction theory was introduced in 1913 by Robert Woodworth who stated that energy or drive, as opposed to habits, impels an organism into action. Walter Cannon, in 1932, added the concept of homeostasis, which contends that a state of disequilibrium is set up in the body whenever internal conditions deviate from the normal steady state. Primary drives are hunger, thirst, sexual desires, and avoidance of pain. Secondary drives arise when a neutral stimulus is paired with a primary drive. Motivation is defined as the response to drives arising out of homeostatic imbalance or tension. Hull's learning theory (1943) stated that all rewards are based on reduction of primary homeostatic drive. Secondary rewards are effective because they have been associated with primary rewards in the past. An example would be that social approval is an effective motivator because social approval was associated with food in the past. The following is the motivational sequence in the drive-reduction theory: need/drive, instrumental behavior (disequilibrium), goal/reward, drive reduction, relief of need, behavior stops (equilibrium) (Kaluger and Unkovic, 1969, p. 71).

Psychoanalytical theory, based on Freudian theory, states that humans are motivated by innate sexual and aggressive instincts: psychosexual energy is released directly in actions or indirectly by suppression and reduction into socially accepted behavior. Psychoanalytical theory is influenced by Darwin's instinct theories, that is, certain actions are inherited, such as reflexes (suckling) and instincts arising through natural selection.

The hedonistic theorists claim that humans seek pleasure and avoid pain; all motives are learned. Behavior tends to maximize delight and minimize distress. An example would be David McClelland, who stated that motivation consists of learned anticipations of a goal, which arouses positive or negative emotional reaction; anticipation of pleasure leads to approach behavior, while anticipation of pain leads to avoidance.

Effectance theorists claim that motivation comes from the human urge for effectance or competence. Robert White (1959) postulated that within all people there is an urge toward mastery of the environment. Bruner (1960) and Sears (1963) have done studies that support the idea that motivation comes with self-reinforcement and intrinsic motivation.

Self-actualization theories state that people desire self-actualization or self-fulfillment. Abraham. Maslow 1954) suggested that people have a number of primary, instinctive motives ranging from lower motives to higher ones. These motives are arranged in a hierarchy that corresponds to the assumed evolutionary level of the motive. First there are physiological motives like hunger, then safety motives like fear, then love motives, esteem motives, and finally the motive for self-actualization. A higher motive does not usually appear until the ones below it are satisfied.

Curiosity and exploratory behaviors have been noted to motivate the behaviors of animals and humans; in the 1950's various investigators reported on this phenomenon. Harlow's famous monkeys explored and handled mechanical puzzles and produced puzzle solutions in the absence of hunger drives; they appeared to be curious and seeking stimulation (Harlow, Harlow, and Meyer, 1950). David Berlyne (1957) studied exploratory behavior in humans; as in Harlow's experiments, the subjects appeared to be seeking stimulation, in this case preferring complex pictures to simple ones. Fowler (1965) studied curiosity and explorative behaviors and viewed curiosity as an acquired expectation.

The preceeding is a concise overview of the historical background of some theories of motivation: drive-reduction, psychoanalytical, hedonistic, effectance, self-actualization, and curiosity, and exploratory. This is by no means a complete overview; the reader may notice that these theories overlap as well as conflict.

It may be helpful at this point to look at motivation in learning from two different approaches: functional and theoretical. One might state that the basic function of a motive is an energizing one. Motives energize behavior, arouse activity, or provide the energy of movement. It is assumed that they interact with learned or innate habits to produce overt behavior. An example would be that most adults know how to write their names (a learned behavior response), but it is not until this response is energized (motivated) that the overt behavior takes place. Theoretically, one might accept the energizing function, but then try to reason that the function arises from or is related to a specific class of internal or external conditions; thus, the learning theories.

Basic theory

According to DeCecco and Crawford (1974), there are four factors that account for motivation: arousal, expectancy, incentives, and punishment (discipline). These four factors are the basis on which the teacher's motivational role is delineated.

AROUSAL

Arousal refers to the general state of excitability of the individual. The level of arousal may be viewed as the level of activity, wakefulness or vigilance, alertness, and responsiveness. According to Hebb (1955), the level of arousal ranges from deep sleep (no arousal) to the optimal level to extreme arousal, which is characterized by emotional disturbance and anxiety (Fig. 28-1).

To be alive is to be active; activity is an intrinsic aspect of human nature. One can imagine a student's behavior ranging from inert, near-hibernation states to alert, infor-

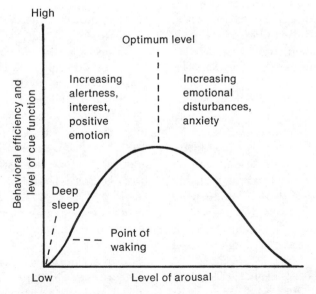

Fig. 28-1. Hypothetical, inverted U-shaped relationship between behavior efficiency, or level of cue function, and level of arousal. (From Hebb, D. O. Drives and C.N.S. (conceptual nervous system). *Psychological Review*, 1955, **62**:250. Copyright 1955 by the American Psychological Association. Reprinted by permission.

mation-seeking to the other extreme of being in a state of panic.

Humans have both internal and external sources of arousal. External sources are the stimuli provided by the environment. Internal sources of arousal come from the cortex and may be in the form of thought, symbol, or fantasy. The student who daydreams to keep aroused in a boring class is utilizing an internal source of arousal.

Factors influencing level of arousal. Some of the factors that influence the individual's level of arousal are curiosity, boredom, anxiety, and frustration.

Curiosity. An individual maintains an arousal level that avoids both boredom, or a lack of stimulation, and intense excitement, or excessive stimulation. Through curiosity and exploratory behavior, the individual seeks optimal stimulation to maintain a suitable level of arousal. Harlow, Harlow, and Meyer (1950), in their experiment with monkeys, demonstrated that adult monkeys explore and handle mechanical puzzles and derive solutions to the puzzles in the absence of food reward. Also, Nissen's (1953) study with sexually naive monkeys indicated a preference for grooming behavior instead of sexual intercourse during the breeding and mating season. Berlyne (1957) studied exploratory behavior in human subjects and found that humans preferred incongruous pictures to normal pictures and also preferred pictures that were more complex and had an element of surprise. Also, Maria Montessori's school children preferred to explore and play with items that were novel and unknown to them. An impressive amount of research shows that humans perform some acts only because they produce novel and unfamiliar situations, experiences, and stimulation.

Boredom. Boredom refers to stimulus deprivation and isolation. Boredom arises when the environment is monotonous and when the task being performed is repetitive.

It often leads to inattentiveness. The study by Bexton, Heron, and Scott (1954) on boredom illustrated that human beings have an inability to stand boredom for extended periods of time. Their subjects were college students. They paid each subject $20.00 a day to remain all day in a lighted, sound-proof room. The students lay on cots and wore transluscent goggles that prevented them from seeing objects. They also wore gloves that reduced their sense of touch. The students were free to terminate the experiment anytime they wanted. The students slept most of the time. After 2 to 3 days they became restless and were even eager to listen to stock-market quotations. They looked forward to taking the difficult tests. They tried to occupy themselves with fantasies of self-induced stimulation. One subject terminated the task very early in the study. This and similar studies (Fowler, 1965) indicate that organisms seek stimulation and also that they respond not only to a change in stimulation but also to create a change. Fowler calls curiosity *incentive motivation.*

DeCecco and Crawford (1974) pointed out that boredom may be the basis for curiosity. Boredom produces drive motivation in normal people. It occurs when the individual or animal is deprived of change in stimulation by long exposure to the same environmental conditions. This is the condition often observed in long-term psychiatric patients, who often sit in the same chair within the same walls year after year. Some stimulate themselves by hallucinations, others by self-stimulating movement.

Therefore, in order for us to maintain an optimal level of arousal, avoid boredom, and experience slight discrepancies, we become motivated to seek novelty, adventure, and stimulation.

Anxiety. Anxiety, as a motivational variable, has been studied by many researchers, and the results of the research can be applied to classroom or patient-teaching settings.

Spence (1956) found that anxiety appeared to facilitate performance in relatively simple types of learning, such as conditioning, but interfered with performance in more complex learning tasks. Spence viewed anxiety as a motivational variable that increases the probability of various responses possible; anxiety tends to increase the likelihood of a correct response. If many responses are possible, however, anxiety tends to increase the likelihood of one or more incorrect responses.

Mandler and Sarason (1952) developed a questionnaire—the Test Anxiety Scale—to measure anxiety in test situations. The findings that emerged from the various studies were that:

1. Low-anxiety students perform better when challenged by the task and by the prospect that their performance will be assessed

2. High-anxiety students perform worse under these same conditions and perform better when they are not threatened with evaluation when faced with a challenging or difficult task

Spielberger (1966) studied anxiety as a state with feelings of apprehension and tension. In a series of studies on the relationship of arousal or an anxiety state to complex learning. Spielberger observed that:

1. High-anxiety students obtained better scores on tests when few recall errors were possible; low-anxiety students obtained better scores when high recall errors were possible

2. Low-anxiety students, in the broad middle range of IQ, performed better than the high-anxiety students; high anxiety had no effect on the performance of low-ability students, but tended to facilitate the performance of the brightest students

3. In concept-learning situations high-anxiety, high-I.Q. students performed better than low-anxiety, high-I.Q. students; also, low-anxiety, low-I.Q. students performed better than high-anxiety, low-I.Q. students.

One cannot conclude from these studies that anxiety must be avoided or reduced in teaching situations. Findings indicate that in general, able students may profit more from anxiety than do less able students.

An issue might be whether to promote anxiety in the classroom or not; in patient teaching, the problem would be to assess the level of anxiety and in some cases to increase it so that the learner could perceive the need to learn. Assessing the level of anxiety in a classroom situation is important and difficult, since individuals vary in levels of anxiety and in performance with anxiety.

Frustration. DeCecco and Crawford (1974, p. 147) defined frustration as "a conflict situation in which the individual must complete one task or turn to another." Lawson's (1965) study on the effect of frustration on learning has shown that frustrating situations may increase the subject's efforts to complete a task. It becomes a challenge to finish the task. Dollard and associates (1939) speculated that this increased vigor of response may account for the possibility that frustration leads to aggression.

Whether frustration will help the student achieve the instructional objectives depends on the student's entering behavior. It is known that frustration will invigorate the student, but it is not certain whether that extra effort will go in studying and in achieving the instructional objectives. Frustration will elicit those behaviors in the student that have the greatest strength. It is, therefore, the role of the teacher to channel this extra vigor that is caused by frustration to achieve relevant goals rather than to achieve irrelevant objectives.

For some students frustrating, new, and challenging situations rekindle their investment of extra effort in accomplishing the task. William James (1892) referred to this as pugnacity. The teacher must enable less pugnacious students to strengthen weaker task-relevant responses (DeCecco and Crawford, 1974, pp. 147-148).

EXPECTANCY

Vroom (1964, p. 17) defined expectancy as "a momentary belief that a particular outcome will follow a particular act." Expectancies range from the subjective certainty that something will either occur or will not occur. Expectancy can be a source of arousal, especially when there is a manageable disagreement or discrepancy between what we see and what we expect to see. As pointed out by DeCecco and Crawford (1974), instructional objectives are the expectancies that are the teacher's main concern, but the teacher must also be concerned with the student's expectancies and valences. A valance is defined as "the individual's anticipated satisfaction, or his emotional preference for certain outcomes" (Vroom, 1964, p. 15). The actual satisfaction a student derives from an experience is called a *value*. For example, a student nurse may look forward to the first trip to the patient's units (valence). After going to the patient's bedside the actual satisfaction or dissatisfaction experienced is the *value*.

With regard to educational outcomes or objectives (valences), students must be made to want or desire these objectives, which they have a good chance of reaching (expectancy). The vigor with which students act or pursue instructional objectives is a product of both expectancy and valence. Underachievers are students who expect little satisfaction in academic achievement (low valence), even though they possess the ability that assures them of academic success (high expectancy).

The relationship of expectancy and valence has been extensively investigated by McClelland and associates (1953). He called it the *motive to achieve*, or *achievement motivation*. Achievement motivation is defined as "the expectancy of finding satisfaction (valence) in mastering difficult and challenging performances" (DeCecco and Crawford, 1974, p. 152).

From their extensive studies McClelland and associates (McClelland, and others, 1953; Atkinson, 1958) have identified the following conditions under which the motive to achieve is best developed:

1. When the student gives a rationale or reason for developing a motive
2. When the student understands that the motive is realistic and reasonable
3. When the student can describe the various aspects of the motive
4. When the student can link the motive to related actions or daily events in life
5. When the student is committed to a concrete goal
6. When the student keeps records of progress
7. When the student perceives the motive as an improvement in self-image
8. When the student perceives and experiences the motive as an improvement on the prevailing cultural values
9. When the student has an honest and warm support from others and is respected by others for possessing the capability of guiding and directing own future behavior
10. When the student engages in study alone
11. When the student has a sense of belonging to a successful group

(DeCecco and Crawford, 1974, p. 151)

INCENTIVES

Incentives are actual goal objects or rewards that incite, arouse, and move to action when they are associated with certain stimuli that signal their presence. For example, one may be motivated by the promise of a raise for good work or by various signs that one will obtain money, as well as by the money itself. Incentives are among the factors that increase the vigor of behavior; one will work harder for $10,000 than for $10.

Incentives are among the factors that increase the vigor of behavior. Incentives operate in two ways: (1) "they are goals or pleasant anticipations of repeating past experiences in the near future" and (2) "they strengthen responses which precede their delivery" (De-Cecco and Crawford, 1974, p. 154). Positive and negative reinforcers can be viewed as incentives (Skinner, 1953). Bandura (1962) studied the relationship of incentives to imitative learning in children and found out that children identify with the adult who is rewarded (for aggressive behavior) in their presence and are alienated from the adult who is punished or left unrewarded (for aggressive behavior).

PUNISHMENT

Solomon (1964) defined punishment as a stimulus the individual seeks to avoid. Under particular conditions, a punishment procedure may suppress undesirable responses, especially when the individual is permitted to make an alternative response to the one that is punished.

DeCecco (1968) pointed out that as in the case of anxiety and frustration, the experimental evidence does not warrant the exclusion of punishment procedure from the repertory of techniques the teacher may use to control the behavior of students and discipline them.

Whiting and Mowrer (1943) used the procedure of punishment where the animal was permitted to make an alternative response that was desirable and incompatible with the punished response. They used this technique successfully to housebreak a dog. Similar principles apply to training and disciplining a child. DeCecco and Crawford (1974) also pointed out that the practical implications of the experimental findings on punishment are within the realm of the teacher's disciplinary function.

Types of motives

There are several different types of motives that affect learning and instruction: social, task, and achievement motives.

SOCIAL MOTIVES

The existence of social motivation is often related to affiliative needs of the learner. Working with other students and relating appropriately to the teacher become essential for learning. The student becomes motivated by a desire to gain the approval of others, to avoid disapproval, and to establish a position of social esteem among classmates and peers. There is also evidence that warmth and nurturance expressed by the teacher toward the learner (especially children) clearly relate to performance of the young learner on concept formation and memory and affect the imitation of irrelevant behavior performed by adults and picked up through vicarious learning (Hartup, 1958; Rosenblith, 1959, Bandura and Huston, 1961; Gewirtz, 1956). Cogan (1958) also found that warm and considerate teachers got an unusual amount of original poetry. Reed (1962) found that warm teachers affected pupil's interest in sciences.

TASK MOTIVATION

Task motivation is also referred to as desire for mastery. It involves the learning of intellectual skills that enables the learner to function independently. Reinforcement for such learning is provided by the accuracy and completeness of accomplishment of tasks the learner undertakes. According to Ausubel (1968), such "cognitive" motives may be considered to be the most important kind of motivation in school learning. He stated that the casual relationship between motivation and learning is reciprocal rather than unidirectional; therefore, it is not necessary to hold instruction until the learner is ready and motivated. Ausubel suggested that the teacher proceed with the instruction. Even though not motivated, the student will learn something, and from this initial satisfaction of learning the student will, hopefully, develop the motivation to learn more. Ausubel further proposed that under some circumstances, the most appropriate way of arousing motivation is by learning to focus on the cognitive rather than the motivational aspect of learning and to rely on motivation that is generated from successful educational achievement and by learning to energize further learning (Ausubel, 1968, pp. 365-366).

Skinner (1968) holds a similar view. He noted that the problem of motivation in school situations is not a matter of imparting motivation, but of arranging the conditions for study and learning (contigencies of reinforcement) so that they will be reinforcing.

ACHIEVEMENT MOTIVE

Achievement motive is also referred to by Sears and Hilgard (1964) as *ego-integrative motive*. By ego-integrative motive Sears and Hilgard mean the group of motives that serve to maintain self-confidence and self-esteem. The motivation to achieve goes beyond task mastery. As mentioned previously, in achievement motivation individuals may acquire a persisting trait of striving to achieve that provides motivation for their activities, including those that pertain to school learning. It is McClelland's (1965) view that a combination of techniques, such as clear delineation of personal goals, perception of self-improvement, assuming responsibility for one's own actions, and having a supportive social environment, can lead to the acquisition of achievement motivation.

Another theory about achievement was advanced by White (1959). He referred to it as *competence motivation*. White viewed it as having a biological origin, related to such sources of motivation as exploration, activity, and manipulation, as they have been studied in animal experiments. White maintained that child's activities can be explained not by means of need satisfaction (such as hunger and thirst), but through the persistence of activities that constitute effective interaction with the environment and that are accompanied by the "feeling of efficacy" (Gagne, 1970, pp. 287-288).

Gagne pointed out the theoretical issue that is inherent in describing what constitutes motivation and how it operates and whether it is intrinsic to the person or closely related to the performance of learning tasks. Gagne (1970, p. 288) further speculated that "perhaps such motivation is simply an example of the shifting of control from one task activity to another through reinforcement contingencies; perhaps it is learned as a persisting general state of motivation to achieve, or perhaps it is an innately determined drive for competence." Even though the explanations of these approaches are different, their practical implications are somewhat similar. For instance, the learner can be rewarded, and subsequent learning can be facilitated by the achievement of learning tasks that are within the learner's capabilities. Achievement, successful interaction within the learning environment, and mastery of educational objectives can lead to persisting satisfaction on the part of the learner and, therefore, can be a source of motivation (Gagne, 1970, pp. 288-289).

Another important issue in motivation that was already touched on very briefly is in the area of uncertainty about the relationship between motivation and learning. Sears and Hilgard (1964) pointed out that some extreme positions assert that motivation affects only performance, not learning; another viewpoint is that motivation is an irrelevant category and that all learning is eventually under the control of the stimuli. Yet another view is that learning (habit formation) arises through simple contiguous association, independent of motivation, while motivation affects utilization of habit, that is, performance.

Application to nursing education and practice
Motivational function of the teacher

There are some general functions the teacher should perform to increase student motivation. These are arousal, expectancy, incentive, and disciplinary functions.

AROUSAL FUNCTION

The arousal function involves the initial responsibility of winning the students' attention and the continuing responsibility of regulating the level of arousal to avoid both sleep and emotional eruption. The arousal function of the teacher is mainly concerned with enabling the students to engage in learning. Learners will perform best when neither sleepy nor frantic, but alert. Therefore, one thing the nurse-teacher can do is to guard against monotony and boredom. The teacher should provide students with enough to think about and to do. In order to keep the learners alert, instruction must provide a certain measure of freedom to wander from one aspect of the subject to another. Learning-by-discovery and brainstorming techniques provide this freedom. Teaching methods can capitalize on the students' need for novel stimulation, their curiosity, and their desire for exploration. Bruner (1961) suggested the learning-by-discovery technique, because learners will engage in learning with the autonomy of self-reward. In this situation students provide their own stimulation and keep themselves aroused. White (1959, p. 318) called the child's "intrinsic need to deal with the environment" competence motivation. It arouses curiosity and increases exploratory behavior.

Torrance's (1962) study on brainstorming showed that the freer, or more open conditions of brainstorming and the originality of responses produce greater motivation or response vigor than the more closed conditions of responding for prizes and simple quantity of responses.

Regulation of the level of arousal includes being aware of the student's, patient's, or client's level of anxiety and frustration, assessing reaction to anxiety and frustration, and intervening to increase or decrease the level of arousal (DeCecco and Crawford, 1974).

EXPECTANCY FUNCTION

The expectancy function of the teacher requires making explicit to the students, what they (the students) will be able to do at the completion of instruction. Instructional objectives are expectancies. They must be concrete enough for the learners to know what is expected. Behaviors expected of students should be stated in terms (words) that are measurable and/or observable. Furthermore, the teacher should take into consideration the learner's entering behavior. Whatever behavior that the objective (expectancy) is asking, the teacher must make sure that the learner has the capability of doing it, that is, it must be within the range of the capability of the learner.

Instructional objectives are intermediate-level expectancies. Whenever these objectives require considerable time and effort on the part of the student, the teacher should set up subtasks and describe them concretely, so that the student's effort does not wane along the way. The student must feel a continued sense of accomplishment. Most students get impatient quickly when things drag on, or with errors and slight gains.

Remote goals refer to the student's long-range life expectancies for, career, home, family, and friends. The choice of these goals, and they way in which the student pursues these goals indicates basic beliefs about what will bring happiness and satisfaction. The inspiring teacher is the one who relates what the student does today to what the student desires to do later in life.

Since expectancies are learned anticipations of the consequences of behavior, De-Cecco and Crawford (1974) suggested two ways in which expectancies can be modified. First, the actual past experience of success and failure is the primary basis for predicting future chances of success and failure. Since success breeds success and failure breeds failure, the teacher must be alert to and work with those students who have never experienced success in order to modify their expectancies. For such students teachers must provide academic success at the level of their entering behavior before they will raise their expectancies to include more difficult future outcomes. Second, the teacher also can control students' expectancies by telling them what their chances of success or failure will be. Teachers often do this with the students during their counseling or advising sessions. Teachers look at each student's previous grades, general intelligence, past performances, and course choice to make some estimates of the student's probable success. Students usually expend most of their energy where they expect the most success.

Since expectancy is dependent on valence, or anticipated satisfactions, Vroom (1964, p. 23) suggested two ways of increasing the student's valence: (1) giving information that increases the desirability of one outcome over the other when students are unfamiliar with the possible results that can be attained, and (2) arousing appropriate motives by telling students that on completion of instruction they will be able to do things they cannot do now. This often provides great incentive.

Bachman's (1964) study found that expectation of success is greatest when a person thinks he has the appropriate training and when free to use it (DeCecco and Crawford, 1974).

Hunt (1961, pp. 267-272) suggested still another way of increasing the learner's motivation by mismatching expectancies. The discrepancy hypothesis states that a moderate amount, a positive degree of discrepancy between what we experience and what we expect to experience can be a source of satisfaction and motivation. Hunt believes that a perfect match between what is expected and what is experienced results in boredom. To avoid boredom of this type teachers can introduce incongruity, complexity, and "suprisingness" into their lessions. The new teaching material must have a proper mixture of familiar and unfamiliar items to attract and maintain the student's attention. Gewirtz's (1959) study in school settings supports the idea of increased motivation through mismatching.

INCENTIVE FUNCTION

A teacher is said to exercise an incentive function by rewarding the students' achievement in a way that encourages them to exert further effort. Incentives are goal objects or symbols that the teacher uses to produce increased vigor in learners. Examples of incentives are feedback of test results, spoken or written praise and encouragement, grades, or results of successful competition. There are several ways the teacher can use each of these rewards effectively.

Feedback. DeCecco and Crawford (1974) indicated that knowledge of results is a very useful incentive because it not only will increase the students' vigor, but also will play an important part in learning procedures and in performance assessments. Test results must be fed back to the students with sufficient frequency and in a form that will confirm their expectancies. Test results that exceed the students' expectation give them a tremendous feeling of satisfaction and become a source of motivation. The teacher, therefore, must provide immediate feedback to the students. Teachers can also arrange instructional materials and procedures in ways that permit students to do their own checking and assess their own performances. Programmed instruction provides such feedback.

Praise and blame or reproof. The fact that human beings psychologically crave recognition or approval renders encouragement and discouragement, praise and reproof effective as incentives. Heidgerken (1953) pointed out that the level of a person's self-esteem is very definitely affected by what others say about the person's competency, beauty, intelligence, and other qualities.

A number of studies have been conducted to determine the effectiveness of praise, reproof, and encouragement in learning and performance. Brigg's (1927) and Hurlock (1924) both demonstrated that children in praised groups gained the most in their performances, in reproved groups gained some, and in ignored groups who heard the praise and the reproof gained a little; but the control group, who received neither praise nor reproof, did not gain at all.

It has also been found that the relative effectiveness of praise and reproof varies with age, sex, and ability. For example, average students usually make the greatest gains as a result of praise; bright students usually make the least gain (Heidgerken, 1953). Therefore, teachers must be very careful in the use of praise and reproof. Mere usage of these incentives does not make a good teacher. Unwise use can create undesirable traits in the students. Overuse can weaken their effectiveness. The teacher should use praise and reproof to build a sense of achievement within the students, that is, to give them a

feeling of satisfaction because they have attained worthwhile objectives. Heidgerken asserted that the teacher should not use praise merely for the sake of praising. It is far better for the teacher to encourage the students by recognition of their progress than to praise them indiscriminately.

Grades as incentives. Grades are and should be used as feedback. Strength and weakness must be pointed out so that students can benefit from their tests. Page (1958) conducted a very extensive study with 2139 junior and senior high school students. He tested the effects of three methods of grading: During the first phase he had three groups, and each group received a different grading strategy:

Group 1—*No comment* group, received only their test score and equivalent letter grade
Group 2—*Free comment* group, received personalized comments that conformed to the teacher's own feelings and practices
Group 3—*Specified comment* group, received the following stereotyped comments for each letter grade:
A—Excellent, keep it up
B—Good work, keep it up
C—Perhaps try to do still better
D—Let's bring this up
E—Let's raise this grade

During the second phase of the experiment, the students were given a second test to determine the effects of the previously mentioned three grading practices. Results showed that both the free comment group and the specified comment group did better than the no comment group. The free comment group did better (but not significantly better) than the specified comment group. The "E" students who received the free comment showed greatest improvement. The effect of the comments did not depend on student ability or school year.

Page concluded from this study that

teachers should take the time to write encouraging comments on student's papers.

Competition and rivalry. There are three types of competition and rivalry:

1. Competition in which an individual is one of a group competing with another group
2. Competition in which an individual is competing with other individuals within the same group
3. Self-competition in which an individual is competing against own self

Competition can be held against absent or imaginery rivals. It can be either intentional and explicit or implicit. As evidenced by a number of studies (Deutsch, 1960; Coleman, 1961), group competition produces substantial gains. However, group competition is not always desirable because it often substitutes the wrong motives for objectives of education. In addition, activity under such conditions does not yield permanent outcomes. Achievement subsides when competition is removed. However, group competition may be used occasionally and effectively to bring a class of students out of boredom and to restore morale (Heidgerken, 1953, p. 152).

Because of the wide range of abilities between individuals in an average class, the teacher must be very careful in using group competition. The slower students cannot keep up with the brighter students and, as a result, they become discouraged and bored or resort to dishonest means of keeping up with the group. Still another factor to be considered in using group competition is that the quality of work suffers under such conditions. Heidgerken concluded by saying that the best use of group competition is to stimulate and teach cooperation.

Self-competition yields the greatest amount of learning. It is the fairest type because the individual is not competing with someone of greater ability. Its stimulative and motivational power does not wear out.

The teacher should facilitate self-competition by acquainting the student with results. Self-competition without knowledge of results is pointless.

DISCIPLINARY FUNCTION

The disciplinary function of the teacher requires the use of restitution and ripple effect in order to control deviant behavior.

Restitution. Restitution refers to the disciplinary technique where the student performs properly what was originally performed improperly. It combines the supression of one response (deviant) with the substitution of another (desirable response). The latter behavior must be rewarded. DeCecco and Crawford (1974) pointed out that the restitution technique, which involves both reward and expression, is preferrable to suppression technique (punishment) alone because it focuses on learning new, acceptable social behaviors rather than on stamping out undesirable responses. Restitution technique creates a situation where there is response competition (the deviant behavior competes with the desirable behavior), with the hope that the desirable behavior will win out.

Any disciplinary technique involves two operations: the presentation of an aversive stimuli (punishment) and the withdrawal of the positive reinforcer. Bandura and Walters (1963) suggested that disciplinary techniques should emphasize rewards that are withdrawn until the child (or the student) complies with the demand or makes restitution. When disciplinary methods are used by warm, affectionate parents (or teachers) children seem to develop self-control and social conscience. When punishment alone is used, children learn to avoid the person who does the punishing.

The ripple effect. Kounin and Gump (1958) described the ripple effect as the way students are affected as a result of witnessing a disciplinary technique used against their classmates.

Gnagey (1965) suggested several ways in which the teacher can arrange the conditions that cause the ripple effect to increase control over the class:

1. Using nonthreatening techniques to avoid negative reactions to the teacher and the lesson
2. Making clear who the student is that performed a deviant act, what the misbehavior is, and what the proper alternative response should be
3. Increasing firmness by lowering or raising the voice and by getting close to the student and looking at the student directly
4. Focusing attention on the learning task and not on teacher approval
5. Being knowledgeable and having well-prepared lessons in the subject area, since students are less likely to misbehave when they are engaged in learning

These techniques have beneficial effects on both the misbehaving student and classmates because of the ripple effect (DeCecco and Crawford, 1974, p. 171).

Observed teacher-student interactions resulting in motivation

Sears and Hilgard (1964) identified three types of teacher-student interactions that affect student performance and motivation. They are: (1) affective, (2) evaluative, and (3) cognitive interactions.

AFFECTIVE INTERACTION

Affective interactions between the teacher and the students are influenced by the emotional-attitudinal variables.

Kounin and Gump (1961) and Kounin, Gump, and Dyan (1961) studied the effects of different types of disciplinary techniques and found three things. (1) *Punitive technique* resulted in the subjects rating the deviancy as "most serious" and the degree of interference with attention to the task the greatest. (2) *Simple reprimand* resulted in students rating the teacher's fairness highest, and students paid more attention to the lesson after witnessing the event (ripple effect). (3) In *ignoring condition* students rated the teacher as highest in her liking for children, but they thought the misbehavior would most likely recur.

Spaulding (1963) found strong negative correlation between the expression of creativity in elementary school–aged children and teacher behavior that is characterized by formal group instruction and using shame as a punitive technique.

Sears (1963) showed a positive correlation between creativity and the teacher rewarding by showing personal interest in the child's ideas, accompanied by high frequency of listening to the child.

Sarason and Mandler (1952) related anxiety to achievement and performance and found: (a) low-anxiety college students did better (in general) on laboratory tasks than high-anxiety students; (b) pressure to complete the task improved the performance for low-anxiety subjects, but did not do so for high-anxiety students.

EVALUATIVE INTERACTION

Evaluation can be done individually in such a manner as to threaten self-esteem, or it can be done according to group standards and thus be less threatening.

A teacher's evaluative activities go far beyond marking papers. They include attention to many experiences of success and failure, of expanded or restricted autonomy, of immediate or long-term goal setting, of recognition of individual progress, and of attitudinal response to divergent behavior. These evaluative behaviors have the characteristics of positive and negative reinforcers (incentives) and, as such, are motivationally relevant to learning.

COGNITIVE INTERACTION

Some plausible conjectures about autocratic and democratic atmospheres do not appear to be supported by studies (Lewin, Lippitti, and White, 1939; Spaulding, 1963). Ryans (1961) found that a businesslike approach, a matter-of-fact method, and warmth had an effect on student achievement and creativity. Also, support was given to nondirective approaches—apparently they kept alive the searching behavior of the student that is important for divergent thinking.

Variables influencing learner's motivation and performance

Such variables as the learner's personality, the teacher's personality, socioeconomic background of the student, and instructional procedures all affect the learner's level of motivation and performance.

Learner's personality

The learner's own personality affects ability to profit from a particular kind of teaching. For example, highly compulsive and anxious children do well (overachieve) in structured teaching situations. Highly anxious but low-compulsive children do poorly (underachieve) in unstructured situations (Sears and Hilgard, 1964).

Dependency tendencies of the children also affect the profit that they derive from teaching techniques. For example, Kagan and Mussen (1956) and Liveson and Mussen (1957) found that dependent-prone children are more likely to comply with an authority figure and conform to group pressure than less dependent children. Their results suggest that dependent-prone children might become overly concerned with following the suggestions and directions of a teacher and more dependent on support and encouragement. Hence, teachers must know their students and must be flexible in their approaches if they are to have the most favorable results.

Teacher personality

Heil, Powell, and Feifer (1960) conducted a study and compared the effects of different types of teacher personality (self-controlling versus fearful versus turbulent) on achievement behavior of children. Results of this study showed that self-controlled teachers positively affected the achievement behavior of students.

Another dimension—that of teacher warmth—appears to affect creativity in students. The warmer and more supportive teacher encourages divergent behavior in students. Bandura and Huston (1961) also pointed out that teacher personality has an influence on teaching effectiveness because of the importance of the teacher as a "model" for pupil behavior.

Socioeconomic variable

The socioeconomic background of the student effects achievement motivation. Kahl (1957) found that by the time a student reaches junior high school, achievement is more related to the father's profession than to the child's intelligence.

School environment and instructional procedures

School environment and atmosphere contribute to the arousal and support of particular motives. The way in which students are grouped may affect their receptivity to teaching by given teachers. Furthermore, the way in which the school is set up will determine whether or not creativity will be encouraged (Sears and Hilgard, 1964).

Instructional procedures have a definite affect on the motivation of the students. For example, Suchman's (1961) program with inquiry training in skills, with reference to science instruction, recommends that some dissonance is necessary for development of inquiry skills.

As mentioned previously, Hunt (1961) has suggested that controlling intrinsic motivation is a matter of providing circumstances of the proper level of incongruity with the residues of previous encounters.

Gallagher (1964), furthermore, pointed out that when students are free to work out their own solution to problems, that is, when they have an opportunity for divergent rather than convergent thinking, intrinsic motivation appears to be readily aroused.

Smedslund also asserted that the type of teaching material used will decide the arousal of orienting response (Sears and Hilgard, 1964).

Researchable questions

Further research is necessary in the area of accommodating individual differences in motivation. In other words, how can instruction be so structured as to promote intrinsic motivation in students. Research is also needed in comparing the effects of different teaching strategies on student motivation, scholastic achievement, and affective behavior. For example, what is the effect of making contracts (about achievement of course objectives) as opposed to using the traditional lecture-discussion method of instruction on the affective behavior of students (that is, desire for more learning and attitudes toward the subject matter)? Also, what is the effect of the size of the classroom, as between the seminar-type of instruction with 8 to 10 students and the traditional lecture-discussion method with 20 to 30 students on the achivement and affective behaviors of the students.

ADDITIONAL LEARNING EXPERIENCES—RECOMMENDED READING LIST

DeCecco, J. P., and Crawford, W. *The psychology of learning and instruction: educational psychology.* (2nd Ed.) Englewood Cliffs, N.J.: Prentice-Hall, Inc., 1974, p. 136-173.

Gagne, R. M. *The conditions of learning.* (2 Ed.) New York: Holt, Rinehart and Winston, Inc., 1970, pp. 281-289.

Sears, P. S., and Hilgard, E. R. The teacher's role in the motivation of the learner. In E. R. Hilgard (Ed.), *Theories of learning and instruction.* The 63rd Yearbook of N.S.S.E., Chicago: The University of Chicago Press, 1964, pp. 182-209.

INSTRUCTIONS TO THE LEARNER REGARDING POSTTEST

Having completed studying the content of this module, you are now ready to take the posttest to determine the extent to which you have achieved the objectives. Return to the pretest and take it over again as the posttest. Correct your answers using the same answer key found on this page and the next. You need to achieve 38 points to be considered as having mastered the module at the 95% level. If your score is less than 38 points, correct your errors, study the content of this module over again more carefully, and read some of the articles in the recommended reading list. Study in this fashion until you achieve the 95% mastery level or better on the posttest.

ANSWER KEY TO PRETEST AND POSTTEST

1. c (DeCecco and Crawford, 1974, p. 137)
2. c (Sears, 1967, p. 35)
3. d (DeCecco and Crawford, 1974, p. 139)
4. b (DeCecco and Crawford, 1974, p. 140)
5. c (DeCecco and Crawford, 1974, pp. 141-144)
6. c (DeCecco and Crawford, 1974, pp. 140-148)
7. c (DeCecco and Crawford, 1974, pp. 140-144, 149)
8. c (DeCecco and Crawford, 1974, pp. 148-153)
9. c (DeCecco and Crawford, 1974, p. 150)
10. b (DeCecco and Crawford, 1974, p. 152)
11. b (DeCecco and Crawford, 1974, pp. 148-152)
12. b and c (DeCecco and Crawford, 1974, pp. 153-154)
13. c (Solomon, 1964; DeCecco and Crawford, 1974, p. 192)
14. b (DeCecco and Crawford, 1974, pp. 156-159)
15. c (DeCecco and Crawford, 1974, pp. 159-161)
16. a (DeCecco and Crawford, 1974, pp. 164-169)
17. b (DeCecco and Crawford, 1974, pp. 169-171)
18. c (DeCecco and Crawford, 1974, pp. 170-171)

19. b (DeCecco and Crawford, 1974, p. 140)
20. g (DeCecco and Crawford, 1974, pp. 152-153)
21. d (DeCecco and Crawford, 1974, p. 148)
22. f (DeCecco and Crawford, 1974, p. 150)
23. e (DeCecco and Crawford, 1974, p. 153)
24. c (DeCecco and Crawford, 1974, p. 151)
25. a (Solomon, 1964; DeCecco and Crawford, 1974, p. 192)
26. f, D (Kaluger and Unkovic, 1969, p. 71)
27. e, A (White, 1959, pp. 297-333)
28. d, B (Maslow, 1954, pp. 149-180)
29. a, C (Berlyne, 1957, pp. 399-404)
30. b, F (McClelland, and others, 1953)
31. c, E (Berlyne, 1957, pp. 399-404)
32. Answers will vary. Some of the criteria that may have been discussed are that the client:
    a. Can give reasons for belonging to the group (developing a motive)
    b. Understands the motive is realistic and can link the motive to deeds and to daily events in own life
    c. Commits self to concrete goals
    d. Keeps a record of progress
    e. Has honest and warm support
    f. Engages in self-study
    g. Has a feeling of belonging to a successful group

    (DeCecco and Crawford, 1974, pp. 151-153)

REFERENCES

Atkinson, J. W. (Ed.) *Motives in fantasy, action, and society.* New York: Van Nostrand Reinhold Co., Inc., 1958.

Ausubel, D. P. *Educational psychology: a cognitive view.* New York: Holt, Rinehart and Winston, Inc., 1968.

Bachman, J. G. Motivation in a task situation as a function of ability and control over task. *Journal of Abnormal and Social Psychology,* 1964, **69:**272-281.

Bandura, A. The influence of rewarding and punishing models on the acquisition and performance of imitative responses. An unpublished manuscript. Stanford University, Stanford 1962.

Bandura, A., and Huston, A. C. Identification as a process of incidental learning. *Journal of Abnormal and Social Psychology,* 1961, **63:**311-318.

Bandura, A., and Walters, R. H. *Social learning and personality development.* New York: Holt, Rinehart and Winston, Inc., 1963.

Berlyne, D. E. Conflict and information-theory variables as determinants of human perceptual curiosity. *Journal of Experimental Psychology,* 1957, **53:**399-404.

Bexton, W., Heron, W., and Scott, T. H. Effects of decreased variation in the sensory environment. *Canadian Journal of Psychology,* 1954, **8:**70-76.

Briggs, T. H. Praise and censure as incentives. *School and Society,* 1927, **26:**597-598.

Bruner, J. *The process of education.* Cambridge, Mass.: Harvard University Press, 1960.

Bruner, J. The act of discovery. *Harvard Educational Review,* 1961, **31:**21-32.

Cogan, M. L. The behavior of teachers and the productive behavior of their pupils. *Journal of Experimental Education,* 1958, **27:**89-124.

Coleman, J. S. *The adolescent subculture.* New York: The Free Press of Glencoe, Inc., 1961.

DeCecco, J., and Crawford, W. *The psychology of learning and instruction: educational psychology.* (2nd Ed.) Englewood Cliffs, N.J.: Prentice-Hall, Inc., 1974.

Deutsch, M. The effects of cooperation and competition on group process. In D. Cartwright and A. Iander (Eds.), *Group dynamics: research and theory.* Evanston, Ill.: Row and Peterson, 1960, pp. 414-448.

Dollard, J., and others. *Frustration and agression.* New Haven, Conn.: Yale University Press, 1939.

Fowler, H. *Curiosity and exploratory behavior.* New York: The Macmillan Co., 1965.

Gagne, R. M. *The conditions of learning.* (2nd Ed.) New York: Holt, Rinehart and Winston, Inc., 1970.

Gallagher, J. J. *Teaching the gifted child.* Boston: Allyn & Bacon, Inc., 1964.

Gewirtz, H. B. Generalization of children's preferences as a function of reinforcement and task similarity. *Journal of Abnormal and Social Psychology,* 1959, **58:**111-118.

Gewirtz, J. L. A program of research on the dimensions and antecedents of emotional dependence. *Child Development,* 1956, **27:**206-211.

Gnagey, W. J. *Controlling classroom misbehavior.* Department of Classroom Teachers, American Educational Research Association, National Education Association, Washington, D.C., 1965.

Harlow, H. F., Harlow, M. K., and Meyer, D. R. Learning motivated by a manipulation drive. *Journal of Experimental Psychology,* 1950, **40:**228-234.

Hartup, W. W. Nurturance and nurturance-withdrawal in relation to the dependency behavior of pre-school children. *Child Development,* 1958, **29:**191-203.

Hebb, D. O. Drives and C.N.S. (conceptual nervous system). *Psychological Review,* 1955, **62:**243-254.

Heidgerken, L. E. *Teaching in schools of nursing and principles and methods.* (2nd Ed.) Philadelphia: J. B. Lippincott Co., 1953.

Heil, L. M., Powell, M., and Feifer, I. *Characteristics of teacher behavior related to the achievement of children in several elementary grades.* U.S. Department of Health, Education and Welfare, Office of Education, Cooperative Research Branch, Washington, D.C., 1960.

Hunt, J. McV. *Intelligence and experience.* New York: The Ronald Press Co., 1961.

Hurlock, E. B. The value of praise and reproof as incentives for children. *Archives of Psychology,* 1924, **11**(71):1-78.

James, W. *Talks to teachers on psychology and to students on some of life's ideals.* New York: W. W. Norton & Co., Inc., 1892 (1958).

Kagan, J., and Mussen, P. H. Dependency themes on the TAT and group conformity. *Journal of Consulting Psychology,* 1956, **20**:19-27.

Kahl, J. A. *The American class structure.* New York: Holt, Rinehart and Winston, Inc., 1957.

Kaluger, G., and Unkovic, C. M. *Psychology and sociology: an integrated approach to understanding human behavior.* St. Louis: The C. V. Mosby Book Co., 1969.

Kounin, J. S., and Gump, P. V. The ripple effect in discipline. *Elementary School Journal,* 1958, **59**:158-162.

Kounin, J. S., and Gump, P. V. The comparative influence of punitive and nonpunitive teachers upon children's concepts of school misconduct. *Journal of Educational Psychology,* 1961, **52**:44-49.

Kounin, J. S., Gump, P. V., Ryan, J. J. Exploration in classroom management. *Journal of Teacher Education,* 1961, **12**:235-246.

Lawson, R. *Frustration: the development of a scientific concept.* New York: The Macmillan Co., 1965.

Lewin, K., Lippitti, R., and White, R. K. Patterns of aggressive behavior in experimentally created 'social climates.' *Journal of Social Psychology,* 1939, **10**:271-299.

Liveson, N., and Mussen, P. H. The relation of control to overt agression and dependency. *Journal of Abnormal and Social Psychology,* 1957, **55**:66-71.

Mandler, S. B., Mandler, G., and Craighill, P. G. The effect of differential instructions on anxiety and learning. *Journal of Abnormal and Social Psychology,* 1952, **47**:561-565.

Maslow, A. *Motivation and personality.* New York: Harper and Row, Publishers. 1954.

McClelland, D. O., Atkinson, J. W., Clark, R. A., and Lowell, E. L. *The achievement motive.* New York: Appleton-Century-Crofts, 1953.

Nissen, H. W. Instinct as seen by a psychologist. *Psychological Review.* 1953, **60**:291-294.

Page, E. B. Teacher comments and student performance. *Journal of Education Psychology,* 1958, **49**:173-181.

Reed, H. B. Implications for science education of a teacher competence research. *Science Education,* 1962, **46**:473-486.

Risk, T. M. *Principles and practices of teaching in secondary education.* New York: American Book Co., 1941.

Rosenblith, J. F. Learning by imitation in kindergarten children. *Child Development,* 1959, **30**:69-80.

Ryans, D. G. Some relationships between pupil behavior and certain teacher characteristics. *Journal of Educational Psychology,* 1961, **52**:82-90.

Sarason, S. B., and Mandler, G. Some correlates of test anxiety. *Journal of Abnormal and Social Psychology,* 1952, **47**:810-817.

Sears, P. S. *The effect of classroom conditions in strength of achievement motive and work output of elementary school children.* Stanford, Calif.: Stanford University Press, 1963.

Sears, P. S. Implications of motivational theory for independent learning. In G. Gleason (Ed.), *The theory and nature of independent learning.* Scranton, Pa.: International Textbook Co., 1967, pp. 35-50.

Sears, P. S., and Hilgard, E. R. The teacher's role in the motivation of the learner. In E. R. Hilgard (Ed.), *Theories of learning and instruction.* The 63rd Yearbook of N.S.S.E. Chicago: The University of Chicago Press, 1964, pp. 182-209.

Skinner, B. F. *Science and human behavior.* New York: Macmillan Co., 1953.

Skinner, B. F. *The technology of teaching.* New York: The Macmillan Co., 1968.

Solomon, R. L. Punishment. *American Psychologist,* 1964, **19**:239-253.

Spaulding, R. Achievement, creativity and self-concept correlates of teacher-pupil transactions in elementary schools. U.S. Office of Education, Cooperative Research Project, No. 1352. Urbana, Ill.: University of Illinois Press, 1963.

Spence, K. W. *Behavior theory and conditioning.* New Haven, Conn.: Yale University Press, 1956.

Spielberger, C. *Anxiety and behavior.* New York: Academic Press, Inc., 1966.

Suchman, J. R. Inquiry training: building skills for autonomous discovery. *Merrill Palmer Quarterly,* 1961, **7**:147-169.

Torrance, E. P. (Ed.) *Guiding creative talent.* Englewood Cliffs, N.J.: Prentice-Hall, Inc., 1962.

Tyler, R. *Basic principles of curriculum and instruction.* Chicago: University of Chicago Press, 1971.

Vroom, V. H. *Work and motivation.* New York: John Wiley & Sons, Inc., 1964.

White, R. W. Motivation reconsidered: the concept of competence. Psychological Review, 1959, **66**:297-333.

Whiting, J. W. M., and Mowrer, O. H. Habit progression and regression—a laboratory study of some factors relevant to human socialization. *Journal of Comparative Psychology,* 1943, **36**:229-253.

MODULE 29

Evaluation

DESCRIPTION OF MODULE

This module is an independent and complete unit of instruction on evaluation in general and evaluation of instruction in specific. In addition to the learner objectives, instructions to the learner, and a pre- and posttest; the module contains the basic text, which is the instructional material. This basic content covers five basic areas that are presented in an integrated form. They are: (1) theoretical framework, (2) relevant research studies, (3) issues, (4) application to nursing education and nursing practice, and (5) research areas. The content of this module is presented in sequential order. References for additional learning experiences in the form of recommended readings are also suggested at the end.

MODULE OBJECTIVES

At the completion of this module and having studied the additional recommended reading list, the student will be able to accomplish the following behavioral objectives at the 95% level of mastery. The student will be able to:

1. Operationally define Wittrock's approach to the evaluation of instruction
2. Identify the purposes for evaluating instruction
3. Distinguish between formal and informal evaluation
4. Identify the three fundamental components of the evaluation of instruction
5. Recognize examples of how the environment of learning is evaluated
6. Recognize examples of how learners are evaluated
7. Distinguish between general goals of education and behavioral objectives
8. List the five steps of the process for evaluating learning
9. Distinguish between formative and summative evaluation
10. Cite research studies that are relevant to evaluation of instruction
11. Identify an issue relevant to the evaluation of instruction
12. Raise a researchable question and identify both the independent and dependent variables

PRETEST AND POSTTEST

Circle the correct answers. Each question is worth 1 point. The 95% level of mastery for this test is 22 correct points. Take the test and correct your answers using the answer key found at the end of this module (p. 479). If you score 22 points or better, you need not study this module.

Multiple choice

1. The purpose of evaluating instruction is:
   a. to evaluate students

b. to evaluate teachers

c. to evaluate environments

d. to make decisions about the instruction

e. to make judgments about the instruction

2. Norm-referenced method of evaluation refers to those situations where:

a. established tests are used

b. an individual's performance score is compared with an established and/or standard norm group

c. means and standard deviations are used to offer intragroup and intergroup comparisons

d. an individual's performance is compared against own past performance

e. the degree of the student's mastery of the subject matter is measured

3. Criterion-referenced evaluation refers to those situations where:

a. performance scores are compared against a set target

b. absolute behavioral objectives are used to evaluate performance

c. student's standing in the group is measured

d. grading is done utilizing the normal curve

e. the use of formative evaluation is a must

4. The degree of learning is measured by means of:

a. giving a summative test and determining the amount of learning that has taken place

b. the grade the student receives in the course

c. assessing the student's behavior before and after instruction has taken place

d. standard achievement tests

5. When evaluation is done during the planning and implementation phases of the project, task, or program, it is referred to as:

a. pretest

b. summative evaluation

c. formative evaluation

d. criterion-referenced evaluation

e. norm-referenced evaluation

6. Judgments are passed under the circumstances of:

a. formative tests

b. summative tests

c. cumulative evaluation

d. achievement test scores

7. A final examination is an example of which type of evaluation:

a. formative

b. summative

c. cumulative

d. comprehensive

8. According to Tyler (1950), the first step in the evaluation process is:

a. listing the situations that will provide for the expression of the desired behavior

b. examining available evaluation instruments

c. identifying and clearly defining objectives for learning

d. constructing an evaluation instrument

9. The type of evaluation system that provides the learner with feedback, pacing of learning, reinforcement, and identification of strengths and weaknesses is referred to as:

a. criterion-referenced evaluation

b. formative evaluation

c. norm-referenced evaluation

d. summative evaluation

10. The following statements that pertain to behavioral objectives are:

a. developing good citizenship

b. encouraging interest in the fine arts

c. being able to define in writing . . .

d. listing seven steps in the performance of a procedure

e. identifying the safety precautions important to a procedure

f. developing high standards of morality

11. The important elements that have to be specified in the statement of behavioral objectives are:

a. content

b. behavior

c. the type of instrument used

d. learner characteristics

12. Evaluation of instruction, according to Wittrock, is:

a. focusing on the qualities of the student's learning environment

b. testing the student's abilities, interests, and achievement after instruction

c. determining explicit changes in the student's behaviors as a result of instruction

d. evaluating the interaction of these three variables: learner, learning, and environment

13. Standardized achievement tests can adequately indicate
   a. how a student has learned
   b. what the relative state of the student's learning is
   c. what the student actually has learned
   d. why a student has learned what he has

14. The following examples that illustrate items that could be used for measuring the learning environment are:
   a. ranking student I.Q. levels
   b. counting the number of books in the library
   c. counting the number of times the student has instructed patients on insulin injection
   d. perusing course objectives
   e. studying evaluation tools
   f. counting the number of hours the student cared for premature babies

15. The following items that can be used to evaluate learners are:
   a. the student's standing in the group
   b. the student's score on standardized tests
   c. the number of hours the student spends in the library
   d. the intellectual merits of the student's teachers
   e. the number of homework problems the student does

16. The components of the evaluation of instruction are:
   a. evaluation of teachers
   b. evaluation of environments
   c. making norms explicit
   d. evaluation of learning
   e. testing components
   f. evaluation of learners

Matching

Part A

_____ 17. Evaluation of instruction
_____ 18. Norm-referenced evaluation
_____ 19. Evaluation
_____ 20. Measurement
_____ 21. Criterions reference evaluation
_____ 22. Formative evaluation
_____ 23. Summative evaluation

Part B

a. The process of appraisal that involves securing evidence on the attainment of specific objectives, acceptance of specific values, and the use of a variety of measuring instruments as a basis for value judgement

b. The type of evaluation where the learner's performance is compared against a specific behavioral objective

c. The type of evaluation that enables the learner's achievement to be compared with other learners in the group

d. Measuring the cause-and-effect relations among the learner, the learning environment, and the learning

e. A method of measurement that is implemented during the developmental, or the fluid stage, of the project

f. Assessment of a program of study at the completion of the program

g. A method of measuring individual differences

h. A method of evaluation that is often used with mastery learning and that acts as a diagnostic measure

i. Process of assigning quantitative values to observed phenomena

TEXT
Theoretical framework
Evaluation: nature, types, and procedures
NATURE OF EVALUATION

Evaluation refers to the process of appraisal, which involves securing evidence on the attainment of specific objectives, acceptance of specific values, and the use of a variety of measuring instruments as a basis for value judgments (Tyler, 1951).

Evaluation serves several purposes and functions. The basic purpose of evaluation is to make decisions and judgments. Stake (1967) pointed out the two main functions of evaluation: (1) to ascertain the nature and the size of the effects of the treatment, and (2) to decide whether or not the observed effects attain acceptable standards of excellence. He has termed these two components "description" and "judgment" respectively. The use of value judgments cannot be overemphasized in evaluation. Value judgments are made at many phases in the development and assessment of instructional systems. Judgments determine the anticipated behavioral outcomes, how they are to be achieved, the components to be measured, and the selection of instruments to assess the components. At a later stage, judgments are used to reach decisions from the outcome data.

Since evaluation is concerned with securing evidence on the achievement of objectives, methods of measurement must be found to judge the extent to which objectives have been attained. The standards against which the evidence is appraised may be the normative data on particular samples; it may also include the absolute criterion-referenced standards.

Norm-referenced and criterion-referenced methods of evaluation are designed to accomplish different purposes. Whether data is appraised by means of one of these methods or the other is determined by what is done with the data derived from the measurement. For instance, when an individual's performance score is compared with an established and/or standard norm group, then *norm-referenced* evaluation is utilized. An example, is the National League for Nursing (NLN) achievement tests, which are norm-referenced tests that compare the student with a national population. Grading on a normal-curve is another example of norm-referenced evaluation. Furthermore, when data is manipulated by the use of means, standard deviations, and the like, they offer intragroup and intergroup comparisons and are again examples of norm-referenced evaluation. The main purpose of norm-referenced evaluation is to compare where an individual stands in relation to others. It tells very little about the individual's degree of competence or capability, or the amount of learning that has actually taken place (Arndt and Huckabay, 1975).

Criterion-referenced methods of evaluation refer to those testing situations where an individual's performance is compared against a set target behavior objective. This type of evaluation enables the teacher or the learner to determine whether or not the student has achieved the specific objective and the degree of achievement of a set of objectives. This type of evaluation is particularly valuable in teaching-learning situations where active learning on the part of the learner is stressed. Furthermore, it indicates how well the student has mastered the given task. It also gives the student a sense of achievement and tends to decrease competitiveness with peers as well as creating the kind of climate where cooperative learning can take place (Arndt and Huckabay, 1975; Bevis, 1978).

Another purpose of evaluation is interpretation of data. For example, various patterns of outcomes may be interpreted to determine the kinds of changes taking place in the student or in a program, the kinds of errors that are made, and the reasons underlying the achievement or lack of achievement of the specified objective.

Within a teaching-learning situation, evaluation involves the systematical collection of evidence to determine the extent to which certain desirable changes in behavior are occurring in the individual. Bloom, Hastings, and Madaus (1971) pointed out that this concept of evaluation has two important aspects: (1) to assess the behavior of the individual, since it is change in the student's behaviors that is taught in education, and (2) to involve more than a single appraisal at any one time. In order to determine the extent of change that has taken place, appraisal at an early point in time and then at later points indicates changes that may have occurred.

TYPES OF EVALUATION

There are two types of evaluation; formative and summative. They differ in terms of purposes, functions, and timing.

Formative evaluation is concerned with the collection of appropriate evidence during the planning and implementation phases of a project, a course or curriculum, or a new learning task, so that revisions can be made based on this type of evidence.

Summative evaluation is used to assess a project or a plan, a course, or a learning task as its completion, when no changes in treatment can be made. The results of summative evaluation are used to make judgments and decisions about the task or project that is being evaluated.

In formative evaluation, no judgments are passed. The information obtained by means of formative evaluation is used to contribute to the individual's learning process and achievement of the objectives. One of the chief aims of formative evaluations is to determine the degree of mastery of a specified objective, such as a learning task, and to identify the part of the task that has not yet been mastered. This helps both the learner and the teacher. Successful communication of information to the learner about progress constitutes the very essence of formative evaluation.

Fundamental to the use of formative evaluation is the specification of a unit of learning or performance of a task. A unit of learning can be determined by natural breaks in the subject matter or by the content that makes a meaningful whole. For example, a unit of learning may be a chapter or a section in a book. It can also be specified in relation to a given period of time; for example, content covered during 1- or 2-week periods.

Once the unit of learning is identified, the unit is analyzed into its component parts. The *content* and the *behavior* aspects of objectives constitute the components of a learning unit. For example, if one of the objectives is stated: "At the completion of the first unit of learning on the anatomy of the human body, the student will be able to identify correctly the names of the bones of the body," the content aspect of this objective (learning unit) is "names of the bones of the body" and the behavior aspect of this unit refers to the response of the student, that is, what the student is supposed to do. In this case, the student has to *identify* correctly the names of the bones. Therefore, "identify" is the behavior expected of the student.

Formative evaluations serve several functions:

1. *Learner diagnosis* is done through formative tests by pointing out the degree of achievement of a specific objective. The tests reveal the particular points of difficulty that the learner is having. Diagnosis in this situation shows the elements in the learning task that the student has not mastered. The study by Bloom, Hastings, and Madaus (1971) has shown that students undergoing difficulties respond best to the diagnostic results when they are referred to specific instructional materials or remedial learning situations. The teacher's task then is to provide the student with specific prescriptions. Bloom, Hastings, and Madaus (1971) also proposed that formative evaluations should be considered as part of the learning process and should not be used to judge the capability of the student nor as a part of final evaluation for grading purposes.

2. *Feedback* to the learner and the teacher is the second major function of formative evaluation. It provides feedback with regard to the mastery of the various objectives in a given unit of learning and information about what the student still needs to learn. It also provides guidance to the student with regard

to the location of the difficulty, so that if motivated, the student can do additional learning in these areas. Feedback is valuable to the teacher in that particular points in the instruction can be identified as being in need of modification. The teacher can also compare the performance of one group of students with an earlier group and assess whatever changes that may have been incorporated in the instructional process with the objective of improvement (Arndt and Huckabay, 1975).

3. *Pacing* is another function of formative evaluation. Frequent formative tests pace the learning of the students and motivate them to put forth the necessary effort at the proper time.

4. *Reinforcing effect* is the fourth function of formative tests. For the person who has mastered a learning unit, formative evaluations positively reinforce this learning and assure that the progress is satisfactory and the present strategy for learning is on target. Knowledge of results is a form of feedback, and it produces a feeling of achievement and satisfaction in the student and, consequently, is very motivating and reinforcing for the individual.

5. *Initial assessment* can be done using formative tests. This is done at the beginning of instruction, prior to learning. It enables the teacher to find out the entering behavior of the student. It serves the same purpose as a pretest.

Forecasting constitutes the sixth function of formative evaluation. Formative tests forecast, or predict, the probable outcome of the summative test. This occurs when both formative and, a few months later, summative tests are given to the student. Since there is overlap between the tests with regard to content area, behavior, and evaluative procedures, the two types of test results will be related. Bloom, Hastings, and Madaus (1971) have found that predictions about the

results of later summative tests can be made. Thus, if teachers and learners wish, they can change the direction of a given forecast (Arndt and Huckabay, 1975).

The major function of *summative* evaluation is to make judgments about the progress and the final product. Certification, grading, and accreditation may be involved here. It is a more comprehensive form of evaluation than formative evaluation.

Timing is an obvious difference between the two types of evaluation. Summative tests are given at the end or completion of a task, or plan, or project. Formative tests are given at more frequent intervals, during the early phases of development of a project or during the learning process.

In this next section, a brief overview of evaluation procedure will be presented. A detailed explanation of each of the steps of the evaluation procedure is provided by Arndt and Huckabay (1975, pp. 136-151).

PROCEDURES OF EVALUATION

It is important that evaluation procedures give evidence about each of the behaviors implied in the major objectives. For example, if one of the objectives is "to identify the names of the bones of the human body," then it is necessary that evaluation give some evidence that the student has correctly identified the names of the bones of the human body. Therefore, the *content* and the *behavior* specified in the objective are the elements that have to be sampled in the evaluation.

The next step in the evaluation procedure is to identify the situations that not only will give the student the chance to express the behavior that is specified in the objective, but will encourage it. The teacher will then be in a position to observe the extent to which the objectives are being achieved. For example, if the objectives states: "the student will be able to identify orally or in written form the names of the bones of the human body," then the teacher must look into situations where oral or written expressions are exhibited.

Therefore, before selecting a procedure to appraise a learning task or an educational program, it is necessary first to identify both the objectives that need to be achieved and the kinds of situations that will evoke the proper behavior. Once these have been accomplished, it is then necessary to devise a means of getting a record of the individual's behavior in the test situation. In the case of a written test, the student keeps a personal record. If it is an oral expression or an interview, tape recordings of the sopken words can be obtained. If it is a motor performance, such as making a bed or catheterizing a patient, either a video-tape recording of the procedure is taken or an observer checklist is utilized.

The essential characteristics of evaluation tools are specification of the terms or units that are used to summarize or appraise the record of behavior, objectivity, the reliability of the tool, sampling, and validity.

Gathering of data is the next step in the process of evaluation. Once data is collected and statistically analyzed, it is then interpreted for the following purposes:

1. to determine the extent to which each of the objectives have been accomplished
2. to identify the strengths and weaknesses of the student to know where the student may need help
3. to make hypotheses about the reasons for the particular pattern of strengths and weaknesses

Evaluation procedures have other values as well. Utmost among them is the clarification of objectives. Since it is not possible to make an evaluation until objectives are clearly defined (enabling one to recognize the behavior that is being sought), evaluation is a powerful device for clarifying objectives. It is also useful in the individual guidance of the learner. Finally, evaluation becomes one of the important ways of providing information about the success of the learner, the program, or whatever else is being evaluated.

Thus, evaluation procedures should be used to determine what and where desirable changes are actually taking place in the individual learner or within an educational program and where still further modifications must be made in order to get optimal learning or an effective educational program. So far, what has been discussed are basic concepts and principles about evaluation in general. In this next section, evaluation of learners, learning, the learning environment, and instruction will be stressed more specifically.

Evaluation of instruction

Evaluation of instruction refers to the appraising of the effects of interaction between the learner, the learning environment, and the learning. Wittrock (1970) pointed out that instruction consists of three elements: the learner, the environment, and the learning. He maintained that to evaluate instruction, the relationships among these components must be quantitatively estimated. This is a new, uncommon, and complex type of evaluation. Wittrock believes that this approach is feasible now that multivariate statistical procedures are becoming available for estimating the cause-and-effect relations in evaluation studies.

One of the purposes of evaluation of instruction is to make decisions about it. Teachers, administrators, and evaluators ask different questions to make decisions about instruction and its effects. For example, they want to know what the effect of assignment, curricula, and experiences are on learners of different abilities and interests. They also want to know what effects similar treatments for different learners are likely to have in the future? To answer these types of questions, Wittrock (1970) proposed that data about the cause-and-effect relations among learners, their environment, and learning are needed.

The second purpose of evaluation is to make judgments and generalizations about instruction and about the cause-and-effect relations within it. Wittrock noted that evaluation studies have contributed very little in this respect. One reason for this lack of help is that researchers have designed studies to evaluate learners, learning, or the learning environment, but they have not attacked the more comprehensive problem of relating these three components with each other to study instruction. Another reason for this lack of help, according to Wittrock, is that evaluation studies, specifically those performed by differential and experimental psychologists, have extrapolated evaluation of instruction far from its origins. For instance, differential psychologists are mostly concerned about individual difference among learners. They utilize mostly norm-referenced evaluation. They are not concerned with the evaluation of the interaction of the learner, the environment, and learning. As a result, when teachers, administrators, and others try to evaluate instruction with standardized tests of student achievement, they find themselves struggling with the properties of the normal curve. They are unable to determine the type of change in behavior the student has undergone, how much the student has learned or improved. All they can tell is how a specific student compares with others in the group.

Wittrock also criticized the experimental psychologist's approach to evaluation of instruction. He states that even though experimentation is designed to obtain the probable causes of learning, it is not often realistic because in such studies the treatments are applied uniformly to two or more students.

Therefore, it is not often useful to solve the common problems of teachers and administrators. What is needed by teachers, Wittrock says, is the evaluation of the "day-to-day teaching and instruction occurring in the natural context of their schools without resorting to techniques of random assignments and manipulated treatments" (Wittrock, 1970, pp. 5-6). These problems of evaluation studies and issues are still unresolved. Until the different types of researchers get together to develop a more comprehensive approach to evaluating instruction, such issues will keep on being debated. Wittrock's model of evaluation of instruction is one approach to bridging the gap between the different schools of thought on evaluation of instruction.

Wittrock's model calls for explicitness of the variables and behaviors and requires a conceptual approach to evaluation that make these variables and behaviors explicit. This explicitness of the variables and behaviors distinguishes formal from informal evaluation.

Informal evaluation consists of judgments that do not necessarily involve an explicit statement of their bases, values, experiences, variables, and data. It is a part of our daily lives. We evaluate informally when we say something is good, bad, or indifferent. Informal evaluations are statements only of our decisions and judgments.

In formal evaluation, judgments and decisions are again made explicit, but in addition, explicit statements and objective measures of the evaluation are required. In evaluation studies, the selection and objective measurement of the bases of the judgments and decisions are the focus.

THE THREE COMPONENTS OF THE EVALUATION OF INSTRUCTION

The three fundamental components of the evaluation of instruction as conceptualized by

Wittrock (1970) that are presented in this module are: the evaluation of environment, the evaluation of learners, and the evaluation of learning.

Evaluation of environments. One of the major quests in evaluation is for the identification of learning experiences and educational environments that produce significant changes in individuals.

Evaluation of environments occurs when we make explicit the physical and the human characteristics of the learners' environments. This can be done by counting the number of books in libraries, the hours spent in instruction in the classroom, the dollars spent per pupil, the college credits of teachers in their majors, the textbooks used, the sequence of instruction, the number of homework problems assigned to the class, and the number of hours students spend studying. These are examples of environmental characteristics commonly measured by teachers and administrators to index learning. In nursing, the number of patients with specific conditions cared for and the number of hours spent in the laboratory, in caring for patients in instructing patients and their families, in studying and administering medications through different routes, and in team conferences and ward conferences are examples of environmental characteristics that can be measured. These measurements are meant to illustrate a few environmental variables; it is recognized that there may be more meaningful environmental characteristics and the environmental factors *alone* are *not* sufficient to enable one to make objective inferences about their effect on learners. Other measures about the intellectual and social processes in learners and also measurement of their learning and the interaction of these three components are needed to effectively evaluate instruction.

Characteristics of instructional environments must be made explicit in evaluation studies. Since the teacher's primary function

is to provide environments best suited to the learner to enhance learning and development as an individual, a teacher must make decisions and inferences about the educational value of environments and their probable effects on individuals. The teacher must be able to identify and appraise those crucial qualities of environments that can be manipulated and also must be able to relate them objectively to individual learners and to changes in behaviors of learners (Wittrock, 1970).

Evaluation of learners. Evaluation of learners focuses on making explicit the behavior and characteristics of learners. Usually this means the focus is on the individual differences among students. Individual differences in student behavior are usually measured by achievement and ability tests, usually for the purposes of selection and placement of learners. This approach has come from the study of individual differences and its psychometric problems. Some of the best work in educational evaluation has come from studies in this area.

Scores on standardized tests of interests, abilities, and achievements are useful for measuring individual differences in learning to select students for more advanced study or for special treatment and also to predict student performance. These tests cannot enable us to make inferences about what the students have learned nor about the role of environments and intellectual processes in producing the learning. Data on the relative achievement status of children do not tell us what, how, or why students have learned, nor what the roles of antecedent learner and environmental factors are in learning.

To measure what the student has learned, it is necessary to measure changes in behavior. To learn why and how the student has learned, it is necessary to quantify the salient characteristics of the environments and measure their relationships to intellectual and social processes, as well as to student achievement.

The basic issues in this area that are explicitly pointed out by Wittrock (1970, p. 10) are "the relationships between the learner's aptitudes, achievements, and interests and the instruction, not only whether there are individual differences among the learners."

Evaluation of learning. Until recent years, our concentration on measuring individual differences among students has overshadowed the evaluating the individual student's learning. For many years tests were constructed and interpreted using the normal curve as the reference. Bloom (1968), noting that educators have used the normal grading curve for so long that they have come to believe in it, stated that the normal curve is not sacred. It is wrong to expect 10% to fail, when failure is determined by a student's ranked position within the class rather than inability to grasp the central ideas of the subject matter. The success of the educational efforts may be measured to the extent that student achievement is not normally distributed. The primary task in education is to develop learning experiences that will take into account individual differences to promote the fullest development of the individual.

Wittrock (1970) also pointed out that it is better to vary instruction with individuals to enable them to learn, rather than to change the criteria until we find some individual differences among their achievements that may be trivial. This type of instruction or evaluation avoids the basic issue of individualizing instructions to meet individual needs and to produce learning.

Individualized instruction is the key to mastery learning. To design different types of instruction for each individual or each group of individuals, to vary instruction with individuals, to help individuals learn, and to include in achievement tests only those items that indicate the learning of defined objectives and content are tasks that are far more valuable than is focusing on differences among individuals.

Essential to evaluation of learning is identification of the learning objectives, that is, the expected changes in the student. Education is a process that helps the learner to change in many ways. One of the principal tasks of teachers is to decide how they want the student to change and what part they can play in assisting in this process. A second task, which arises as instruction unfolds and terminates at its completion, is to determine whether the student has changed in the ways desired and then to define the outcomes achieved (Bloom, Hastings, and Madaus, 1971).

The ways the teacher would like to see the student change make up the educational objectives, or goals, of instruction. Careful consideration must be given to decide the possible and desirable outcomes that will be systematically sought. At the same time, it must be realized that not all outcomes can be anticipated and recognized.

Statements of objectives are attempts by teachers to clarify within their own minds and to communicate to others the sought-for-changes in the learner. Statements of objectives should be couched in terms that convey the same meaning to all readers. The expected changes in behaviors must be explicitly defined in observable and measurable terms. Once the objectives are defined clearly, they can become plans that shape and guide the instruction and evaluation processes.

According to Wittrock (1970), measuring change in student behavior toward behaviorally defined objectives is a relatively new approach to evaluation. It is only during the last several years that curriculum evaluation has become widely viewed as the evaluation of change in behavior toward behaviorally defined goals. Evaluation of learning is conducted by taking two or more measures of the behavior of the learner—before and after instruction. The difference between the two measures is the amount learned, or the amount of change in behavior.

The process of evaluation of learning may be viewed as a six-step process:

1. Developing the behavioral objectives or make explicit the change in behavior desired.
2. Developing an evaluation tool to measure the behavioral objectives
3. Measuring the entering behavior by a pretest using the evaluation tool
4. Implementing the instructional plan by developing learning experiences and teaching strategies
5. Measuring the terminal behavior by a posttest using the evaluation tool developed (Popham and Baker, 1970).
6. Interpreting test results, including assigning grades and identifying strengths and weaknesses of the student as well as of the instruction

In developing evaluation tools, the ways of selecting test items differ depending on whether the goal is comparing learners or measuring learning, which is concerned with changes in behavior. To measure learners, which is mostly concerned with measuring individual differences, test items are largely selected for their use in discriminating among individuals. On the other hand, to measure changes in behavior produced by instruction, the test items are selected based on their usefullness in discriminating among learners (Wittrock, 1970). For instance, to measure whether a nursing student learned the names of the bones of the human body in anatomy class, an item that sampled that information would be included in a test of behavior change. As pointed out by Wittrock, the fact that all or none of the nursing students gave the correct answer is not as relevant to the measuring of learning as is the validity of the content of the item. Wittrock, (1970, p. 13) also makes a very important point that "if all the students got a valid and reliable item wrong on a post-test, the instruction, not the test, would be changed."

The criterion-referenced method of evaluating learning has advantages over the more traditional norm-referenced evaluation. In the former case, the objectives lead to test items that are written for their content validity and not for their ability to discriminate among students. As a result of this focus, evaluations are becoming more concerned with learning by students than with discriminating among students. Teachers are also becoming more free to conceive of mastery learning by students as a reality that is available to most students rather than to a few. Wittrock also pointed out that evaluation studies should include changes in behavior of students, teachers, and others.

Evaluation of instruction. One method of evaluating instruction that is proposed by Wittrock is relating the characteristics of the learning environment, learner characteristics, and the learning. This is a comprehensive approach to evaluation of instruction that requires making explicit and relating to each other the salient characteristics of the three variables as they occur in naturalistic settings: (1) individual learners, (2) their instructional environment, and (3) their learning. The cause-and-effect relations can be estimated by using appropriate multivariate statistical tools, and conclusions and judgments about instruction can be made that were not possible before.

This comprehensive approach to evaluation of instruction is relatively new. The concept of causal relationships between the learner, his environment, and his learning still awaits researching. Wittrock (1970) pointed out that for many years researchers in the areas of sociology, political science, economics, and statistics have been developing quantitative methods for estimating cause-and-effect relations in nonexperimental data. Now that these methods are being used with some success in these fields, it seems time to apply them further to educational problems, such as evaluation of instruction.

Several relevant research studies have been conducted and articles written about the possibilities and limitations of conducting research that test cause-and-effect relationships in naturalistic settings. For instance, Blalock (1964), Simon (1957), and Wold (1956, 1963) pointed out the general problems of obtaining causal inferences in nonexperimental research. The studies of Yee and Gagi (1968), Duncan (1966), Boudon (1965), and many others indicate the possibility of measuring cause-and-effect relations in nonexperimental settings, which have relevance to evaluation of instructions. These studies are too complex to discuss in this chapter. The interested reader is advised to refer to the original articles that are cited in the references.

Many other research studies have been conducted to test the different concepts of evaluation. For example, the positive effects of the use of formative evaluation and statement of behaviorally stated objects on cognitive and affective behaviors of the learners has been amply demonstrated in Bloom's (1968) study in which he eloquently argues for the possibility of mastery learning for 95% of the students. His findings have been supported by the studies of Airasian (1967) and Block (1971).

The effect of classroom environment on academic achievement has been evaluated in studies by Antony (1967). Using observational and interview techniques. Antony identified aspects of classroom environment (such as variety of instructional material and techniques used, types of feedback, frequency and variety of reinforcements, and so on that affect learning. Results indicated positive relationships between these environmental variables and learning.

The evaluation study of Huckabay and Arndt (1976) utilized pre- and posttests to measure the amount of cognitive learning that had taken place in graduate nursing students. Results showed that (1) mastery learning produced the most amount of learning, as compared to the traditional lecture-discussion method of instruction, and (2) in general, students tended to overestimate what they thought they knew about subject matter in the course on theories of learning when asked to evaluate themselves using the Likert Rating Scale as an evaluation tool.

Other studies and articles (Bare, 1967; Cronbach, 1963; Metz and Grissold, 1966; O'Shea, 1967; Moritz and Sexton, 1970; Nichols, 1968; Simpson, 1969) have been conducted and written about evaluation that demonstrate different methods of evaluation and the effect of behavioral change and course improvement through evaluation.

Issues in evaluation of instruction

Wittrock (1970) identified some of the criticisms that have been aimed at the current use of the evaluation of learning. Critics claim that if one measures only behavioral changes toward objectives, significant changes in students resulting from the instruction will be ignored. Since not all important dimensions of change in student behavior can be foreseen, areas of behavior should not be ignored because they were not included in the objectives before instruction began.

Changes in behavior of people other than students, such as teachers, parents, and so forth, are not looked at in the evaluation of learning. There is a need to incorporate this kind of data into evaluation.

Another concern is that precisely worded behavioral objectives tend to become narrow and trivial and to lose the essence of the instruction. Narrowness might be overcome by writing hierarchical sets of more specific objectives to sample more general, imprecisely worded but significant objectives.

Another criticism of evaluation of learning is that the characteristics of the environment of instruction, the intellectual and social characteristics of the learner interacting with the environment, and the characteristic of the school as a social system are not made explicit.

Many issues can be raised from the study of instruction, most of which hinge on the subject of evaluation in general. Wittrock's concept of the evaluation of instruction might be thought of as an issue because his is one approach to evaluation of instruction as opposed to other schools of thought. Furthermore, his approach still awaits further testing. Also, whether cause-and-effect relations can be correctly estimated in nonexperimental settings is another area of concern.

The grading of formative evaluation is another issue that has not been resolved yet. The opponents of grading (Bloom, 1968; Block, 1971) argue that since formative evaluation is a diagnostic test, and it is an aid to learning and thus part of the process of learning, it should not be graded and used for judgmental and decision-making purposes. The advocates do not discuss it within the context of formative evaluations. The effect of grading versus nongrading of formative evaluation on cognitive and affective behaviors of learners was tested by Huckabay (1979). Results showed that subjects enrolled in a nongraded formative evaluation course learned (cognitively) more than those whose formative evaluations were graded. There were no significant differences between the groups on affective behaviors.

Application to nursing education and practice

Many of the concepts of evaluation have already been applied to aspects of nursing education. This section stresses some of the major points and concepts that are applicable to both nursing education and practice.

Evaluation of instruction, as Wittrock defined it, is for the purposes of making decisions about instruction, making judgments about it, and gaining an understanding of it. When instruction can be evaluated in the way Wittrock proposed, nursing educators and nursing administrators will stand on more substantive grounds as they make those judgments and decisions about instruction. As in other areas of education, this approach necessitates the measuring of the three essential components of evaluation of instruction—the evaluation of the environment of learning, the evaluation of the intellectual and social processes of the learner, and the evaluation of the learning. Then to evaluate the instruction, the interaction among these three must be quantitatively estimated.

The appropriate use of norm-referenced versus criterion-referenced evaluation is of the utmost importance. If the nursing teacher is interested in knowing how students compare against the national sample, then norm-referenced evaluation is appropriate. However, if the teacher is interested in knowing how much students have learned (an evaluation of learning), then the absolute standard of criterion-referenced evaluation is appropriate. The teacher has to keep in mind that in order to measure learning and utilize criterion-referenced evaluation, the following are needed: (1) specific behaviorally stated objectives, (2) a valid and reliable evaluation tool that measures the stated objectives, (3) a pretest to evaluate the entering behavior of the student, (4) implementation of the teaching strategy, (5) a posttest to determine the amount of learning (change in behavior) that has taken place, and (6) interpretation of data to identify strengths and weaknesses of the student and the teacher and to offer an appropriate prescription to correct these weaknesses.

Formative evaluations are essential for the implementation of mastery learning. If the teacher subscribes to this school of thought, then appropriate implementation of formative evaluation is a must.

The basic concepts that are presented here are equally applicable to the teaching and evaluation of a patient in patient-teaching situations or to a nurse employee. The principles are the same, only the circumstances are different. The concepts presented in this module about evaluation in general can be applied to a myriad of situations in nursing education and practice.

The discussion utilizing the concepts of mastery learning, the process of constructing objectives, formative and summative evaluation, criterion-referenced versus norm-referenced evaluation, and others can be applied to the building of modules, lesson plans, curriculum planning, patient-teaching programs, and evaluation tools as well as to the evaluation of the forenamed operations.

Researchable questions

Wittrock's concept of the evaluation of instruction, a relatively new approach, is a by-product of research in learning. The realization of Wittrock's concept is dependent on further research and awaits the refinement of multivariate statistical procedures, which estimate the cause-and-effect relations in evaluation studies.

There is also a great need for the quantification of the three components of his model—the evaluation of the environment, the evaluation of the learner, and the evaluation of the learning—and much research is being conducted in these areas. Explicit identification of the characteristics of the learning environment, the social and intellectual capabilities of the learners, and learning are needed. Valid and reliable tools to measure the three components of evaluation of instruction are also needed.

One can raise even more specific questions that still await investigating; for example, what is the effect of formative evaluation on the self-concept of the student?

ADDITIONAL LEARNING EXPERIENCES—RECOMMENDED READING LIST

Arndt, C., and Huckabay, L. M. D. *Nursing administration: theory for practice with a systems approach.* St. Louis: The C. V. Mosby Book Co., 1975, pp. 136-151.

Wittrock, M. C. The evaluation of instruction: cause and effect relations in naturalistic data. In M. C. Wittrock and D. Wiley (Eds.) *Evaluation of instruction: issues and problems.* New York: Holt, Rinehart and Winston, Inc., 1970, pp. 3-21.

Wittrock, M. C., and Wiley, D., (Eds.) *Evaluation of instruction: issues and problems.* New York: Holt, Rinehart and Winston, Inc., 1970.

INSTRUCTIONS TO THE LEARNER REGARDING POSTTEST

At this stage of your learning process you are ready to take the posttest to determine the extent to which you have achieved the objectives of this module. Return to the pretest and take it over again as the posttest. Correct your answers using the answer key that is found at the end of this module (p. 479). You need to score 22 points to achieve the 95% mastery level. If your score is less than 22 correct points, correct your errors, study the content of this module over again more carefully, and read some of the articles in the recommended reading list. You need to study in this fashion until you achieve the 95% mastery level or better.

ANSWER KEY TO PRETEST AND POSTTEST

1. d and e (Wittrock, 1970, pp. 4-5)
2. b and c (Arndt and Huckabay, 1975, pp. 136-151; Bevis, 1978, pp. 192-196)
3. a and b (Arndt and Huckabay, 1975, pp. 136-151)
4. c (Bloom, Hastings, and Madaus, 1971, pp. 53-54)
5. c (Arndt and Huckabay, 1975, pp. 136-151)
6. c (Arndt and Huckabay, 1975, pp. 136-151)
7. b (Block, 1971, p. 79)
8. c (Tyler, 1950, pp. 106-125)
9. b (Bloom, 1968, pp. 1-12; Arndt and Huckabay, 1975, pp. 136-151)
10. c, d, and e (Popham and Baker, 1970, pp. 8-12)
11. a and b (Arndt and Huckabay, 1975, pp. 136-151)
12. d (Wittrock, 1970, p. 4)
13. b (Wittrock, 1970, p. 9)
14. b, c, and f (Wittrock, 1970, pp. 8-9)
15. a, b (Wittrock, 1970, pp. 9-10)
16. b, d, and f (Wittrock, 1970, p. 4)
17. d (Wittrock, 1970, p. 4)
18. c and g (Bevis, 1978, pp. 192-196; Arndt and Huckabay, 1975, pp. 136-151; Wittrock, 1970, p. 5)
19. a (Tyler, 1951, p. 48)
20. i (Arndt and Huckabay, 1975, pp. 136-151)
21. b (Bloom, pp. 1-12, 1968; Arndt and Huckabay, 1975, pp. 136-151)
22. e and h (Bloom, 1968, pp. 1-12; Arndt and Huckabay, 1975, pp. 136-151)
23. f (Bloom, 1968, pp. 1-12; Arndt and Huckabay, 1975, pp. 136-151)

REFERENCES

Airasian, Peter, W. The role of evaluation in mastery learning In. J. H. Block (Ed.), *Mastery learning: theory and practice.* New York: Holt, Rinehart and Winston, Inc., 1971, pp. 77-78.

Anthony, B. C. M. *The identification and measurement of classroom environmental process variables related to academic achievement.* Unpublished doctoral dissertation, University of Chicago, 1967.

Arndt, C., and Huckabay, L. M. D. *Nursing administration: theory for practice with a system's approach.* St. Louis: The C. V. Mosby Book Co., 1975.

Bare, Carol E. Behavioral change through effective evaluation. *Journal of Nursing Education,* 1967, 6(4):7.

Barritt, E. R., and Trion, L. A. Advantages and disadvantages of nongrading. *Nursing Outlook,* 1970, 18:40-41.

Bevis, E. O. *Curriculum building in nursing: a process.* (2nd Ed.) St. Louis: The C. V. Mosby Co., 1978.

Blalock, J. M., Jr. *Causal inferences in nonexperimental research.* Chapel Hill, N. C.: University of North Carolina Press, 1964.

Block, J. H. (Ed.) *Mastery learning: theory for practice.* New York: Holt, Rinehart and Winston, Inc., 1971.

Bloom, B. S. Learning for mastery. *Evaluation Comment,* 1968, 1(2):1-12.

Bloom, B. S., Hastings, J. T., and Madaus, G. F. *Handbook on formative and summative evaluation of student learning.* New York: McGraw-Hill Book Co., 1971.

Boudon, R. Methodes l'analyse causale. *Revue Francaise de Sociologie,* 1965, 6:24-43.

Cronbach, L. J. Evaluation for course improvement. *Teachers College Record,* 1963, 64:672-683.

Duncan, O. D. Path analysis: sociological examples. *The American Journal of Sociology,* 1966, 72(1):671-684.

Goldberg, L. Grades as motivants. *Psychology in the Schools,* 1965, 2:(1):17-23.

Huckabay, L. M. D. Cognitive-affective consequences of grading versus nongrading of formative evaluations. *Nursing Research,* 1979, 28(3):173-178.

Huckabay, L. M. D., and Arndt, C. The effect of acquisition of knowledge on self-evaluation, and the relationship of self-evaluation to perception of real and ideal self-concept. *Nursing Research,* 1976, 25(4):244-251.

Metz, E., and Grissold, G. K. Evaluation: a tangible process. *Nursing Outlook,* 1966, 14:41-45.

Moritz, D. A., and Sexton, D. L. Evaluation: a suggestion for appraising quality. *Journal Nursing Education,* 1970, 9(1):17-21.

Nichols, G. A. Clinical observations and actions of nursing students. *Journal of Nursing Education,* 1968, 7(4).

O'Shea, H. S. A guide to evaluation of clinical performance. *American Journal of Nursing,* 1967, 67(9):1877-1879.

Popham, J. W., and Baker, I. I. *Establishing instructional goals.* Englewood Cliffs, N.J.: Prentice-Hall, Inc., 1970.

Simon, H. A. *Models of man: social and rational.* New York: Wiley and Sons, Inc., 1957.

Stake, R. C. The countenance of educational evaluation. *Teachers College Record,* 1967, 68:523-540.

Tyler, R. W. *Basic principles of curriculum and instruction.* Chicago: University of Chicago Press, 1950.

Tyler, R. W. The functions of measurement in improving instruction. In E. F. Lindquist (Ed.), *Educational measurement*. Washington, D. C.: American Council on Education, 1951, pp. 47-67.

Wittrock, M. C. The Evaluation of instruction: cause-and-effect relations in naturalistic data. In M. C. Wittrock and D. Wiley (Eds.), *The evaluation of instruction: issues and problems*. New York: Holt, Rinehart and Winston, Inc., 1970, pp. 3-21.

Wold, H. O. Causal inference from observational data: a review of ends and means. *Journal of the Royal Statistical Society (London)*, Series A (General), 1956, 119:28-50.

Wold, H. O. The approach of model building and the possibilities of its utilization in the human sciences. Manuscript for *Entretion de Monaco en Sciences Humaines*. Monaco: Centre International d'Etude des Problèmes Humaines, 1963.

Yee, A. H., and Gagi, N. L. Techniques for estimating the source and direction of causal influence in panel data. *Psychological Bulletin*, 1968, **70**:115-126.

Index